Hepatitis C Protocols

METHODS IN MOLECULAR MEDICINE™

John M. Walker, SERIES EDITOR

19. **Hepatitis C Protocols,** edited by *Johnson Yiu-Nam Lau,* 1998
18. **Tissue Engineering,** edited by *Jeffrey R. Morgan and Martin L. Yarmush,* 1998
17. **HIV Protocols,** edited by *Nelson Michael and Jerome II. Kim,* 1998
16. **Clinical Applications of PCR,** edited by *Y. M. Dennis Lo,* 1998
15. **Molecular Bacteriology:** *Protocols and Clinical Applications,* edited by *Neil Woodford and Alan Johnson,* 1998
14. **Tumor Marker Protocols,** edited by *Margaret Hanausek and Zbigniew Walaszek,* 1998
13. **Molecular Diagnosis of Infectious Diseases,** edited by *Udo Reischl,* 1998
12. **Diagnostic Virology Protocols,** edited by *John R. Stephenson and Alan Warnes,* 1998
11. **Therapeutic Application of Ribozymes,** edited by *Kevin J. Scanlon,* 1998
10. **Herpes Simplex Virus Protocols,** edited by *S. Moira Brown and Alasdair MacLean,* 1998
9. **Lectin Methods and Protocols,** edited by *Jonathan M. Rhodes and Jeremy D. Milton,* 1998
8. *Helicobacter pylori* **Protocols,** edited by *Christopher L. Clayton and Harry L. T. Mobley,* 1997
7. **Gene Therapy Protocols,** edited by *Paul D. Robbins,* 1997
6. **Molecular Diagnosis of Cancer,** edited by *Finbarr Cotter,* 1996
5. **Molecular Diagnosis of Genetic Diseases,** edited by *Rob Elles,* 1996
4. **Vaccine Protocols,** edited by *Andrew Robinson, Graham H. Farrar, and Christopher N. Wiblin,* 1996
3. **Prion Diseases,** edited by *Harry F. Baker and Rosalind M. Ridley,* 1996
2. **Human Cell Culture Protocols,** edited by *Gareth E. Jones,* 1996
1. **Antisense Therapeutics,** edited by *Sudhir Agrawal,* 1996

METHODS IN MOLECULAR MEDICINE™

Hepatitis C Protocols

Edited by
Johnson Yiu-Nam Lau, MD
Schering-Plough Research Institute, Kenilworth, NJ

Forewords by
T. Jake Liang
Gary L. Davis
Michael Houghton, Q. L. Choo, and George Kuo

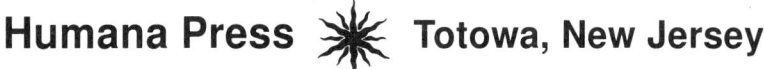

Humana Press ✳ Totowa, New Jersey

© 1998 Humana Press Inc.
999 Riverview Drive, Suite 208
Totowa, New Jersey 07512

All rights reserved. No part of this book may be reproduced, stored in a retrieval system, or transmitted in any form or by any means, electronic, mechanical, photocopying, microfilming, recording, or otherwise without written permission from the Publisher. Methods in Molecular Medicine™ is a trademark of The Humana Press Inc.

All authored papers, comments, opinions, conclusions, or recommendations are those of the author(s), and do not necessarily reflect the views of the publisher.

This publication is printed on acid-free paper. ∞
ANSI Z39.48-1984 (American Standards Institute) Permanence of Paper for Printed Library Materials.

Cover illustration:

Cover design by Patricia F. Cleary.

For additional copies, pricing for bulk purchases, and/or information about other Humana titles, contact Humana at the above address or at any of the following numbers: Tel.: 973-256-1699; Fax: 973-256-8341; E-mail: humana@mindspring.com; Website: http://humanapress.com

Photocopy Authorization Policy:
Authorization to photocopy items for internal or personal use, or the internal or personal use of specific clients, is granted by Humana Press Inc., provided that the base fee of US $8.00 per copy, plus US $00.25 per page, is paid directly to the Copyright Clearance Center at 222 Rosewood Drive, Danvers, MA 01923. For those organizations that have been granted a photocopy license from the CCC, a separate system of payment has been arranged and is acceptable to Humana Press Inc. The fee code for users of the Transactional Reporting Service is: [0-89603-521-2/98 $8.00 + $00.25].

Printed in the United States of America. 10 9 8 7 6 5 4 3 2 1

Library of Congress Cataloging in Publication Data

Main entry under title:

Methods in molecular medicine™.

Hepatitis C protocols/edited by Johnson Y. N. Lau; forewords by Q. L. Choo, Gary L. Davis, Michael Houghton, George Kuo, T. Jake Liang.
   p.   cm.—(Methods in molecular medicine; 19)
   Includes index.
   ISBN 0-89603-521-2 (alk. paper)
   1. Hepatitis C virus—Research—Methodology. I. Lau, Johnson Y. N. (Johnson Yiu-Nam)   II. Series.
   [DNLM: 1. Hepatitis C—diagnosis. 2. Hepatitis C—genetics. 3. Hepatitis C Antibodies. 4. Hepatitis C Antigens.   WC 536 H53363   1998]
   QR201.H46H447   1998
   616.3'623—dc21
   DNLM/DLC
   for Library of Congress   98-24896
   CIP

Foreword

The identification of hepatitis C virus by Michael Houghton and his colleagues at the Chiron Corporation nearly 10 years ago represented a technical tour de force of modern molecular medicine. This breakthrough not only unearthed the causative agent of non-A non-B hepatitis that had eluded the best of scientists for more than 20 years, but also was symbolic of another chapter in the changing paradigm of modern science and medicine. The revolutionary concept of identifying a pathogen without actually visualizing or detecting it will forever redefine the way we approach pathogenesis of diseases whose cause is unknown. It is benefitting that this discovery treads on the heels of the human immunodeficiency pandemic, and parallels the alarming emergence of various microbial pestilences in the world. Despite the rapid advances in our understanding of the virus, there is much remaining to learn about it. This book highlights some of the important areas yet to be unraveled. As illustrated in this book, the marriage between basic science and clinical medicine is essential in our quest for these unknowns. The last decade has focused on the fundamentals of the virus; the next decade must underscore translational research, bridging clinical medicine and basic science with realization of fundamental knowledge to improve prevention, diagnosis, and treatment of viral hepatitis C. Undoubtedly in the next millenium, we will develop a much better strategy to combat this virus and have a much brighter outlook on the disease for the millions of people infected with the virus.

T. Jake Liang
Liver Diseases Section
National Institute of Diabetes and Digestive
and Kidney Diseases
National Institutes of Health
Bethesda, MD

Foreword

After agreeing to write the foreword to this volume of highly technical reviews of the basic science of hepatitis C virus (HCV) research, I found myself wondering what I had gotten myself into. Why would a clinician and clinical researcher be asked to provide an introduction to such a "high tech" reference book? However, as I read these excellent chapters and reflected on how I might use the information in my own practice, the answer became clear.

Throughout most of our history, physicians have been comforters and, until relatively recently, they offered little to the patient that the family could not provide. Thus, physicians had a very limited role in the practice of medicine, such as it was at that time. The widespread marriage of science and medicine occurred later than one might think. The discoveries of Pasteur, Koch, Ehrlich, and others beginning in the 1860s fueled the public's view that science could be utilized for the public good and offer at least the potential of a meaningful treatment for the patient. But science was not something that the family and community could provide without the services of a physician. However, physicians did not achieve significant credibility in society until they began to apply science in their training and practice. Licensing of physicians did not start in earnest until 1877. Before this time, there were few prerequisites to establishing a medical practice. Johns Hopkins, the prototype of modern medical schools, was not established until 1893. The application of science was directly responsible for the legitimization of medicine in the United States; technology provided substance and value to the practice.

The impact of science on the practice of medicine is even more evident today and becomes increasingly important each year. Yet it has become such an integral part of our practices that many of us take the evolution for granted. It is simply astounding to stop and consider the role that technology plays in the daily office and hospital practices of clinicans today. Little of the technology that we use in our practices today was available 20, or even 10, years ago. Diagnostic tests based on molecular hybridization and amplification, magnetic resonance imaging, cytokine therapies, modern synthetic and recombinant pharmaceuticals, and computer-based informatics are just a few examples.

The impact of science is obvious in the diagnosis and treatment of viral diseases. This is perhaps most apparent in the case of HIV, where major research discoveries have occurred at an incredible pace. Recent developments have led to the ability to diagnose infection when even low levels of viremia are present, to characterize the virus, to design therapeutic tools directed at specific targets in the virus, and to predict and monitor the outcome of treatment. The understanding of the hepatitis C virus has also grown at a rapid pace since it was identified in 1989. However, despite the fact that nearly 4 million people in the United States have this infection, research funding has been limited and we have not yet come as far as we have with HIV. Political issues aside, the chapters in this volume reflect the state-of-the-art in the research and understanding of the virology of the hepatitis C virus. It is these tools and this knowledge that will allow us, as scientists, to better understand the inner working of this agent and design better ways to diagnose and treat the infection. This science of today will become the clinical practice of tomorrow.

Several of the chapters review issues that are immediately valuable to gastroenterologists, hepatologists, infectious disease physicians, and those working in laboratory medicine. They tell us where we are and where we are going in this field. First, the chapters dealing with different methodologies and quality control for the detection and quantitation of HCV are particularly timely. Qualitative and quantitative tests have already become commercially available, even though most lack standardization and we as clinicians are still struggling with how to use them. These articles point out the benefits and limitations of the current methodology and tell us how improved sensitivity and standardization can be accomplished. This is essential before the assays can be widely applied in clinical practice. Second, the discussion of viral heterogeneity is quite relevant. Viral heterogeneity will certainly be important in unraveling the interaction between the virus and the host. Although information on heterogeniety is currently most useful in basic research in immunodiagnostics and immuno-pathogenesis, epidemiologic surveys, and designing virus-targeted treatments, it may also have a role in clinical practice. It is now evident that viral genotype and the degree of viral heterogeneity have an impact on the response to interferon therapy. Genotype assays are already commercially available, but once again, the role of these tests in the clinic is not yet clear. Finally, the chapters on the biological characterization of the virus, in vitro culture techniques, and animal models provide us with a glimpse of the future of HCV research, particularly with respect to therapeutics. As with HIV, future therapies for HCV are likely to target the replicative machinery of the virus. Some of the targets of these agents, e.g., proteases, can currently be isolated, inserted, and expressed in artificial systems in order to screen potential new agents.

Today's high technology will become tomorrow's work horse. The incredible science described in this book today will provide the basis for the design of the tools that we will use in the diagnosis, management, and treatment of our patients with HCV infection tomorrow.

Gary L. Davis, MD
University of Florida College of Medicine
Gainesville, FL

Foreword

Almost 10 years have now passed since the application of molecular cloning methods resulted in the identification and characterization of the hepatitis C virus. During this time, significant medical advances have been made in the areas of immunodiagnosis and blood screening as well as methods determining viral load, which have facilitated the clinical management of patients. In addition, valuable information has been obtained concerning genome organization, viral polyprotein processing, and viral heterogeneity and its role in disease progression and sensitivity to interferon treatment. However, many important objectives still remain. Most importantly, given the high disease burden associated globally with the hepatitis C virus and the continued high incidence of infection in many countries, the development of more effective antivirals as well as the introduction of vaccines represent key goals. In addition, a clearer understanding of those factors influencing the progression of liver disease as well as nonhepatic diseases remains very important. Apart from these key medical objectives, a number of fundamental areas of viral biology also remain to be defined. These include viral replication strategies, virion structure, and mechanisms of virion assembly and release. In particular, since this virus has a well-known propensity to cause chronic, persistent infections and disease, the identification of those mechanisms responsible for such persistence and evasion of the host immune response represents a substantial but most intriguing challenge.

It is with these issues in mind that the current volume has been assembled from many of the leading researchers in the field and describes state-of-the-art methods and tools that are being used to address these important medical and scientific questions. We can look forward, therefore, over the next decades of hepatitis C research to acquiring a greater knowledge of this unique RNA virus and its interactions with the host as well as, hopefully, the development of specific therapeutics and vaccines.

Michael Houghton
Qui-Lim Choo
George Kuo

Preface

Since the report on the cloning of the hepatitis C virus (HCV) genome in 1989, an explosion of information on the epidemiology and natural history of the virus load has evolved. HCV infection afflicts 170 million people worldwide. Most people who acquire HCV progress to develop chronic infection and hepatitis; a proportion of them will have their liver disease advance to liver cirrhosis and end-stage liver disease in one to three decades. At present, HCV-related end-stage liver disease is a major indication for liver transplantation. The health impact of HCV worldwide is enormous.

With the use of molecular biology, immunology, and cell biology techniques, important information has been gathered on the virologic and immunologic aspects of HCV infection. Certainly, much more data are needed to further our knowledge on the clinical, virologic, and immunopathogenic aspects of HCV infection. This information may provide the foundation for the development of new therapies and better therapeutic strategies for patients with HCV infection. *Hepatitis C Protocols* contains a collection of research techniques used for the study of HCV. The authors were chosen based on their expertise in their respective areas. The chapters are written in a fashion that allows investigators to use them as manuals. A few reviews were included in some specialized areas. There is also a chapter that discusses the use of liver transplant recipients with HCV infection as a model for the study of pathogenesis. It is our hope that researchers will find this manual useful in their pursuit of HCV research, and clinical investigators will find this book helpful for their understanding of the principles involved in laboratory research on HCV.

I would like to take this opportunity to extend my gratitude to my teachers and friends: Professor P. C. Wu, Professor C. L. Lai, Dr. H. J. Lin, Professor Roger Williams, Dr. Graeme J. M. Alexander, Professor James E. McGuigan, Professor Philip P. Toskes, Professor Gerold Schiebler, Professor Richard W. Moyer, Professor Gary L. Davis, and Professor Sum Lee. Without their guidance and support, I would not have the opportunity of presenting this highly practical manual to you today.

Johnson Yiu-Nam Lau

*To my wife, Jane, for her unfailing support,
and our daughters Grace (Ling-Ling) and Gillian (Gi-Gi),
for keeping us rejuvenated*

Contents

Forewords
    T. Jake Liang v
    Gary L. Davis vi
    Michael Houghton, Qui-Lim Choo, and George Kuo viii
Preface ix
Contributors xvii

PART I. DETECTION OF ANTI-HCV IN SERUM 1
1 Detection of Anti-GOR Antibodies in HCV Infection
    Michael P. Manns and Gerd Michel 3
2 Confirmation of HCV Antibodies by the Line Immunoassay INNO-LIA HCV Ab III
    Geert Maertens, Filip Dekeyser, Anja Van Geel, Erwin Sablon,
    Fons Bosman, Maan Zrein, and Dirk Pollet 11

PART II. DETECTION AND QUANTITATION OF HCV IN SERUM 27
3 Detection of HCV RNA in Serum by Reverse Transcriptase-PCR and Radiolabeled Liquid Hybridization
    Richard L. Hodinka 29
4 Detection of HCV RNA in Serum by Reverse Transcription Polymerase Chain Reaction (RT-PCR)
    KePing Qian 47
5 The AMPLICOR® HCV Tests for the Detection and Quantitation of Serum or Plasma HCV RNA
    Karen A. Gutekunst, Joanne P. Spadoro, Elizabeth A. Dragon,
    and Maurice Rosenstraus 55
6 Quantification of HCV RNA in Clinical Specimens by Branched DNA (bDNA) Technology
    Judith C. Wilber and Mickey S. Urdea 71
7 Quality Control of the Polymerase Chain Reaction
    Maurice Rosenstraus, Joanne P. Spadoro,
    Diane McGovern-Wolfe, and Elizabeth A. Dragon 79

8 Preparation of Genotype-Specific HCV RNA Transcripts for Assessing HCV Detection and Quantification Assays
Jill J. Detmer, Janice A. Kolberg, Crystle L. K. Zayati, and Mark L. Collins 99

PART III. DETECTION OF HCV IN LIVER TISSUE 113

9 Detection of HCV RNA in Formalin-Fixed, Paraffin-Embedded Liver Tissue by RT-PCR
Johnson Y. N. Lau 115

10 Quantification of HCV RNA in Liver Tissue by bDNA Assay
Peter J. Dailey, Mark L. Collins, Mickey S. Urdea, and Judith C. Wilber 119

PART IV. HCV GENOTYPES 131

11 Hepatitis C Virus: *Types, Subtypes, and Beyond*
Donald B. Smith and Peter Simmonds 133

12 Molecular Evolutionary Analysis: *Its Application in the Study of Hepatitis C Virus*
Masashi Mizokami and Johnson Y. N. Lau 147

13 Genotyping by Type-Specific Primers That Can Type HCV Types 1–6
Tomoyoshi Ohno and Masashi Mizokami 159

14 Genotyping Hepatitis C Virus by Type-Specific Primers for PCR Based on NS5 Region
Kazuaki Chayama 165

15 Determination of HCV Genotypes by RFLP
Fiona Davidson and Peter Simmonds 175

16 HCV Genotyping by the Line Probe Assay INNO-LiPA HCV II
Geert Maertens and Lieven Stuyver 183

17 Serological Genotyping Using Synthetic Peptides Derived from the NS4 Region
Linda E. Prescott and Peter Simmonds 199

18 Determination of HCV Quasispecies by Cloning and Sequencing
Masashi Mizokami and Tomoyoshi Ohno 207

19 Detection of Hepatitis C Virus Quasispecies Heterogeneity by Single-Strand Conformational Polymorphism
Regino P. González-Peralta 213

20 Hepatitis C Virus Heteroduplex Tracking Assay:
 Application to Genotype Determination, Quasispecies Analysis,
 and Molecular Evolution Studies
 **Amy J. Weiner, Piero L. Calvo, Joe Kansopon,
 David Gretch, Ferruccio Bonino, Maurizia Brunetto,
 and Michael Houghton** 221

PART V. DETECTION OF HCV IN SITU 235

21 In Situ Detection of HCV: An Overview
 Francesco Negro and Johnson Y. N. Lau 237
22 In Situ Detection of Hepatitis C Viral Antigens
 Regino P. González-Peralta and Krzysztof Krawczynski 249
23 In Situ Hybridization and the Detection and Localization of HCV RNA
 Francesco Negro, Donatella Pacchioni, and Gianni Bussolati .. 257
24 The In Situ Detection of PCR-Amplified Hepatitis C RNA
 Gerard J. Nuovo and Maria Lynn Alfieri 263
25 Immunoelectron Microscopic Characterization of HCV
 Shozo Watanabe, Masahiko Kaito, and Michinori Kohara 279

PART VI. MOLECULAR BIOLOGIC CHARACTERIZATION 287

26 Cloning and Assembly of Complex Libraries of Full-Length HCV
 cDNA Clones
 Alexander A. Kolykhalov, Karen E. Reed, and Charles M. Rice 289
27 Use of the Vaccinia Virus/T7 Expression System for Studying HCV
 Protein Processing
 Eugene V. Agapov, Karen E. Reed, and Charles M. Rice 303
28 Use of a Discistronic Vector for the Quantitation of HCV IRES Activity
 Joyce A. Feller and Johnson Y. N. Lau 315
29 Expression and Dimerization of Hepatitis C Virus Core Protein in E. coli
 Shih-Yen Lo and Jing-Hsiung Ou 325
30 Expression and Characterization of the HCV NS2 Protease
 Karen E. Reed and Charles M. Rice 331
31 Expression and Characterization of HCV NS3 Protease
 **Eric D'Souza, Norman Gray, Malcolm Ellis,
 and Berwyn E. Clarke** 343
32 Expression and Characterization of the HCV NS3 Helicase Domain
 **Frank Preugschat, Mary H. Hanlon, Martin J. Rink,
 Berwyn E. Clarke, and David J. T. Porter** 353

33 Hepatitis C Virus RNA-Dependent RNA Polymerase
   (NS5B Polymerase)
   Curt H. Hagedorn 365

34 Detection and Molecular Cloning of the Extreme 3'-End of HCV
   Torahiko Tanaka and Kunitada Shimotohno 373

35 In Vitro Stability of Hepatitis C Virus RNA
   Jane W. S. Fang 381

36 Methods for the Study of Sequence-Specific Binding of Proteins
   to the HCV RNA Genome
   Lee M. Kaplan and Raymond T. Chung 385

PART VII. HCV-SPECIFIC IMMUNOLOGIC RESPONSE 405

37 Role of Immune Response in HCV
   Marion Peters 407

38 Determination of Hepatitis C Virus-Specific CD4+ T-Cell Activity
   in PBMC
   J. Tilman Gerlach, Helmut Diepolder, and Gerd R. Pape 413

39 Measurement of HCV-Specific CD8+ Cytotoxic T-Cell Activities
   in the Peripheral Blood by Europium Release Assay
   Michio Imawari 423

40 Determination of HCV-Specific Bulk CD8+ Activity in Liver
   David R. Nelson 431

41 Characterization of HCV-Specific Cytotoxic T-Lymphocytes
   from Liver Tissue
   Margaret James Koziel 439

42 Production of Human Monoclonal Antibodies to Hepatitis C Virus
   and Their Characterization
   Mario U. Mondelli and Antonella Cerino 451

PART VIII. IN VITRO CULTURE MODEL 463

43 Specific Detection of Negative Strand RNA of Hepatitis C Virus Using
   Chemical RNA Modification
   Toshiaki Gunji and Kunitada Shimotohno 465

44 Strand-Specific rTth RT-PCR for the Analysis of HCV Replication
   Robert E. Lanford and Deborah Chavez 471

45 Cell Culture Systems for the Detection of HCV Infection
   Yohko K. Shimizu and Hiroshi Yoshikura 483

46 Replication and Detection of Hepatitis C Virus in Liver-Derived Cell
   Lines
   Regino P. González-Peralta 489

47 Primary Human Hepatocyte Culture for the Study of HCV
*John F. O'Connell, Stuart Cox, Peter Buontempo,
Angela Skelton, Liubomir A. Pisarov, Kenneth Dorko,
and Stephen C. Strom* 495

48 A Cultivation Method for Highly Differentiated Primary Chimpanzee
Hepatocytes Permissive for Hepatitis C Virus Replication
Robert E. Lanford and Larry Estlack 501

PART IX. CONSTRUCTION OF RECOMBINANT VIRAL VECTORS FOR THE EXPRESSION
OF HCV GENES 517

49 Construction of Recombinant Vaccinia Virus Expressing HCV Genes
Joyce A. Feller 519

50 Construction of Recombinant Adeno-Associated Virus (AAV)
Markus Reiser and Sergei Zolotukhin 533

51 Production of Replication-Deficient Adenovirus Recombinants
*Gavin W. G. Wilkinson, Carole Rickards,
and Berwyn E. Clarke* 539

52 Generation of Recombinant Herpes Simplex Virus Amplicons
Zhi Hong and Ann D. Kwong 553

53 Construction of Recombinant Sindbis-Based Expression Vectors
for the Study of HCV Genes and Their Products
Brett D. Lindenbach, Ilya Frolov, and Charles M. Rice 565

PART X. IN VIVO MODELS 575

54 The Chimpanzee Model: *Contributions and Considerations*
Elizabeth Muchmore 577

55 Liver Transplantation as a Model to Study Hepatitis C Virus Infection
Howayda M. Hassoba and Teresa L. Wright 589

Index 609

Contributors

EUGENE V. AGAPOV • *Department of Molecular Microbiology, Washington University School of Medicine, St. Louis, MO*
MARIA LYNN ALFIERI • *MGN Medical Research Laboratories, Setauket, NY*
FERRUCCIO BONINO • *University of Torino, Italy*
FONS BOSMAN • *Hepatitis Program, Innogenetics, Gent, Belgium*
MAURIZIA BRUNETTO • *Nucleic Acid Diagnostics and New Markers, Chiron Diagnostics, Emeryville, CA*
PETER BUONTEMPO • *Department of Antiviral Therapy, Schering-Plough Research Institute, Kenilworth, NJ*
GIANNI BUSSOLATI • *Division of Gastroenterology and Hepatology, University Hospital, Geneva, Switzerland*
PIERO L. CALVO • *Nucleic Acid Diagnostics and New Markers, Chiron Diagnostics, Emeryville, CA*
ANTONELLA CERINO • *Istituto di Clinica delle Malattie Infettive, IRCCS Policlinico San Matteo, Pavia, Italy*
DEBORAH CHAVEZ • *Department of Virology and Immunology, Southwest Foundation for Biomedical Research, San Antonio, TX*
KAZUAKI CHAYAMA • *Department of Gastroenterology, Memorial Institute for Medical Research, Toranomon Hospital, Tokyo, Japan*
RAYMOND T. CHUNG • *Gastrointestinal Unit, Massachusetts General Hospital and Harvard Medical School, Boston, MA*
BERWYN E. CLARKE • *Virology Research Unit, Glaxo Wellcome PLC, Stevenage, UK*
MARK L. COLLINS • *Nucleic Acid Diagnostics and New Markers, Chiron Diagnostics, Emeryville, CA*
STUART COX • *Department of Antiviral Therapy, Schering-Plough Research Institute, Kenilworth, NJ*
PETER J. DAILEY • *Nucleic Acid Diagnostics and New Markers, Chiron Diagnostics, Emeryville, CA*
FIONA DAVIDSON • *Department of Medical Microbiology, University of Edinburgh Medical School, Edinburgh, UK*
FILIP DEKEYSER • *Hepatitis Program, Innogenetics, Gent, Belgium*

JILL J. DETMER • *Nucleic Acid Diagnostics and New Markers, Chiron Diagnostics, Emeryville, CA*
HELMUT DIEPOLDER • *Department of Medicine, University of Munich, Germany*
KENNETH DORKO • *Cell and Molecular Pathology, University of Pittsburgh, PA*
ELIZABETH A. DRAGON • *Department of Diagnostics Development, Roche Molecular Systems, Branchburg, NJ*
ERIC D'SOUZA • *Virology Research Unit, Glaxo Wellcome PLC, Stevenage, UK*
MALCOLM ELLIS • *Virology Research Unit, Glaxo Wellcome PLC, Stevenage, UK*
LARRY ESTLACK • *Department of Virology and Immunology, Southwest Foundation for Biomedical Research, San Antonio, TX*
JANE W. S. FANG • *Department of Antiviral Therapy, Schering-Plough Research Institute, Kenilworth, NJ*
JOYCE A. FELLER • *Department of Molecular Genetics and Microbiology, University of Florida, Gainesville, FL*
ILYA FROLOV • *Department of Molecular Microbiology, Washington University School of Medicine, St. Louis, MO*
J. TILMAN GERLACH • *Department of Medicine, University of Munich, Germany*
REGINO P. GONZÁLEZ-PERALTA • *Division of Gastroenterology and Hepatology, Department of Pediatrics, and Section of Hepatobiliary Diseases, Division of Gastroenterology, Hepatology, and Nutrition, Department of Medicine, University of Florida, Gainesville, FL*
NORMAN GRAY • *Enzyme Pharmacology Research Unit, Glaxo Wellcome Medicines Research Center, Stevenage, UK*
DAVID GRETCH • *Viral Hepatitis Laboratory, University of Washington, Seattle, WA*
TOSHIAKI GUNJI • *Third Department of Internal Medicine, Tokyo University, Tokyo, Japan*
KAREN A. GUTEKUNST • *Department of Diagnostics Development, Roche Molecular Systems, Branchburg, NJ*
CURT H. HAGEDORN • *Department of Medicine, Genetics Program of the Winship Cancer Center, and the Program in Biochemistry, Cell, and Developmental Biology, Emory University School of Medicine, Atlanta, GA*
MARY H. HANLON • *Division of Biochemistry, Glaxo Wellcome, Research Triangle Park, NC*
HOWAYDA M. HASSOBA • *Department of Gastroenterology, Veterans Affairs Medical Center and the University of California, San Francisco, CA*
RICHARD L. HODINKA • *Departments of Pathology and Pediatrics, Clinical Virology Laboratory, Children's Hospital of Philadelphia and University of Pennsylvania School of Medicine, Philadelphia, PA*

Contributors

ZHI HONG • *Department of Antiviral Therapy, Schering-Plough Research Institute, Kenilworth, NJ*

MICHAEL HOUGHTON • *Chiron Corporation, Emeryville, CA*

MICHIO IMAWARI • *Liver Study Laboratory, Jichi Medical School, Tochigi, Japan*

MASAHIKO KAITO • *Third Department of Internal Medicine, Mie University School of Medicine, Mie, Japan*

JOE KANSOPON • *Nucleic Acid Diagnostics and New Markers, Chiron Diagnostics, Emeryville, CA*

LEE M. KAPLAN • *Gastrointestinal Unit, Massachusetts General Hospital and Harvard Medical School, Boston, MA*

MICHINORI KOHARA • *Department of Microbiology, The Tokyo Metropolitan Institute of Medical Science, Tokyo, Japan*

JANICE A. KOLBERG • *Nucleic Acid Diagnostics and New Markers, Chiron Diagnostics, Emeryville, CA*

ALEXANDER A. KOLYKHALOV • *Department of Molecular Microbiology, Washington University School of Medicine, St. Louis, MO*

MARGARET JAMES KOZIEL • *Infectious Disease Division, Beth Israel-Deaconess Medical Center, Boston, MA*

KRZYSZTOF KRAWCZYNSKI • *Section of Experimental Pathology, Hepatitis Branch, Centers for Disease Control and Prevention, Atlanta, GA*

ANN D. KWONG • *Vertex Pharmaceuticals, Boston, MA*

ROBERT E. LANFORD • *Department of Virology and Immunology, Southwest Foundation for Biomedical Research, San Antonio, TX*

JOHNSON Y. N. LAU • *Department of Antiviral Therapy, Schering-Plough Research Institute, Kenilworth, NJ*

BRETT D. LINDENBACH • *Department of Molecular Microbiology, Washington University School of Medicine, St. Louis, MO*

SHIH-YEN LO • *Department of Medical Technology, Tzu-chi College of Medicine, Hualian, Taiwan*

GEERT MAERTENS • *Hepatitis Program, Innogenetics, Gent, Belgium*

MICHAEL P. MANNS • *Department of Gastroenterology and Hepatology, Zentrum Innere Medizin und Dermatologie, Medizinische Hochschule, Hannover, Germany*

DIANE MCGOVERN-WOLFE • *Department of Diagnostics Development, Roche Molecular Systems, Branchburg, NJ*

GERD MICHEL • *European Research and Development Unit, Abbott Laboratories, Wiesbaden-Delkenheim, Germany*

MASASHI MIZOKAMI • *Second Department of Medicine, Nagoya City University Medical School, Nagoya, Japan*

MARIO U. MONDELLI • *Istituto di Clinica delle Malattie Infettive, IRCCS Policlinico San Matteo, Pavia, Italy*
ELIZABETH MUCHMORE • *Tuxedo, NY*
FRANCESCO NEGRO • *Division of Gastroenterology and Hepatology, University Hospital, Geneva, Switzerland*
DAVID R. NELSON • *Section of Hepatobiliary Diseases, Division of Gastroenterology, Hepatology, and Nutrition, University of Florida, Gainesville, FL*
GERARD J. NUOVO • *MGN Medical Research Laboratories, Setauket, NY*
JOHN F. O'CONNELL • *Wyeth-Ayerst Research, Pearl River, NJ*
TOMOYOSHI OHNO • *Second Department of Medicine, Nagoya City University Medical School, Nagoya, Japan*
JING HSIUNG OU • *Department of Molecular Microbiology and Immunology, University of Southern California, Los Angeles, CA*
DONATELLA PACCHIONI • *Division of Gastroenterology and Hepatology, University Hospital, Geneva, Switzerland*
GERD R. PAPE • *Department of Medicine, University of Munich, Germany*
MARION PETERS • *Department of Medicine, Washington University School of Medicine, St. Louis, MO*
LIUBOMIR A. PISAROV • *Cell and Molecular Pathology, University of Pittsburgh, PA*
DIRK POLLET • *Hepatitis Program, Innogenetics, Gent, Belgium*
DAVID J. T. PORTER • *Division of Biochemistry, Glaxo Wellcome, Research Triangle Park, NC*
LINDA E. PRESCOTT • *Department of Medical Microbiology, University of Edinburgh Medical School, Edinburgh, UK*
FRANK PREUGSCHAT • *Division of Biochemistry, Glaxo Wellcome, Research Triangle Park, NC*
KEPING QIAN • *Section of Hepatobiliary Diseases, Department of Medicine, University of Florida, Gainesville, FL*
KAREN E. REED • *Department of Molecular Microbiology, Washington University School of Medicine, St. Louis, MO*
MARKUS REISER • *Medizinische Universitätsklinik, Knappschattskrankenhaus, Bochum, Germany*
CHARLES M. RICE • *Department of Molecular Microbiology, Washington University School of Medicine, St. Louis, MO*
CAROLE RICKARDS • *Department of Medicine, University of Wales College of Medicine, Cardiff, UK*
MARTIN J. RINK • *Division of Biochemistry, Glaxo Wellcome, Research Triangle Park, NC*

Contributors

MAURICE ROSENSTRAUS • *Department of Diagnostics Development, Roche Molecular Systems, Branchburg, NJ*
ERWIN SABLON • *Hepatitis Program, Innogenetics, Gent, Belgium*
YOHKO K. SHIMIZU • *Department of Bacteriology, Faculty of Medicine, University of Tokyo, Japan*
KUNITADA SHIMOTOHNO • *Institute for Virus Research, Kyoto University, Kyoto, Japan*
PETER SIMMONDS • *Department of Medical Microbiology, University of Edinburgh Medical School, Edinburgh, UK*
ANGELA SKELTON • *Department of Antiviral Therapy, Schering-Plough Research Institute, Kenilworth, NJ*
DONALD B. SMITH • *Department of Medical Microbiology, University of Edinburgh, UK*
JOANNE P. SPADORO • *Department of Diagnostics Development, Roche Molecular Systems, Branchburg, NJ*
STEPHEN C. STROM • *Department of Cell and Molecular Pathology, University of Pittsburgh, PA*
LIEVEN STUYVER • *Hepatitis Program, Innogenetics, Gent, Belgium*
TORAHIKO TANAKA • *Virology Division, National Cancer Center Research Institute, Tokyo, Japan*
MICKEY S. URDEA • *Nucleic Acid Diagnostics and New Markers, Chiron Diagnostics, Emeryville, CA*
ANJA VAN GEEL • *Hepatitis Program, Innogenetics, Gent, Belgium*
SHOZO WATANABE • *Health Administration Center, Mie University, Mie, Japan*
AMY J. WEINER • *Chiron Corporation, Emeryville, CA*
JUDITH C. WILBER • *Nucleic Acid Diagnostics and New Markers, Chiron Diagnostics, Emeryville, CA*
GAVIN W. G. WILKINSON • *Department of Medicine, University of Wales College of Medicine, Cardiff, UK*
TERESA L. WRIGHT • *Department of Gastroenterology, Veterans Affairs Medical Center and the University of California, San Francisco, CA*
HIROSHI YOSHIKURA • *Department of Bacteriology, Faculty of Medicine, University of Tokyo, Japan*
CRYSTLE L. K. ZAYATI • *Nucleic Acid Diagnostics and New Markers, Chiron Diagnostics, Emeryville, CA*
SERGEI ZOLOTUKHIN • *Gene Therapy Center, University of Florida, Gainesville, FL*
MAAN ZREIN • *Hepatitis Program, Innogenetics, Gent, Belgium*

I

DETECTION OF ANTI-HCV IN SERUM

1

Detection of Anti-GOR Antibodies in HCV Infection

Michael P. Manns and Gerd Michel

1. Introduction

The interactions of the hepatitis C virus (HCV) with the immune system are numerous. As one of the many results, a considerable number of autoantibodies occur in serum. This chapter describes methods to detect anti-GOR antibodies *(1–3)*. Anti-GOR are autoantibodies that are specifically associated with replicating HCV infection. Anti-GOR antibodies were first described by Mishiro et al. *(1)*. These authors had tried to isolate the HCV from chimpanzees infected with serum from a patient with posttransfusion hepatitis non-A, non-B. Screening a cDNA library prepared from RNA isolated from a chimpanzee that was infected with serum from a hepatitis non-A, non-B patient resulted in the isolation of several cDNA clones. Expressed protein of one of such clones specifically reacted with serum from patients with non-A, non-B posttransfusion hepatitis, which later became known as the HCV. Interestingly, this cDNA clone reacted with the liver of uninfected chimpanzees.

The term GOR was given, since this clone was isolated in New York when Gorbachev, president of the former Soviet Union at that time, visited the US. The GOR antigen is expressed in the nucleus of liver cells and seems to be overexpressed in tissue from hepatocellular carcinoma compared to normal liver tissue *(2)*.

Immunoassays based on a linear synthetic GOR peptide were developed *(1,3)*, one of them is described in detail in this chapter *(3)*. Analyses of anti-GOR antibodies in patients' sera have shown that anti-GOR develops early in the course of HCV infection *(1)*, and disappears once HCV replication stops—either spontaneously or after interferon treatment *(4–9)*. Anti-GOR was followed in relation to the spectrum of anti-HCV antibodies in blood donors and post transfusion hepatitis C *(8–11)*. Anti-GOR does not occur in autoimmune liver diseases without HCV infection. In 1992, it became evident that a significant proportion of patients with liver kidney microsomal antibodies type 1 (LKM-1), which are markers of autoimmune hepatitis type 2, are positive for anti HCV. These patients were later confirmed to be HCV RNA-positive *(3)*. When testing patients with autoimmune liver diseases for anti-GOR antibodies only LKM-1 antibody positive patients who were anti-HCV positive were anti-GOR positive *(3)*. This led to the term type 2a for genuine autoimmune hepatitis type 2 without evidence of hepatotropic virus infection. In contrast, the term type 2b was given to anti-HCV, HCV-RNA, and anti-GOR positive patients with LKM-1 antibody associated liver disease *(3)*. Since patients with autoimmune hepatitis type 2b share the clinical characteristics of chronic hepatitis C and corticosteroids are not effective as treatment, these patients are nowadays no longer classified as autoimmune hepatitis type 2 b but as chronic hepatitis C with associated autoimmunity *(12)*. Further studies have shown that anti- GOR antibodies occur in hepatocellular carcinoma if this condition is caused by hepatitis C *(13)*. Furthermore, they are detectable in hepatitis C associated glomerulonephritis *(14)*. In hepatitis D, anti-GOR is only detectable if there is coinfection with HCV *(15)*.

The nature of the cellular GOR antigen is still unclear. There is sequence homology between the hepatitis C core antigen and a protein of the nucleus of liver cells *(2)*. Therefore, anti-GOR may be regarded as antibodies against the hepatitis C core antigen crossreacting with a thus far poorly defined nuclear autoantigen. Thus, anti-GOR does not represent a true marker of autoimmunity. T-cells were shown to proliferate in the presence of the GOR peptide *(16–18)*. Further studies report on the occurrence of anti-GOR in relation to HCV reinfection after liver transplantation *(19)* and other markers of autoimmunity, like antithyroid antibodies *(20)*. Recently, a possible pathogenetic role for the GOR antigen was again postulated.

We have developed an indirect enzyme-linked immunosorbent assay (ELISA) for the detection of antibodies to the human autoantigen GOR utilizing a highly purified synthetic peptide, designated spGOR-2 *(2,3)*, attached to a polystyrene solid phase. After incubation with human serum or plasma specifically bound anti-spGOR-2, IgG class antibodies are detected by use of goat antihuman-IgG covalently conjugated to horseradish peroxidase (HRP) as the reporter enzyme. Results are quantified by colorimetric measurement employing *o*-phenylenediamine as the substrate.

2. Materials

1. spGOR-2 peptide was synthesized at Abbott Laboratories Pharmaceutical Division (North Chicago, IL) (*see* **Notes 1** and **2**). Bovine serum albumin (BSA, fatty acid-free), phosphate buffered saline (PBS, ready-to-use buffer tablets), and

sodium dodecyl sulfate (SDS) were purchased from Sigma Chemicals (Munich, Germany). Sodium bicarbonate (Na_2CO_3 anhydrous), sodium hydrogencarbonate ($NaHCO_3$, anhydrous), 10 M NaOH, 1 N sulfuric acid, Tween 20, and sodium azide (NaN_3) were analytical-grade and came from Merck AG (Darmstadt, Germany).

2. Goat antihuman–IgG–HRPO conjugate concentrate (#4A1 4B02), conjugate diluent (#4A1 4C02), HCV specimen diluent (#4A1 4F02), (o-phenylenediamine × 2HCl) (OPD) (#718198), and OPD diluent (#569502) are commercial products from Abbott Laboratories.
3. Negative control serum (#4A14E) for the anti-GOR assay was taken from Abbott second-generation. HCV screening assay. A selected patient serum was used as a positive control. Sera were stored in aliquots at –20°C.
4. Sodium carbonate coating buffer (0.1 M): mix 300 mL of stock solution A (Na_2CO_3, 0.1 M) and 700 mL stock solution B ($NaHCO_3$, 0.1 M). NaN_3 was added to give a final concentration of 0.2 mg/mL, and pH was adjusted to 9.6 with 10 M NaOH.
5. Washing solution: 0.01 M PBS (prepared from buffer tablets), Tween 20 (0.05% v/v), and SDS (0.01% w/v). Store at 4°C for a maximum of 2 wk.
6. Blocking solution: 1% (w/v) BSA in coating buffer, pH 9.6, sterility filtered. Store at 4°C. Because of the risk of microbial contamination, extended storage of this solution is not recommended.
7. An ATC 340 ELISA reader with a 81 2SW1 microtiter plate washing station (SLT Instruments, Germany) was used to process microtiter plates. Peptides were weighed on a Mettler Toledo MT5 high-precision balance.

   spGOR-2 peptide was coated to polystyrene Maxisorb™ 96-well microtiter plates (NUNC, Roskilde, Denmark). Plate sealer from the same company was used to cover microtiter plates during the EIA procedure and storage.

   Automatic pipets and all other laboratory equipment were regularly checked and maintained under an ISO 9001-certified quality management system at Abbott Laboratories.

3. Methods
3.1. Anti-spGOR-2 IgG Enzyme Immunoassay (Anti-GOR EIA)
3.1.1. Solid Phase Peptide Coating

1. Weigh 10 mg of spGOR-2 peptide in an Eppendorf tube, and dissolve in 1 mL of oxygen-free, double-distilled water (*see* **Note 2**).
2. Immediately serially dilute (3X 1:10) with carbonate coating buffer, pH 9.6, to a final working concentration of 0.01 mg/mL. For practical reasons, to coat one 96-well microtiter plate, prepare 10 mL of working solution.
3. Dispense 0.1 mL of peptide solution/well of the microtiter plate employing an automated pipet (e.g., multichannel or Eppendorf).
4. Cover with seal and incubate without shaking at 37°C for 1.5 h.
5. Discard coating solution, and wash 6 times using washing program #18.
6. Remove residual fluid by blotting plates on filter paper.

7. Dispense BSA blocking solution at 0.2 mL/well.
8. Cover with seal, and incubate without shaking at 37°C for 1.5 h.
9. Wash 6 times using washing program #18.
10. Invert plates, and blot dry on filter paper.
11. Plates can be used readily or covered with plate sealing tape, and stored at 4°C for at least 4 wk.

3.1.2. EIA Procedure

1. Serially dilute 0.02 mL of serum or plasma specimens and the negative control with HCV specimen diluent to a final dilution of 1:1000.
2. Dilute the positive control to a final concentration of 1:5000 with HCV specimen diluent.
3. Remove plate seal. Leave unused wells covered with tape for later use.
4. Pipet 0.1 mL of diluted specimens and controls/well. Use duplicates for patient specimens and triplicates for controls.
5. Seal the plate, and incubate without shaking at 37°C for 3 h.
6. Dilute antihuman–IgG–HRPO conjugate 1:40 with conjugate diluent (*see* **Note 3**). Eleven milliliters are required to process one plate.
7. At the end of the incubation period, wash microtiter plates 6 times with washing solution. Use 0.3 mL/well. Allow filled plates to stand for 2 min between wash cycles. Empty wells by inversion and tap dry.
8. Dispense 0.1 mL of diluted antihuman–IgG–HRPO conjugate/well.
9. Seal plate and incubate without shaking at 37°C for 1 h.
10. Wash as described under **step 7**.
11. Prepare OPD substrate working solution by dissolving one OPD tablet in 5 mL of OPD diluent (*see* **Note 3**). Prepare 10 min prior to use, and keep in the dark. Use within 60 min. Fifteen milliliters are required for one plate.
12. Use 0.1 mL OPD solution/well, and incubate in the dark at room temperature for 30 min without shaking.
13. Stop color reaction by addition of 0.1 mL 1 *N* sulfuric acid, and read absorbance at 492 nm in the ELISA reader.

3.1.3. Expected Results

Typically, in our hands, negative controls read at an optical density (OD_{492nm}) of <0.070. Positive controls should read between 0.60 and 1.70, depending on the sample chosen. A specimen is considered positive if its OD_{492nm} value exceeds 0.230. This cutoff value was calculated as the mean ± 10 SD based on a large series in an apparently healthy control population. Specimens with absorbance values less than the cutoff value are considered negative.

4. Notes

1. Peptide characteristics: The GOR-2 sequence H$_2$N-GRRGQKAKS NPNRPLP-VPRNPCRGPSG-COOH, used in the EIA, is derived from the published GOR47-1 human host sequence (**ref. *1***; DDBJ/EMBL/GenBank accession num-

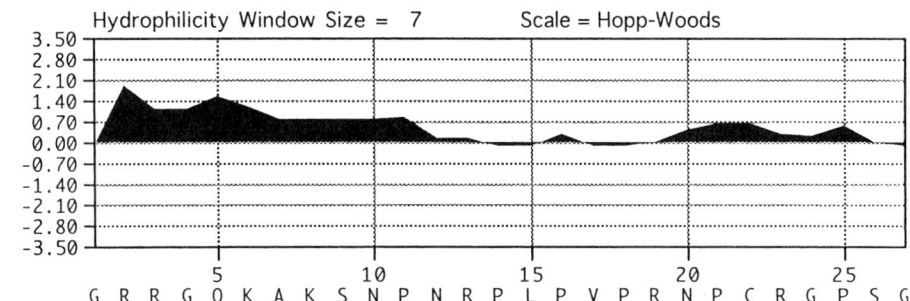

Fig. 1. Hopp and Woods hydrophilicity plot of the spGOR-2 peptide.

ber D1010017). The synthetic peptide is a white, slightly hyproscopic powder with an average molecular mass of 2898.3 and a theoretical isoelectric point (pl) of 12.7. The putative immunoreactive epitope is represented by amino acid residues 18–24 (average molecular mass = 1679.9, pl = 12.9). A hydrophilicity plot of the spGOR-2 sequence is shown in **Fig. 1**.

To date, we have used three different lots of spGOR-2 with a peptide content of >75%. On synthesis, the peptide is delivered as trifluoroacetate salt. Crude peptides were purified by HPLC, and the purity of all three batches was >97%. Synthetic products were verified by amino acid analysis and mass spectrometry.

2. Peptide handling: spGOR-2 can be stored at –20°C in tightly sealed containers without loss of activity for at least 1 yr. Prior to opening and weighing, peptide-containing vials are brought to room temperature in a desiccator. To minimize adsorption of water, portions of the peptide should be weighed rapidly and the storage vial resealed tightly. We use an electrical discharging device (Aldrich Chemicals, Steinheim, Germany) to remove charges from all plastic and glass materials before removing peptide from storage vials.

The peptide trifluoroacetate salt is readily soluble in water. spGOR-2 contains Cys, Asn, and Gln. Peptides containing these amino acids are known to have a limited lifetime when stored in solution. We therefore do not recommend keeping spGOR-2 stock solutions in storage, in particular since we have not generated respective stability data.

3. Anti-GOR EIA: It is important to note that both the conjugate and the OPD reagents are sensitive to light and elevated temperature. Conjugate concentrate and conjugate diluent should be brought to room temperature before mixing. Allow diluted conjugate to equilibrate at room temperature for approx 60 min prior to use. Store at 2–8°C and bring to room temperature before using.

The OPD substrate solution (OPD plus diluent) should be colorless to pale yellow. A yellow or orange color of the solution indicates that the reagent has been contaminated and must be discarded. Bring to room temperature before use. Store reagents at 2–8°C in the dark.

Although other BSA preparations may also work sufficiently well as blocking agents, we have obtained the best results by using fatty acid-free BSA.

In an early development phase, we used covalent peptide coating for the anti-GOR assay. Since passive coating of polystyrene plates as described under **Subheading 3.1.1.** gave comparable results, is more convenient, and is cheaper to perform, the covalent binding approach was discontinued.

In order to evaluate reproducibility of the test results, assay precision was assessed using positive and negative control samples. In a typical set of experiments, both intraassay and interassay CVs ranged from 6 to 10% ($n = 12$ replicates). In our laboratory, anti-GOR results are continuously tracked on respective quality-control charts.

4. Biohazard and laboratory safety: OPD, sodium azide, and sulfuric acid are biohazardous chemicals. Use rubber gloves and eye protection. Avoid contact with skin. Do not eat, drink, or smoke during work. Contact your local biosafety officer to obtain information on respective waste management.

Handling of potentially infectious specimens provides that all laboratory personnel are trained in biosafety and good laboratory practice. Because of the strong association of anti-GOR antibodies and HCV infection, respective biosafety precautions are mandatory.

References

1. Mishiro, S., Hoshi, Y., Takeda, K., Yoshikawa, A., Gotanda, T., Takahashi, K., Akahane, Y., et al. (1990) Non-A, non-B hepatitis specific antibodies direct at host-derived epitope: implication for an autoimmune process. *Lancet* **336,** 1400–1405.
2. Mishiro, S., Takeda, K., Hoshi, Y., Yoshikawa, A., Gotanda, T., and Itoh, Y. (1991) An autoantibody cross-reactive to hepatitis C virus core and host nuclear antigen. *Autoimmunity* **10,** 269–273.
3. Michel, G., Ritter, G., Gerken, G., Meyer zum Büschenfelde, K.-H., Decker, R., and Manns, M. F. (1992). Anti-GOR and hepatitis C virus in autoimmune liver diseases. *Lancet* **339,** 267–269.
4. Mergener, K., Michel, G., Braun, H.-B., Thome-Kromer, B., Korn, A., Müller, R., et al. (1992) Anti-GOR titers in chronic hepatitis C in relation to interferon therapy. *Hepatology* **16,** 213A.
5. Taliani, G., Lecce, R., Badolato, M. C., Boza, A., Poliandri, G., Furlan, C., et al. (1994) Anti-GOR antibodies in anti-hepatitis positive subjects with and without virus replication and liver disease. *J. Hepatol.* **20,** 845.
6. Lau, Y. N., Mizokami, M., Davis, G. L., Kolberg, J. A., Urdea, M. S., Orito, E., et al. (1995) Relationship between the presence of circulating anti-GOR and hepatitis viremia/genotype. *J. Hepatol.* **22,** 707.
7. Lohr, H., Gerken, G., Michel, G., and Meyer zum Büschenfelde, K.-H. (1993) In vitro secretion of anti-GOR antibodies in relation to anti-HCV secreted by mononuclear cells from patients with chronic hepatitis C. *Gastroenterology* **107,** 1443–1448.
8. Hosein, B., Fang X., and Wang, C. Y. (1992) Anti-HCV, anti-GOR, and autoimmunity [Letter]. *Lancet* **339,** 871.

9. Michel, G., Braun, H.-B., Mehta, S., Thome-Kromer, B., Lennartz, L., Klarmann, R., et al. (1993) Anti-GOR2 and anti-GOR346 in acute post-transfusion hepatitis C. *International Symposium on Viral Hepatitis and Liver Disease, Tokyo*. Abstract 193.
10. Michel, G., Bocher, M., Braun, H.-B., Muller, R., Zdebel, R., and Heyermann, H. (1992) Differentiation of HCV specific antibodies in anti-GOR reactive blood donors. *Hepatology* **16**, 72A.
11. Michel, G., Saeed, A. A., Braun, H. B., Thome-Kromer, B., Al-Rasheed, A. M., Rankin, D., et al. (1992) Anti-GOR antibody reactivity in anti-HCV positive Egyptian blood donors, in *Hepatitis C Virus Related Viruses. Molecular Virology and Pathogenesis.* 1st Annual Meeting. Abstract (Houghton, M., Boninio, F., and D'Aquino, M., ed.), Chiron Corp., Venice, Italy, R87.
12. Desmet, V., Gerber, M. A., Hoofnagle, J. H., Manns, M., and Scheuer, P. (1994) Classification of chronic hepatitis: diagnosis, grading and staging. *Hepatology* **19**, 1513–1520.
13. Rehermann, B., Schneider, A., Michel, G., Braun, H. B., and Manns, M. (1995) GOR-antibodies in patients with chronic liver disease and hepatocellular carcinoma. *Z. Gastroenterol.* **32**, 396–398.
14. Lau, J. Y. N., Davis, G. L., Orito, E., Qian, P., and Mizokami, M. (1993) Significance of antibody to the host cellular gene derived epitope GOR in chronic hepatitis C infection. *J. Hepatol.* **17**, 253–257.
15. Durazo, M., Philipp, T., van Pelt, F. N. A. M., Luttig, B., Borgesio, E., Michel, G., et al. (1995). Heterogeneity of microsomal antibodies (LKM) in chronic hepatitis C and D virus infection. *Gastroenterology* **108**, 455–462.
16. Rehermann, B., Schneider, S., Michel, G., and Manns, M. (1993). GORspecific T- lymphcytes: proliferation in chronic hepatitis C. *Z. Gastroenterol.* **30**, 84,85.
17. Mehta, S. U., Mishiro, S., Sekiguchi, K., Leung, T., Dawson, G. J., Pendy, L. M., et al. (1992) Immune response to GOR, a marker for Non-A, Non- B hepatitis and its correlation with hepatitis C virus infection. *J. Clin. Immunol.* **12**, 1–7.
18. Koskinas, J., McFarlane, B. M., Nouri-Aria, K. T., Tibbs, C. J., Mizokami, M., Donaldson, P. T., et al. (1994) Cellular and humoral immune reactions against autoantigens and hepatitis C viral antigens in chronic hepatitis C. *Gastroenterology* **107**, 1436–1442.
19. Rehermann, B., Seifert, U., Tillmann, H. L., Michel, G., Pichimayr, R., and Manns, M. P. (1996) Serological pattern of HCV recurrence after liver transplantation. *J. Hepatol.* **24**, 15–20.
20. Tran, A., Braun, H. B., Benzaken, S., Fredenreich, A., Dreyfus, G., Durant, J., et al. (1995) Anti-GOR and anti-thyroid autoantibodies in patients with chronic hepatitis C. *Clin. Immunol. Immunopathol.* **77**, 127–130.

2

Confirmation of HCV Antibodies by the Line Immunoassay INNO-LIA HCV Ab III

Geert Maertens, Filip Dekeyser, Anja Van Geel, Erwin Sablon, Fons Bosman, Maan Zrein, and Dirk Pollet

1. Introduction
1.1. Hepatitis C Virus (HCV) and Its Disease

HCVs constitute a genus within the Flaviviridae, with closest homology to the hepatitis G and GB viruses, and Pestiviruses. The positive-stranded RNA genome encodes at least nine proteins. Core, E1, and E2 constitute the structural proteins; NS2, NS3, NS4A, NS4B, NS5A, and NS5B are nonstructural (NS) proteins. HCV isolates display high levels of sequence heterogeneity allowing classification into at least 11 types and 90 subtypes *(1)*. HCV infection of the human liver is often clinically benign, with mild icterus in the acute phase; the disease may even go unnoticed in some cases of acute resolving hepatitis C. In the majority (>70%) of cases, however, HCV infection leads to chronic persistent or active infection, often with complications of liver cirrhosis and auto-immune disorders. Hepatocellular carcinoma may occur after about 20–35 yr *(2)*; sometimes even without the intermediate phase of cirrhosis. No prophylaxis is available today and treatment with interferon-alpha (IFN-α) only leads to long-term resolution in about 4–36% of treated cases, depending on the HCV genotype *(1)*.

1.2. Screening and Confirmation of HCV Antibodies

Since productive culture methods for HCV are currently not available, and since only minute amounts of HCV antigens circulate in the infected patient, direct detection of HCV particles cannot be performed routinely, and indirect diagnosis is only possible using cumbersome amplification techniques for HCV RNA detection. Unlike with many other viral infections, HCV particles generally persist in the blood, liver, and lymphocytes, despite the presence of cellular and humoral immune response to most of the HCV proteins. HCV antibodies can be conveniently detected by ELISA techniques, which allow high-throughput screening in blood banks and clinical laboratories. Supplementary antibody testing is required and is now mandatory in most countries. True HCV reactivity is thus discriminated from false reactivity, which may be caused by nonspecific binding of serum or plasma immunoglobulines or anti-idiotypic components to coating or blocking reagents, to contaminants present in HCV antigen preparations, or even to fusion parts or nonspecific regions of the recombinant antigens themselves *(3)*. HCV RNA detection by PCR or bDNA techniques has recently been introduced to monitor chronic HCV disease, especially during therapy. Surprisingly, HCV RNA detection is sometimes employed to confirm HCV antibody screening tests, despite the fact that only ~70–94% of repeatedly HCV antibody positive patient samples are positive by nested polymerase chain reaction (PCR) *(4)*. Of HCV antibody positive blood donors, who usually present with milder forms of the disease and low HCV RNA levels, confirmation by nested PCR is usually on the order of ~40% *(5,6)*. Strip-based assays therefore provide the only reliable alternative for HCV antibody confirmation. Even in the case of an indeterminate result in the confirmatory assay, serological follow-up of the patient rather than HCV RNA detection is advisable. Since native HCV antigens are not available, such confirmatory assays incorporate synthetic peptides and/or recombinant fragments of HCV proteins.

1.3. The Line Immunoassay (LIA)

Innogenetics (Gent, Belgium) introduced the concept of strip technology in which usually a combination of synthetic peptides and recombinant proteins are applied as discrete lines in an ordered and easily readable fashion. The INNO-LIA HIV antibody tests have proven to be superior to routinely used Western blots *(7)*. The Line Immunoassay allows multiparameter testing, and thus, enables incorporation of cutoff and other rating systems, sample addition control, as well as testing for false reactivity to non-HCV proteins used as carrier or fusion partner required for some antigens in the ELISA test. In principle, the test format allows the combination of antigens of different etiological agents or phenotypically linked conditions into a single test.

1.4. Test Principle

The INNO-LIA HCV Ab III is a third-generation Line Immunoassay, which incorporates HCV antigens derived from the Core region, the E2 hypervariable region (HVR), the NS3 helicase region, and the NS4A, NS4B, and NS5A regions. **Table 1** gives an overview of the polyprotein positions of HCV anti-

Table 1
HCV Polyprotein Regions of the INNO-LIA HCV Ab III

INNO-LIA HCV Ab III test			
I and II	III	Position	HCV subtype
c1		1–20	1a/b
c2		13–32	1a/b
c3		37–56	1a/b
c4		49–68	1a/b
	C1	1–32	1a/b
	C2	31–74	1a/b
	E2 HVRI	386–409	1a + 1b
	NS3	1188–1465	1b
NS4		1696–1739	1a
	NS4A + B	1696–1739	1a
	NS4B	1916–1944	1a/b
NS5A	NS5A	2263–2318	1a

gens in first-, second-, and third-generation INNO-LIA HCV antibody tests. The first generation test was launched in 1991 and already incorporated Core and NS5 peptides in addition to NS4 antigens. In the second generation test, sensitivity was considerably improved by introducing biotin-coupled peptides. In the third-generation assay, highly purified recombinant subtype 1b NS3 protein and E2 peptides enabled superior sensitivity while safeguarding the reliable specificity, which is characteristic of peptide-based tests *(8)*. Perhaps one of the most important features of this assay is its unprecedented correlation with HCV RNA positivity *(9–11)* (*see* **Note 1**).

The antigens were coated as six discrete lines on a nylon strip with plastic backing. In addition, four control lines are coated on each strip: antistreptavidin, 3+ positive control (antihuman Ig), 1+ positive control (human IgG), and the ± cutoff line (human IgG). A diluted test sample is incubated in a trough together with the LIA III strip. If present in the sample, HCV antibodies will bind to the HCV antigen lines on the strip. Subsequently, an affinity-purified alkaline phosphatase-labeled goat antihuman IgG (H + L) conjugate is added and reacts with specific HCV antigen/antibody complexes if previously formed. Incubation with enzyme substrate produces a chestnut-like color, the intensity of which is proportionate to the amount of HCV-specific antibody captured from the sample on any given line (**Fig. 1**). Color development is stopped with sulfuric acid. If no HCV-specific antibodies are present, the conjugate only binds to the ±, 1+, and 3+ control lines. If the addition of sample is omitted, only the ± and 1+ control lines will be stained.

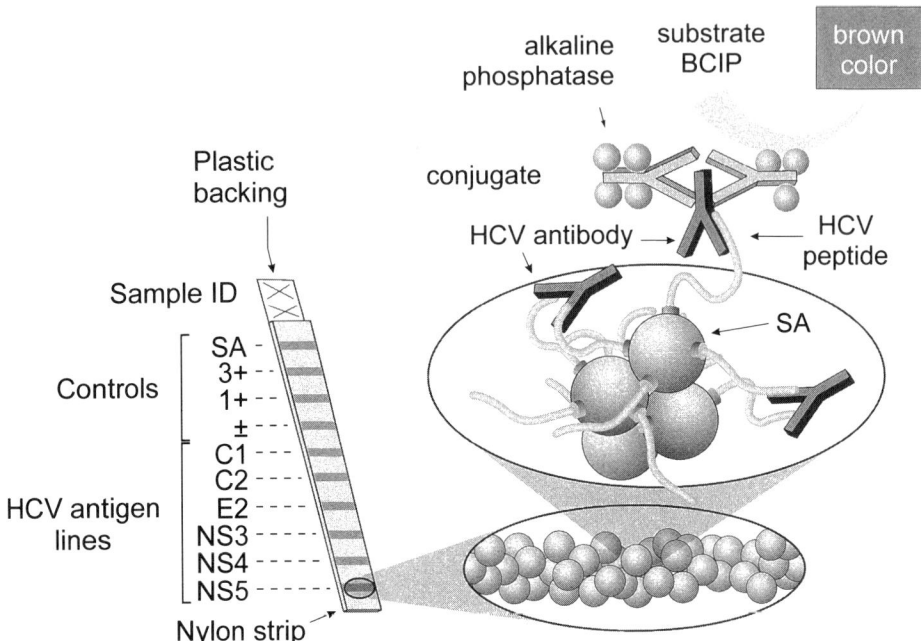

Fig. 1. Schematic representation of the INNO-LIA HCV Ab III procedure.

2. Materials
2.1. Antigens Applied on the INNO-LIA HCV Ab III Strip
2.1.1. The Core Region

The native HCV Core protein is translated from codons 1–191 of the HCV genome. On expression of this region in *Escherichia coli*, however, poor levels of intact protein are obtained owing to the presence of the hydrophobic carboxy-terminal region. Many laboratories therefore generated recombinant core proteins that encompass the region from amino acids (aa) 1–2 to 120–150. Recombinant core proteins expressed and purified from *E. coli* are known to exhibit false reactivity *(11)*. These proteins have been replaced by more specific synthetic peptides in third-generation HCV confirmation tests. We employed Core peptides already from the first-generation HCV assays onward. We determined the immunodominant epitope regions of the HCV Core region by means of overlapping 20-mer and 9-mer peptides. The most important B-cell epitopes localize in 2 clusters near the amino-terminal part of the Core protein. One extends from aa 7–25, the other from aa 35–67. Each in turn can be separated in two epitope regions (aa 7–16 and aa 19–25; aa 35–49 and 56–67). Overall, eight different epitopes could be mapped between aa 7 and 67. We incorporated synthetic peptides encompassing the two immunodominant epitope clusters and, in order to increase sensitivity and specificity, applied these as two different lines C1 and C2 (**Table 1**). Since a separate epitope cluster is represented in each line, crossreactivity between the two LIA III core lines is excluded. The epitopes located between aa 7–16 and 56–67 have not been incorporated in some third-generation confirmatory assays. Almost all HCV antibody-positive sera react with one or both of the LIA III Core lines (*see* **Note 2**).

2.1.2. The E2 HVR I

Detection of E2Ab has been shown to be important for confirmation of HCV antibodies *(12)*. When the HCV E2 region is scanned for B-cell epitopes using 20- to 25-mer peptides, only the HVRI region shows important reactivity. Several peptides derived from HVRI sequences of different isolates belonging to HCV subtypes 1a and 1b were incorporated into LIA III (*see* **Note 3**). Reactivity to the LIA III E2 line is seen with approx 50–60% of HCV antibody-positive sera, and shows a strong correlation with HCV RNA positivity *(9)*.

2.1.3. The NS3 Helicase Region

The amino-terminal part of the helicase region (hepatitis C clone 19b [HCCl19b], **Table 1**) was cloned from a European subtype 1b isolate IG8309. Subtype 1b infections show the highest prevalence worldwide. In Europe, they represent ~50–60% of HCV infections, whereas subtype 1a HCV strains prevail in ~0–35% of European infections, roughly averaging ~10% *(1)*. From most studies investigating genotype-specific antibody reactivities, it was reported that the HCV NS3 helicase region does not display complete crossreactivity between major genotypes. For example, Dow et al. reported reduced sensitivities for the c33 and c100 antigens in RIBA 3.0 for HCV type 2 and 3 samples *(13)*. Based on aa sequences available from the Genbank, one can deduce that subtype 1a and 1b NS3 proteins differ by 7 (2.5%) to 21 (7.6%) aa in the region incorporated in diagnostic assays. We have encountered several cases to be positive only with the subtype 1b NS3 protein incorporated in the LIA III, but not with subtype 1a NS3 proteins (*see* **Note 4**). These observations are of particular importance in early diagnosis of HCV infection where detection of NS3 antibodies is crucial. Since the majority of HCV antibody screening is performed with tests incorporating subtype 1a NS3 proteins, it is not known how many subtype 1b HCV infections, the most life-threatening of all, are currently missed. With the exception of NS4, variability in the other regions does not seem to influence detection of HCV antibody *(13)*.

The NS3 protein was synthesized as a murine tumor necrosis factor (mTNF) fusion protein in *E. coli*. The mTNF fusion partner allows extremely high expression levels, a prerequisite for obtaining ultrapure recombinant antigen preparations. Here, the fusion partner does not interfere with specificity, since human anti-mTNF antibodies are only encountered very infrequently. Several RIBA-3 NS3-only cases have been reported to be LIA III-negative. Although some of these cases may represent specific reactivities (*see* **Note 4**), most of such reactivities, even when accompanied by c100 or NS5 reactivities on RIBA 3.0, could not be confirmed by other antibody tests, by PCR, nor were these associated with risk factors of the subject, and could consequently be classified as false positive cases *(13,14)* (*see* **Note 4**).

2.1.4. The NS4A and NS4B Regions

NS4 peptides were included from the first-generation LIA onward. The small NS4A protein is now known to be associated with the NS3 protease as a cofactor. NS4A contains one epitope region, which is incorporated in the NS4 line. The NS4B protein displays strongly reactive linear epitopes at its N- and C-terminus, and these epitopes were also incorporated as synthetic peptides in the LIA III NS4 line. The NS4A and amino-terminal NS4B regions form a discontinuous linear epitope region, which is often referred to as 5-1-1. We previously located the major epitope of NS4A between aa 1696 and 1701, whereas the N-terminus of NS4B contains five epitopes, two of which are located between aa 1714 and 1724, and three of which extend from aa 1725–1739. The epitope from aa 1733–1739 is not incorporated in third-generation confirmatory assays other than LIA III (for example, the 5-1-1 region extends from aa 1694–1735). Extreme genotypic variability is observed in this region *(1)*, allowing, to a certain extent, serological determination of HCV types *(15)*. For screening and confirmatory tests, however, such variability (up to 60% dissimilarity) poses important challenges with respect to sensitivity of detection of NS4 antibodies. Although NS4 antibodies are generated in about 80% of HCV infections, only 10% of subtype 3a sera react with the 5-1-1 peptide, which is derived from subtype 1a *(16)*. The sequences of the LIA III NS4 peptides have been shown to be less liable to genotypic variations *(16,17)*. The NS4B C-terminal epitope lies within a conserved region and thus presents a crossreactive epitope region (aa 1916–1944), which is sometimes referred to as c100, but which is not incorporated in the recombinant C100-3 region (aa 1569–1931). The epitope has therefore only recently been introduced in some third-generation confirmatory assays, such as LIA III. An extended hydrophobic region connects the N- and C-termini of the NS4B protein. It is devoid of specific B-cell epitopes and caused the notorious false reactivities of the formerly used C100-3 protein (*see* **Note 5**). Recombinant

NS4 proteins have now been replaced by synthetic peptides in most third-generation tests.

2.1.5. The NS5A Region

By scanning the NS5 region, we detected a major epitope cluster between aa 2260 and 2330 in NS5A, composed of four different epitopes. The NS5B region also contains some minor epitopes, but unlike the NS5A region, NS5B displays marked homology to other RNA viruses *(18)*. Proteins incorporating both NS5A and NS5B regions are prone to nonspecific reactivities *(9,12–14)*. We therefore omitted NS5B antigens from the LIA III strip; several peptides from the HCV-specific NS5A region were also applied on a single NS5 line. The LIA III NS5 reactivity has indeed shown to be specific *(9,13)* (*see* **Note 6**). Although the usefulness of NS5 antibodies in HCV antibody screening is often debated, Zaaijer et al. clearly demonstrated that NS5 reactivity is sometimes needed to achieve positive confirmation of HCV antibody *(9)*. Also Dow and coworkers reported a PCR-positive case with isolated strong NS5A reactivity on LIA III, which reacted negatively in screening tests not incorporating NS5 *(19)*. Furthermore, NS5 antibody may be a useful marker for monitoring disease or treatment. Lunel and coworkers recently detected an association between the presence of NS5 antibodies (especially antibody reacting with the LIA III NS5A) before treatment with sustained response to IFN-α treatment.

In conclusion, samples that show a negative result when tested with alternative HCV screening or confirmatory assays can still be reactive to HCV when tested in the INNO-LIA HCV Ab III owing to the presence of unique HCV epitopes.

2.2. Reagents Provided with the Kit

1. Twenty LIA HCV antigen-coated test strips with plastic backing, ID number, sample addition control, and rating controls.
2. Human negative control serum, prediluted.
3. Human positive control serum containing HCV antibody to each of the 6 LIA III antigen lines, prediluted.
4. Sample diluent.
5. Concentrated solution of alkaline phosphatase-conjugated goat antihuman IgG (H + L chain), to be diluted 1:100 in conjugate diluent prior to use.
6. Conjugate diluent.
7. Concentrated solution of 5-bromo-4-chloro-3-indolylphosphate in dimethyl formamide, to be diluted 1:100 in substrate buffer prior to use.
8. Substrate buffer.
9. Stop solution (0.1 N sulfuric acid).
10. Five times concentrated wash solution.
11. Two incubation trays with 11 troughs each, in a plastic minigrip bag.
12. Five adhesive plate sealers.

2.3. Materials Required, But Not Provided

1. Distilled or deionized water.
2. Precision pipets (with disposable tip) capable of delivering 10 µL, 20–200 µL, and 200–1000 µL. To avoid contamination, the use of cotton-plugged (aerosol-resistant) tips is advisable if the same sample is intended to be used for HCV RNA determination.
3. An orbital or longitudinal shaker or rocker (*see* **Note 7**).
4. Vortex mixer or equivalent.
5. Graduated cylinders; 10, 25, 50, and 100 mL.
6. Tweezers for handling of the strips.
7. Hot-air fan (hair dryer) or dry 37°C incubator.

3. Method

3.1. Manual Procedure

1. Use the required number of test troughs, taking a positive and negative control test into account. Identify each test trough for controls and specimens, and place into the tray.
2. Add 1 mL of sample diluent to each specimen test trough. Note that the positive and negative controls are already prediluted in sample diluent.
3. Add 10 µL of the appropriate specimen or 1 mL of each control to the corresponding labeled troughs.
4. Remove the required number of LIA strips from their container, identify the strips, and add one strip to each of the test troughs. Using the tweezers, completely submerge the strip, membrane-side up, in the trough containing sample diluent.
5. Cover the troughs with an adhesive sealer. Incubate the samples by placing the tray on a shaker or rocker, and agitate overnight (16 ± 2 h) at room temperature (the test has been validated to operate well between 15 and 30°C).
6. Prepare conjugate solution 10 min prior to the end of the incubation.
7. Wash each test strip three times with washing solution (*see* **Note 8**).
8. Add 1 mL of prepared conjugate solution to each test trough.
9. Incubate with the conjugate by placing the test tray on the shaker or rocker and agitate for 30 min at room temperature.
10. Prepare substrate solution 10 min prior to the end of the incubation.
11. Wash each test strip twice with wash solution and once with substrate buffer.
12. Add 1 mL of prepared substrate solution to each test trough.
13. Incubate at room temperature on the shaker or rocker and agitate for 30 min.
14. Aspirate liquid. Add 1 mL of stop solution to each trough.
15. Incubate with the stop solution on the shaker or rocker for 10–30 min at room temperature.
16. Remove the strips from the test troughs, and place on absorbent paper using a pair of tweezers. Results can be interpreted after complete drying. Developed strips will retain color if protected from light.

Table 2
Interpretation of the INNO-LIA Strip

Reactivity of the HCV antigen line	Result[a]
$<\pm$ Cutoff line	–
$\geq\pm$ Cutoff line, <1+ control	±
= 1+ Control	1+
>1+ Control, <3+ control	2+
=3+ Control	3+
>3+ Control	4+

[a]Different interpretation criteria may be requested by different registration authorities.

3.2. Automated Procedure Using the Auto-LIA™ System

The *Auto*-LIA procedure enables automated processing of up to 30 strips. After addition of the sample, the system allows full walk-away processing and excludes manipulation errors. Combined with the LIA-Scan™ software package, it allows highly standardized and reliable HCV antibody confirmation.

3.3. Interpretation of the LIA III Strip

1. For each of the six HCV antigen lines, rating is judged relative to the intensities of the control lines 3+, 1+, and ± as presented in **Table 2**.
2. Interpretation criteria.
    HCV antibody negative: all HCV antigen lines are negative.
    HCV antibody positive: one of the following possibilities: one HCV antigen line shows a reactivity of 2+ or higher, or at least two HCV antigen lines show reactivities of 1+ or higher.
    HCV antibody indeterminate: 1+ or ± reactivities are present on one antigen line, whereas other antigen lines do not display reactivities higher than ±. A follow-up sample should be tested.
    A sample showing reactivity to the streptavidin control line may crossreact with other HCV antigens lines and cannot be interpreted. A follow-up sample should be tested. Alternatively, streptavidin antibodies may be competed by repeating the test and adding 10 µL of a solution of 5 mg/mL streptavidin to 1 mL of sample diluent prior to the addition of sample.
3. Validation: For the test to be valid, the following criteria must be met:
    a. The positive control strip must show a reaction of at least 1+ on all antigen lines, except for the E2 line, which may show a reaction of ±.
    b. The negative control strip must show no reactivity or reactivities inferior to the cutoff line ± on all antigen lines.
    c. The control level 1+ as well as the strong positive control level 3+ should be visible on all strips with control level 3+ > control level 1+.
    d. The antistreptavidin control line should be invisible.

3.4. Semiquantitative Determination of HCV Antibody Levels

Objective semiquantification and interpretation can be obtained by scanning of the LIA strips. Conventional scanners, such as Hewlett Packard or Apple, are compatible with a specific software program (LIA-Scan™ Infectious Diseases). Such semiquantitative analysis of six different HCV antibody levels can be conveniently used for monitoring of treatment or natural evolution of hepatitis C disease (*see* **Note 9**). Each line is scanned by means of 8 vertical and 24 horizontal measurements yielding 192 readings/line or 1920 data per strip. A value of 0 is given to the cutoff line, and 100 corresponds to the 3+ control. Since the 3+ control intensity varies according to the immunoglobulin content of the sample, this variable is balanced. Using the control lines and a system recognizing spots, complete test validation, interpretation, and indication of possible errors are reported in the form of a hard copy (**Fig. 2**). An interassay coefficient of variation of <5% could be demonstrated, rendering the system suitable for monitoring of HCV antibodies over prolonged periods, such as in IFN-α treatment (*see* **Note 9**).

4. Notes

1. In a comparative analysis of five HCV confirmatory tests, Zaaijer et al. *(9)* reported 94% of RIBA-2 indeterminate/PCR-positive samples to be positive by LIA III (as compared with 39–90% for the four other tests); 77% of RIBA-2 indeterminate/PCR-negative samples were also negative by LIA III (compared with 15–67% in other tests). A very low number of indeterminate results is thus generated by LIA III, allowing fast referral of patients, without the need to request follow-up samples for the sole purpose of confirmation of HCV infection.
2. The use of two different core epitope regions is often questioned, especially since a 2+ single-line reactivity yields a positive result. Several cases only reacting with the LIA III C1 or C2 regions in the absence of any other HCV antibody have been encountered in our laboratories (**Table 3**) and by others *(20–22)*. Such cases were confirmed to be HCV RNA-positive, but scored negative in other commercial confirmatory assays. Cases showing isolated core antibody reactivity correlated well with PCR positivity, unlike isolated NS3, NS4, or NS5 reactivities *(10,11,14)*, and are often associated with infection by HCV types other than type 1 *(13)*. In a panel of samples obtained from Egyptian blood donors and cancer patients, Attia et al. detected isolated core reactivities by LIA II, which were not detectable in other assays *(21)*. The Middle East is known to be endemic for HCV type 4 *(1)*. Dussaix et al. demonstrated similar patterns in French patients *(22)*. Furthermore, in a panel of 1613 negative control samples, none showed positive reactivity to either one of the core lines. We therefore believe the HCV core antigens to be highly sensitive and specific tools in HCV antibody confirmation, justifying the use of two completely separated epitope clusters.

Line Immunoassay INNO-LIA HCV Ab III

```
Assay print out                                          LIA-Scan version 2.3a
```

```
                    Sample ID : PC 3
                   Assay Name : Inno-Lia HCV Ab III
                 Assay Result : HCV positive
                Assay Lot no. : 61216666
                   Assay Date : 31/01/97
                   Assay Time : 13:30:50
                 Patient name :

                     Sheet ID : T262a
                     Position : 3
                     Operator : First time user

        Software licenced to  : innogenetics
                                ontwikkeling
```

Assay Picture :

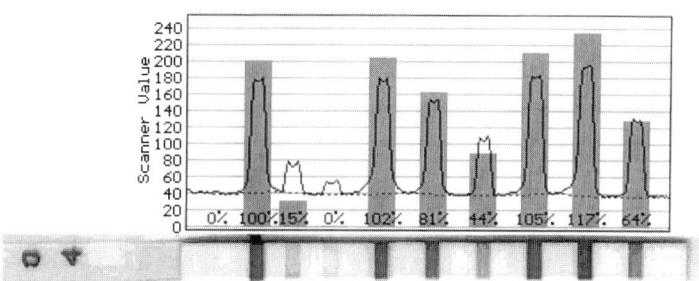

Evaluation Data :

Antigen band	Int.	Rating	Qual.	Conclusion
Core 1+2	102%	+++	Good	Strong Reactive
Core 3+4	81%	+++	Good	Strong Reactive
NS1	44%	++	Good	Strong Reactive
NS3	105%	+++	Good	Strong Reactive
NS4	117%	+++	Good	Strong Reactive
NS5	64%	++	Good	Strong Reactive
Streptadivin	0%		Good	
anti-Ig	100%		Good	
IgG Medium COV	15%		Good	
IgG Low COV	0%		Good	

Fig. 2. The LIA-Scan system.

3. Although >90% of infected subjects develop anti-E2 antibodies, the majority of these are directed against conformational epitopes that can only be detected using E2 purified for mammalian cells. Recombinant E2 was not available until recently and was not yet incorporated in any HCV test.
4. As a consequence of the use of a subtype 1b NS3 protein in our screening and confirmation assays, we have been able to gather samples showing unique reactivities to this NS3 protein. Some of these cases are presented in **Table 3**. Most c33 only reactivities are thought to represent false-positive reactivities. Dow and

Table 3

Sample	ELISAs INNOTES HCV Ab III	Ortho 3.0	CONFIRMATORY ASSAYS INNO-LIA HCV Ab III C1	C2	E2	NS3	NS4	NS5	result	RIBA-3 C100p	C33c	C22p	NS5	Result	Western Blot*	PCR	LIPA	Origin	
Core																			
IG28660	4.4	0.42	2	+/-	0	0	0	0	Pos	0	0	0	0	Neg	Pos	Neg	na	France	Donor
IG15561	1.6	0	2	0	+/-	0	0	0	Pos	+/-	+/-	3	0	Ind	na	Pos	na	Brazil	Patient
IG13577	4.8	2.5	0	2	0	0	0	0	Pos	0	0	0	0	Neg	na	na			
E2																			
IG20117	na	na	0	0	2	0	0	0	Pos					na	na	Pos	7a	France	Patient
IG21743	na	na	+/-	+/-	+/-	0	0	0	Ind					na	na	Pos	4c	Egypt	Donor
IG21890	na	na	4	4	4	0	0	0	Pos					na	na	Pos	2c	France	Patient
NS3																			
IG28659	1.3	1.01	0	0	0	2	0	0	Pos	0	0	0	0	Neg	Pos	Neg		France	Donor
IG28668	0.9	0.06	0	0	0	2	0	0	Pos	0	0	0	0	Neg	Pos	Neg		France	Donor
IG28675	0.3	0.05	0	0	0	2	0	0	Neg	0	3	0	0	Ind	Pos	Neg		France	Donor
IG28695	1	1.02	0	0	0	3	0	0	Pos	0	4	0	0	Ind	Pos	Neg		France	Donor
IG21923	Pos	na	0	+/-	0	4	0	0	Pos	0	0	0	0	Neg	Pos**	Pos	1b	France	Donor
IG21925	Pos	na	0	0	0	0	0	0	Neg	0	2	0	0	Neg	Pos**	Pos	1b	France	Donor
IG28691	1	2.5	0	0	0	0	0	0	Neg	0	3	0	0	Ind	Neg	Neg		France	Donor
D1***	na	Pos	0	0	0	0	0	0	Neg	0	1	0	1	Pos	Neg	Neg		Holland	Donor
IG28708	0.2	3.5	0	0	0	0	0	0	Neg	0	1	0	0	Ind	Neg	Neg		France	Donor
NS4																			
IG28669	0.2	2.84	0	0	0	0	0	0	Neg	2	0	0	0	Ind	Neg	Neg		France	Donor
NS5																			
T11755 G	na	Pos	0	0	0	0	0	0	Neg	0	0	2	2	Pos	na	Neg		Scotland	Donor
D4***	na	Pos	0	0	0	0	0	0	Neg	1	0	2	2	Pos	Neg	Neg		Holland	Donor
na****	na	4.65	0	0	0	0	0	3	Pos	1	3	0	4	Pos	na	Pos	3a	Scotland	Donor

coworkers, for example, only confirmed 1 out of 220 RIBA-3 c33 indeterminate cases by PCR *(13)*, and ascribe the improved specificity of RIBA-3 over RIBA-2 to the use of core and NS4 peptides, with little improvement of specificity for the RIBA-3 c33 band *(19)*. On the other hand, also cases with unique reactivity to the c33 antigen have been reported from commercially available panels originating from the US, but they are thought to be overrepresented, because most of the HCV screening is performed using this subtype 1a antigen. Interestingly, NS3 reactivities do not always agree between screening and confirmatory assays either (**Table 3**).

5. Isolated LIA III NS4 reactivities are rare, but specific (**Table 3**). False-positive c100 reactivities are not confirmed on LIA III *(13,14,22)*.
6. Tests incorporating NS5A and NS5B regions often show isolated reactivities to the NS5 band. All such cases have been shown to be HCV RNA-negative and LIA III-negative *(9,13,14,22)*. Conversely, NS5 reactivity patterns were comparable between LIA III and other tests in PCR-positive samples *(9,19,20)*.
7. Sufficient agitation during all incubation steps of the INNO-LIA procedure is essential to obtain high-quality strips. Orbital shakers should have an orbit of ≥13 mm. Recommended speeds are 90 (24-mm orbit) to 160 (13-mm orbit) rpm. Longitudinal shakers with back and forth agitation should be adjusted to 120 movements/min. For rockers, vertical agitation should not exceed 30 mm to avoid spilling of liquid; recommended speed is 55 movements/min.
8. Directions for washing: After overnight incubation, carefully remove the adhesive plate sealer. The liquid is aspirated from the trough with a pipet, preferably attached to a vacuum device. Hold the tray at an angle sufficient to allow the liquid to flow to one side of the trough. Use the side of the tray at which the plastic ID area of the strips is located. This will prevent damaging of the nylon strips. One milliliter of diluted wash solution is added to each trough, and the tray is agitated for 1 min on an orbital mixer. These steps are repeated as many times as indicated in the assay procedure. The strips should not be allowed to dry in between washing steps. The use of a clean aspiration device with disinfectant trap is recommended. Care should be taken to submerge the entire strip completely during each washing step.
9. Using the LIA-Scan system, we monitored antibodies to the 6 LIA III antigens before, during, and after treatment. Only in long-term responders to treatment, did we find a significant decrease in E2 HVR, NS3, and NS4 antibodies during and after treatment, with NS4 antibodies decreasing most significantly. Lunel and coworkers (personal communication) detected the presence of NS5 antibodies in close to 100% of responders before IFN treatment, both in RIBA and LIA. In nonresponders, NS5 antibodies were detected in 50% of cases by RIBA and only in 30% by LIA. NS5A antibody detection before treatment may therefore aid in the prediction of response to interferon-α.

Acknowledgment

This work was supported in part by the Flemish government, Ministry of Economics (grants FIOV/IWT/91/007.tv1 and ADV/94072/Innogenetics) as part of Eureka Project EU680 "hepatitis C."

References

1. Maertens, G. and Stuyver, L. (1996) Genotypes and genetic variation of hepatitis C virus, in *Molecular Medicine of Hepatitis* (Zuckerman, A. and Harrison, T., eds.), *Molecular Medical Science Series* (James, K. and Morris A., eds.), John Wiley, Chichester, UK, pp. 183–233.
2. Saito, I., Miyamura, T., Ohbayashi, A., Harada, H., Katayama, T., Kikuchi, S., et al. (1990) *Proc. Natl. Acad. Sci. USA* **87,** 6547–6549.
3. McFarlane, I., Smith, H., Johnson, P., Bray, G., Vergani, D., and Williams, R. (1990) Hepatitis C virus antibodies in chronic active hepatitis: pathogenic factor or false-positive result? *Lancet* **335,** 754–757.
4. Marin, M., Bresciani, S., Puoti, M., Rodella, A., Gussago, A., Ravaggi, A., et al. (1994) Clinical significance of serum HCV RNA as marker of HCV infection. *J. Clin. Microbiol.* **32,** 3008–3012.
5. Stuyver, L., Fretz, C., Esquivel, C., Boudifa, A., Jaulmes, D., Azar, N., et al. (1996) HCV genotype analysis in apparently healthy anti-HCV positive Parisian blood donors. *Transfusion* **36 (6),** 552–558.
6. Waumans, L., Claeys, H., Verhaert, H., Mertens, W., and Vermylen, C. (1993) Hepatitis C virus confirmation in blood donor screening. *Vox Sang.* **64,** 145–149.
7. Pollet, D., Saman, E., Peeters, D., Warmenbol, H., Heyndricks, L., Wouters, C., et al. (1990) Confirmation and differentiation of antibodies to human immunodeficiency virus 1 and 2 with a strip-based assay including recombinant antigens and synthetic peptides. *Clin. Chem.* **37,** 1700–1707.
8. Peeters, D., Dekeyser, F., DeLeys, R., Maertens, G., and Pollet, D. (1993) Confirmation of anti-hepatitis C virus antibodies using the INNO-LIA HCV Ab III including Core, E2/NS1, NS3, NS4, and NS5 epitopes. International Symposium on Viral Hepatitis and Liver Disease, Tokyo, abstract 413.
9. Zaaijer, H., Vrielink, H., van Exel-Oehlers P., Cuypers, H., and Lelie, P. (1994) Confirmation of hepatitis C infection: a comparison of five immunoblot assays. *Transfusion* **34,** 603–607.
10. De Beenhouwer, H., Verhaert, H., Claeys, H., and Vermylen, C. (1992) Confirmation of hepatitis C virus positive blood donors by immunoblotting and polymerase chain reaction. *Vox Sang.* **63,** 198–203.
11. Claeys, H., Volkaerts, A., Verhaert, H., De Beenhouwer, H., and Vermylen C. (1992) Evaluation of anti-HCV capsid indeterminate samples. *Lancet* **340,** 249.
12. Zaaijer, H., Vallari, D., Cunnigham, M., Lesniewski, R., Reesink, H., van der Poel C., et al. (1994) E2 and NS5: new antigens for detection of hepatitis C virus antibodies. *J. Med. Virol.* **44,** 395–397.
13. Dow, B., Buchanan, I., Munro, H., Follett, E., Prescott, L., Yap, P., et al. (1996) Relevance of RIBA-3 supplementary test to HCV PCR positivity and genotypes for HCV confirmation of blood donors. *J. Med. Virol.* **49,** 132–136.
14. Damen, M., Vrielink, H., Lelie, P., Zaaijer, H., and Reesink, H. (1995) Incorrect Diagnosis of hepatitis C with RIBA-3. *Vox Sang.* **69,** 358.

15. Stuyver, L., van Arnhem, W., Wyseur, A., DeLeys, R., and Maertens, G. (1993) Analysis of the putative E1 envelope and NS4A epitope regions of HCV type 3. *Biochem. Biophys. Res. Comm.* **192,** 635–641.
16. McOmish, F., Chan, S.-W., Dow, B., et al. (1993) Detection of 3 types of hepatitis C virus in blood donors: investigation of type-specific differences in serologic reactivity and rate of alanine aminotransferase abnormalities. *Transfusion* **33,** 1357–1359.
17. Chan, S.-W., Simmonds, P., McOmish, F., Yap, P.-L., Mitchell, R., Dow, B., et al. (1991) Serological responses to infection with three different types of hepatitis C virus. *Lancet* **338,** 1391.
18. Miller, R., and Purcell, R. (1990) Hepatitis C virus shares amino acid sequence similarity with pestiviruses and flaviviruses as well as members of two plant virus supergroups. *Proc. Natl. Acad. Sci. USA* **87,** 2057–2061.
19. Dow, B., Follett, E., Jordan, T., McOmish, F., Davidson, J., Gillon, J., et al. (1994) Testing of blood donations for hepatitis C virus. *Lancet* **343,** 477–478.
20. Vernelen, K., Claeys, H., Verhaert, H., Volkaerts, A., and Vermylen, C. (1994) Significance of NS3 and NS5 antigens in screening for HCV antibody. *Lancet* **343,** 853.
21. Attia, M., Zekri, A.-R., Goudsmit, J., Boom, R., Khaled, H., Mansour, M., et al. (1996) Diverse patterns of hepatitis C virus core and nonstructural antigens by antibodies present in Egyptian cancer patients and blood donors. *J. Clin. Microbiol.* **34,** 2665–2669.
22. Dussaix, E., Charnaux, N., Laurent-Puig, P., Chopineau, S., Laurian, Y., and Buffet, C. (1994) Analysis of sera indeterminate by Ortho RIBA-2 by using three confirmatory assays for anti-hepatitis C virus antibody. *J. Clin. Microbiol.* **32,** 2071–2075.

II

DETECTION AND QUANTITATION OF HCV IN SERUM

3

Detection of HCV RNA in Serum by Reverse Transcriptase-PCR and Radiolabeled Liquid Hybridization

Richard L. Hodinka

1. Introduction

Hepatitis C virus (HCV) possesses a single-stranded, positive-sense RNA that is 9.4 kb in length. The complete HCV genome has been cloned and sequenced and encodes for a nucleocapsid, an envelope, and five nonstructural proteins *(1,2)*. The 5' untranslated region of the virus is highly conserved among the HCV genotypes that have been identified to date *(3–5)* and has been selected by most investigators as the site for developing oligonucleotide primers and probes for the polymerase chain reaction (PCR) *(6–9)*. PCR has proven to be a rapid, sensitive, and useful method for the detection of HCV infections *(6–16)*. The assay can detect HCV in HCV antibody-negative individuals suspected of having hepatitis and can discriminate chronic HCV infections from resolved acute infections in patients who are positive for HCV antibody. The procedure can also be used to:

1. diagnose HCV infections in newborns of HCV-infected women;
2. resolve indeterminate serologic results;
3. monitor antiviral therapy, and
4. identify HCV infection in high-risk, seronegative individuals.

The reverse transcriptase (RT)-PCR protocol that follows has been adapted and modified from **refs.** *6* and *8* and uses a combination of RNA extraction, cDNA synthesis, PCR amplification, gel electrophoresis, and autoradiography to detect HCV RNA from human serum, plasma, or tissue. The primers used are from the highly conserved 5' untranslated region of the viral genome. For RT-PCR analysis by this method, HCV RNA is extracted from specimens by

Table 1
Oligonucleotide Primer and Probe Sequences for PCR Detection of HCV RNA

Function	Sequence name[a]	Nucleotide sequence, 5' to 3'	Nucleotide position
cDNA synthesis antisense primer	5PUTc1-a	CCC AAC ACT ACT CGG CTA G	–74 to –92
Sense primer	5PUT 1-s	AAC TAC TGT CTT CAC GCA GAA AGC	–266 to –289
Probe	5PUT p1-s	GCC ATG GCG TTA GTA TGA GTG TC	–238 to –260

[a] 5PUT, 5' untranslated; c, cDNA synthesis; a, antisense; s, sense.

using RNAzol B *(17)* and chloroform:isoamyl alcohol (24:1). The RNA is then precipitated using isopropanol and an MS2 RNA carrier molecule, washed in ethanol, dried, and resuspended in RNase-free water. Double-stranded cDNA synthesis is conducted with the antisense primer 5PUTc1-a (**Table 1**) by using Moloney Murine Leukemia Virus-RT (MMLV-RT). The PCR is performed under mineral oil in a solution containing Taq polymerase, $MgCl_2$ each deoxynucleoside triphosphate, and primers 5PUTc1-a and 5PUT 1-s (sense primer). After an initial denaturation step at 94°C for 5 min, 35 cycles at 94°C for 1.5 min, 60°C for 2.0 min, and 72°C for 3.0 min are followed by an additional cycle at 72°C for 7 min. Detection of amplified product is accomplished by liquid hybridization with ^{32}P-labeled oligonucleotide probe (5PUT p1-s) followed by 10% polyacrylamide gel electrophoresis and autoradiography.

2. Materials
2.1. Reagents
2.1.1. Probe Labeling

1. The oligonucleotide probe 5PUT p1-s (*see* **Table 1**) can be synthesized in-house or obtained commercially. Make a 330 ng/μL stock solution of the probe and store aliquots indefinitely at –20°C before use. When needed, dilute the stock solution 1:100 in sterile distilled, deionized water (ddH_2O) to make a working solution of 3.3 ng/μL of probe. Make single-use 100 μL aliquots of the working dilution in sterile 1.5 mL Eppendorf tubes and store indefinitely at –20°C until use. The probe should be labeled with ^{32}P-γATP as described in **Subheading 3.2.**
2. T4 Kinase (Gibco-BRL Life Technologies, Grand Island, NY). Store at –20°C before use.
3. Sephadex G-25 columns (Boehringer Mannheim Biochemicals, Indianapolis, IN). Store at 4°C and bring to room temperature before use.
4. 10X PNK Buffer. All reagents for this buffer can be purchased from Sigma Chemical Co., St. Louis, MO: 0.61 g Tris (TRIZMA Base), 0.10 g $MgCl_2$, 0.08 g

dithiothreitol (DTT), 0.002 g spermidine (free base), and 0.004 g EDTA. Bring the volume of the buffer to 10.0 mL with ddH$_2$O and stir to dissolve the ingredients. Prepare multiple 100 µL aliquots of 10X PNK buffer in 500 µL Eppendorf tubes and store for no longer than 1 yr at –20°C before use. The preparation yields a final concentration of 0.5 M Tris-HCl, 0.1 M MgCl$_2$, 50 mM DTT, 1 mM spermidine, and 1 mM EDTA.
5. 10% Orange-G dye (Sigma). Prepare 0.1 g of Orange-G dye in 1.0 mL sterile ddH$_2$O. Store at room temperature for no longer than 1 yr.
6. STE buffer. All reagents for this buffer can be purchased from Sigma: 0.58 g NaCl, 0.12 g Tris (TRIZMA Base), and 0.04 g EDTA. Bring the volume of the buffer to 100 mL with ddH$_2$O and stir to dissolve the ingredients. Filter the solution using a 0.45 µm membrane filter and store at room temperature for no longer than 1 yr before use. The preparation yields a final concentration of 0.1 M NaCl, 10 mM Tris, and 1 mM EDTA.
7. Distilled, deionized water.
8. ^{32}P-γATP (Boehringer Mannheim).
9. Scintillation fluid (Amersham, Arlington Heights, IL).
10. All purpose radioactive decontamination fluid (NEN Research Products, Boston, MA).

2.1.2. RNA Extraction

1. RNAzol B (Tel-Test, Inc., Friendswood, TX): Prepare 900 µL aliquots in 1.5 mL RNase-free Eppendorf tubes and store at 4°C before use.
2. Chloroform:Isoamyl alcohol (24:1): Make 100 mL of stock solution in a sterile bottle. Wrap the bottle in aluminum foil and keep in the dark at room temperature for no longer than 3 mo.
3. MS2 RNA (Boehringer Mannheim): Make a 1:40 dilution to obtain a working solution of 20 µg/mL of MS2 RNA (e.g., 50 µL MS2 RNA into 1950 µL RNase-free water). Prepare 50 µL aliquots in RNase-free Eppendorf tubes and store at 4°C for no longer than 3 mo before use.
4. Isopropanol: Store indefinitely at room temperature.
5. 75% Ethanol: Add 25 mL RNase-free water to 75 mL of 200 proof ethanol. Make 1 mL aliquots in RNase-free Eppendorf tubes and store at –20°C for no longer than 3 mo before use.
6. RNase-free water. Buy commercially (Promega Corp., Madison, WI) or DEPC diethyl pyrocarbonate (Sigma)-treated ddH$_2$O.

2.1.3. PCR Amplification

1. Enzymes:
   a. Murine Moloney Leukemia Virus-Reverse Transcriptase (MMLV-RT; Gibco-BRL): Place 2.5 µL aliquots of MMLV-RT into 500 µL RNase-free Eppendorf tubes and store at –20°C before use. Do not leave this enzyme at room temperature any longer than is absolutely necessary.
   b. Taq DNA polymerase. Obtain this enzyme as part of PCR Core Reagent Kit, Perkin Elmer (Branchburg, NJ). Place 5 µL aliquots into 500 µL RNase-free

Epppendorf tubes and store at –20°C before use. Do not leave this enzyme at room temperature any longer than is absolutely necessary.

2. RNase Inhibitor (RNasin, human placenta, Promega Corp.): Place 5 µL aliquots into 500 µL RNase-free Eppendorf tubes and store at –20°C before use.
3. Oligonucleotide primers (see **Table 1**). 5PUTc1-a (antisense) and 5PUT 1-s (sense) can be synthesized in-house or obtained commercially. Make a 20 µM/mL stock solution of each primer in RNase-free water. Prepare 75 µL aliquots in RNase-free Eppendorf tubes and store indefinitely at –20°C before use.
4. PCR Core Reagent Kit (Perkin Elmer). Store at –20°C.
5. PCR Buffer II (Perkin Elmer). Store at –20°C.
6. 25 mM MgCl$_2$ solution (Perkin Elmer). Store at –20°C.
7. RT-Master Mix for cDNA synthesis:

PCR Buffer II (500 mM KCl, 100 mM Tris, pH 8.3 stock)	200 µL
MgCl$_2$ (25 mM stock)	400 µL
RNase-free water	250 µL
dATP (10 mM stock)	200 µL
dTTP (10 mM stock)	200 µL
dGTP (10 mM stock)	200 µL
dCTP (10 mM stock)	200 µL
5PUTc1-a primer (20 µM)	75 µL
Total	1725 µL

   Divide the RT-Master Mix into 10 aliquots of 172.5 µL each in 500 µL RNase-free Eppendorf tubes. Expose the tubes to short and long wavelength UV light for 30 min each and store at –20°C for no longer than 3 mo before use.
8. Taq-Master Mix for PCR:

MgCl$_2$ (25 mM stock)	400 µL
PCR Buffer II	800 µL
RNase-free water	6675 µL
5PUT 1-s primer (20 µM)	75 µL
Total	7950 µL

   Divide the Taq-Master Mix into 10 aliquots of 795 µL each in 1.5 mL Eppendorf tubes. Expose the tubes as above to short and long wavelength UV light and store at –20°C for no longer than 3 mo before use.
9. RNase-free water: Buy commercially (Promega Corp.) or DEPC (diethyl pyrocarbonate)-treated water.
10. Mineral oil: Prepare aliquots of mineral oil in 1.5 mL RNase-free Eppendorf tubes and expose to short and long wavelength UV light for 30 min. Aliquots are for single use only.
11. Positive patient control. Serum from a serologically positive patient with chronic HCV hepatitis.
12. Negative patient control. Serum from an HCV-uninfected patient.
13. Negative amplification control. Use 2 µL of RNase-free water as a substitute for extracted RNA at the reverse transcriptase step.

Detection of HCV RNA in Serum

2.1.4. Solution Hybridization

1. 5 M NaCl. Prepare by weighing 0.292 g of NaCl and adding to 1.0 mL of sterile ddH$_2$O. Store at room temperature for no longer than 1 yr before use.
2. ^{32}P-labeled 5PUT p1-s probe.
3. Sterile ddH$_2$O.

2.1.5. Detection of Amplified Product

1. 10X TBE buffer. All reagents for this buffer can be purchased from Sigma: 60.0 g TRIZMA Base, 30.9 g boric acid, and 3.7 g EDTA. Dissolve ingredients into 300 mL of ddH$_2$O with stirring. Bring the volume of the solution to 500 mL. The pH of the buffer should be 8.19. Filter the solution using a 0.45 µm membrane filter and store at room temperature for no longer than 3 mo before use. This buffer is used to make loading buffer and polyacrylamide gels, and as an electrophoresis running buffer.
2. 1X TBE running buffer: Just prior to use, mix 50 mL of 10X TBE and 450 mL of ddH$_2$O to make 1X TBE running buffer.
3. 40% Polyacrylamide (for 10% gels): 57.0 g acrylamide (Bio-Rad Laboratories, Hercules, CA) and 3.0 g bis-acrylamide (Bio-Rad). Wear mask, gloves, and a laboratory coat while weighing ingredients. Polyacrylamide is a neurotoxin as a powder or a liquid. Dissolve in 90 mL of ddH$_2$O with stirring and gentle heat (if necessary). Be careful not to heat any more than is needed because polyacrylamide may polymerize violently when heated. Bring the volume of solution to 150 mL and filter using a 0.45 µm membrane filter. Protect the reagent from light and store for no longer than 6 mo at 4°C before use.
4. 10% gel for electrophoresis. For preparation, see **Subheading 4.6.**
5. Ammonium persulfate (Bio-Rad: for gel polymerization). Make a 10% solution by weighing 0.5 g of ammonium persulfate and adding to 5 mL of ddH$_2$O. Protect the solution from light and store at 4°C for no longer than 6 mo before use.
6. Loading buffer: 1.25 mL 10X TBE buffer (*see above*), 0.50 mL 1% xylene cyanole (XC; Sigma) solution (weigh 0.05 g XC and add to 5 mL ddH$_2$O for a 1% solution), 0.50 mL 1% bromophenol blue (BPB; Sigma) solution (weigh 0.05 g BPB and add to 5 mL ddH$_2$O for a 1% solution), 2.50 mL 40% sucrose (Sigma) solution (weigh 2.0 g sucrose and add to 5 mL ddH$_2$O for a 40% solution), and 0.25 mL ddH$_2$O. For daily use, store at room temperature. Store at –20°C for no longer than 1 yr before use. Yields 5.0 mL of loading buffer in the following concentration: 2.5X TBE, 0.1% XC and BPB, and 20% sucrose.
7. TEMED (Bio-Rad; for gel polymerization).

2.2. Supplies and Equipment

1. 500 µL and 1.5 mL Eppendorf tubes (DEPC-treated, RNase free). For DEPC treatment, place the tubes in a large beaker and soak the tubes overnight at 37°C in 0.2% DEPC (e.g., 2.0 mL of DEPC into 1000 mL of ddH$_2$O). After soaking, empty the DEPC solution from the beaker and autoclave the tubes for 15 min at

121°C, 15 psi followed by 30 min on the dry cycle. If necessary, evaporate the remaining moisture from the tubes by placing the beaker in a biological safety cabinet with the aluminum foil lid resting on top of the beaker and the cabinet's UV light on.
2. Micropipeters with aerosol barrier filter tips or positive displacement pipets and tips (Rainin Instrument Co., Woburn, MA).
3. Sterile 1.0, 5.0, 10.0, and 25 mL serological pipets and safety pipetting devices.
4. Disposable protective gowns, latex gloves, and safety glasses.
5. Appropriate tube racks.
6. Suitable containers for ice.
7. Photographic intensifying screens (Cronex; NEN Research Products).
8. Beta shields.
9. GeneAmp reaction tubes (Perkin Elmer).
10. Eppendorf tube cap openers.
11. Sterile cotton-plugged Pasteur pipets.
12. Disposable plastic pipets.
13. Sterile cryovials (Sarstedt, Newton, NC).
14. 15 and 50 mL polypropylene centrifuge tubes (Corning Glass Works, Corning, NY).
15. 0.5% hypochlorite solution and 70% ethanol for cleaning work surfaces.
16. Infectious- and radioactive-waste disposal containers.
17. Adequate sterilization facilities.
18. Whatman paper.
19. 30 mL syringe with 21-gage butterfly needle.
20. 13 × 18 cm XOMAT AR-5 film (Eastman Kodak Company, Rochester, NY).

2.3. Equipment

1. Refrigerator at 2–8°C.
2. Freezer at –70°C.
3. Class II biological safety cabinet.
4. High speed microcentrifuge (Eppendorf, Fisher Scientific, Malvern, PA).
5. DNA Speed-Vac (Savant Instruments, Inc., Farmingdale, NY).
6. Dry baths (Thermolyne Dri-baths, Fisher Scientific).
7. Water baths.
8. Vortex mixers.
9. Thermal cycler (Perkin Elmer Model 480).
10. Polyacrylamide gel apparatus (Mini-Protean II Dual Slab Cell; Bio-Rad).
11. Electrophoresis power supply (Bio-Rad).
12. Timers.
13. Ultraviolet transilluminator (Fisher Scientific).
14. Beta counter.
15. Light box.

2.4. Preliminary Comments and Precautions

1. Bring all reagents to appropriate temperatures before use and return them to the recommended storage temperatures immediately after use.

2. Do not smoke, eat, or drink in areas where specimens or reagents are handled.
3. Appropriate precautions should be taken when handling infectious and radioactive materials. Do not mouth pipet samples or reagents. Avoid contact with broken skin or mucous membranes. Wear latex gloves, disposable laboratory gowns, and other appropriate protective devices. Wash hands thoroughly after handling these materials.
4. Use radioactive material only in designated work areas and cover laboratory bench surfaces with an absorbent material.
5. Use an absorbent material and suitable detergent to clean radioactive spills from involved surfaces and 0.5% sodium hypochlorite to wipe all areas before and after processing of infectious material. Dispose of all infectious and radioactive materials properly.
6. Expiration dates should be indicated on the labels of all reagents, or observe the expiration date established by the manufacturer. Do not use materials and reagents beyond the assigned expiration dates and do not interchange or mix different lots of reagents.
7. Arrange materials and equipment to provide easy access and minimize the number of manipulations.
8. Accurate processing of specimens and careful preparation of reagents is required for quality performance of this procedure.
9. Use appropriate aseptic technique throughout the procedure.

3. Methods
3.1. Specimen Collection and Handling

1. Serum is the specimen of choice, although plasma and tissue specimens can also be used. A minimum of 3–5 mL of blood should be collected in a tube without anticoagulant.
2. Allow the blood to clot and separate the serum from the clotted blood by centrifugation at 400g for 10 min at room temperature. This should be done as soon as possible, within 1–6 h of collection to avoid degradation of the HCV RNA.
3. The serum should be immediately transferred to sterile screw-capped tubes (Sarstedt, Newton, NC), placed on ice, or appropriately stored at 2–8°C, and transported within 24 h to the processing laboratory. If a delay in transport of more than 24 h is anticipated, the specimen should be rapidly frozen to at least –60°C (dry ice) and transported to the laboratory on dry ice.
4. Following receipt of specimens in the laboratory, those stored at 4°C should be processed for PCR within 24 h or they should be frozen at –70°C until tested.
5. For plasma, collect blood in tubes with nonheparin or non-EDTA anticoagulants (e.g., sodium citrate or acid citrate dextrose), centrifuge at 400g for 10 min at room temperature, and remove the plasma. Store as for serum.
6. Tissue specimens should be placed in viral transport medium, transported as above, and processed using the following protocol.
   a. Using a disposable 15 mL tissue grinder, aseptically homogenize a small piece (approx 1–3 mm^2) of tissue in 2.0 mL of sterile PBS without Ca^{2+} or Mg^{2+} to achieve an even cell suspension.

b. Transfer the homogenate to a 15 mL conical centrifuge tube. Add 8.0 mL of PBS to the tube and mix by inverting the tube several times.
c. Centrifuge the cell suspension for 10 min at 400g at room temperature.
d. After centrifugation, aspirate the supernatant and resuspend the cell pellet in 10 mL of PBS. Repeat the centrifugation as above.
e. Following the final wash, aspirate the supernatant and resuspend the cell pellet in 250 µL of PBS.
f. The cells can be immediately extracted for RNA or placed in labeled cryovials and stored at –70°C before use.

3.2. Probe Preparation (5' End-Labeling of Probe)

1. Heat a 100 µL aliquot of probe 5PUT p1-s in a 65°C water bath for 5 min. Pulse spin the tube for 10 s at maximum speed in a microcentrifuge to pull down condensation. Keep tube on ice until ready to use.
2. For each aliquot of probe to be labeled, prepare a labeled 1.5 mL Eppendorf tube containing 5 µL 10X PNK buffer, 2 µL T4 kinase (yields 20 U), 3 µL sterile ddH$_2$O, and 30 µL of 3.3 ng/µL of probe 5PUT p1-s.
3. Following all radioactive precautions, add 10 µL of ^{32}P-γATP to the Eppendorf tube. Incubate the tube for 30 min in a 37°C water bath.
4. Remove the tube from the water bath and pulse spin as above to pull down condensation.
5. Add an additional 1 µL of T4 kinase and incubate the tube for another 30 min at 37°C.
6. Equilibrate a Sephadex G-25 column:
    a. Gently invert the column to resuspend the Sephadex beads in the buffer. Gentle tapping may be required. Once fully resuspended, remove the top and bottom cap of the column and place the column in the provided Eppendorf tube. Allow the column buffer to drain by gravity into the tube.
    b. Remove the liquid from the Eppendorf tube and discard. Place the column into the Eppendorf tube and put both the column and the tube into the provided larger snap-capped tube.
    c. Spin the column inside the snap capped tube at 2000g for 2 min at room temperature. Use maximum brake to stop the centrifuge.
    d. After centrifugation, remove the liquid from the Eppendorf tube. Replace the column in the Eppendorf tube and slowly pipet 400 µL of STE buffer onto the top of the column without disturbing the Sephadex beads. Spin as in **step c**.
    e. Measure the liquid in the Eppendorf tube as it is removed and discarded following centrifugation. If the volume is not 400 µL, repeat **step d** until it is approx 400 µL. This will usually require 2–3 repeated additions of buffer and centrifugations to equilibrate the column.
7. When the end-labeling incubation in **step 5** is completed, pulse spin the Eppendorf tube (now containing labeled probe) briefly to pull down condensation and then add 1 µL of 10% Orange-G dye to the probe solution.
8. Drop by drop, gently pipet the probe solution onto the Sephadex beads in the equilibrated column. Spin the column for 2 min as described above in **steps 6b** and **6c**.

9. The Orange-G dye should remain at the top or within the column. If any dye comes through the column, then the probe solution will have to be purified again using a freshly equilibrated column.
10. Approximately 50 µL of labeled probe should now be in the Eppendorf tube. Store at –20°C for no longer than 5–6 wk before use.
11. To determine the counts per minute of radiolabeled probe, dilute the labeled probe 1:10 in ddH$_2$O. Add 1 µL of this dilution to 5 mL of scintillation fluid in a scintillation vial. Count the vial in a Beta counter. Calculate the volume of probe required to yield 200,000 counts per minute per sample.
12. The radiolabeled probe should be stored in the original container in a specially designated area of the laboratory in accordance with federal, state, and local regulations.

3.3. Specimen Preparation (RNA Extraction)

1. Add 100 µL of patient serum, plasma, or homogenized tissue and 100 µL of positive and negative control sera to 900 µL of RNAzol B in individual Eppendorf tubes and vortex vigorously for 15 s.
2. Add 100 µL chloroform:isoamyl alcohol (24:1) to each Eppendorf tube. Vortex for 15 s.
3. Place the tubes on ice for 5 min.
4. Spin in a microcentrifuge at 12,000g for 15 min at 4°C. While samples are centrifuging, label 1.5 mL Eppendorf tubes with patient name and date on the side and specimen number on the top.
5. Add 500 µL of anhydrous isopropanol and 5 µL of MS2-RNA to each labeled Eppendorf tube.
6. After centrifugation, place the samples on ice. With a 200 µL pipet set to 125 µL, carefully transfer only the aqueous phase to the labeled 1.5 mL Eppendorf tubes. This will take 4–5 transfers. Gently invert the labeled tubes six times to mix.
7. Place tubes at –70°C for 60 min to precipitate the RNA. **Note:** This is a good stopping point. If necessary, samples can remain at –70°C overnight.
8. After the 60 min incubation, remove the Eppendorf tubes from the freezer. Gently invert the tubes six times and place on ice.
9. Centrifuge the tubes at 12,000g for 15 min at 4°C. Position the tubes in the centrifuge with the hinge of each tube cap facing upward as a point of reference.
10. After centrifugation, aspirate the isopropanol using a sterile cotton plugged Pasteur pipet. Be very careful not to aspirate the precipitated RNA pellet. The pellet will not be visible but will be positioned on the same side of the tube as the cap hinge. Therefore, aspirate the liquid from the opposite side of the tube.
11. Add 250 µL of 75% ethanol and gently invert the tubes six times. Place the tubes on ice. **Note**: Extracted specimens can be stored at –70°C at this point, if necessary.
12. Centrifuge the tubes at 12,000g for 10 min at 4°C. Position the tubes in the centrifuge as described in **step 9**.
13. Aspirate the ethanol as in **step 10**.
14. Leaving the caps open, place the Eppendorf tubes into a DNA Speed-Vac set on high heat. Centrifuge the tubes for 6 min.

15. Remove the tubes from the Speed-Vac and observe for white crystalline pellets. If no pellet is visible, centrifuge the tubes again for 1 min. Continue to centrifuge the tubes in 1 min increments until a pellet is observed.
16. When pellets are dried sufficiently, resuspend them with 20 µL of RNase-free water. Specimens can be placed on ice at this point for RT-PCR or stored at –70°C for future testing.

3.4. HCV RT-PCR

1. Remove from the –20°C freezer aliquots of Taq DNA polymerase, MMLV-RT, RNAsin, RT master mix, Taq master mix, positive and negative controls, and samples to be amplified. Pulse-spin the thawed reagents, specimens, and controls to pull down condensation before opening the tubes.
2. Obtain the appropriate number of 500 µL GeneAmp reaction tubes. In addition to each specimen, set up at least one positive control, one negative control, and one reagent (DNA-free) control per assay. Label each tube cap with the date, "HCV", and specimen number. Do not cap the tubes tightly at this point because the caps are difficult to open.
3. Add 2.5 µL of MMLV-RT and 5 µL of RNAsin to 172.5 µL of RT master mix. Vortex and pulse spin. Add 18 µL of the freshly prepared master mix solution to each labeled Eppendorf tube. **Note**: 1 prepared aliquot of reagent is sufficient for 10 tests.
4. Using a plastic disposable transfer pipets, place two drops of UV-treated mineral oil over the RT master mix in each reaction tube, and then close the tube caps.
5. One by one, reopen the tubes and transfer 2 µL of resuspended specimen and control RNA to each prepared tube. Substitute 2 µL of RNase-free water for the nucleic acid-free reagent control. Be sure to carefully go through the layer of mineral oil and add the RNA directly to the master mix.
6. Transfer the reaction tubes to a plastic or styrofoam float and incubate for 15 min in a 42°C water bath to allow for reverse transcription of RNA to cDNA.
7. While the samples are incubating, transfer 5 µL of Taq DNA polymerase to 795 µL of Taq master mix. Vortex and pulse spin. **Note**: 1 prepared aliquot of reagent is sufficient for 10 tests. Place the prepared master mix on ice until ready to use.
8. After incubation, transfer the reaction tubes to a 99°C heat block for 5 min to inactivate the MMLV-RT.
9. Then place the reaction tubes in a 80°C heat block positioned in a biological safety cabinet.
10. Carefully add 80 µL of prepared Taq master mix to each tube.
11. Turn on the thermal cycler and preheat the block to 94°C.
12. Spin the samples in a microcentrifuge at 14,000g for 30 s at room temperature.
13. Place the samples in the thermal cycler for 35 cycles of amplification. Set the temperature and time cycles as follows:

1 cycle	5.0 min, 94°C
35 cycles	1.5 min, 94°C
	2.0 min, 60°C
	3.0 min, 72°C
1 cycle	7.0 min, 72°C
	Indefinite at 15°C

Detection of HCV RNA in Serum

14. Following amplification, pulse-spin the reaction tubes to pull down condensation. The samples are ready for hybridization or they may be stored frozen at −20°C.

3.5. Solution Hybridization

1. Complete the remaining steps in an area designated for post amplification work and radioactive use.
2. After checking the water level, activate circulating 56 and 95°C water baths and allow them to come to temperature. Place a piece of absorbent bench mat on the work surface. Set up radioactive shielding over the bench mat. Line the area behind the shield with a small piece of absorbent bench mat. Use double plastic bags in appropriate containers for disposal of radioactive waste.
3. For solution hybridization of the amplified products to the ^{32}P-labeled probe, combine appropriate amounts of 5 M NaCl with probe and ddH$_2$O for each sample to be hybridized. The volumes of probe and ddH$_2$O will vary according to the age/activity of the probe. Use sufficient probe diluted in water to yield 200,000 counts per minute per sample. Remember that ^{32}P has a physical half-life of 14.3 d.
4. There should always be a total of 5 µL of probe/water/NaCl solution for each specimen. This may be prepared in a single tube for the entire run and aliquoted into the individual specimen tubes for the hybridization. For example, if using freshly labeled probe, you might use this recipe:

Per sample	Per 10 samples
2 µL of a 1:10 probe dilution in ddH$_2$O	20 µL of a 1:10 probe dilution in ddH$_2$O
2.5 µL ddH$_2$O	25 µL ddH$_2$O
0.5 µL 5 M NaCl	5 µL 5 M NaCl

    Then aliquot 5 µL into each labeled 500 µL Eppendorf tube.
5. Pulse spin the amplified samples. Proceeding slowly through the mineral oil, remove 10 µL of amplified specimen and add to a correspondingly labeled hybridization tube that contains the probe solution. Mix by pipetting up and down several times. Cap tightly and transfer the tubes to a plastic or styrofoam float. Keeping the tubes shielded, transfer the tubes to the 95°C waterbath for 5 min.
6. Then transfer the tubes in a shielded fashion to the 56°C water bath for 30 min incubation. Upon removal from the water bath, pulse-spin the tubes to pull down condensation. The hybridized samples may be held at 4°C until ready for visualization.
7. Discard all radioactive waste in a manner consistent with established federal, state, and local policies.

3.6. Visualization

1. Electrophorese the hybridized samples on a 10% polyacrylamide gel, and then perform autoradiography. The gel electrophoresis is essentially the same as detailed by Bio-Rad.

2. Follow the Bio-Rad Instruction Manual for the set up of the Mini Protean II Dual Slab Cell. Use one or two slab cells as needed.
3. 10% polyacrylamide gel preparation:
    a. To make a 10% polyacrylamide gel, mix the following cold (keep on ice in bucket) reagents without generating bubbles: 14.0 mL ddH$_2$O, 1.0 mL 10X TBE, 5.0 mL 40% polyacrylamide and
    b. Add the above reagents to a 50 mL conical centrifuge tube. Cap the tube and invert gently twice.
    c. Working quickly but without making bubbles, add 0.4 mL of 10% ammonium persulfate. Cap and invert gently twice.
    d. Add 12 µL of TEMED. Cap and invert gently twice.
    e. Place the solution on ice. The described volume is sufficient for making two gels. Generating no bubbles, draw the solution into a 30 mL syringe. Attach a 21-gage butterfly needle to the syringe and fill each side of the prepared slab cell apparatus.
    f. Insert a Teflon comb (10 well × 0.75 mm) at an angle into each side of the slab cell setup. Adjust the combs and allow the gels to polymerize for 45 min to 1 h. Work quickly but carefully while preparing the gels.
    g. When the gels have polymerized, remove one slab cell apparatus from the casting stand. Remove the comb and quickly rinse the wells using a squeeze bottle containing ddH$_2$O.
    h. Dry each well using precut strips of absorbent Whatman paper.
    i. Repeat procedure with the second gel.
    j. Mark the smaller glass plate with the location of the wells using a black permanent marker. Doing this will make it easier to visualize the wells during loading of processed specimens.
4. Upper buffer chamber:
    a. Assemble the upper buffer chamber as described in the Bio-Rad Instruction Manual.
    b. After assembly of the chamber, fill the inner chamber of the electrophoresis apparatus with 1X TBE running buffer to just below the large glass plate. Fill the outer chamber with approx 200 mL of buffer.
5. Loading samples (Follow federal, state, and local precautions for use of radioactive material):
    a. Place a piece of absorbent bench mat on the work surface. Set up radioactive shielding over the bench mat. Line the work area of the shield surface with a small piece of absorbent bench mat. Use double plastic bags in appropriate containers for the disposal of radioactive waste.
    b. Add 7 µL of loading buffer to each sample. Mix by gently pipetting up and down.
    c. Transfer the entire volume to the corresponding well of the gel. Load the wells slowly and be careful to avoid cross contamination of adjacent wells. The order of loading of samples should be actual clinical specimens first, followed by positive and then negative controls.
    d. When all of the samples are loaded, check the level of running buffer in the chamber. Add more if needed.

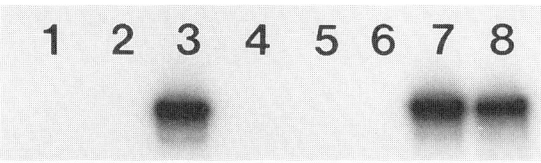

Fig. 1. Reverse-transcriptase-polymerase chain reaction for the detection of HCV RNA in serum. Amplification of a 194 bp HCV cDNA sequence was performed using a set of primers specific for the 5'-untranslated region of the HCV genome. Detection of amplified product was done by liquid hybridization with a ^{32}P-labeled oligonucleotide probe followed by polyacrylamide gel electrophoresis and autoradiography. lane 1, negative reagent control (DNA-free); lane 2, negative serum control; lanes 3–7, clinical specimens, with lanes 3 and 7 representing positive patient results; lane 8, HCV-positive serum control.

    e. Place lid on the gel apparatus, making certain that the electrical connections are red to red and black to black. Run at 150 V for 35 min.
    f. Disassemble the gel apparatus in the reverse sequence that it was assembled. Place the gel on a small piece of Whatman filter paper (paper should be slightly larger than the gel and of an appropriate size to fit into the intensifying screen). Wrap the gel in plastic wrap and place it into the intensifying screen. Tape the edges of the gel to the cassette so the gel remains stationary. Move to a photographic dark room and insert a piece of XOMAT AR-5 film (Kodak) into the cassette. Expose the film for a minimum of 60 min and a maximum of 120 min, depending on the activity of the radiolabeled probe for the run. Develop the film and read the results on a standard light box.

3.7. Interpretation and Reporting of Results

1. In a valid run of samples, the positive control will demonstrate a distinct band of diagnostic significance (**Fig. 1**). Negative and DNA-free reagent controls will show no band. A patient sample should be compared to the positive and negative controls for result interpretation. Any specimen showing no band is considered to be negative for HCV by PCR. A specimen is considered to be positive for HCV by PCR if the banding pattern is consistent with that observed for the positive control.
2. Specimens can be initially tested in singlet. The PCR process should be repeated in duplicate for specimens giving weak or questionable reactions on the gels and results reported based on an interpretation of the three testings. If specimen results cannot be resolved by repeat testing, the specimen should be reported as indeterminate for HCV by PCR. If clinically indicated, a second specimen should be submitted for repeat testing by RT-PCR.
3. A PCR run should be considered invalid and repeated if the negative controls appear positive or the positive controls give no band.
4. The significance of results should be evaluated with respect to the clinical situation.

4. Notes

1. Because of the extreme sensitivity of PCR and the potential for product carry over, strict adherence to appropriate guidelines *(18,19)* for the use of nucleic acid amplification techniques is mandatory when performing HCV RT-PCR.
    a. Separate areas should be designated for preamplification reagent preparation (area 1) and specimen processing (area 2), amplification (area 3) and postamplification (area 4) work. Strictly maintain these areas. **Always** work in a unidirectional flow from the preamplification areas to the postamplification area. Amplified products are reportedly carried on skin, hair, and clothing.
    b. Each area should have its own designated equipment, materials, and reagents. Do not mix or use these items in other areas.
    c. To decrease the risk of product carry over, always pulse-spin all reaction tubes prior to opening and complete all specimen preparation steps in an area free of target sequence contamination.
    d. Disposable gown and gloves must be worn in all PCR areas. Never reuse a gown or gloves and never wear a gown or gloves from one area while in another area. Do not hesitate to change gowns and gloves frequently, especially if there is any possible aerosol, splash, or spill on these items.
    e. Whenever possible, use positive displacement pipets or filter barrier pipet tips for **all** work.
    f. **Never** bring amplified samples into the preamplification areas.
    g. DNA may be denatured by using bleach or UV light treatment. Use both liberally to decrease the risk of nucleic acid contamination. Clean each PCR area thoroughly with a 1.0% solution of bleach, making certain to wipe the bench tops, hoods, and other equipment. Remove the bleach residue using 70% ethanol. The potential for product carryover can also be minimized by sterilizing the nucleic acid in samples for PCR. This can be accomplished by using the bacterial enzyme uracil-N-glycosylase to selectively degrade amplified strands of uracil-containing DNA that have been carried over from previous amplifications. Alternatively, the compounds, psoralen or isopsoralen, can be added to samples to photoinactivate amplified products, rendering them unavailable for subsequent amplifications.
    h. Multiple reagent and template-free negative controls should be assayed with each PCR reaction to assist in detecting contamination.
    i. Do not enter into the amplification or postamplification detection areas before doing preamplification work on the same day. A technologist that has handled amplified product should not then process samples for PCR on that day.
    j. Where possible, reagents for PCR should be stored in single-use aliquots and the remainder discarded after a single PCR run. Reagents should be stored separately away from all specimens (unamplified or amplified) and unamplified specimens must be stored separately from those that have been amplified.
    k. If a UV box is used to treat reagents, turn off the UV light in the box before placing your arms and hands into the working area. Do not expose eyes directly to UV light. Wear protective goggles if needed.

1. When performing RT-PCR for HCV, appropriate quality control and quality assurance programs should be established for reagents, equipment, and instruments, and for the recording and reporting of results. Laboratories should also participate in a formal external proficiency testing program, if available, and should implement procedures to test for internal consistency in results.
2. Because RNA is especially vulnerable to degradation, improper collection, handling, and/or storage of serum or plasma samples can seriously effect the results obtained using HCV RT-PCR *(20–22)*. It is critical to remove the serum or plasma from the blood as soon as possible and preferably within 1–6 h of collection. It is also important to avoid holding the serum or plasma at room temperature for extended times, to avoid hemolysis of blood during collection and processing, and to avoid freeze-thawing of samples that have been frozen.
3. The primers and probes used in the described RT-PCR will detect all known genotypes of HCV. The sensitivity of this assay is 10–100 copies per 10 µL and the use of a radiolabeled probe to detect the PCR product eliminates the need for nested PCR. The specific detection of the product is also enhanced using a hybridized probe.
4. The detection of amplified product can be accomplished using one of many methods. A procedure of solution hybridization with a radiolabeled probe followed by separation and detection of the hybridized product using polyacrylamide gel electrophoresis and autoradiography is described here. Although quite sensitive, this procedure is relatively labor-intense and involves radioactive material. Several nonisotopic detection systems in a 96-well microplate-based format similar to that used for enzyme immunoassays are now commercially available.
5. Useful clinical information regarding the detection of HCV RNA by RT-PCR includes:
    a. Since HCV culture or antigen detection methods are not available to clinical laboratories, detection of RNA in serum is used as a marker for the virus itself. Although detecting HCV-specific antibody by enzyme immunoassay and recombinant immunoblots *(23–25)* remain the first choice for diagnosis of HCV infection, only molecular amplification assays, such as PCR, can detect HCV-infected individuals prior to antibody production and differentiate acute and chronic HCV infection in an individual who is antibody positive.
    b. With RT-PCR, HCV viremia is detected within a few days after infection and generally persists throughout chronic infection.
    c. HCV RNA may not be detectable in serum during all stages of infection, becuase fluctuating levels of RNA are commonly observed. Therefore, a single negative HCV RNA test does not always indicate that an individual is uninfected or has responded to appropriate antiviral therapy. Sustained loss of detectable HCV RNA in serum may indicate response to treatment.
    d. HCV RNA can be detected in 50–75% of serum samples from random, seropositive blood donors *(10,11)* and can be detected in as many as 100% of sera from seropositive symptomatic patients and from seropositive blood donors with elevated alanine aminotransferase (ALT) levels *(9,12–14,16)*.

References

1. Choo, Q.-L., Kuo, G., Weiner, A. J., Overby, L. R., Bradley, D. W., and Houghton, M. (1989) Isolation of a cDNA clone derived from a blood-borne non-A, non-B viral hepatitis genome. *Science* **244,** 359–362.
2. Houghton, M., Weiner, A., Han, J., Kuo, G., and Choo, Q.-L. (1991) Molecular biology of the hepatitis C viruses: implications for diagnosis, development and control of viral disease. *Hepatology* **14,** 381–388.
3. Han, J., Shyamala, V., Richman, K. H., Brauer, M. H., Tekamp-Olson, P., Irvine, B., Urdea, M. S., Kuo, G., Choo, Q.-L., and Houghton, M. (1991) Characterization of the terminal regions of hepatitis C viral RNA: identification of conserved sequences in the 5'- untranslated region and poly A tails at the 3'-end. *Proc. Natl. Acad. Sci. USA* **88,** 1711–1715.
4. Cha, T.-A., Beall, E., Irvine, B., Kolberg, J., Chien, D., Kuo, G., and Urdea, M. S. (1992) At least five related, but distinct, hepatitis C viral genotypes exist. *Proc. Natl. Acad. Sci. USA* **89,** 7144–7148.
5. Simmonds, P., Holmes, E. C., Cha, T. A., Chan, S. W., McOmish, F., Irvine, B., Beall, E., Yap, P. L., Kolberg, J., and Urdea, M. S. (1993) Classification of hepatitis C virus into six major genotypes and a series of subtypes by phylogenetic analysis of the NS-5 region. *J. Gen Virol.* **74,** 2391–2399.
6. Cha, T.-A., Kolberg, J., Irvine, B., Stempien, M., Beall, E., Yano, M., Choo, Q.- L., Houghton, M., Kuo, G., Han, J. H., and Urdea, M. S. (1991) Use of a signature nucleotide sequence of hepatitis C virus for detection of viral RNA in human serum and plasma. *J. Clin. Microbiol.* **29,** 2528–2534.
7. Bukh, J., Purcell, R. H., and Miller, R. H. (1992) Importance of primer selection for the detection of hepatitis C virus RNA with the polymerase chain reaction assay. *Proc. Natl. Acad. Sci. USA* **89,** 187–191.
8. Wilber, J. C., Johnson, P. J., and Urdea, M. S. (1993) Reverse transcriptase-PCR for hepatitis C virus RNA, in *Diagnostic Molecular Microbiology: Principles and Applications* (Persing, D. H., Smith, T. F., Tenover, F. C., and White, T. J., eds.), American Society for Microbiology, Washington, DC, pp. 327–331.
9. Okamoto, H., Okada, S., Sugiyama, Y., Yotsumoto, S., Tanaka, T., Sugai, Y., Akahane, Y., Machida, A., Mishiro, S., Yoshizawa, H., Miyakawa, Y., and Mayumi, M. (1990) Detection of hepatitis C virus RNA by a two stage polymerase chain reaction with two pairs of primers and deduced from the 5'-noncoding region. *Jpn. J. Exp. Med.* **60,** 215–222.
10. Weiner, A. J., Truett, M. A., Rosenblatt, J., Han, J., Quan, S., Polito, A. J., Kuo, G., Choo, Q.-L., Houghton, M., Agius, C., Page, E., and Nelles, M. J. (1990) HCV testing in a low-risk population. *Lancet* **336,** 695.
11. Garson, J. A., Preston, F. E., Makris, M., Tuke, P., Ring, C., Machin, S. J., and Tedder, R. S. (1990) Detection by PCR of hepatitis C virus in factor VIII concentrates. *Lancet* **335,** 1473,1474.
12. Ulrich, P. P., Romeo, J. M., Lane, P. K., Kelly, I., Daniel, L. J., and Vyas, G. N. (1990) Detection, semiquantitation, and genetic variation in hepatitis C virus

sequences amplified from the plasma of blood donors with elevated alanine aminotransferase. *J. Clin. Invest.* **86,** 1609–1614.
13. Kaneko, A., Unoura, M., Kobayashi, K., Kuno, K., Murakami, S., and Hattori, N. (1990) Detection of serum hepatitis C virus RNA (letter). *Lancet* **335,** 976.
14. Garson, J. A., Tedder, R. S., Briggs, M., Tuke, P., Glazebrook, J. A., Trute, A., Parker, D., Barbara, J. A. J., Contreras, M., and Aloysius, S. (1990) Detection of hepatitis C viral sequences in blood donations by "nested" polymerase chain reaction and prediction of infectivity. *Lancet* **335,** 1419–1422.
15. Weiner, A. J., Kuo, G., Bradley, D. W., Bonino, F., Saracco, G., Lee, C., Rosenblatt, J., Choo, Q.-L., and Houghton, M. (1990) Detection of hepatitis C viral sequences in non-A, non-B hepatitis. *Lancet* **335,** 1–3.
16. Gretch, D. R., Wilson, J. J., Carithers, R. L., dela Rosa, C., Han, J. H., and Corey, L. (1993) Detection of hepatitis C virus RNA: Comparison of one-stage polymerase chain reaction (PCR) with nested-set PCR. *J. Clin. Microbiol.* **31,** 289–291.
17. Chomczynski, P. and Sacchi, N. (1987) Single-step method of RNA isolation by acid guanidinium thiocyanate-phenol-chloroform extraction. *Anal. Biochem.* **162,** 156–159.
18. Kwok, S. and Higuchi, R. (1989) Avoiding false positives with PCR. *Nature* **339,** 237,238.
19. National Committee for Clinical Laboratory Standards. (1995) Molecular diagnostic methods for infectious diseases; Approved Guideline. NCCLS Document MM3-A, Villanova, PA.
20. Busch, M. P., Wilber, J. C., Johnson, P., Tobler, L., and Evans, C. S. (1992) Impact of specimen handling and storage on detection of hepatitis C virus RNA. *Transfusion* **32,** 420–425.
21. Wang, J.-T., Wang, T.-H., Sheu, J.-C., Lin, S.-M., Lin, J.-T., and Chen, D.-S. (1992) Effects of anticoagulants and storage of blood samples on efficacy of the polymerase chain reaction assay for hepatitis C virus. *J. Clin. Microbiol.* **30,** 750–753.
22. Cuypers, H. T. M., Bresters, D., Winkel, I. N., Reesink, H. W., Weiner, A. J., Houghton, M., van der Poel, C. L., and Lelie, P. N. (1992) Storage conditions of blood samples and primer selection affect the yield of cDNA polymerase chain reaction products of hepatitis C virus. *J. Clin. Microbiol.* **30,** 3220–3224.
23. Kuo, G., Choo, Q.-L., Alter, H. J., Gitnick, G. L., Redeker, A. G., Purcell, R. H., Miyamura, T., Dienstag, J. L., Alter, M. J., Stevens, C. E., Tegtmeier, G. E., Bonino, F., Colombo, M., Lee, W.-S., Kuo, C., Berfer, K., Shuster, J. R., Overby, L. R., Bradley, D. W., and Houghton, M. (1989) An assay for circulating antibodies to a major etiologic virus of human non-A, non-B hepatitis. *Science* **244,** 362–364.
24. Ebeling, F., Naukkarinen, R., and Leikola, J. (1990) Recombinant immunoblot assay for hepatitis C antibody as predictor of infectivity. *Lancet* **335,** 982,983.
25. McHutchison, J. G., Person, J. L., Govindarajan, S., Valinluck, B., Gore, T., Lee, S. R., Nelies, M., Polito, A., Chien, D., DiNello, R., Quan, S., Kuo, G., and Redeker, A. (1992) Improved detection of hepatitis C virus antibodies in high risk population. *Hepatology* **15,** 19.

4

Detection of HCV RNA in Serum by Reverse Transcription Polymerase Chain Reaction (RT-PCR)

KePing Qian

1. Introduction

In the field of biological science, the development of new techniques (e.g., Southern blotting, molecular cloning, pulsed-field gel electrophoresis) often led to better understanding of fundamental and applied biological problems. The polymerase chain reaction (PCR) is among the techniques that led to change in the way of detecting viral sequences in minute quantity.

The PCR is a technique for in vitro amplification of specific DNA sequences by simultaneous copying of complementary strands of DNA. Despite the development of the PCR in early 1980, it was not widely adopted until the discovery of heat-stable DNA polymerase, which significantly simplified this procedure. PCR has since been developed to be used in different biological settings, which are beyonnd the scope of this chapter. Here, the protocol that is routinely used for the qualitative detection of HCV in our laboratory is described. Using synthetic HCV RNA as the standard, the sensitivity of this RT-PCR assay is routinely <10 copies/sample (<5 copies/sample in most runs).

2. Materials

2.1. Reagents for Extraction of Small Quantity of RNA in Serum

1. Water: sterile, nuclease-free (biotechnology grade; Amresco [Solon, OH], E476) (*see* **Note 1**).
2. 2-mercaptoethanol: Store at 4°C.
3. 0.75 M Sodium citrate, pH 7: dissolve 22.1 g trisodium citrate dihydrate (FW 294.1) in approx 80 mL deionized water, pH to 7.0 with citric acid. Bring volume to 100 mL and autoclave.
4. 10% (w/v) Sarcosyl: dissolve 10 g sarcosyl in approx 80 mL deionized water with gentle stirring. Bring volume to 100 mL and pass through a 0.45 µm filter.

From: *Methods in Molecular Medicine, Vol. 19: Hepatitis C Protocols*
Edited by: J. Y. N. Lau © Humana Press Inc., Totowa, NJ

5. Chomczynski's solution D *(1)*:
    a. Stock solution: dissolve 250 g guanidinium thiocyanate in a pre-autoclaved battle with 293 mL water, 17.6 mL 0.75 M sodium citrate, pH 7.0, and 26.4 mL 10% sarcosyl at 65°C. Can be stored at room temperature for at least 3 mo.
    b. Chomczynski's solution D: prepared by adding 0.36 mL 2-mercaptoethanol in 50 mL the stock solution. Can be store at room temperature for 1 mo.
6. 0.5% (w/v) Bromphenol blue (BPB): dissolve 50 mg BPB blue in 10 mL water.
7. Chomczynski's solution D-BPB: Chomczynski's solution with 0.02 mg/mL BPB. To 50 mL stock Chomczynski's solution D, add 0.20 mL 0.5% BPB.
8. 2 M Sodium acetate, pH 3.0: dissolve 27.2 g NaAc · 3H$_2$O in ~50 mL deionized water, pH to 4.0 with acetic acid. Bring volume to 100 mL, autoclave, and store at –20°C.
9. 3 M Sodium acetate, pH 6.5: dissolve 40.8 g NaAc · 3H$_2$O in 40 mL deionized water, pH to 6.5 with acetic acid. Bring volume to 100 mL, autoclave, and store at –20°C.
10. 1% (w/v) Glycogen: dissolve 1 g glycogen (oyster) in 100 mL deionized water with gentle stirring, and pass through a 0.45 μm filter. Store at –20°C.
11. Glycogen-acetate mixture: mix 1 mL 1% glycogen and 7 mL 3M sodium acetate, pass through a 0.45 μm filter. Store at –20°C. Aliquot in small volumes and discard after thawing.
12. Saturated phenol, pH 4.3 (biotechnology grade; Amresco, X981): store at 4°C.
13. Chloroform/isoamyl-alcohol 24:1 (biotechnology-grade; Amresco, X205).
14. 0.1 M DTT (Dithiothreitol): (*see* **Note 2**) dissolve 1.54 g DTT (Sigma [St. Louis, MO] D8161) in 100 mL water and aliquot in small volumes. Store at –20°C.
15. Blue TKTRID buffer:
    a. Blue TKT buffer: mix 895 μL water with 100 μL 10X reaction buffer w/o MgCl$_2$ (Promega [Madison, WI] M1661) and 5 μL BPB (5 mg/mL).
    b. Add 50 μL 0.1 M DTT and 12.5 μL Ribonuclease inhibitor (RNasin, Promega N2111) to 1 mL of blue TKT buffer to make blue TKTRID buffer. For best results, make fresh before use.
16. Absolute ethanol (200 proof): store at –20°C.
17. 75% Ethanol: add 250 mL water in 750 mL absolute ethanol. Store at –20°C.
18. HCV RNA-positive scrum (with level of around 1000 copies/mL made by dilution of samples with known quantities) and HCV RNA-negative serum from healthy blood donors with no known risk factors and with confirmed negative serological profiles, and previously shown to be negative by RT-PCR.

2.2. Reagents for RT-"Nested" PCR

1. 1 M Tris-HCl, pH 8.3: dissolve 12.1 g Tris (hydroxymethyl) aminomethane in approx 70 mL deionized water, adjust pH to 8.3 with concentrated HCl. Bring volume to 100 mL and autoclave.
2. 1 M KCl: Dissolve 74.55 g potassium chloride in to approx 900 mL water. Bring volume to 1000 mL and autoclave.
3. 1 M MgCl$_2$: Dissolve 20.3 g magnesium chloride hexahydrate in approx 90 mL water. Bring volume to 100 mL and autoclave.

4. 100 mM dNTPs, pH 7.5: (deoxynucleotide triphosphates) (Promega, U1240): store at $-20°C$.
5. RNasin (ribonuclease inhibitor, RI) (Promega N2111): store at $-20°C$.
6. *Taq* DNA polymerase (*Taq*) (Promega, M1661): store at $-20°C$.
7. Moloney Murine Leukemia Virus Reverse Transcriptase (M-MLV RT [RT]) (Promega, M1701): store at $-20°C$.
8. Primers (*See* **Note 3**):
   a. Outer primers: Store at $-20°C$.
      Antisense GTGCTCATGGTGCACGGTCTACGAGACCT
      Sense CTGTGAGGAACTACTGTCTT
   b. Inner primers: Store at $-20°C$.
      Anti-sense CACTCGCAAGCACCCTATCAGGCAGT
      Sense TTCACGCAGAAAGCGTCTAG
9. Mineral oil.
10. PCRa mix: make 10 mL PCRa solution. Add 100 µL 1 M Tris-HCl, pH 8.3, 500 µL 1 M KCl, 25 µL each dNTPs, 40 µL 1 M MgCl$_2$, 0.5 µM each outer primers (*See* **Note 4**) and 50 µL BPB (5 mg/mL) in ~7 mL water. Mix and bring volume to 10 mL. Store at $-20°C$ in 160 and 320 µL aliquots for 10 and 20 samples, respectively.
11. PCRb mix: Make 20 mL PCRb solution. Add 200 mL 1 M Tris-HCl, pH 8.3, 1000 µL 1 M KCl, 40 µL each dNTPs, 20 µL 1 M MgCl$_2$, and 1.25 µM each inner primers in ~15 mL water. Mix and bring volume to 20 mL. Store at $-20°C$ in 420 and 840 µL aliquots for 10 and 20 samples, respectively.

2.3. Reagents for Electrophoresis

1. 40X TAE buffer: dissolve 193.8 g (1.6 M) Tris, 108.9 g (0.8 M) NaAc.3H$_2$O, and 14.9 g (40 mM) EDTA-Na$_2$ · 2H$_2$O in ~800 mL deionized water. Adjust pH to 7.6 with acetic acid. Bring volume to 1000 mL.
2. Ethidium bromide (10 mg/mL): dissolve 100 mg ethidium bromide in 10 mL deionized water with gentle stirring.
3. 10% (w/v) SDS: dissolve 10 g SDS in ~75 mL deionized water with gentle stirring. Bring volume to 100 mL. Solution may be autoclaved or filter with a 0.2 mm filter. Store at room temperature; if stored in the cold, the SDS will precipitate out.
4. 1 M EDTA, pH 8.0: dissolve 37.2 g EDTA-Na$_2$ · 2H$_2$O in ~80 mL deionized water. Adjust pH to 8.0 with acetic acid. Bring volume to 100 mL.
5. 6X Loading buffer: add 50 mg BPB (0.05% w/v), 40 g sucrose (40% w/v), 10 mL 1 M EDTA (0.1 M), pH 8.0, and 5 mL 10% SDS (0.5% w/v) in ~40 mL deionized water with gentle stirring. Bring volume to 100 mL.
6. Agarose: SEAKEM LE agarose (FMC 50004).
7. Running buffer: (1X TAE buffer with 0.5 µg/mL ethidium bromide): add 25 mL 40X TAE buffer and 50 µL ethidium bromide (10 mg/mL) to ~900 mL deionized water. Bring volume to 1000 mL. Make fresh before use.
8. ØX174 DNA/*Hae*III Marker (Promega, G1751).

2.4. Equipment

1. A set of pipets: 0.5–10, 10–50, 40–200, and 200–1000 µL.
2. Incubator: (Boekel Industries Inc., Model 133000).
3. Perkin Elmer thermal cycler.
4. Electrophoresis system: horizontal slab.
5. Polaroid camera with UV illuminator.

3. Methods
3.1. Extraction of Small Quantity of RNA in Serum

See general precautions (*see* **Note 5**).

1. Into a 2.0 mL sterile screw-capped microcentrifuge tube (Fisher 05-664-66), add:
   450 µL D-BPB solution.
   100 µL serum (*see* **Note 6**), mixing by pipeting up and down.
   50 µL 2 M NaAc, pH 4.0 buffer, mix by swirling the tube.
   500 µL saturated phenol, pH 4.3.
   100 µL chloroform/isoamyl alcohol 24:1.
2. Screw caps on tightly and shake the tubes on high speed for 30 min.
3. Chill the tubes on ice for 15 min.
4. Centrifuge for 15 min, 13,000g in a refrigerated microcentrifuge at 4°C.
5. Remove 400 µL aqueous layer to a 2.0 mL sterile screw-capped microcentrifuge tube containing 40 uL glycogen–acetate mixture and 1 mL absolute ethanol.
6. Mix well and place the tubes in –20°C freezer overnight or –80°C freezer for ~1 h. This is a good point to stop and continue on the next day. Samples can be frozen at –80°C.
7. Centrifuge for 45 min, 13,000g in a refrigerated microcentrifuge at 4°C.
8. Pour off supernatant, and blot each tube lightly on Kimwipes Ex-L paper. Take care not to cross-contaminate specimens.
9. Add 1 mL 75% ethanol without disturbing the pellet. Do not shake the tube. Extraction can be stored at –80°C at this point.
10. Centrifuge for 10 min, 13,000g in a refrigerated microcentrifuge at 4°C.
11. Pour off supernatant.
12. Swab the sides of the tube using a sterile cotton applicator. Do not touch the pellet.
13. Resuspend in 18 µL blue TKTRID buffer, and flick the tube to dissolve pellet.
14. Place the tube in an incubator at 37°C for 15 min and spin briefly. The RNA sample can be used immediately for PCR, or stored at –20°C until sample is taken for PCR. Before each use, place the tube in an incubator at 37°C for 15 min and spin briefly. PCR should be carried out within 7 d.

3.2. RT-PCR (Reverse Transcription Polymerase Chain Reaction)

See general precautions (**Note 7**).

1. Thaw out one vial of PCRa aliquot (320 µL), and add 16 µL 0.1 M DTT, 200 U RI, 10 U *Taq*, and 300 U RT (M-MLV) (for 20 sample).

2. Cap the vial tightly and invert gently several times. Spin briefly.
3. Dispense 16 µL **step 1** mixture to 20 0.5-mL microtubes (autoclaved).
4. Add 4 µL RNA sample to the appropriately labeled tube, and mix by pipeting up and down. Microcentrifuge tubes briefly.
5. Drop 40 µL mineral oil into each tube, and carefully cap each tube firmly. Make sure that there is no space between the rim of the vial and the cap. Thermal cyclers that have heating plates on top of the reaction tubes do not require mineral oil.
6. Microcentrifuge tubes briefly.
7. Place tubes in thermal cycler. Set temperature cycles of the first round PCR as follows:
   37°C 45 min
   94°C 4 min
   35 Cycles (*See* **Note 8**)
      94°C   1 min
      50°C   1 min
      72°C   1 min
      72°C   7 min
   4°C Indefinitely
8. Thaw out a vial of PCRb aliquot (840 µL), and add 20 U *Taq*. Mix contents by inverting gently and spin briefly for 20 samples.
9. Dispense 40 µL **step 8** mixture to 20 0.5-mL microtubes (autoclaved).
10. Add 4 µL of the first-round PCR product to appropriate tube, and mix by pipeting up and down. Microcentrifuge tubes briefly.
11. Drop 40 µL mineral oil into each tube, carefully cap each tube firmly, and spin briefly.
12. Place in thermal cycler. Set temperature cycles of the second round PCR as follows:
    94°C 4 min
    30 Cycles
       94°C   1 min
       55°C   1 min
       72°C   1 min
    72°C 7 min
    4°C Indefinitely

3.3. Electrophoresis

1. Mix 2 µL 6X loading buffer with 8 µL of the each second-round PCR product and 8 µL of pre-diluted ØX174 DNA/*Hae*III Marker (0.05 µg/µL) by pipetting up and down.
2. Heat the tubes at 65°C for ~5 min.
3. Electrophorese using a 2% agarose gel in 1X TAE buffer with 0.5 µg/mL ethidium bromide at 80 V for about 1 h.
4. Photograph the gel with UV illumination.

4. Notes

1. As with any RNA preparative procedure, care must be taked to ensure that solutions are free of ribonuclease. Solutions that come into contact with the RNA after the addition of guanidinium solution are all made with nuclease-free sterile water. Most investigators treat the solutions with diethylpyrocarbonate (DEPC), with the exception of the Tris solution, which may degrade in the presence of DEPC. We found that using commerically available nuclease-free, sterile water was easier and reduced the risk of crosscontamination, especially in the process of autoclaving, which is essential to remove DEPC.
2. DTT is not used by some investigators.
3. The primers are synthetic oligonucleotides of 20–30 bases long. For characteristics of good primers, please refer to any standard molecular biology textbook. For HCV with high level of genetic variations, the primers should be chosen from the most highly conserved region. Our primers are derived from the conserved regions within the 5' untranslated region (5'UTR) of HCV.
4. The concentration of the primer should not be too much to interfere with molecular biology reaction.
5. Wear gloves at all time, and change them often when working with RNA solutions, as the hands are one of the most common sources of ribonuclease contamination.
6. To determine the optimal conditions for the preparation of serum specimens for HCV RNA determination, we have conducted the following experiments. Patient samples were processed such that differences in time from clot formation to centrifugation, centrifugation to separation of serum, and collection of serum until freezing were assessed independently. The effects of multiple cycles of freezing and thawing were also determined. These optimal conditions are given in **ref. 2**.
7. PCR is sensitive to contamination by amplified products from target sequences cloned in plasmid vectors, transferred through pipetes, reagents, hands, or even air current. It has been suggested that different stages of PCR should be done in separate rooms and with a different set of equipment. In the laboratory at the University of Florida, sample preparation, RNA extraction, RT-PCR, and gel electrophoresis are all done in different laboratories with different sets of equipment.
8. The target DNA is denatured at 94–98°C to allow the primer to bind to the separated single strands when the temperature is lowered. The lower denaturation temperature (94°C) is less harmful to the enzyme. The denaturation temperature is usually 1 min, although in our experience, 20 s is usually enough. The new version of the PCR machines claimed that this step can be even shorter. The temperature for primer annealing is usually between 50 and 60°C, and is dependent on the T_m of the primers. The higher temperature ensures greater specificity of the PCR, but may not allow efficient annealing of primers to targets with base mismatches, which may be important in the amplification of HCV.

Acknowledgments

This protocol was adapted from the protocol originally described by Lin et al. *(3)* and modified by Johnson Y. N. Lau. The author would like to thank Dr. Lau for his unfailing support during his leadership in the laboratory at the University of Florida.

References

1. Chomczynski, P., and Sacchi, N. (1987) Single-step method of RNA isolation by Guanidinium thiocyanate-phenol-chloroform extraction. *Anal. Biochem.* **162,** 156–159.
2. Davis, G. L., Lau, J. Y. N., Urdea, M. S., Neuwald, P. D., Wilber, J. C., Lindsay, K., et al. (1994) Quantitative detection of hepatitis C virus RNA with a solid-phase signal amplification method: definition of optimal condition for specimen collection and clinical application in interferon-treated patients. *Hepatology* **19,** 1337–1341.
3. Lin H. J., Hollinger F. B., Mizokami, M., and Shi, N. (1992) A polyemrase chain reaction assay for hepatitis C virus RNA using a single tube for reverse transcription and serial rounds of amplification with nested primers. *J. Med. Vir.* **3,** 220–225.

5

The AMPLICOR® HCV Tests for the Detection and Quantitation of Serum or Plasma HCV RNA

Karen A. Gutekunst, Joanne P. Spadoro, Elizabeth A. Dragon, and Maurice Rosenstraus

1. Introduction

Clinical diagnosis of HCV infection is generally accomplished by using immunoserological assays to detect the presence of anti-HCV antibodies. Such immunoserological assays have been approved for blood donor screening, thereby reducing the incidence of post-transfusion hepatitis in the United States. Although useful, immunoserological assays have several limitations. Recent evaluations have shown that interpretation of these immunological tests often is difficult, since 25–90% (depending on the risk group under evaluation) of samples repeatedly reactive in the screening assay are negative on supplemental evaluation with a recombinant immunoblot assay (RIBA) *(1,2)*. Also, the presence of anti-HCV antibodies indicates prior exposure to HCV infection, but cannot be considered a marker for current infection. Nor can anti-HCV antibody levels be used to monitor response to therapeutic agents. Finally, in cases of acute HCV infection resulting from accidental needlestick exposure, many patients fail to produce antibody to HCV *(3)*, which makes diagnosis of HCV infection impossible using immunoserological techniques. At the present time, an immunological assay for direct detection of HCV antigen is unavailable.

The limitations of immunoserological tests can be overcome by using amplification technologies, such as the polymerase chain reaction (PCR), to detect HCV RNA in serum or plasma and thus provide direct evidence for current infection. Because of its ability to specifically amplify minute quantities of nucleic acid, PCR has been applied with great success in clinical diagnostics *(4–6)*. Recent technological advances in specimen processing, automation, and standardization of reagents have made PCR suitable for routine clinical diagnosis. PCR assays that can quantitate the amount of nucleic acid in a specimen have also been developed. Using PCR, it has been possible to detect HCV viremia prior to immunological sero-conversion *(7,8)*. Recent studies have established the validity of early changes in serum or plasma HCV RNA levels as a surrogate marker for prediction of long-term response to interferon therapy *(9,10)*. Since PCR is able to amplify HCV RNA directly, independent of the patient's immunological status, a PCR-based assay also is valuable in detecting HCV RNA in immunocompromised patients.

Roche Molecular Systems (Branchburg, NJ) has developed a family of PCR tests for the detection and quantitation of HCV RNA in serum or plasma. The AMPLICOR® HCV and the fully automated COBAS AMPLICOR™ HCV Tests are in vitro nucleic acid amplification tests for the detection of HCV RNA in human serum or plasma. These tests can be used in conjunction with clinical presentation and other laboratory markers to implicate HCV as the cause of disease in patients with non-A, non-B hepatitis. The AMPLICOR HCV MONITOR™ and COBAS AMPLICOR HCV MONITOR™ tests can be used to assess loss of or changes in serum or plasma HCV RNA levels in response to antiviral treatment.

2. Materials
2.1. AMPLICOR Kits
2.1.1. For Qualitative COBAS AMPLICOR or AMPLICOR HCV Tests

Common kits:

1. AMPLICOR HCV specimen preparation kit.
2. AMPLICOR HCV controls kit.
3. AMPLICOR HCV amplification kit.

For AMPLICOR microwell plate detection:

1. AMPLICOR HCV detection kit.
2. AMPLICOR internal control detection kit.

For automated COBAS AMPLICOR:

1. COBAS AMPLICOR HCV detection kit.
2. COBAS AMPLICOR internal control detection kit.
3. COBAS AMPLICOR detection kit.
4. COBAS AMPLICOR wash buffer kit.

2.1.2. Material Needed for Quantitative AMPLICOR HCV MONITOR Test

1. AMPLICOR HCV MONITOR kit (contains all specimen preparation, amplification, and detection reagents).

AMPLICOR HCV Tests 57

For quantitative COBAS AMPLICOR HCV MONITOR test:

1. COBAS AMPLICOR HCV MONITOR specimen preparation kit.
2. COBAS AMPLICOR HCV MONITOR controls kit.
3. COBAS AMPLICOR HCV MONITOR amplification kit.
4. COBAS AMPLICOR HCV MONITOR detection kit.
5. COBAS AMPLICOR detection kit.
6. COBAS AMPLICOR wash buffer kit.

2.2. Laboratory Supplies and Equipment

2.2.1. Preamplification–Reagent Preparation Area

Common equipment:

1. Plastic resealable bag.
2. Eppendorf® Repeater™ pipet with 1.25 mL Combitip® reservoir (sterile, individually wrapped).
3. Micropipets (adjustable volume, 20–200 µL) with plugged (aerosol barrier) RNase-free tips (50 and 200 µL).
4. Latex gloves, powderless.
5. Vortex mixer.

For AMPLICOR tests:

1. Perkin-Elmer MicroAmp® reaction tubes.
2. Perkin-Elmer MicroAmp caps.
3. Perkin-Elmer MicroAmp tray/retainers.
4. Perkin-Elmer MicroAmp tray base.

For COBAS AMPLICOR tests:

1. COBAS AMPLICOR A-ring fitted with 12 A-tubes.
2. COBAS AMPLICOR A-ring holder.

2.2.2. Preamplification–Specimen Preparation Area

1. VACUTAINER® blood collection tubes either with EDTA (Becton Dickinson #6454) or ACD (Becton Dickinson #4606) or SST® Tube for Serum Separation (Becton Dickinson #367784 or #367789).
2. Microcentrifuge (maximum RCF 16,000g, minimum RCF 12,500g).
3. 60 ± 2°C dry heat block.
4. 1.5 mL screw-cap tubes, sterile (Sarstedt 72.692.105, or equivalent).
5. Tube racks (Sarstedt 93.1428).
6. 95% ethanol (freshly diluted to 70% using deionized water).
7. Isopropanol, reagent grade.
8. Fine RNase-free tips, sterile transfer pipets.
9. Vortex mixer.
10. Latex gloves, powderless.

11. Sterile disposable, polystyrene pipets (5, 10, and 25 mL).
12. Micropipets with plugged (aerosol barrier) or positive displacement RNase-free tips (50, 100, 200, 400, 600, 800, and 1000 µL).

2.3. Postamplification Area

For AMPLICOR tests:

1. Perkin-Elmer GeneAmp PCR System 9600 or GeneAmp PCR System 2400 thermal cycler.
2. Perkin-Elmer GeneAmp PCR System 9600 or GeneAmp PCR System 2400 MicroAmp base and cap installing tool.
3. Multichannel pipeter (25 and 100 µL).
4. Plugged (aerosol barrier) RNase-free micropipet tips (25 and 100 µL) and unplugged tips (100 µL).
5. Microwell plate washer.
6. Microwell plate reader.
7. Disposable reagent reservoirs.
8. Microwell plate lid.
9. Incubator 37°C ± 2°C.
10. Graduated vessels.
11. Distilled or deionized water.

For COBAS AMPLICOR tests:

1. COBAS AMPLICOR and printer.
2. COBAS AMPLICOR operator's manual.
3. COBAS AMPLICOR method manual.
4. COBAS AMPLICOR D-cups.
5. Distilled or deionized water.
6. 5-mL Serological pipets.
7. Graduated cylinder (minimum 1 L).
8. Vortex mixer.
9. Latex gloves.

3. Methods

The AMPLICOR HCV tests are based on five major processes: specimen preparation; reverse transcription (RT) of target RNA to generate cDNA, PCR amplification of target cDNA using HCV-specific complementary primers; hybridization of the amplified products (amplicon) to oligonucleotide probes specific to the target(s), and detection of the probe-bound amplified products by colorimetric determination. For the AMPLICOR HCV tests, the user programs a thermal cycler to perform reverse transcription and amplification automatically; hybridization, detection, and calculations (for MONITOR tests) are performed manually. For the COBAS AMPLICOR HCV tests, the user simply enters the test name and specimen identification codes; the COBAS AMPLICOR system then uses preprogrammed parameters to automatically perform reverse transcription, amplification, detection, and results interpretation (for the qualitative test) or calculations (for the MONITOR test) without user intervention.

To achieve selective amplification of target nucleic acid from the clinical specimen, the amplification reaction mixtures for all HCV tests contain AmpErase® and deoxyuridine triphosphate (dUTP) *(11)*. To identify processed specimens containing substances that may interfere with PCR amplification, the qualitative AMPLICOR and COBAS AMPLICOR HCV tests utilize an internal control (HCV IC) *(12)*. The quantitative AMPLICOR and COBAS AMPLICOR HCV MONITOR Tests utilize a quantitation standard (HCV QS) as a reference for calculating the HCV RNA concentration in the specimen.

3.1. Selective Amplification

AmpErase (uracil-*N*-glycosylase, UNG) recognizes and catalyzes the destruction of DNA strands containing deoxyuridine, but not DNA containing thymidine *(11)*. Deoxyuridine is not present in naturally occurring DNA, but is always present in amplicon because of the use of deoxyuridine triphosphate as one of the dNTPs in the Master Mix reagent; therefore, only amplicon contains deoxyuridine. Deoxyuridine renders contaminating amplicon susceptible to destruction by AmpErase prior to amplification of the target DNA. AmpErase, which is included in the Master Mix reagent, catalyzes the cleavage of deoxyuridine containing DNA at deoxyuridine residues by opening the deoxyribose chain at the C1-position. When heated in the first thermal cycling step at the alkaline pH of Master Mix, the amplicon DNA chain breaks at the position of the deoxyuridine, thereby rendering the DNA nonamplifiable. AmpErase is inactive at temperatures above 55°C, i.e., throughout the thermal cycling steps, and therefore does not destroy target amplicon. Following amplification, any residual enzyme is denatured by the addition of the denaturation solution, thereby preventing the degradation of target amplicon. AmpErase in the AMPLICOR HCV family of tests has been demonstrated to inactivate at least 10^3 copies of deoxyuridine-containing HCV amplicon per PCR.

3.2. Internal Control/Quantitation Standard

The HCV IC is an in vitro transcribed RNA transcript with primer binding regions identical to those of the HCV target sequence, a randomized internal sequence of similar length and base composition as the HCV target sequence, and a unique probe binding region that differentiates the HCV IC from the target amplicon *(12)*. The HCV IC is introduced into each amplification reaction and is coamplified with the target RNA from the clinical specimen.

The HCV QS is a noninfectious RNA transcript that contains the identical primer binding sites as the HCV target and a unique probe binding region that allows HCV QS amplicon to be distinguished from HCV amplicon. The HCV QS is incorporated into each individual specimen at known copy number and is carried through the specimen preparation, reverse transcription, PCR amplification, hybridization, and detection steps along with the HCV target. HCV RNA levels in the test specimens are determined by comparing the HCV signal to the HCV QS signal for each specimen. Therefore, the HCV QS compensates for any effects of inhibition and controls for variation in the specimen preparation, amplification, and detection processes to allow the accurate quantitation of HCV RNA in each specimen.

3.3. Specimen Preparation (see Notes 1–12)

As described in detail below, HCV RNA is extracted from viral particles with HCV lysis reagent, and the extracted RNA is then recovered by alcohol precipitation. The HCV lysis reagent contains the chaotropic reagent guanidine isothiocyanate.

1. For the HCV MONITOR test, vortex the HCV MONITOR quantitation standard (QS) and add 70 µL HCV MONITOR QS to one bottle of HCV lysis reagent and mix well. For the original COBAS AMPLICOR and AMPLICOR HCV Tests, use the HCV lysis reagent as supplied. For the newer, more sensitive versions of the qualitative HCV tests, vortex the HCV IC, add 100 µL to one bottle of HCV lysis reagent, and mix well.
2. Label a 1.5-mL screw cap microcentrifuge tube for each specimen and control.
3. Thaw specimens at room temperature and vortex for 3–5 s.
4. Dispense 400 µL lysis reagent into each tube.
5. Add 100 µL (or 200 µL for the newer qualitative tests) of each patient specimen to appropriate tubes. Cap the tubes and vortex for 3–5 s.
6. For each negative and positive control, add 100 µL (or 200 µL for the newer qualitative tests) negative plasma (human) to the appropriate tubes. Cap the tubes and vortex for 3–5 s, then add 100 µL of each control to the appropriate tubes. Cap the tubes and mix thoroughly.
7. Incubate the tubes for 10 min at 60°C.
8. Remove the caps from the specimen and control tubes and add 500 µL (or 600 µL for the newer qualitative tests) 100% isopropanol to each tube. Recap the tubes and vortex for 3–5 s. Incubate the tubes for 2 min at room temperature.
9. Centrifuge specimens at maximum speed (13,000–16,000g) for 15 min at room temperature.
10. Using a new, fine-tip disposable transfer pipet for each tube, carefully remove and discard the supernatant from each tube, being careful not to disrupt the pellet (which may not be visible).
11. Add 1.0 mL 70% ethanol to each tube, recap, and vortex for 3–5 s.

12. Place the tubes into a microcentrifuge and centrifuge the tubes for 5 min at maximum speed (13,000–16,000g) at room temperature.
13. Carefully remove the supernatant using a new, fine-tip disposable transfer pipet for each tube without disturbing the pellet. The pellet should be clearly visible at this step. Remove as much of the supernatant as possible because residual ethanol can inhibit the amplification.
14. For the original COBAS AMPLICOR and AMPLICOR HCV tests only, vortex the HCV IC and add 50 µL to one bottle of HCV specimen diluent. For the HCV MONITOR and newer qualitative HCV tests, specimen diluent is used as supplied.
15. Add 1000 µL (or 200 µL for the newer qualitative tests) HCV specimen diluent to each tube. Break apart the pellet as much as possible with a P200 pipeter fitted with a P200 plugged pipet tip. Vortex for 10 s. Some insoluble material may remain.
16. Amplify the processed specimens within 2 h of preparation or store frozen at –20°C or colder for up to 1 mo.
17. Pipet 50 µL of each prepared control and patient specimen to a MicroAmp reaction tube (or COBAS AMPLICOR A-tube) containing 50 µL of HCV master mix.

3.4. Reverse Transcription and PCR Amplification (see Notes 13–17)

All HCV tests amplify and detect a 244 base target sequence located in a highly conserved 5' untranslated region of the HCV genome *(8)*, defined by the primers KY78 and KY80. Primer KY78 is biotinylated and the primer KY80 is not.

The reverse transcription and amplification reactions are performed with the thermostable recombinant enzyme *Thermus thermophilus* DNA polymerase (r*Tth* pol). In the presence of manganese and under the appropriate buffer conditions, r*Tth* pol has both reverse transcriptase (RT) and DNA polymerase activity *(13)*. This allows both reverse transcription and PCR amplification to occur in the same reaction mixture.

3.4.1. Reverse Transcription

The downstream or antisense primer (KY78) is biotinylated at the 5' end. The reaction tubes are placed in a thermal cycler that automatically performs the heating and cooling steps required for reverse transcription and amplification. First the reactions are heated to allow the downstream primer to anneal specifically to the HCV and HCV IC (or HCV QS) target RNA. In the presence of excess deoxynucleoside triphosphates (dNTPs), including deoxyadenosine, deoxyguanosine, deoxycytidine, and deoxyuridine triphosphates, r*Tth* pol extends the annealed primer forming a complementary (cDNA) strand.

3.4.2. PCR Amplification

Following reverse transcription of the HCV and HCV IC (or HCV QS) target RNA, the reaction mixture is heated to denature the RNA:cDNA hybrid and expose the HCV and HCV IC (or HCV QS) target sequences. As the mixture cools, the upstream primer (KY80) anneals to the cDNA strand and the r*Tth* pol catalyzes the extension reaction, yielding a double-stranded DNA copy of the target region of each HCV and HCV IC (or HCV QS) RNA. This completes the first cycle of PCR. The reaction mixture is heated again to separate the double-stranded DNA and expose the primer target sequences. As the mixture cools, the primers anneal to the target DNA. In the presence of excess dNTPs, r*Tth* pol extends the annealed primers along the target templates to produce a 244 base-pair double-stranded DNA molecule termed an amplicon. This process is automatically repeated for the appropriate number of cycles, each cycle effectively doubling the amount of amplicon DNA. Amplification occurs only in the region of the HCV genome between the primers.

3.4.3. Performing Reverse Transcription/PCR Amplification

1. For the AMPLICOR HCV (qualitative) test, program the Perkin-Elmer GeneAmp PCR System 9600 or GeneAmp PCR System 2400 thermal cycler as follows: hold program: 5 min at 50°C; hold program: 30 min at 60°C; hold program: 1 min at 95°C; cycle program (2 cycles): 15 s at 95°C, 20 s at 60°C; cycle program (38 cycles): 15 s at 90°C, 20 s at 60°C; and hold program: 15 min at 72°C.
2. For the newer AMPLICOR HCV (qualitative) Test, program the thermal cycler as follows: hold program: 5 min at 50°C; hold program: 30 min at 62°C; cycle program (37 cycles): 10 s at 95°C, 25 s at 58°C; and hold program: up to 2 h at 91°C.
3. For the AMPLICOR HCV MONITOR (quantitative) test, program the thermal cycler as follows: hold program: 5 min at 50°C; hold program: 30 min at 60°C; hold program: 1 min at 95°C; cycle program (2 cycles): 15 s at 95°C, 20 s at 60°C; cycle program (33 cycles): 15 s at 90°C, 20 s at 60°C; and hold program: 15 min at 72°C.
4. For the newer version of the AMPLICOR HCV MONITOR test, program the thermal cycler as follows: hold program: 5 min at 50°C; hold program: 30 min at 62°C; cycle program (32 cycles): 10 s at 95°C, 25 s at 58°C; and hold program: up to 2 h at 91°C.
5. For the COBAS AMPLICOR tests, the COBAS AMPLICOR system will automatically perform the correct thermal cycling program after the user enters the correct test name.
6. After the thermal cycling is complete, remove the caps from the tubes and immediately pipet 100 µL of denaturation solution into each reaction tube using a multichannel pipeter and mix by pipetting up and down five times. The COBAS AMPLICOR system will automatically perform this step.

7. The denatured amplicon can be held at room temperature no more than 2 h before proceeding to the detection reaction. If the detection reaction cannot be performed within 2 h, recap the tubes and store the denatured amplicon at 2–8°C for up to 1 wk.

3.5. Hybridization Reaction (see Notes 18–21)

Following PCR amplification, the HCV and HCV IC (or HCV QS) amplicons are chemically denatured to form single-stranded DNA by adding denaturation solution to the reaction tubes. For the quantitative MONITOR tests, the denatured amplicon is serially diluted. Aliquots of undiluted and diluted amplicon are hybridized to HCV-specific (KY150) and HCV IC-specific (or HCV QS-specific) oligonucleotide probes that are bound to a solid phase. Microwell plates (MWPs) serve as the solid phase for the AMPLICOR tests and magnetic microparticles (MP) serve as the solid phase for the COBAS AMPLICOR tests. In manual AMPLICOR tests, MWPs are incubated at 37°C for 60 min. The COBAS AMPLICOR system performs all of these steps automatically without user intervention. The following specific instructions apply to the manual AMPLICOR assays:

1. Allow the MWP to warm to room temperature before removing from the foil pouch. Set the required number of 8-well MWP strips into the MWP frame. Unused strips may be returned to the pouch for later use. Reseal the pouch, making sure the desiccant pillow remains in the pouch.
2. a. For qualitative detection of the amplicon, add 100 µL hybridization buffer to each well to be tested. Add 25 µL of denatured amplicon to the corresponding well on the microwell plate. Tap the plate gently to mix. Cover the plate and incubate for 1 h at 37°C.
   b. For quantitative detection of the amplicon (AMPLICOR HCV MONITOR), one column of wells is used for each specimen being tested. Add 100 µL hybridization buffer to each well required for testing. Add 25 µL of the denatured amplicon to the HCV wells in row A of the MWP, and mix up and down 10 times with a 12-channel pipeter with plugged tips. Make serial fivefold dilutions in the HCV wells in rows B through E as follows. Transfer 25 µL from row A to row B and mix as before. Continue through row E. Mix row E as before, then remove and discard 25 µL. Discard pipet tips. Add 25 µL of the denatured amplicon to the QS wells in row F of the MWP and mix up and down 10 times with a 12-channel pipeter with plugged tips. Transfer 25 µL from row F to row G. Mix as before, then transfer 25 µL to row H. Mix as before, then remove 25 µL from row H and discard.
3. Cover the MWP and incubate for 1 h at 37 ± 2°C.
4. Wash the MWP five times with the working wash solution using an automated MWP washer. Program the MWP washer as follows:
   a. Aspirate contents of the well.
   b. Fill each well to top (400–450 µL). Let soak for 30 s and aspirate dry.

c. Repeat **step b** four additional times.
   d. After automated washing is completed, tap the plate dry.

3.6. Detection Reaction (see Notes 22–27)

Following the hybridization reaction, the MWPs (or tubes of MP) are washed to remove any unbound material. An avidin–horseradish peroxidase conjugate (Av-HRP) is added to each well of the MWPs (or to tubes of MP) and incubated at 37°C for the appropriate amount of time. Av-HRP binds to the biotin-labeled amplicon captured by the plate-bound oligonucleotide probes. The MWPs (or tubes of MP) are washed again to remove unbound Av-HRP and a substrate solution containing hydrogen peroxide and 3,3',5,5'-tetramethylbenzidine (TMB) is added to the MWPs (or tubes of MP). In the presence of hydrogen peroxide, the bound horseradish peroxidase catalyzes the oxidation of TMB to form a colored complex. In the AMPLICOR tests, the reaction is stopped by addition of a weak acid, and the optical density at 450 nm is measured using an automated microwell plate reader. In the COBAS AMPLICOR tests, the reaction is not stopped; after a precisely timed incubation, the optical density of the reaction at 660 nm is measured by a spectrophotometer integrated in the COBAS system. The COBAS AMPLICOR system performs all of these steps automatically without user intervention. The following specific instructions apply to the manual AMPLICOR assays:

1. Add 100 µL Avidin-HRP conjugate to each well. Cover the MWP and incubate for 15 min at 37 ± 2°C.
2. Wash the MWP as described in **step 4** of **Subheading 3.5.**
3. Prepare working substrate solution. For each MWP, measure 12 mL substrate A and 3 mL substrate B. Mix together to prepare working substrate. Protect working substrate from direct light. Working substrate must be at room temperature and used within 3 h of preparation.
4. Pipet 100 µL working substrate solution into each well.
5. Allow color to develop for 10 min at room temperature in the dark.
6. Add 100 µL stop reagent to each well.
7. Measure the optical density at 450 nm (single wavelength) within 10 min of stop reagent addition.

3.7. Interpretation of Qualitative Results

For the qualitative tests, the results are interpreted by comparing the HCV and HCV IC absorbance values to established cutoffs. The COBAS system performs this comparison automatically and reports the interpretation along with the actual absorbance values. For the manual AMPLICOR tests, results are interpreted as in **Table 1**.

**Table 1
Interpretation of AMPLICOR HCV Test Results**

HCV specimen result (A_{450})	HCV IC specimen result (A_{450})	Interpretation
<0.25	≥0.6	No HCV RNA detected
<0.25	<0.6	Invalid negative result; process another aliquot of specimen
≥0.6	Any value	Positive for HCV
≥.25 but <0.6	Any value	Equivocal for HCV; repeat in duplicate

3.8. HCV RNA Quantitation

For the MONITOR tests, viral load is quantitated by utilizing the HCV QS, which is added to the test sample at a known concentration. The following calculations are performed manually (AMPLICOR tests) or automatically (COBAS tests):

1. For each reaction, select the dilution giving the lowest HCV signal having an optical density that is ≥0.20 and ≤2.0 absorbance units.
2. Subtract the background absorbance (0.07 for the AMPLICOR tests) from this value.
3. Calculate the HCV total OD by multiplying the background corrected HCV absorbance by the dilution factor used to generate the selected sample.
4. For each reaction, select the dilution giving the lowest HCV QS signal having an optical density that is ≥0.20 and ≤2.0 absorbance units.
5. Subtract the background absorbance (0.07 for the AMPLICOR tests) from this value.
6. Calculate the HCV QS Total OD by multiplying the background corrected QS absorbance by the dilution factor used to generate the selected signal.
7. Calculate the amount of HCV RNA in each specimen using the following equation:

HCV RNA copies/mL of specimen = (Total HCV OD/Total QS OD) × Input copies HCV QS × 200

Where 200 is the specimen dilution factor (the equivalent of 5 µL of serum or plasma is added to each amplification reaction).

3.9. Test Performance Characteristics

The qualitative AMPLICOR HCV test exhibited a sensitivity of 83% and a specificity of 100% compared to HCV serology. The qualitative COBAS AMPLICOR HCV Test exhibited a sensitivity of 78% and a specificity of 98% compared to HCV serology. The sensitivity of the AMPLICOR tests may actually be higher. A positive EIA test for anti-HCV antibody indicates prior exposure, but does not serve as a marker for current infection. Thus, HCV RNA-negative, anti-HCV antibody-positive specimens may be anti-HCV antibody false-positive rather than HCV RNA false-negative. Similarly, the specificity of the AMPLICOR tests may also be higher. Some HCV RNA-positive, anti-HCV-negative specimens may have been obtained from infected, nonseroconverting patients and, thus, should be anti-HCV false-negative rather than HCV RNA false-positive.

The AMPLICOR HCV MONITOR test has a dynamic range of approx 2000–500,000 copies of HCV RNA/mL of serum or plasma. The COBAS AMPLICOR HCV MONITOR Test has a dynamic range of approx 1000–1,000,000 copies of HCV RNA/mL of serum or plasma.

4. Notes
4.1. Specimen Preparation

1. For the manual assays, soak all Perkin-Elmer amplification trays, retainers, and bases in 10% bleach and rinse thoroughly with deionized water before reuse.
2. Before initiating specimen preparation, clean the work surface with 10% bleach followed by 70% alcohol (isopropanol or ethanol). This process will destroy bacteria and viruses and will denature DNA or RNA. Ultraviolet (UV) lighting should be used to irradiate nucleic acid that may be on the work surface. It is a good practice to turn on the UV light 20–30 min prior to starting.
3. Use dedicated pipets for specimen preparation to protect reagents and specimens from amplicon contamination. Use aerosol barrier tips for all liquid transfers to prevent reagent contamination and crosscontamination of nucleic acid from specimen to specimen. Aerosol barrier tips also prevent RNases from being introduced that will destroy RNA.
4. Use powder-free gloves. Glove powder can nonspecifically inhibit each of the major steps of the PCR assay.
5. Dissolve the lysis buffer completely before adding the well-vortexed HCV QS. Lysis buffer may be warmed at a temperature of 37°C, but no warmer, for up to 30 min. Always bring warmed lysis reagent to room temperature before adding the HCV QS.
6. The HCV QS must never be heated to 37°C. The HCV QS must be well vortexed before addition to the lysis reagent. Original vials of all AMPLICOR controls and standards should be vortexed as follows: upright: 5 s, upside down: 5 s, upright: 10 s, finish by tapping the vial on the counter to remove any liquid inside the cap.
7. Use only sterile screw-cap tubes for storing and preparing specimens. Flip cap tubes can cause specimen aerosols when tubes are opened. Flip cap tubes can cause splashes that can result in crosscontamination or a biosafety hazard.
8. To avoid crosscontamination when transferring aliquots of specimen to tubes containing lysis reagent, uncap one specimen tube and one lysis reagent tube at a

time. After transferring the specimen aliquot, recap the both the specimen tube and the lysis reagent tube before proceeding to the next specimen. Use a new aerosol barrier pipet tip for each specimen. Replace gloves immediately if they become contaminated with specimen.
9. When preparing controls, add negative human plasma (NHP) to the lysis buffer in the control tubes and vortex well before adding the control. This will destroy possible RNase activity in the NHP that could degrade control RNA. It is best to add the control last and then start the 10-min RT incubation.
10. Use fine tip transfer pipets to aspirate all supernatants.
11. Use only 70% ethanol to wash precipitated RNA; use of other alcohol solutions will compromise reproducibility.
12. After adding specimen diluent to the pellet, use the pipet tip to scrape the pellet off the side of the screw-cap tube. Because the HCV RNA is very sticky, scraping is essential for consistent, reproducible results.

4.2. Reverse Transcription and PCR Amplification

13. Arrange tubes of processed specimens, amplification tubes, and waste containers so that the pipet does not have to pass over open reaction tubes.
14. Uncap one tube of processed specimen at a time. After transferring an aliquot of specimen to the amplification tube, recap the tube before proceeding to the next specimen.
15. Use aerosol barrier tips when transferring aliquots of processed specimens to prevent pipeters from becoming contaminated with nucleic acid.
16. To avoid crosscontamination between samples, cap each A-tube (for COBAS tests) or each column of MicroAmp® tubes (for AMPLICOR tests) immediately after adding the processed specimens.
17. Use only Perkin Elmer 9600 or 2400 thermal cyclers for performing manual AMPLICOR tests. The amplification parameters have been optimized for these systems and may yield suboptimal results when performed on other thermal cyclers.

4.3. Hybridization Reaction

The following hints apply to the manual AMPLICOR tests:

18. Remove caps from amplification tubes slowly and with extreme care just prior to adding denaturation solution. If caps are opened too rapidly, droplets of reaction mixture may splash into neighboring tubes. Because reaction tubes may contain extremely high levels of amplicon, introduction of a small amount of contaminating reaction mixture into a negative tube may be sufficient to produce a false-positive result.
19. Use plugged tips and a multichannel pipeter (range 50–300 µL) to add denaturation solution to the wells. Change tips for each row or column. Pipet up and down to mix well.
20. Use plugged tips and a multichannel pipeter (range 5–50 µL) to transfer aliquots of reaction mixture to the MWP. Work carefully to avoid splashing

that could result in crosscontamination of neighboring wells. Change tips for each row or column.
21. Recap reaction tubes with new caps immediately after transferring reaction mixture to the MWP. This will help to prevent accidental spillage that could contaminate equipment and work surfaces with large amounts of amplicon.

4.4. Detection Reaction

The following hints apply to the manual AMPLICOR tests:

22. Clean disposable reagent reservoirs should be used for detection reagents. If reagent reservoirs are reused they must be labeled for specific reagents and cleaned thoroughly between each use with deionized water. Do not reuse reagent reservoirs more than five times.
23. Working wash buffer must be prepared by measuring the 10X-wash concentrate and then adding nine equal parts of deionized water. As a result of overfill, there may be up to 120 mL of wash buffer concentrate per bottle. Wash buffer preparation: 100 mL 10X- Wash Concentrate + 900 mL deionized water; mix well.
24. Substrates A and B must be measured when preparing the working substrate. All vials are over filled so that the exact amount of reagents may be pipetted from the bottle. The overfill between substrate A and B may not be proportional.
25. Mix substrate A and B no more than 3 h before use. Store protected from light. Excessive storage or exposure to light may cause high background signals and false-positive results.
26. Microwell plates are measured at 450 nm without a reference filter. All AMPLICOR test have been optimized for this measurement. Using a reference filter will falsely depress the sensitivity and results.
27. For the qualititative test, measure the absorbance within 60 min of adding stop reagent to the MWP. For the MONITOR test, measure the absorbance within 10 min of adding stop reagent to the MWP.

References

1. McHutchison, J., Person, J., Govindarajan, S., et al. (1992) Improved detection of hepatitis C virus antibodies in high-risk populations. *Hepatology* **15,** 19–25.
2. Chaudray, R. K., Andonov, A., and MacLean, C. (1993) Detection of hepatitis C virus infection with recombinant immunoblot assay, synthetic immunoblot assay, and polymerase chain reaction. *J. Clin. Lab. Anal.* **7,** 164–167.
3. Mitsui, T., Iwano, K., Masuko, K., et al. (1992) Hepatitis C virus infection in medical personnel after needlestick accident. *Hepatology* **16,** 1109–1114.
4. Dale, B. and Dragon, E. A. (1994) Polymerase chain reaction in infectious disease diagnosis. *Lab. Med.* **25,** 637–641.
5. DiDomenico, N., Link, H., Knobel, R., Caratsch, T., Weschler, W., Loewy, Z. G., and Rosenstraus, M. (1996) COBAS AMPLICOR™: A fully automated RNA and DNA amplification and detection system for routine diagnostic PCR. *Clin. Chem.* **42,** 1915–1923.

6. White, T. J., Madej, R., and Persing, D. H. (1992) The polymerase chain reaction: clinical applications. *Adv. Clin. Chem.* **29,** 161–196.
7. Puoti, M., Zonaro, A., Ravagil, A., et al. (1992) Hepatitis C virus RNA and antibody response in the clinical course of acute hepatitis C virus infection. *Hepatology* **16,** 877–881.
8. Young, K., Resnick, R., and Myers, T. (1993) Detection of hepatitis C virus RNA by a combined reverse transcriptase-polymerase chain reaction assay. *J. Clin. Microbiol.* **31,** 882–886.
9. Orito, E., Mizokami, M., Nakano, T., Terashima, H., Nojiri, O., Sakakibara, K., Mizuno, M., Ogino, M., Nakamura, M., Matsumoto, Y., et al. (1994) Serum hepatitis C virus RNA level as a predictor of subsequent response to interferon-α therapy in Japanese patients with chronic hepatitis. *C. J. Med. Virol.* **44,** 410–414.
10. Orito, E., Mizokami, M., Suzuki, K., Ohba, H., Ohno, T., Mori, M., Hayashi, K., Kato, K., Iino, S., and Lau, J. (1995) Loss of serum HCV RNA at week 4 of interferon-α therapy is associated with more favorable long-term response in patients with chronic hepatitis. *C. J. Med. Virol.* **46,** 109–115.
11. Longo, M. C., Beringer, M. S., and Hartley, J. L. (1990) Use of uracil DNA glycosylase to control carry-over contamination in polymerase chain reactions. *Gene* **93,** 125–128.
12. Rosenstraus, M., Wang, Z., Chang, S.-Y., DeBonville, D., and Spadoro J. P. (1998) An internal control for routine diagnostic PCR: design, properties and effect on clinical performance. *J. Clin. Microbiol.* **36,** 191–197.
13. Myers, T. W. and Gelfand, D. H. (1991) Reverse transcription and DNA amplification by a thermus thermophilus DNA polymerase. *Biochemistry* **3,** 7661–7666.

6

Quantification of HCV RNA in Clinical Specimens by Branched DNA (bDNA) Technology

Judith C. Wilber and Mickey S. Urdea

1. Introduction

The diagnosis and monitoring of hepatitis C virus (HCV) infection have been aided by the development of HCV RNA quantification assays. A direct measure of viral load, HCV RNA quantification has the advantage of providing information on viral kinetics and provides unique insight into the disease process. Branched DNA (bDNA) signal amplification technology provides a novel approach for the direct quantification of HCV RNA in patient specimens. The bDNA assay measures HCV RNA at physiological levels by boosting the reporter signal, rather than by replicating target sequences as the means of detection, and thus avoids the errors inherent in the extraction and amplification of target sequences. Inherently quantitative and nonradioactive, the bDNA assay is amenable to routine use in a clinical research setting, and has been used by several groups to explore the natural history, pathogenesis, and treatment of HCV infection.

The bDNA assay for quantification of HCV RNA is based on a series of specific hybridization reactions and chemiluminescent detection of hybridized probes in a 96-well microplate format (**Fig. 1**). A series of probes that are complementary to sequences in the 5'-untranslated and 5'-third of the core gene of the HCV genome capture the HCV RNA to the microwell surface. A second series of complementary probes link the HCV RNA to synthetic bDNA molecules. Each bDNA molecule has 15 arms, each of which is designed to hybridize to three alkaline phosphatase molecules. With up to 18 bDNA molecules bound to each HCV RNA, as many as 810 separate alkaline phosphatase molecules/HCV RNA can be hybridized, thus providing tremendous enhancement of the signal. The new probes for the bDNA assay have been designed to

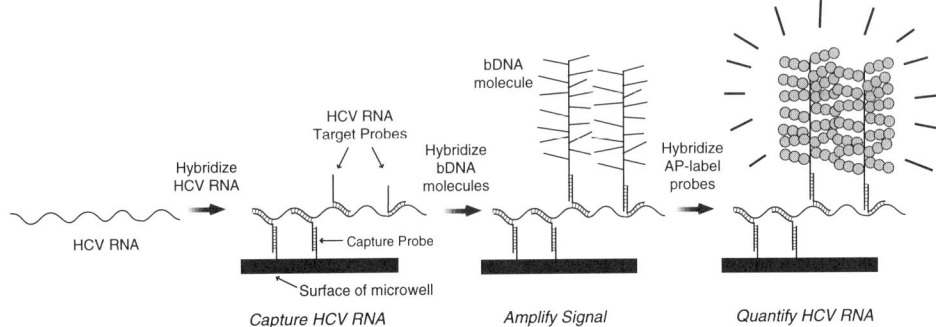

Fig. 1. Schematic of the bDNA assay for HCV RNA quantification.

ensure that each of the HCV genotypes is detected equally *(1)*. The overall clinical sensitivity is over 95%, and reproducibility is excellent.

Technological and practical features of the bDNA assay facilitate its routine use in a clinical or research laboratory setting. There is no sample preparation for serum and plasma specimens, and there are no special handling procedures necessary for containment of potential contaminants. The bDNA assay uses a 96-well microplate format that is familiar to most laboratories, which allows many samples to be processed: 2–4 plates, each with 42 samples in duplicate plus standards and controls, can easily be processed by 1 person in 1 d. The probes for the bDNA assay (Quantiplex™ HCV RNA 2.0) have been designed to measure RNA from all major genotypes of HCV equally. Also, because the bDNA assay uses a chemiluminescent detection system, it does not suffer from the limited shelf-life of radioactive assays.

A complement to serological, biochemical, and histological measures of disease, the bDNA assay for HCV RNA quantification may be a useful tool for the management of patients chronically infected with HCV. Several studies have used the bDNA assay to show that pretreatment HCV RNA levels may be predictive of response in patients undergoing interferon (IFN) therapy *(2–7)*. Indeed, a gradation of response to IFN therapy has been found in an analysis of combined patient populations from throughout the world with varying pretreatment serum HCV RNA levels *(8)*. In addition, HCV RNA quantification using the bDNA assay has revealed that, although viral load in chronic HCV patients is generally stable, in a subset of patients, HCV RNA levels can fluctuate considerably, particularly posttherapy *(9,10)*. It may be possible to obtain improved efficacy if treatment or retreatment is initiated at a time-point when a patient's viral load is at its lowest. This possibility is especially important for patients who have already received IFN therapy and have suffered relapse, since these individuals are more likely to relapse again *(11)*. The results of these and other studies demonstrate that accurate quantification of HCV RNA using the bDNA assay cannot only help to predict the likelihood of a patient's response to IFN, but also may aid in decisions regarding the timing of initiation of treatment or retreatment in HCV-infected individuals.

In addition to HCV RNA quantification in serum specimens, use of the bDNA assay to quantify HCV RNA in liver biopsy specimens may help to establish the efficacy of therapy. At the end of therapy, it can be problematic to determine whether a patient has truly cleared the virus, since residual HCV replication may occur in the liver. If a follow-up liver biopsy is performed to assess improvement in histology, then quantification of HCV RNA in liver biopsy material could provide a means of establishing true viral clearance. A modification of the bDNA assay has been developed to measure HCV RNA in liver tissue *(12,13)*. The advantage of using the bDNA assay in measuring liver HCV RNA is that unlike RT-PCR methods, which are inhibited by the high concentrations of heme present in liver tissue, the bDNA assay does not require highly purified nucleic acid preparations. A simple RNA extraction (described in Chapter 10) that has been optimized for recovery of HCV RNA is all that is required to obtain HCV RNA quantification results with the bDNA assay that accurately reflect the concentration of virus in the liver.

Quantification of HCV RNA as a measure of viral load is being used increasingly to follow disease progression and monitor therapeutic response in HCV-infected patients. By providing unique insight into viral dynamics, HCV RNA quantification should be useful in the evaluation of new therapeutic regimens. A unique and powerful tool for reliable quantification of HCV RNA in clinical specimens, the bDNA assay provides researchers and clinicians with valuable information to define and refine antiviral therapy for HCV-infected individuals.

2. Materials
2.1. Reagents for Day 1

1. HCV capture wells: polystyrene capture wells coated with synthetic oligonucleotides.
2. HCV lysis diluent: buffered solution containing protein and synthetic oligonucleotides, which is used to make specimen working reagent (*see* **Subheading 3.2.1.**).
3. HCV lysis reagent: Stabilized proteinase K solution, which is used to make specimen working reagent (*see* **Subheading 3.2.1.**).
4. HCV target probes: synthetic oligonucleotides to mediate capture and to bind bDNA amplifier in distilled water containing 0.05% sodium azide and 0.05% ProClin 300 as preservatives.
5. Specimen working reagent: 627.5 mM LiCl, 157 mM HEPES, pH 7.5, 12.5 mM EDTA, 1.6% lithium lauryl sulfate, 19 µg/mL sonicated salmon sperm DNA,

0.05% sodium azide, 0.05% Proclin 300 (Supelco, Inc., Bellefonte, PA), 2.2 mg/mL proteinase K, 0.17 pmol/mL HCV target probes to mediate capture, 1.34 pmol/mL HCV target probes to bind amplifier.
6. Specimens: A 100-μL serum or plasma specimen is required to perform the assay in duplicate—50 μL/replicate.
7. Standards: recombinant single-stranded DNA at 120 MEq/mL (standard A), 12 MEq/mL (standard B), 1.2 MEq/mL (standard C), 0.2 MEq/mL (standard D), and 0 MEq/mL (standard E) in normal human serum containing 0.05% sodium azide and 0.05% ProClin 300 as preservatives.
8. Controls: a known concentration of recombinant single-stranded DNA in normal human serum (HCV high control) and β-propiolactone-treated HCV in human serum (HCV low control) with 0.05% sodium azide and 0.05% ProClin 300 as preservatives.

2.2. Reagents for Day 2

1. HCV label diluent: 0.5% blocking reagent (Boehringer Mannheim, Indianapolis, IN), 0.1% sodium dodecyl sulfate (SDS), 5X standard saline citrate (SSC), 0.05% sodium azide, 0.05% Proclin 300.
2. HCV amplifier reagent: 2.0 pmol/mL bDNA amplifier in HCV label diluent.
3. HCV label working reagent: 4 pmol/mL alkaline phosphatase-conjugated label probe in HCV label diluent.
4. HCV wash A: 0.1X SSC, 0.1% SDS, 0.05% sodium azide, 0.05% Proclin 300.
5. HCV wash B: 0.1X SSC, 0.05% sodium azide, 0.05% Proclin 300.
6. Substrate solution: 99.7% Lumiphos™ 530 (Lumigen, Detroit, MI), 0.03% sodium dodecyl sulfate.

2.3. Equipment

1. Chiron plate heater ($53 \pm 0.5°C$) equipped with 8×12 microwell holder.
2. Chiron plate-reading luminometer maintained at $37 \pm 2.5°C$ to read a 96-microwell plate.

3. Methods
3.1. Specimen Preparation

One of the advantages of the bDNA assay is that it can be applied to a number of specimen types, since it does not require highly purified nucleic acid preparations. The bDNA assay yields reliable quantification of HCV RNA in both crude serum and plasma specimens, as well as extracts from liver biopsy specimens.

1. Serum: Collect blood in a sterile tube with no anticoagulants. Serum separator tubes are recommended. Allow blood to clot at room temperature, and centrifuge within 2 h to separate serum from cells. Use standard laboratory procedures to remove serum aseptically from the clot within 4 h of blood collection. Store serum specimens at −60 to −80°C in sterile tubes. Avoid repeated freezing and thawing.

bDNA Technology

2. Plasma: Collect blood in sterile tubes containing K_3 EDTA (0.15% [v/v] final concentration). Store whole blood at room temperature before separating plasma from cells. Use standard laboratory procedures to remove plasma from cells aseptically within 2 h of collection. Do not clarify plasma by filtration or further centrifugation. Store the plasma at –60 to –80°C in sterile tubes. Avoid repeated freezing and thawing.
3. Cell extracts: The procedure for processing liver biopsy specimens for use in the bDNA assay is described in Chapter 10.

3.2. Plate Setup for Day 1

1. Prepare specimen working reagent immediately before use. Warm HCV lysis diluent to 37°C for 10–15 min and mix gently. Bring HCV lysis reagent and HCV target probes to room temperature. Vortex HCV lysis reagent, and vortex and centrifuge (500g, <5 s) HCV target probes. In a sterile-packaged polypropylene tube, prepare sufficient specimen working reagent using a 60:5:0.4 ratio of HCV lysis diluent:HCV lysis reagent:HCV target probes.
2. Add 150 µL specimen working reagent to each HCV capture well.
3. Add 50 µL of serum or plasma specimens, standards, and controls to the appropriate HCV capture wells, in duplicate.
4. Seal the microwells with Mylar® film.
5. Incubate the microwells overnight at 53°C in the Chiron plate heater.

3.3. Plate Processing for Day 2

1. Take the plate from the Chiron plate heater, and let stand 10 min at room temperature.
2. While the plate is cooling down, prepare the HCV amplifier reagent by diluting the amplifier concentrate at 40 pmol/mL into HCV label diluent. The final concentration should be 2.0 pmol/mL.
3. Wash the microwells twice with HCV wash A.
4. Pipet 50 µL of diluted amplifier into each well. Incubate the microwells for 30 min at 53°C in the Chiron plate heater.
5. Take the plate from the Chiron plate heater, and let it stand for 10 min at room temperature.
6. While the plate is cooling down, prepare the HCV label working reagent by diluting the label probe concentrate at 100 pmol/mL into HCV label diluent. The final concentration should be 4.0 pmol/mL.
7. Wash the microwells twice with HCV wash A.
8. Pipet 50 µL of the HCV label working solution into each microwell. Incubate the microwells for 15 min at 53°C in the Chiron plate heater.
9. Take the plate from the Chiron plate heater, and let it stand for 10 min at room temperature.
10. While the plate is cooling down, prepare the substrate solution by combining 3 µL 10% SDS for each 1.0 mL Lumiphos™ 530.
11. Wash the microwells twice with HCV wash A and then three times with HCV wash B. Add 50 µL of the substrate solution into each microwell.

12. Pipet 50 µL of the substrate solution into each microwell. Incubate the microwells for 30 min at 37°C.
13. Measure the chemiluminescence in the plate-reading luminometer.
14. Calculate the amount of HCV RNA in each specimen from the standard curve, defined by a quadratic curve function.

4. Notes

1. All of the reagents described in **Subheadings 2.** and **3.** are manufactured materials available as research reagents under the name Quantiplex™ HCV RNA 2.0 (bDNA), Chiron Diagnostics.
2. The bDNA assay is intended for research use only.
3. It is recommended that specimens and controls be handled using established good laboratory working practices, as if capable of transmitting an infectious agent. The HCV low control contains β-propiolactone-treated HCV and human serum. The normal human serum used to manufacture all standards and controls was shown to be below the quantification limit of the Quantiplex™ HCV RNA 2.0 assay, and nonreactive for hepatitis B surface antigen, anti-HIV-1/anti-HIV-2, and anti-HCV.
4. Assay steps may be performed on an open bench covered with plastic-backed absorbent paper to contain possible spills. Spills should be disinfected promptly with a 0.5% sodium hypochlorite solution (a freshly prepared 1:10 dilution of liquid household bleach) or equivalent disinfectant. Contaminated materials should be disposed of as biohazardous waste.
5. Personal protective apparel, including disposable gloves, should be worn throughout the test procedure. Hands should be washed afterward, and gloves should be disposed of as biohazardous waste.
6. Do not pipet by mouth. Do not eat, drink, smoke, or apply cosmetics in areas where reagents or specimens are handled.
7. Assay all specimens, HCV standards, and HCV controls in duplicate.
8. Add all specimens and reagents to HCV capture wells by touching the pipet tip to the wall near the midpoint of the well, above the surface of the fluid in the well.
9. Do not break apart HCV capture well strips into segments. Seal HCV capture wells securely with a fresh plate sealer to prevent evaporation during incubations. When removing the plate sealer following incubations, use care not to pull the HCV capture wells out of the microwell holder.
10. Bring all reagents to the temperature specified in the assay procedure before use. Room temperature is defined as 15–30°C.
11. Use of lipemic or turbid specimens may yield inconclusive results.
12. The results from the Chiron luminometer are reported in relative luminescence (RL) units, which are a measurement of the amount of light emitted from each HCV capture well. Light emission is proportional to the amount of HCV RNA present in the specimen. To generate a standard curve, a quadratic equation is used to fit the RL values of the standards (A–D). HCV RNA quantitative results are obtained by comparing the mean RL units of each specimen to the standard

curve. The final result is reported in megaequivalents per milliliter (MEq/mL) where one HCV RNA MEq/mL in the bDNA assay (Quantiplex™ HCV RNA 2.0) is equal to the luminescence generated by 10^6 molecules of a 3.2-kb HCV RNA transcript.
13. The quantification limit of the bDNA assay (Quantiplex™ HCV RNA 2.0) is 0.2 HCV RNA MEq/mL. Specimens with RL values equal to or greater than Standard D (0.2 MEq/mL) contain HCV RNA in the quantity indicated. Specimens with RL values less than that of standard D (0.2 MEq/mL) fall below the quantification limit of the assay and are reported as <0.2 HCV RNA MEq/mL.
14. Specimens with mean RL values greater than that of standard A (120 MEq/mL) are above the upper limit of the standard curve, and must be diluted and retested to obtain a quantitative value. Dilute the specimen 1:10 or 1:100 in either serum or plasma, depending on the matrix of the original specimen, that has been shown not to contain measurable HCV RNA by the bDNA assay (Quantiplex™ HCV RNA 2.0), and is not hemolyzed, lipemic, or turbid. Retest the diluted specimen following the standard procedure, and multiply the resulting quantification value by the dilution factor to obtain the HCV RNA MEq/mL in the original specimen.
15. Specimens with mean RL values equal to or greater than standard D (0.2 MEq/mL) and with RL percent coefficient of variance >25% must be retested. Specimens with one duplicate RL value above the quantification limit and one below the quantification limit that also have an RL percent coefficient of variance >25% must be retested.

Acknowledgments

We thank Kristina Whitfield for graphics and Linda Wuestehube for editorial assistance.

References

1. Detmer, J., Lagier, R., Flynn, J., Zayati, C., Kolberg, J., Collins, M., et al. (1996) Accurate quantification of HCV RNA from all HCV genotypes using branched DNA (bDNA) technology. *J. Clin. Microbiol.* **34,** 901–907.
2. Iino, S., Komata, M., Kumada, H., Akane, T., Kiyosawa, S., Hayashi, N., et al. (1993) Quantification of HCV-RNA by branched DNA probe assay. *J. Med. Pharm. Sci.* **30,** 327–334.
3. Lau, J. Y. N., Davis, G. L., Kniffen, J., Qian, K. P., Urdea, M. S., Chan, C. S., et al. (1993) Significance of serum hepatitis C virus RNA levels in chronic hepatitis C. *Lancet* **341,** 1501–1504.
4. Magrin, S., Craxi, A., Fabiano, C., Simonetti, R. G., Fiorentino, G., Marino, L., et al. (1994) Hepatitis C viremia in chronic liver disease: relationship to interferon-alpha or corticosteroid treatment. *Hepatology* **19,** 273–279.
5. Orito, E., Mizokami, M., Nakano, T., Terashima, H., Nojiri, O., Sakakibara, et al. (1994) Serum hepatitis C virus RNA level as a predictor of subsequent response to interferon-alpha therapy in Japanese patients with chronic hepatitis C. *J. Med. Virol.* **44,** 410–414.

6. Toyoda, H., Nakano, S., Kumada, T., Takeda, I., Sugiyama, K., Osada, T., et al. (1996) Comparison of serum hepatitis C virus RNA concentration by branched DNA probe assay with competitive reverse transcription polymerase chain reaction as a predictor of response to interferon-alpha therapy in chronic hepatitis C patients. *J. Med. Virol.* **48,** 354–359.
7. Yuki, N., Hayashi, N., Kasahara, A., Hagiwara, H., Takehara, T., Oshita, M., et al. (1995) Pretreatment viral load and response to prolonged interferon-alpha course for chronic hepatitis C. *J. Hepatol.* **22,** 457–463.
8. Urdea, M. (1995) The use of branched DNA (bDNA) assays to monitor the clinical course and therapy of HCV infections and the development of molecular standards, in *Program and Abstracts of the Fifth International Symposium on Hepatitis C Virus and Related Viruses,* Gold Coast, Australia.
9. Alter, H. J., Sánchez-Pescador, R., Urdea, M.S., Wilber, J. C., Lagier, R. J., Di Bisceglie, A. M., et al. (1995) Evaluation of branched DNA signal amplification for the detection of hepatitis C virus RNA. *J. Viral Hepatitis* **2,** 121–132.
10. Lau, J. Y. N., Mizokami, M., Ohno, T., Diamond, D. A., Kniffen, J., and Davis, G. L. (1993) Discrepancy between biochemical and virological responses to interferon-a in chronic hepatitis C. *Lancet* **342,** 1208–1209.
11. Arase, Y., Kumada, H., Chayama, K., Naoya, N., Tsubota, A., Koida, I., et al. (1995) Usefulness of HCV-RNA counts by the method of HCV-bDNA probe in interferon retreatment for patients with HCV-RNA positive chronic hepatitis C. *Int. Hepatol. Commun.* **4,** 19–25.
12. Coelho-Little, E., Jeffers, L. J., Bartholomew, M., Reddy, K. R., Schiff, E. R., and Dailey, P. J. (1995) Correlation of HCV-RNA levels in serum and liver of patients with chronic hepatitis C. *J. Hepatol.* **22,** 508.
13. Idrovo, V., Dailey, P. J., Jeffers, L. J., Coelho-Little, E., Bartholomew, M., Alvarez, L., et al. (1996) Hepatitis C virus RNA quantification in right and left lobes of the liver in patients with chronic hepatitis C. *J. Viral Hepatitis* **3,** 239–246.

7

Quality Control of the Polymerase Chain Reaction

Maurice Rosenstraus, Joanne P. Spadoro, Diane McGovern-Wolfe, and Elizabeth A. Dragon

1. Introduction

The polymerase chain reaction (PCR) has revolutionized both the basic and the applied aspects of the biomedical field with more than 40,000 papers having been published employing this technique. PCR has become an indispensable tool for basic research applications, such as cloning *(1)*, sequencing *(2)*, mRNA analysis *(3)*, DNA and RNA quantitation *(4–6)*, mutagenesis *(7)*, and gene detection *(8)*. Because of its ability to amplify minute quantities of nucleic acid specifically, PCR has also been applied with great success in clinical diagnostics *(9–11)*, genetic testing *(12–15)*, forensics *(16,17)*, and environmental testing *(18,19)*.

Several methodological enhancements have enabled PCR to progress from a research tool to a technology that can be used for performing routine analyses in a clinical setting. These include simplified protocols for extracting nucleic acids from specimens *(20)*, thermostable polymerases *(21–23)*, instrumentation to automate amplification and detection *(10,24,25)*, and techniques for quantitating the amount of target nucleic acid in a specimen *(4–6)*. Of equal importance is the development of quality-control measures that enable PCR to meet the rigorous standards required for routine clinical testing. False-negative results can be minimized by optimizing assay reagents and by using an internal control (IC) to detect specimens inhibitory to amplification. False-positive results can be minimized by careful design of laboratory facilities, attention to laboratory technique, and the incorporation of enzymatic or chemical methods for controlling carryover contamination of previously amplified nucleic acid. As a result of these measures, the clinical laboratory can exploit the exquisite sensitivity and specificity of PCR, and assure the integrity of the test results.

From: *Methods in Molecular Medicine, Vol. 19: Hepatitis C Protocols*
Edited by: J. Y. N. Lau © Humana Press Inc., Totowa, NJ

2. Operation of a PCR Laboratory
2.1. Equipment

A molecular diagnostic laboratory performing PCR requires equipment for extracting nucleic acids from specimens, amplification, and detection. The equipment required to perform PCR-based tests depends on the assay formats being used. A thermal cycler is required for all assay formats.

Manual PCR assays require equipment for detecting amplified products. A microwell plate washer and microwell plate reader are required for assays, such as AMPLICOR tests, in which amplification products are detected by hybridization to probe-coated microwell plates. Gel electrophoresis equipment is required for assays that employ Southern blotting to detect amplification products. Equipment for preparing dot blots is required when detection involves hybridizing probes to immobilized amplification products or hybridizing amplification products to immobilized probes (reverse dot blot). Equipment for handling radioisotopes and visualizing autoradiograms is required when radioactive probes are used to detect amplification products.

Fully automated PCR assays, such as the COBAS AMPLICOR tests, are performed using a single instrument that performs amplification and then detects the products generated. The COBAS AMPLICOR system contains a single thermal cycler with two independently regulated heating/cooling blocks, an incubator, a magnetic particle washer, a pipet, and a photometer *(10)*. Amplified products are captured on oligonucleotide-coated paramagnetic microparticles and detected using an avidin–horseradish peroxidase (HRP) conjugate. The COBAS AMPLICOR simplifies laboratory setup, consolidates work stations, and decreases hands-on labor. In addition, COBAS AMPLICOR tests exhibit better reproducibility and precision than their manual counterparts, because all reagent transfers during the detection portion of an assay are performed by a fully automated, highly reproducible pipet. The COBAS AMPLICOR also minimizes the amount of DNA introduced into the laboratory environment. The operator closes reaction tubes after the specimen is added and does not reopen them (closed, contained amplification). Because all amplification and detection operations are automatically performed within the COBAS AMPLICOR, laboratory personnel, surfaces, and equipment are protected from contamination with amplified DNA.

2.2. Lab Design

A PCR laboratory should contain two functional work areas: a preamplification area and a postamplification area. These two areas can be in separate rooms, or when space constraints exist, separate work stations in a single room. Regardless of whether one or two rooms are used, supplies and equipment should be dedicated to each work area and should not be moved to other areas. One convenient and easy way to assure that supplies and equipment are exchanged between areas is to use a color-coding system.

2.3. Preamplification Area

The preamplification area should contain one work area for preparing reagents and a second work area for preparing specimens. A separate tabletop or laminar flow hood should be used to define each work area. Amplification reaction mixtures and specimen preparation reagents should be made in the reagent preparation area. Specimens should be prepared using the appropriate biosafety precautions and added to amplification reaction tubes in the specimen preparation area. Preamplification activities should begin with reagent preparation and proceed to specimen preparation. Supplies and equipment should be dedicated to each preamplification activity and not be used for other activities or be moved between areas. Equipment and supplies used for reagent preparation should not be used for specimen preparation activities or for pipeting or processing amplified DNA or other sources of target DNA.

2.4. Postamplification Area

Amplification and analysis of the resulting PCR product are performed in the postamplification area. When manual PCR assays are performed in this area, work surfaces and equipment are usually contaminated with high levels of amplified DNA (amplicon). After working in a potentially contaminated postamplification area, one should avoid entering the preamplification area. One may, however, shuttle between pre- and postamplification areas when postamplification activity is restricted to loading samples and reagents onto a fully automated PCR assay system, such as the COBAS AMPLICOR. When doing so, lab coats, gloves, and safety glasses worn in the postamplification area must be removed, and must not be brought into the preamplification area. Supplies and equipment should be dedicated to the postamplification area and not be used for other activities or be moved to the preamplification area.

2.5. Laboratory Techniques and Practices

Laboratory personnel should be completely aware of the consequences of sloppy technique. Because of the sensitivity of PCR, even an aerosol contamination can result in the generation of false-positive results. Once a reagent or supply is contaminated with amplicon, it is extremely difficult to locate the source of contamination and to eliminate it completely. As a result, one is usually forced to discard most reagents and begin again. The consequences of sloppy technique, therefore, are lost time, lost experiments, and extreme frustration.

Laboratory coats, gloves, and safety glasses should be worn at all times. Separate laboratory coats should be dedicated to each area and coats should be color-coded to avoid mix-up between pre- and postamplification areas. Gloves should be changed frequently. Work surfaces should be wiped down with 10–50% bleach followed by 70% ethanol after each work session. The ethanol inactivates residual bleach, which could potentially poison assay components. Aerosol-resistant plugged pipet tips or positive displacement pipets should be used to transfer any solution containing nucleic acid. Procedures specific for each work area are discussed below.

2.6. Preamplification Area—Reagent Preparation

Newly prepared reagents should be aliquoted to minimize the chance of contamination by repeated use. Premanufactured amplification mixtures and reagents should be dispensed to reaction tubes in the reagent preparation area. Reaction tubes should then be capped and moved to the specimen preparation area for addition of sample. Of critical importance is the absolute exclusion of amplicon and target DNA (such as plasmids, phage-containing target sequences, or clinical specimens) from the reagent preparation area at all times. One should never bring nucleic acid-containing reagents (with the exception of the IC reagent), or supplies from the sample preparation and postamplification areas into the reagent preparation area. Laboratory coats dedicated to reagent preparation should be worn and stored only in the reagent preparation area.

2.7. Preamplification Area—Specimen Preparation

Pipets with plugged tips or positive displacement pipets should be used for adding specimen preparation reagents to specimens and dispensing prepared specimens to amplification reaction tubes. To prevent crosscontamination between specimens, each tube should be uncapped prior to each reagent addition and immediately recapped before proceeding to the next specimen. When transferring specimens to amplification reaction tubes, position the samples so that the pipet does not have to pass over open reaction tubes. Amplification reaction tubes should be capped immediately after adding specimen. When handling specimens, take care to avoid contaminating gloves with specimen. If gloves do become contaminated, they should be replaced with a clean pair before proceeding to the next specimen. If any specimen droplets fall onto the work area, immediately wipe the surface with a paper towel soaked with bleach, and then rinse the surface with a paper towel soaked with 70% ethanol. Before and after each work session, containment hood surfaces and pipeters should be wiped down with freshly prepared 10% bleach followed by 70% ethanol. When not in use, the containment hood should be closed, and the UV lamp should be turned on.

2.8. Postamplification Area

Always wear laboratory coats and gloves, and remove them whenever leaving the area. Reaction tubes, which may contain extremely high levels of amplicon, should be opened with extreme care to avoid spillage and aerosolization. Pipets with aerosol-resistant plugged tips must be used when adding reagents to or transferring aliquots from reaction tubes. Pipet tips must be changed after each reagent addition or aliquot withdrawal. Reaction tubes should be recapped immediately after use. Capped reaction tubes may be stored at 2–8°C or –20°C if additional postamplification analyses may need to be performed. All pipet tips, used reagents, gloves, and reaction tubes that are no longer needed should be placed in biohazard bags and autoclaved.

3. Quality Control in a PCR Laboratory

To achieve optimal sensitivity, specificity, and reproducibility when performing PCR tests, pay careful attention to the following factors: methods for controlling contamination, types of assay controls used, selection and synthesis of primer oligonucleotides, type of polymerase used, amplification conditions, methods of validating assay performance, and equipment calibration and maintenance. Each of these factors is discussed in detail below.

3.1. Contamination Control

Three sources of contamination afflict all amplification technologies, including PCR: crosscontamination between specimens, contamination of specimens by positive controls, and contamination with previously amplified products (carryover contamination). The first two sources can be controlled by careful technique. Carryover contamination is more problematic because target amplification techniques generate extremely large quantities of product. Amplification reactions may contain up to 5×10^{12} molecules of amplified nucleic acid/100 µL amplification reaction. Contaminating a new reaction with just 1 fL of a previous amplification reaction will introduce up to 50 target molecules; after amplification, these 50 copies will generate enough product to produce a false-positive signal. Successful application of PCR is dependent on effective control of carryover contamination.

Spatial and temporal segregation of pre- and postamplification work as described above provides a primary defense against carryover contamination. Additional biochemical controls can be employed to inactivate amplified DNA, rendering it non-amplifiable and, thereby, further reducing the likelihood of false positives owing to carryover contamination.

Several postamplification inactivation methods have been developed. In one method, a chelated metal complex and an oxidizing agent are added to reaction tubes after the detection assay is completed to inactivate the remaining amplified DNA *(26)*. This system has limited utility, because amplified DNA released while performing the detection assay remains a potential source of carryover contamination. Destroying the amplified DNA remaining in reaction tubes controls the buildup of amplified DNA, reducing the chance that it will find its way to the pre-amplification area, but this can also be achieved by capping amplification reaction tubes and placing them in biohazard bags, which are autoclaved regularly.

More useful are methods that modify amplified DNA prior to performing the detection assay. The chemical modifications alter DNA so that it cannot be reamplified, but can still function in the detection assay. In one method, the DNA-inactivating agent hydroxylamine is added to reaction tubes immediately after amplification *(27)*. In a second method, ribose-containing primers are used for amplification, and the ends of the amplified DNA are inactivated by adding NaOH to reaction tubes immediately after amplification (for review, *see* **ref. 28**). A disadvantage of these procedures is that noninactivated DNA can contaminate personnel, lab surfaces, and equipment when inactivating agents are being added to reaction tubes.

In an alternative postamplification method, amplified DNA can be inactivated without opening the reaction tube. Derivatives of the photosensitizing agent psoralen are included in the amplification reaction mixture. At the conclusion of amplification and before opening tubes to remove samples for detection, the reactions are exposed to long-wavelength UV light *(29,30*, for review *see* **ref. 28**). The psoralen derivative intercalates into the amplified DNA and becomes covalently linked on exposure to light. The covalently modified DNA cannot serve as a template for amplification. Provided that noncrosslinking isopsoralen derivatives are used, the modified DNA can still be detected in hybridization assays. When using this method, the concentration of psoralen must be selected to achieve sufficient sterilization while minimizing any adverse effect on amplification and hybridization efficiency.

In one preamplification control method, PCR reagents are irradiated with UV light prior to the addition of target nucleic acid *(31–33*, for review *see* **ref. 28**). The UV light inactivates any contaminating DNA in the reagents by inducing thymidine dimer formation. The effectiveness of this technique is a function of amplicon size and A-T content. The treatment may adversely affect *Taq* polymerase and nucleotides in the reaction mixture, thereby reducing amplification efficiency.

A second preamplification biochemical control system "immunizes" the amplification reaction to amplicon. This system, which is employed in all AMPLICOR and COBAS AMPLICOR tests, consists of two components: a method for marking amplified DNA so it can be distinguished from naturally occurring DNA, and a method for destroying amplified DNA. DNA synthesized during an amplification reaction is distinguished from naturally occurring DNA by substituting deoxyuridine triphosphate for thymidine triphosphate as one of the deoxyribonucleoside triphosphates in the amplification reaction mixture. Although the ribonucleoside uridine is one of the four nucleosides in naturally occurring RNA, deoxyuridine is never found in naturally occurring DNA. The enzyme Uracil-*N*-glycosylase is included in the amplification reaction mixture to recognize and catalyze specifically the destruction of DNA-containing deoxyuridine, but not DNA-containing thymidine *(34)*. When first loaded into the thermal cycler, amplification reaction mixtures are incubated at 50°C to allow Uracil-*N*-glycosylase to attack deoxyuridine residues by opening the deoxyribose chain at the C1-position. When the thermal cycler heats the reaction mixture to denature DNA and initiate amplification, the damaged DNA chain breaks at the position of the deoxyuridine (strand scission), thereby rendering the DNA nonamplifiable. Throughout the remaining thermal cycling steps, the temperature is maintained above 55°C. Uracil-*N*-glycosylase is inactive at these elevated temperatures and, therefore, does not destroy newly amplified, deoxyuridine-containing DNA. Following amplification, any residual enzyme is denatured by the addition of an alkaline denaturation reagent, thereby preventing the degradation of newly amplified DNA.

3.2. Assay Controls

Various types of controls may be used to ensure that all equipment and reagents are working properly and that all procedures are performed correctly. Negative controls are used to demonstrate the absence of contamination or other problems that could cause false-positive results. Positive controls are used to demonstrate that the assay is capable of detecting target DNA. An IC is used to demonstrate that amplification has occurred in individual specimens and, thus, provides assurance that negative test results are true negative.

The choice of which controls to employ depends on the types of samples being tested, the complexity of the test procedures, the experience of the operator, and whether one is using "home-brew" reagents or standardized commercial kits, which are manufactured and tested in compliance with rigorous quality-control standards. An IC may be required when testing relatively crude clinical specimens that are likely to contain amplification inhibitors. The IC may not be needed if previous experience has demonstrated that the types of specimens being tested are rarely inhibitory. Specimen-processing controls should be considered when employing complex extraction protocols. Positive and negative amplification controls should be included in each assay to make sure all amplification and detection reagents and equipment functioned correctly. Amplification controls will also fail if detection fails. Thus, for assay formats that have an appreciable probability of detection failure, separate detection controls should be used to enable the operator to distinguish amplification from detection failures. To yield meaningful results, all positive and internal controls should be used at concentrations near the limit of the assay sensitivity. If the control concentration is too high, the control may yield an acceptable result even if test performance was suboptimal.

3.3. Internal Control

Because currently available methods for processing clinical specimens do not yield highly purified nucleic acid, a fraction of processed specimens may contain substances that inhibit PCR. Inhibitory specimens can be identified by monitoring amplification of a second target nucleic acid, which serves as an IC. Obtaining a positive signal from the second target demonstrates successful amplification, thereby validating a negative result for the primary target *(35)*.

One approach to monitoring amplification involves using a normal cellular gene sequence, which is expected to be present in all specimens, as the IC. Using an endogenous cellular sequence has the advantage of controlling specimen integrity; if the specimen is not collected (or stored) properly, the endogenous target will be absent (or degraded) and fail to yield a positive result. On the other hand, endogenous sequences, which require a second primer pair specific for the sequence, have several serious limitations. Amplification of the endogenous sequence may not parallel amplification of primary target because of differences in the primer sequences and size of the amplified product. Furthermore, the amount of endogenous sequence in a specimen may be much greater than the amount of the primary target. If amplification is very inefficient in a particular specimen, the high-concentration endogenous sequence may yield a positive signal, whereas a low-concentration primary target does not.

The second approach to monitoring amplification, using a synthetic IC as a proxy for primary target, overcomes the inherent limitations of an endogenous IC. One design of a synthetic IC is a DNA plasmid or RNA transcript with primer binding regions identical to those of the target sequence, a randomized internal sequence of similar length and base composition as the target sequence, and a unique probe binding region that differentiates the IC from amplified target nucleic acid. These features were selected to ensure equivalent amplification of the IC and the target nucleic acid. The IC is introduced into each amplification reaction and is coamplified with target nucleic acid from the clinical specimen. A limited number of IC molecules are added to each reaction; thus, a positive IC signal assures amplification sufficient to generate a positive signal from very small quantities of target. When introduced into an amplification reaction, the IC can monitor amplification and detection. When the IC is introduced into the unprocessed specimen, it can also monitor specimen processing. Although a synthetic IC offers many advantages over using a housekeeping gene as an IC, the former cannot be used to monitor specimen integrity.

When using an IC, one must select a cutoff signal to distinguish inhibitory from noninhibitory specimens. To determine the IC cutoff, one should analyze the distribution of IC signals in a set of specimens that are negative for the target DNA. The set includes all true-negative and false-negative specimens. Specimens that are positive for target DNA (both true and false positives) are not included in this analysis, because the depressed IC signals in these specimens do not necessarily serve as an indicator of amplification (IC amplification may be suppressed by competition from a high concentration of target DNA). One should also determine how test sensitivity increases as the IC cutoff is increased. As the IC cutoff increases, the total number of specimens classified as inhibitory also increases. At some point, increasing the cutoff further does not improve sensitivity, because no additional PCR-negative, infected specimens are classified as inhibitory. This value is chosen as the IC cutoff. Choosing a higher value as the cutoff would increase the number of specimens deemed inhibitory without improving performance.

3.4. Specimen Processing Controls

These controls are designed to monitor the effectiveness of extraction and recovery of nucleic acid from specimens. As such, the state of the target nucleic acid in a specimen-processing control should closely match its state in a specimen. One easy way to accomplish this is to use a known positive specimen. The amount of target in the selected specimen should be determined by end point dilution. The positive specimen should then be diluted with negative specimen to give a target nucleic acid concentration that approaches the limit of the test's sensitivity. By using a low copy number control, the operator will be able to detect subtle deficiencies in specimen processing.

Controls can also be constructed by adding a known quantity of cultured organisms to a negative specimen. Care must be exercised to make sure that the cultured organism will mimic the behavior of the organism in a specimen. Consider, for example, a PCR test designed to detect a virus in a clinical sample where the majority of viral nucleic acid is cell-associated and is recovered by using low-speed centrifugation to sediment cells. Purified viral particles added to a negative clinical specimen would be an inappropriate control. Because they are not cell-associated, recovery of the virions would not simulate recovery of cell-associated virus via low-speed centrifugation. Likewise, during cell lysis steps, release of nucleic acid from virions may not parallel release from cells; for example, a defective cell lysis treatment could be sufficiently potent to release nucleic acid from virions, but may not lyse cells in clinical specimens.

3.5. Amplification Controls

Amplification controls consist of specific (positive control) and nonspecific (negative control) nucleic acids that are added to individual control amplification reactions. These control reactions are amplified and detected in parallel with the test samples. The final concentration of the positive control nucleic acid should be 10–20 copies/amplification reaction. Using a such a low concentration of positive control will provide assurance that the assay system is functioning well enough to achieve maximal analytical sensitivity. The positive and negative control nucleic acids should be diluted in a matrix that is identical to that of the processed specimen.

3.6. Detection Controls

Amplicon generated from target DNA can be used as a detection control. A standardized preparation can be made by pooling multiple amplification reactions and diluting the pooled amplicon to a concentration that gives a low to moderate signal in the detection system. The dilution buffer should be formulated to match the matrix used to prepare test samples for detection. The diluted amplicon should be divided into single-use aliquots and stored frozen. An aliquot should be thawed just before performing the detection assay and tested in parallel with the test samples. Any leftover amplicon should be discarded.

3.7. Primers

Select primers that are 20–30 bases in length and approx 50% G + C content. Avoid sequences with secondary structure or with long stretches of polypurines and polypyrimidines. A primer must not contain sequences that are complementary to those in other primers; take care to monitor all primer combinations for complementarity when designing multiplex PCR assays.

When specificity of amplification is critical, make sure the selected primer sequence is substantially different from related sequences in closely related organisms and includes mismatches near the 3'-end of the primer sequence *(36,37)*. Sequences with a limited number of internal mismatches may partially hybridize to a nonspecific target and will be extended if the 3'-end of the primer perfectly matches the nonspecific target sequence. When a variety of closely related organisms must be amplified, design consensus primers that contain minimal mismatches when compared to each of the target sequences. Select a primer whose 3'-end is identical in all target organisms. If the set of target sequences exhibits enough divergence, it will be difficult to design a single set of primers that amplify all sequences. One solution is to use multiple primer sets, each of which amplifies a subset of the target sequences. Another strategy is to incorporate modified bases, such as inonsine, that can pair with any base at positions of sequence divergence *(38,39)*.

To preserve assay specificity and maximize amplification efficiency, full-length primer sequences must be purified from incomplete "failure" sequences that accumulate during synthesis. Full-length primers can be separated from "failure" sequences by reverse-phase high-pressure liquid chromatography, anion-exchange chromatography, or a combination of the two. Crosscontamination of primer sequences must be avoided by dedicating purification columns to an individual sequence or by stripping columns with a strong acid, base, or both after each use. Primers recovered following preparative chromatography should exhibit purities of 85–95% as determined by high-resolution, anion-exchange chromatography (**Fig. 1**; *40*). Quantitative PCR tests demand 95% primer purity. For qualitative tests that require high analytical sensitivity, use primers of 90% or greater purity. For qualitative tests where analytical sensitivity is less critical, 85% primer purity may be acceptable.

3.8. Polymerases

The choice of polymerase depends on the intended use of the PCR test and whether the target nucleic acid is RNA or DNA. All of the enzymes discussed below are manufactured by Roche Molecular Systems, Branchburg, NJ, and may be purchased from Perkin-Elmer Applied Biosystems, Foster City, CA.

For RNA targets, r*Tth* DNA polymerase is the enzyme of choice. This recombinant enzyme contains both thermostable reverse transcriptase and thermostable DNA polymerase activities, permitting reverse transcription of RNA and amplification of the resulting cDNA to proceed in the same tube without operator intervention *(22,41)*.

Recombinant, thermostabile *Taq* polymerase (AmpliTaq® DNA Polymerase) is the enzyme of choice for DNA targets in most assays. Because it is a recombinant enzyme that is manufactured under carefully controlled conditions, it exhibits excellent reproducibility from vial to vial and lot to lot.

For certain applications, nonspecific amplification of bacterial DNA sequences normally present in AmpliTaq may interfere with assay performance. AmpliTaq DNA Polymerase, LD can be used in such applications; this is the same enzyme as AmpliTaq DNA Polymerase, but is further purified through a proprietary separation process to minimize intrinsic contamination by bacterial DNA sequences.

In certain PCR assays, nonspecific products may form at room temperature prior to the initiation of amplification. For example, multiplex assays may exhibit unacceptable levels of primer oligomer formation. Hot-start PCR *(42,43)* is designed to overcome this problem by withholding a crucial amplification reaction component until the reaction mixture is elevated above the minimum temperature required for specific primer annealing; the missing reactant is then manually added to the reaction mixture, and thermal cycling resumes.

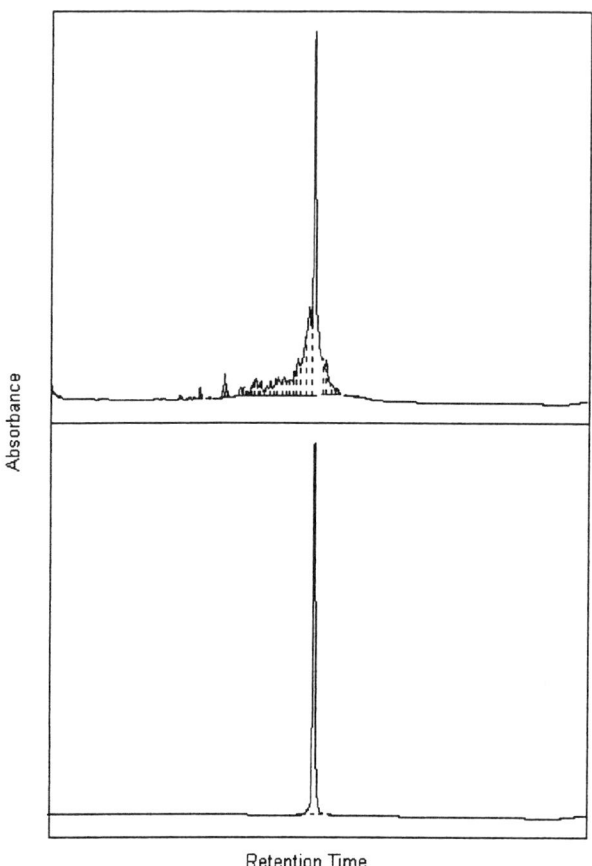

Fig. 1. Recovery of high-purity oligonucleotide following preparative chromatography. A newly synthesized oligonucleotide shows many incomplete "failure" sequences when analyzed by anion-exchange chromatography (upper chromatogram). Selected fractions recovered following preparative chromatography are essentially devoid of failure sequences (lower chromatogram).

By using the enzyme AmpliTaq Gold™ instead of a conventional thermostable DNA polymerase, hot-start PCR can now be performed without resorting to extra steps and manipulations. AmpliTaq Gold is in an inactive state when added to the reaction mixture and is activated by heating the reaction mixture at 94–95°C for 9–12 min prior to initiating thermal cycling.

Several other polymerases can be used for special applications. Use the enzyme rTth DNA Polymerase, XL to amplify target DNA sequences ranging from 5–40 kb. If amplified DNA will be used for cloning, use the enzyme *UlTma* DNA Polymerase to prevent the generation of mutant sequences; this enzyme has a "proofreading" activity that repairs 3'-mismatches that form during amplification. Use AmpliTaq DNA Polymerase, Stoffel Fragment when performing multiplex PCR for targets having different optimum Mg^{2+} concentrations. This recombinant enzyme is a fragment of AmpliTaq DNA Polymerase; it lacks 289 amino acids from the amino-terminus of the native enzyme *(44)*. The Stoffel Fragment should also be used when performing Arbitrarily Primed PCR, a technique in which genomic DNA is amplified using a set of short primers of arbitrary sequence *(45)*.

3.9. Amplification Conditions

Optimized reaction conditions must be identified for each PCR system. First, the composition of the reaction mixture must be determined; this work can be done using general thermal cycling parameters that give adequate results in most systems. After the reaction mixture formulation is selected, thermal cycling parameters should be optimized. Once thermal cycling conditions are established, the concentration of each key reaction mixture component should be varied to ensure that it is still optimal and to determine concentration tolerances.

Optimization should be performed using purified target nucleic acid as well as clinical specimens when appropriate. If closely related nontarget sequences are known, their amplification should also be monitored during optimization to identify and avoid conditions that compromise specificity. Inhibitory specimens, if available, can be used to reveal assay conditions that alleviate or exacerbate inhibition. During optimization, it is very useful to analyze reaction products in ethidium bromide-stained gels as well as with specific probes. Minimal nonspecific amplification (as visualized on a gel) should be evident in an optimized system.

Multiple reaction mixture components and several thermal cycling parameters impact amplification performance. Also, any of these parameters may have discordant effects on different assay end points, especially in multiplex assays, where each target may have different requirements. For example, if low denaturation temperature or short denaturation cycle time were required to minimize inhibition, denaturation itself might be compromised. Using such denaturation conditions would enable amplification of inhibitory specimens at the expense of reduced amplification efficiency for specimens that are not inhibitory. Thus, it may be helpful to use computer-assisted statistical experimental design techniques to identify interactions between variables, while limiting the number of variable combinations tested. Computer-assisted data analysis may also be helpful for identifying sets of parameters that yield acceptable results for all end points. Statistical experimental design software packages are commercially available (e.g., Design-Ease®, available from Stat-Ease Corporation, Minneapolis, MN).

3.10. Reaction Mixture Composition

Determine the optimal concentrations for the following key reaction mixture components: primers, deoxynucleotide triphosphates, divalent cation (Mg^{2+} or Mn^{2+}), and polymerase. Because the deoxynucleotide triphosphate concentration affects the divalent cation requirement, various combinations of concentrations should be tested. Increasing the concentration of polymerase may be helpful for overcoming PCR inhibition. Cosolvents, such as glycerol or dimethylsulfoxide, may enhance amplification efficiency and/or the stability of the reaction mixture. The optimal salt (usually KCl) concentration in the reaction mixture will depend on the salt concentration in processed specimens. Different buffering systems should be evaluated for their effects on analytical sensitivity and assay specificity. During these optimization studies, reaction products should be analyzed by gel electrophoresis to identify conditions that maximize the amount of specific amplification product while minimizing the amount of nonspecific amplification products.

3.11. Thermal Cycling Parameters

The effect of simultaneously varying denaturation time and temperature should be studied. Temperature and time of exposure must be sufficient to melt duplex DNA, but should be kept as short as possible to minimize irreversible damage to polymerase. In one system, we found that lower denaturation temperature coupled with shorter denaturation time overcame PCR inhibition in some specimens. It may be advantageous to use longer denaturation time and/or higher temperatures for the first few amplification cycles when most of the templates are genomic DNA. It may be possible to switch to a shorter denaturation time and/or a lower temperature at later cycles when most of the templates are short amplicon, which may denature more readily than genomic DNA.

Annealing time, annealing temperature, and extension time may interact and, therefore, should be varied simultaneously during optimization experiments. Amplification of related nontarget sequences should be monitored when optimizing annealing temperature. Annealing temperatures below 60°C could compromise assay specificity and should be avoided, especially during early cycles. If an annealing temperature below 60°C dramatically enhances assay sensitivity, it may be possible to use it at later cycles. Nonspecific amplification initiated at later cycles will not interfere with ongoing amplification of the specific target, nor will it generate enough product to give false-positive signals.

The optimal number of cycles should also be determined. Nonspecific products may accumulate when more than 40 cycles are used. For quantitative assays, the number of cycles should be adjusted so that the amount of amplified product varies linearly with input target concentration over the desired dynamic range of the test.

3.12. Validation of Assay Performance

Assay performance should be validated after optimizing reagents and thermal cycling conditions. Specificity, analytical sensitivity, reproducibility, and susceptibility to potentially interfering substances should be evaluated. The performance of the assay should be compared to the performance of an established reference test on a panel of specimens.

The specificity of the assay must be verified by demonstrating that it does not generate positive results from nontarget nucleic acid sequences that might be found in specimens that will be used in the test. Use high concentrations (10^4–10^7 copies/amplification reaction) of nontarget sequences when evaluating specificity. The assay should also be tested for reactivity with various sources of target nucleic acid to verify that it will detect all variants. For example, a diagnostic test for a virus or bacteria must react with all known subspecies or strains.

To determine the analytical sensitivity of the assay, serially dilute a known quantity of target nucleic acid in specimen matrix and identify the lowest concentration that consistently gives a positive signal. The starting concentration of target should be determined by an independent assay. For example, use a virus stock containing a known number of plaque-forming units (PFU)/mL for a diagnostic viral PCR assay. In this example, the analytical sensitivity would be expressed as the number of PFU/mL that consistently yield a positive signal. Of course, the exact number of target sequences required to yield a positive signal cannot be determined without knowing the ratio of infectious to noninfectious virions.

Reproducibility should be assessed by having multiple operators perform the assay over several days as described in the NCCLS Guidelines (EP5-T2), "Evaluation of Performance of Clinical Chemistry Devices." Each operator should test multiple replicates of each test sample at each time-point. The concentration of target sequence in the test samples should approach the limit of assay sensitivity. The test sample matrix should be similar to that of actual specimens. Test samples should be processed just like specimens. Reproducibility of reagents should be evaluated by having a single operator test multiple batches of reagents in parallel.

Specimens may contain endogenous or exogenous substances, or their metabolites, that could interfere with a PCR assay. Generate a list of relevant potentially interfering substances by reviewing the composition of each type of specimen that will be used in the assay. For example, evaluate heparin, bronchial dilators, and feminine hygiene products when testing blood, respiratory, and urogenital specimens, respectively. Each substance identified should be evaluated by adding it at various concentrations to known positive and negative samples. Any substance that generates a false-positive or false-negative result is classified as an interfering substance. The test should not be performed on specimens known to contain such substances.

Finally, the results of PCR testing should be compared to results of an established reference test performed on the same set of specimens. The design of the comparison will depend on the intended use of the PCR assay. When used to distinguish between several variants of a particular target sequence (e.g., forensic analysis, identity testing, genetic screening), PCR should exhibit agreement with the reference test on the subset of variants present in a particular specimen. When PCR has the ability to identify variants not detectable by the reference test (e.g., when PCR can identify variants that are not detectable by immunological tests), the PCR result can be validated by nucleic acid sequencing.

For quantitative PCR tests, use an independent test to measure the target concentration in a set of specimens; examples of independent tests include electron microscopic quantitation of virus particles, colony-forming or plaque-forming assays, quantitative antigen tests, and fluorimetric measurement of DNA concentration (when DNA from the target organism can be separated from host or other microbial DNA). Prepare serial dilutions of each specimen and quantitate the target concentration in each dilution by PCR. The target concentration as measured by PCR should vary linearly with input target concentration, as determined by the independent test, over a range of concentrations; this defines the dynamic range of the assay. Ideally, the target concentration determined by PCR should be within 0.5 log of the concentration determined by the reference test. If the difference is larger, a careful evaluation of the potential biases and limitations inherent to the independent test may help to identify the source of the discrepancy.

For qualitative PCR tests, use 2 × 2 contingency tables to compare PCR and reference test results. Discrepancies between PCR and reference test results may not indicate poor performance of the PCR test; rather, the reference test may be at fault. For example, apparent PCR false positives may occur if PCR is significantly more sensitive than the reference test. Apparent PCR-false negatives may result if the reference test is less specific than PCR. Therefore, all discordant results should be evaluated by additional testing. Apparent PCR false-positive (or false-negative) specimens can be evaluated by performing a third test, such as PCR for an another sequence within the genome of the target organism. A positive (or negative) result in the third test would confirm that the target organism is present, suggesting that PCR was truly positive (or truly negative) and that the reference test was falsely negative (or falsely positive). After resolving discordant results, the accuracy, sensitivity, and specificity of the PCR test should be determined by comparing the initial PCR test results to the resolved result. A good test should exhibit >90% sensitivity (PCR true positives/total resolved positives) and > 99% specificity (PCR true negatives/total resolved negatives). A nearly equal number of PCR false positives and false negatives indicates that there is no systematic problem with the test and suggests that sampling variation is responsible for most PCR discrepancies vs resolved results.

3.13. Equipment Calibration and Maintenance

Proper maintenance and calibration of equipment is critical for achieving accurate, reliable results. Pipeters should be checked for worn parts and calibrated at least annually; properly functioning pipets are especially critical to achieve accurate results in quantitative tests. Biosafety cabinets should be serviced annually to ensure safety and protect against contamination. Centrifuges should be decontaminated periodically or whenever a spill occurs by wiping surfaces and the inside of tube holders with 10% bleach followed by 70% ethanol.

The thermal cycler wells and cover should be periodically cleaned with isopropanol or 70% ethanol. If the thermal cycler should become contaminated with amplification reaction mixture, decontaminate all surfaces by wiping with 10% bleach followed by isopropanol or 70% ethanol. Diagnostic testing and calibration should be performed as per the manufacturer's recommended schedule. History files can be printed after each run to document that parameters were properly executed.

Detection equipment, such as microwell plate washers and readers, should be adjusted as per the manufacturer's recommendations. Equipment should be cleaned at the end of each day or after each use. For example, microwell plate washers should be flushed with deionized water at the end of each day; at the beginning of the next work day, the washer should be primed with wash buffer. To prevent buildup of fungi or other microbes, microwell plate washers should be rinsed with 10% bleach followed by deionized water once a month.

Fully automated PCR systems, such as the COBAS AMPLICOR, must be serviced as per the manufacturer's recommendations. False-positive or false-negative results may occur if instrument parts are not cleaned or replaced as specified in the preventative maintenance schedule. Prior to each instrument run, waste containers should be checked and emptied if necessary; used reaction tubes and empty or expired reagent vials should be discarded.

4. Summary

PCR has evolved into a valuable, reliable tool for routine clinical testing owing in part to advances in quality-control measures. Careful laboratory design and work-flow controls, coupled with assay automation and sophisticated biochemical control systems, have conquered the contamination problems that plagued early PCR users. The clinical labs' stringent requirements for reproducible, reliable results can be attained through the use of meticulously designed controls and standardized, optimized reagents. Accuracy can be assured by subjecting assays to rigorous validation protocols.

References

1. Stoker, A. W. (1990) Cloning of PCR products after defined cohesive termini are created with T4 DNA polymerase. *Nucleic Acids Res.* **18,** 4290.
2. Bevan, I. S., Rapley, R., and Walker, M. R. (1992) Sequencing of PCR amplified DNA. *PCR Methods Appl.* **1,** 222–228.
3. Barnea, E., Zuk, D., Simantov, R., Nudel, U., and Yaffee, D. (1990) Specificity of expression of the muscle and brain dystrophin gene promoters in muscle and brain cells. *Neuron* **5,** 881–888.
4. Kellogg, D. E., Sninsky, J. J., and Kwok, S. (1990) Quantitation of HIV-1 proviral DNA relative to cellular DNA by the polymerase chain reaction. *Anal. Biochem.* **189,** 202–208.
5. Mulder, J., McKinney, N., Christopherson, C., Sninsky, J., Greenfield, L., and Kwok, S. (1994) Rapid and simple PCR assay for quantitiation of human immunodeficiency virus type 1 RNA in plasma: application to acute retroviral infection. *J. Clin. Microbiol.* **32,** 292–300.
6. Wang, A., Doyle, M., and Mark, D. (1989) Quantitation of mRNA by polymerase chain reaction. *Proc. Natl. Acad. Sci. USA* **86,** 9717–9721.
7. Sakar, G. and Sommer, S. S. (1990) The "mega primer" method of site-directed mutagenesis. *BioTechniques* **8,** 404–407.
8. Saiki, R., Scharf, S., Faloona, F., Mullis, K., Horn, G., Erlich, H., et al. (1985) Enzymatic amplification of β-globin genomic sequences and restriction site analysis for diagnosis of sickle cell anemia. *Science* **230,** 1350–1354.
9. Dale, B. and Dragon, E. A. (1994) Polymerase chain reaction in infectious disease diagnosis. *Lab. Med.* **25,** 637–641.
10. DiDomenico, N., Link, H., Knobel, R., Caratsch, T., Weschler, W., Loewy, Z. G., et al. (1996) COBAS AMPLICOR™: A fully automated RNA and DNA amplification and detection system for routine diagnostic PCR. *Clin. Chem.* **42,** 1915–1923.
11. White, T. J., Madej, R., and Persing, D. H. (1992) The polymerase chain reaction: clinical applications. *Adv. Clin. Chem.* **29,** 161–196.
12. Alford, R. L., Rossiter, B. J., and Caskey, C. T. (1994) DNA diagnosis in monogenic diseases. *Int. J. Technol. Assess. Health Care* **10,** 628–643.
13. Begovich, A. B. and Erlich, H. A. (1995) HLA typing for bone marrow transplantation—new polymerase chain reaction-based methods. *JAMA* **273,** 586–591.
14. Bugawan, T. L., Apple, R., and Erlich, H. A. (1994) A method for typing polymorphism at the HLA-A locus using PCR amplification and immobilized oligonucleotide probes. *Tissue Antigens* **44,** 137–147.
15. Muggleton-Harris, A. L. and Braude, P. R. (1993) Preimplantation diagnosis of genetic disease. *Curr. Opinion Obstet. Gynecol.* **5,** 600–605.
16. Buldowle, B., Lindsey, J. A., DeCou, J. A., Koons, B. W., Giusti, A. M., and Comey, C. T. (1995) Validation and population studies of the loci LDLR, GYPA,

HBGG, D7S8, and GC (PM loci), and HLA-DQα using a multiplex amplification and typing procedure. *J. Forensic Sci.* **40,** 45–50.
17. von Beroldingen, C. H., Blake, E. T., Higuchi, R., Sensabaugh, G. F., and Erlich, H. A. (1989) Applications of PCR to the analysis of biological evidence, in *PCR Technology: Principles and Applications for DNA Amplification* (Erlich, H., ed.), Stockton, New York, pp. 209–223.
18. Palmer, C. J., Bonilla, G. F., Roll, B., Paszko-Kolva, C., Sangermano, L. R., and Fujioka, R. S. (1995) Detection of Legionella species in reclaimed water and air with the EnviroAmp Legionella PCR kit and direct fluorescent antibody staining. *Appl. Environ. Microbiol.* **61,** 407–412.
19. Palmer, C. J., Tsai, Y. L., Paszko-Kolva, C., Mayer, C., and Sangermano, L. R. (1993) Detection of Legionella species in sewage and ocean water by polymerase chain reaction, direct fluorescent-antibody, and plate culture methods. *Appl. Environ. Microbiol.* **59,** 3618–3624.
20. Greenfield, L. and White, T. J. (1993) Sample preparation methods, in *Diagnostic Molecular Microbiology: Principles and Applications* (Persing, D. H., Smith, T. F., Tenover, F. C., and White, T. J., eds.), American Society for Microbiology, Washington, DC, pp. 122–137.
21. Abramson, R. D. (1995) Thermostable DNA polymerases, in *PCR Strategies* (Innis, M. A., Gelfand, D. H., and Sninsky, J. J., eds.), Academic, New York, pp. 39–57.
22. Myers, T. W. and Gelfand, D. H. (1991) Reverse transcription and DNA amplification by a *Thermus thermophilus* DNA polymerase. *Biochemistry* **30,** 7661–7666.
23. Saiki, R. K., Gelfand, D. H., Stoffel, S., Scharf, S. J., Higuchi, R., Horn, G. T., et al. (1988) Primer-directed enzymatic amplification of DNA with a thermostable DNA polymerase. *Science* **239,** 487–491.
24. Haff, L., Atwood, J. G., DiCesare, J., Katz, E., Picozza, E., Williams, J. F., et al. (1991) A high-performance system for automation of the polymerase chain reaction. *BioTechniques* **10,** 102–112.
25. Jungkind, D., DiRenzo, S., Beavis, K. G., and Silverman, N. S. (1996) Evaluation of automated COBAS AMPLICOR PCR system for detection of several infectious agents and its impact on laboratory management. *J. Clin. Microbiol.* **34,** 2778–2783.
26. Chernesky, M. A., Jang, D., Lee, H., Burczak, J. D., Hu, H., Sellors, J., et al. (1994) Diagnosis of *Chlamydia trachomatis* infections in men and women by testing first-void urine by ligase chain reaction. *J. Clin. Microbiol.* **32,** 2682–2685.
27. Aslanzadeh, J. (1992) Application of hydroxylamine hydrochloride for post-PCR sterilization. *Ann. Clin. Lab. Sci.* **22,** 280.
28. Persing, D. H. and Cimino, G. D. (1993) Amplification product inactivation methods, in *Diagnostic Molecular Microbiology: Principles and Applications* (Persing, D. H., Smith, T. F., Tenover, F. C., and White, T. J., eds.), American Society for Microbiology, Washington, DC, pp. 105–121.
29. Cimino, G. D., Metchette, K. C., Tessman, J. W., Hearst, J. E., and Isaacs, S. T. (1991) Post-PCR sterilization: a method to control carryover contmination for the polymerase chain reaction. *Nucleic Acids Res.* **19,** 99–107.

30. Isaacs, S. T., Tessman, J. W., Metchette, K. C., Hearst, J. E., and Cimino, G. D. (1991) Post-PCR sterilization: development and application to an HIV-1 diagnostic assay. *Nucleic Acids Res.* **19,** 109–116.
31. Cimino, G. D., Metchette, K. C., Isaacs, S. T., and Zhu, Y. S. (1990) More false-positive problems. *Nature (Lond.)* **347,** 340,341.
32. Fox, J. C., Ait-Khalid, M., Webster, A., and Emery, V. C. (1991) Eliminating PCR contamination: is UV irradiation the answer? *J. Virol. Methods* **33,** 375–383.
33. Ou, C. Y., Moore, J. J., and Schochetman, G. (1991) Use of UV irradiation to reduce false-positivity in the polymerase chain reaction. *BioTechniques* **10,** 442–446.
34. Longo, M. C., Berninger, M. S., and Harley, J. L. (1990) Use of uracil DNA glycosylase to control carry-over contamination in polymerase chain reaction. *Gene* **93,** 125–128.
35. Rosenstraus, M., Wang, Z., Chang, S.-Y., DeBonville, D., and Spadoro, J. P. (1997) An internal control for routine diagnostic PCR: design, properties and effect on clinical performance. Manuscript submitted.
36. Kwok, S., Kellogg, D. E., McKinney, N., Spasic, D., Goda, L., Levenson, C., et al. (1990) Effects of primer-template mismatches on the polymerase chain reaction: Human immunodeficiency virus type 1 model studies. *Nucleic Acids Res.* **18,** 999–1005.
37. Christopherson, C., Sninsky, J., and Kwok, S. (1997) The effects of internal primer-template mismatches on RT-PCR: HIV-1 model studies. *Nucleic Acids Res.* **25,** 654–658.
38. Kwok, S., Chang, S.-Y., Sninsky, J. J., and Wang, A. (1994) A guide to the design and use of mismatched and degenerate primers. *PCR Methods Appl.* **3,** s39–s47.
39. Lin, P. K. T. and Brown, D. M. (1992) Synthesis of oligodeoxyribonucleotides containing degenerate bases and their use as primers in the polymerase chain reaction. *Nucleic Acids Res.* **20,** 5149–5152.
40. Singman, C. N., Brown, D. R., Gupta, A. P., and McGovern-Wolfe, D. (1997) High resolution chromatographic analysis of oligonucleotides. Manuscript in preparation.
41. Young, K., Resnick, R. M., and Myers, T. W. (1993) Detection of hepatitis C virus RNA by a combined reverse transcription-polymerase chain reaction assay. *J. Clin. Microbiol.* **31,** 882–886.
42. Chou, Q., Russell, M., Birch, D. E., Raymond, J., and Bloch, W. (1992) Prevention of pre-PCR mis-priming and primer dimerization improves low-copy-number amplifications. *Nucleic Acids Res.* **20,** 1717–1723.
43. Horton, R. M., Hoppe, B. L., and Conti-Troconi, B. M. (1994) AmpliGrease: "Hot Start" PCR using petroleum jelly. *BioTechniques* **16,** 42–43.
44. Lawyer, F. C., Stoffel, S., Saiki, R. K., Myambo, K., Drummond, R., and Gelfand, D. H. (1989) Isolation, characterization, and expression in Escherichia coli of the DNA polymerase gene from Thermus aquaticus. *J. Biol. Chem.* **264,** 6427–6437.
45. Welsh, J. and McClelland, M. (1990) Fingerprinting genomes using PCR with arbitrary primers. *Nucleic Acids Res.* **18,** 7213–7218.

8

Preparation of Genotype-Specific HCV RNA Transcripts for Assessing HCV Detection and Quantification Assays

Jill J. Detmer, Janice A. Kolberg, Crystle L. K. Zayati, and Mark L. Collins

1. Introduction

Hepatitis C virus (HCV), the etiological agent responsible for the majority of cases of parenterally acquired liver disease, is found throughout the world. HCV is an enveloped virus with a small, single-stranded RNA genome. Because it uses an error-prone, RNA-dependent RNA polymerase, HCV has a high spontaneous mutation rate, and isolates of HCV display significant genetic heterogeneity. Isolates of HCV have been classified into at least six major genotypes and multiple subtypes based on sequencing and phylogenetic analysis (1). These genetic variants of HCV show a diverse geographical distribution. HCV types 1a, 1b, 2b, and 3a are the most prevalent in the US and western Europe (2,3), although all six major genotypes have been noted.

The genetic diversity of HCV poses a challenge to nucleic acid tests for measuring viral load (4). All nucleic acid quantification assays depend on the hybridization of oligonucleotide probes to HCV sequences, and these probes must have equivalent hybridization kinetics in order to measure all genotypes of HCV equally. However, the different HCV genotypes may show as little as 70% overall sequence homology throughout the entire 9.5-kb genome. Even the most highly conserved region of the HCV genome, the 5'-untranslated region, shows significant heterogeneity (5). This sequence heterogeneity can have a major impact on the hybridization efficiency of oligonucleotide probes in nucleic acid quantification assays. For assays that utilize polymerase chain reaction (PCR), this problem is compounded by a requirement for equivalent efficiencies of amplification between a standard and the template of interest in

From: *Methods in Molecular Medicine, Vol. 19: Hepatitis C Protocols*
Edited by: J. Y. N. Lau © Humana Press Inc., Totowa, NJ

order to determine accurately the amount of nucleic acid present. Templates differing in sequence from the standard are unlikely to be amplified with equal efficiency, and thus introduce an additional source of error in quantifying HCV RNA.

As might be expected from these theoretical difficulties, not all nucleic acid quantification assays measure RNA from the different HCV genotypes equally. Independent studies have shown that some PCR-based assays underestimated HCV RNA genotype 3 by as much as 8- to 10-fold *(6)*. Difficulties in the equal quantification of HCV genotypes have been less pronounced with the branched DNA (bDNA) assay, which uses multiple synthetic oligonucleotide probes to measure HCV RNA. Even so, the first-generation bDNA assay (Quantiplex™ HCV RNA 1.0, Chiron Diagnostics, Emeryville, CA) exhibited a variance of threefold between HCV genotypes 1 and 2 *(7)*. With the design of new oligonucleotide probes, based on additional sequence information, an improved bDNA assay (Quantiplex™ HCV RNA 2.0, Chiron Diagnostics) has been introduced, which is virtually unaffected by the genotypic variability of HCV. This improved bDNA assay, described in detail in Chapter 6, has been shown to measure RNA from all six major HCV genotypes equally *(6,7)*. Differences between assays in the efficacy of RNA quantification of HCV genotypes are important to consider for investigations into the clinical relevance of viral load in HCV-infected patients.

Accurate quantification of RNA from all HCV genotypes has become even more vital in light of the mounting evidence for the clinical relevance of viral load measurements for patients considering therapy. Numerous studies have shown that serum HCV RNA levels are prognostic of a patient's likelihood of response to interferon-alpha (IFN-α) treatment, and can be used to predict whether a patient's response to IFN-α treatment is likely to be sustained (for example, *8–11)*. Thus, to be clinically meaningful, HCV RNA measurements must be accurate, irrespective of HCV genotype. It is important to note that studies exploring the clinical significance of viral load measurements are performed by measuring HCV RNA levels in HCV-infected patient populations. Since specimens from different patients may contain different genetic variants of HCV, it is essential that nucleic acid quantification assays accurately measure RNA from all HCV genotypes.

To test the accuracy of quantification of RNA from all HCV genotypes, we have developed a method to prepare highly purified, rigorously quantified genotype-specific HCV RNA transcripts. As illustrated in **Fig. 1**, in this method HCV RNA is isolated from plasma or serum specimens from patients chronically infected with HCV. Clinical specimens are genotyped using the INNO-LiPA HCV Line Probe Assay *(12,13)* and are confirmed by sequence analysis of the NS5 and 5'-untranslated regions of the HCV genome *(1,14)*. The isolated HCV RNA is used to generate 822 nucleotide reverse transcriptase PCR

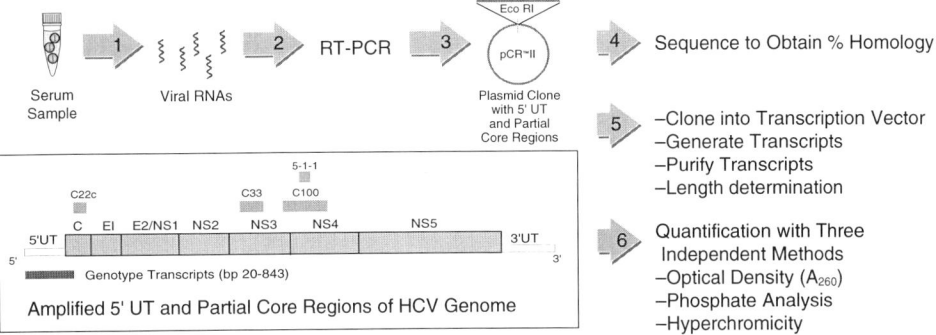

Fig. 1. Procedure for preparing high-quality HCV RNA transcripts from clinical specimens.

(RT-PCR) products (containing the 5'UT and some of the core), which are cloned into an RNA expression vector. The cloned DNA is isolated, linearized, and purified. Genotype-specific run off transcripts are produced using T7 RNA polymerase and are purified over two consecutive NAP-25 columns.

The quality-control procedure used to determine if the HCV RNA transcripts are of sufficiently high quality and purity to be used as reference standards also is presented in **Fig. 1**. First, the length of the transcripts is determined by formaldehyde gel analysis. Then, following phenol extraction and ethanol precipitation, the concentration of the transcripts is determined by several independent methods, including absorbance at 260 nm (A_{260}), phosphate analysis, and hyperchromicity analysis. To qualify for use as reference standards, the HCV RNA transcripts must meet stringent criteria for integrity and purity—transcripts must be >50% full length, and show <20% difference in concentration by the three quantification methods.

The genotype-specific HCV RNA transcripts prepared by the method presented in this chapter have been used in a number of applications. These highly purified transcripts were used to develop and validate the improved bDNA assay (described above), which accurately measures RNA from all major genotypes of HCV *(7)*. They also have been used as standards to compare the performance of additional qualitative and quantitative assays *(6)*. As a reliable reference prepared by well-established and independent techniques, these transcripts have served as an indispensable tool for optimizing assay conditions and testing alternative probe designs. Further, these transcripts have been used as reference standards to ensure the accuracy of HCV RNA quantification in clinical specimens and to facilitate comparison of results.

The availability of highly purified and rigorously quantified genotype-specific HCV RNA transcripts will continue to expand our understanding of the clinical and pathobiological relevance of HCV RNA levels in HCV infection. The method described in this chapter also has been used for preparation of HIV RNA transcripts *(15)* and should be generally useful for quantifying other RNA targets.

2. Reagents and Materials
2.1. Specimens for Study

HCV RNA is obtained from plasma and serum specimens from stable patients chronically infected with HCV. Chronic HCV infection is defined by elevated serum alanine aminotransferase values of at least 1.5 times the upper limit of normal for at least 6 mo and by the presence of anti-HCV antibodies as detected by enzyme-linked immunoassay (EIA-2; Ortho Diagnostic Systems, Raritan, NJ).

1. Plasma specimens are collected by standard procedures with EDTA as the anticoagulant. Serum samples are removed from the clot within 4 h of blood collection and specimens stored at –20°C or colder.
2. The HCV genotype of the clinical specimens is determined using the commercially available INNO-LiPA HCV Line Probe Assay (Innogenetics N.V., Zwijndrecht, Belgium) and verified by nucleotide sequence analysis of the 401-bp NS5 *(14)* and 5' untranslated regions *(1)*.
3. HCV RNA is extracted from 100-μL specimens as described *(5)* and stored in 20 μL of diethyl pyrocarbonate-(DEPC) treated water at –80°C for cDNA synthesis.

2.2. Reagents for RT-PCR and Cloning

1. Sense PCR primers for HCV genotypes 1–6: 5'-GACACTCCACCATGAATCA-CTCCCCTG-3' (nucleotides 21–47).
2. Antisense PCR primers for HCV genotypes 1, 5 and 6: 5'-CCCTGTTGCATAGT-TCACGCCGTC-3' (nucleotides 819–842).
3. Antisense PCR primers for HCV genotypes 2–4: 5'-CCCTGTTGCCGAAATTT-ATCCCGTC-3' (nucleotides 819–842).
4. RT reaction mixture: 10 mM Tris-HCl, pH 8.3, 50 mM KCl, 5 mM MgCl$_2$, 1 mM of each of the four dNTPs (Pharmacia, Piscataway, NJ), 3.75 μM random hexamers (Promega), 40 U RNasin (Promega, Madison, Wisconsin), and 200 U M-MLV Reverse Transcriptase (BRL, Gaithersburg, MD) in a final volume of 20 μL.
5. PCR reaction mixture (final concentration): 10 mM Tris-HCl, pH 8.3, 50 mM KCl, 2 mM MgCl$_2$, 0.4 mM of each of the four dNTPs, 0.2 μM of each primer, and 2.5 U AmpliTaq™ DNA polymerase (Perkin Elmer, Norwalk, CT).
6. Molecular-biology-grade agarose (Fisher Scientific, Fair Lawn, NJ).
7. Prep-A-Gene™ DNA Purification Kit (Bio-Rad Laboratories, Hercules, CA).
8. Transcription vector with a single 3'-thymidine overhang (TA cloning, Invitrogen, San Diego, CA).

2.3. Reagents for Restriction Digestion and Purification of DNA

1. Wizard™ Megapreps DNA Purification System (Promega, Madison, WI).
2. Appropriate restriction enzyme for the plasmid.
3. Proteinase K solution: 200 µg/mL proteinase K, 2 mM CaCl$_2$, 10 mM Tris-HCl, pH 8.0.
4. Phenol/chloroform/isoamyl alcohol (25:24:1).
5. Chloroform/isoamyl alcohol (24:1).
6. 3 M sodium acetate, pH 5.4 (DEPC-treated, RNase-free).
7. Absolute ethanol, Gold Shield; 75% ethanol for washing precipitates.
8. DEPC-treated water.
9. 1X PE buffer: 20 mM phosphate buffer, pH 6.7, 1 mM EDTA.

2.4. Reagents for RNA Transcription

1. MEGAscript™ T7 Transcription kit for large-scale synthesis of RNA (Ambion, Austin, TX). Solutions provided by manufacturer include 10X transcription buffer, ATP solution (75 mM ATP), CTP solution (75 mM CTP), GTP solution (75 mM GTP), UTP solution (75 mM UTP), T7 enzyme mix, RNase-free DNase 1, and RNase-free water.
2. α-^{32}P-GTP, 10 mCi/mL (Dupont NEN, Wilmington, DE).
3. PRIME RNase INHIBITOR, 1 U/µL (5 Prime → 3 Prime, Inc. Boulder, CO).
4. Proteinase K, 20 mg/mL.
5. DEPC-treated water.

2.5. Reagents for NAP-25 Chromatography

1. Autoclaved 1X TE: 10 mM Tris, 1 mM EDTA, pH 7.5.
2. RNA storage buffer #1: Autoclaved 1X TE, treated with 20 µg/mL proteinase K for at least 15 min at 37°C and stored at –20°C in 40 mL aliquots.
3. 4 M NaCl, DEPC-treated and autoclaved, and then treated with proteinase K as above.
4. RNA storage buffer #2: Autoclaved 1X TE, 0.1 M NaCl, treated with proteinase K as above.
5. PCR RNA storage buffer: Autoclaved 1X TE, to which is added DEPC-treated, autoclaved 0.1 M NaCl and 20 µg/mL nuclease-free carrier tRNA, and 10 U/mL prime RNase inhibitor (5 Prime → 3 Prime, Inc., Boulder, CO).

2.6. Reagents for Isotopic Tracer Analysis

1. DE81 filters (Whatman, Maidstone, UK).
2. Wash buffer for DE81 filters: 0.5 M sodium phosphate, pH 6.7, DEPC-treated and autoclaved, then treated with 20 µg/mL proteinase K as above, and stored at –20°C in 40 mL aliquots. (**Note:** All phosphate buffers used in this chapter are at pH 6.7, prepared as a 1:1 mixture of monobasic and dibasic phosphate).
3. Synthesized HCV RNA.

4. ^{32}P-labeled nucleotide solution, γ-^{32}P ATP or α-^{32}P GTP. (**Note:** This is a negative control to show that the unincorporated ^{32}P is >99% removed during the course of the washes.)

2.7. Reagents for Formaldehyde Gel Analysis

1. Running buffer (2 L): Autoclaved DEPC-treated 20 mM sodium phosphate, 1 mM EDTA.
2. Denaturation buffer: 63% formamide, 8% formaldehyde, 26 mM phosphate, 1.3 mM EDTA, and 0.17% bromophenol blue, 0.17% xylene cyanol FF, 10% Ficoll type 400 (Pharmacia, Piscataway, NJ). Formamide and formaldehyde are added just before use to a concentrate of the other ingredients, which is prepared in advance in water, filtered-sterilized, and stored in the dark at 4°C.
3. RNA Molecular Weights Marker Kit (BRL, Gaithersburg, MD).

2.8. Reagents for RNA Digestion

1. 10X One-Phor-All Plus (Pharmacia) and 1 M MgCl$_2$ stock
2. Calf intestinal alkaline phosphatase (CIP, Pharmacia)
3. Snake venom phosphodiesterase (SVPD, Pharmacia)
4. HCV RNA transcripts, approx 40–60 μg each.
5. Control samples (water blanks)
6. α-^{32}P-rGTP or a substitute rNTP.
7. Quench reagent: 20 μg/mL proteinase K in DEPC-treated water.

2.9. Reagents for Phosphate Determination

1. 4, 8, and 16X dilutions (^{32}P-traced) of the US Department of Commerce, National Institute of Standards and Technology (NIST) phosphate reference (SRM 3186) as calibrators.
2. New England Reagent Lab (NERL, East Providence, RI) phosphate standards at 10, 7, 5, 3, and 1 μg/dL.
3. Digests of ribonucleotides as controls (rA, rG, rU, rC).
4. Digests of HCV RNA transcripts.
5. Controls (water blanks).
6. Fast phosphorus reagent (Stanbio, San Antonio, TX).

2.10. Reagents for Hyperchromicity Analysis

1. 1X PE buffer: 20 mM phosphate, pH 6.7, 1 mM EDTA.
2. 1.1X PE buffer: 22 mM phosphate, 1.1 mM EDTA.

3. Methods

3.1. RT-PCR and Cloning

1. HCV cDNA is synthesized from approx 2–4 μL HCV RNA (*see* **Subheading 2.1.**) at 42°C for 15 min in 20 μL of RT reaction mixture. The reaction mixture is

Genotype-Specific HCV RNA Transcripts

inactivated by heating at 99°C for 5 min, and then cooled to 80°C before addition of components for subsequent amplification.

2. PCR is performed in a final volume of 100 µL, with 80 µL of the PCR reaction mixture added to the 20-µL reverse transcription mix. Five cycles of 1 min at 97°C, 1 min at 50°C, and 2 min at 72°C are done, followed by 30 cycles of 1 min at 94°C, 1 min at 50°C, and 3 min at 72°C. Final extension is at 72°C for 10 min.
3. Amplification products are analyzed by agarose-gel electrophoresis and gel-purified if necessary to obtain a single band of the predicted size. The expected size of the RT-PCR fragment is 822 bp, which includes the 5'-noncoding region and most of the core region.
4. The amplified 822-bp fragment is ligated into a transcription vector with a single 3'-thymidine overhang following manufacturer's instructions (TA cloning, Invitrogen, San Diego, CA).

3.2. Preparation of DNA for Transcription

1. Plasmid DNA is purified with the T7 Wizard™ Megapreps DNA Purification System following the instructions supplied with the kit and the concentration determined by A_{260} measurement.
2. Approximately 25 µg of purified plasmid DNA are digested with the appropriate restriction enzyme.
3. Complete digestion is critical and is verified by agarose-gel electrophoresis.
4. The restriction enzyme digest is terminated by addition of 0.5 vol of proteinase K solution, followed by incubation at 37°C for 30 min.
5. Three phenol chloroform extractions and two chloroform extractions are done.
6. The DNA is ethanol-precipitated with 0.3 M DEPC-treated, autoclaved sodium acetate, washed in 75% ethanol, dried under vacuum, resuspended in 30 µL DEPC-treated water, and quantified by A_{260} vs 1X PE.

3.3. Preparation of HCV RNA Transcripts and Size Markers

The amounts indicated below are for a typical transcription reaction using 5 µg of linearized DNA. The protocol may be scaled up or down as needed. A sample of DEPC-treated water (i.e., no template DNA) should be run with the transcription reactions as a control. The transcription reaction described below is adapted from the Ambion protocol.

1. A Megascript Common Reaction Mix (CRM) is prepared at room temperature by combining the following amounts of each reagent for each sample and control to be analyzed. (Note: It is important to assemble materials for the transcription reaction at room temperature since spermidine in the 10X Transcription Buffer can precipitate if the reaction is assembled on ice.)
   Common reaction mix (CRM)
   4 µL α ^{32}P-GTP @ 10 mCi/mL
   10 µL 10X transcription buffer
   10 µL ATP solution

10 µL CTP solution
   6 µL GTP solution
   10 µL UTP solution
   4 µL Prime RNase inhibitor
   10 µL T7 enzyme mix.
2. A DNA template mix is prepared by combining the following amounts of each reagent in separate tubes for each sample and control to be analyzed:
   DNA template mix
   5 µg restricted, purified DNA
   DEPC-treated water to 40 µL
   4 µL Prime RNase inhibitor.
3. Both CRM and DNA template mix are incubated separately for 15 min at 37°C.
4. The transcription reaction is prepared by adding 60 µL of the CRM to each tube containing 40 µL of the DNA template mix. The samples are mixed by pipeting and centrifuged at 12,000g in a microfuge for 10 s.
5. Incubation is for 2 h at 37°C.
6. RNA size markers are prepared according to the manufacturer's instructions.
7. Prior to digestion of the DNA template, RNase-free DNase I is incubated with Prime RNase inhibitor (in a 5:1 v:v ratio) for 15 min at room temperature.
8. Two µL Prime RNase inhibitor-treated DNase are added to each sample, which is mixed by pipeting and centrifuged briefly.
9. After 10 min at 37°C, 2 µL of 20 mg/mL proteinase K are added to each transcription reaction, and the samples are incubated for 10 min at 37°C.

3.4. DE81 Chromatography of the Transcription Reaction

DE81 chromatography is used to determine the percent incorporation of radioactive nucleotide and to estimate the specific activity of the RNA. The procedure described below is an adaptation from *Molecular Cloning, Laboratory Manual* by Sambrook et al. *(16)*.

1. The transcription reactions (100 µL) are diluted with 2.0 mL of RNA storage buffer #1 and incubated at room temperature for 5 min before quadruplicate 20-µL aliquots are spotted on DE81 filters for determination of the percent incorporation (typically >50%), the yield in picomoles, and the specific activity of the RNA in counts per minute (cpm)/pmol.
2. The filters are dried under a hot lamp for 5 min, and two filters for each sample are washed for 3 min in four successive 40-mL aliquots of autoclaved, DEPC-treated 0.5 *M* phosphate buffer, which has been pretreated with proteinase K as described above. Two filters per sample are not washed (controls).
3. The filters are then dried and counted in a scintillation counter to <2% error.
4. The vials are labeled and saved in a dark place to be counted again with later readings of the same sample after phenol extraction and ethanol precipitation.
5. The percent incorporation (P) = average washed sample count ÷ average unwashed sample count × 100. The number of pmol of RNA synthesized =

450,000 × P/G, where G is the number of guanosine residues in the RNA. An initial estimate of the specific activity of the RNA is made as total radioactivity/ pmol of RNA. Total radioactivity = (1000/20) × (100/2) × average wash count.

3.5. NAP-25 Chromatography and DE81 Analysis

The NAP-25 columns serve to exchange the buffer and purify the RNA from the unincorporated nucleotides. For optimal purity, the HCV RNA transcript is applied to two sequential NAP-25 columns. As a control, the no template DNA transcription reaction control can also be run on the NAP-25 columns.

1. Two NAP-25 columns (Pharmacia, Uppsala, Sweden) are equilibrated with 20 mL RNA storage buffer #1 at room temperature.
2. A total of 500 µL proteinase K-treated 4 M NaCl is added to the RNA samples in 2.0 mL of RNA storage buffer #1. After thorough mixing, the samples are incubated at room temperature for 5 min before being added to the column.
3. The RNA transcript mixture in 2.5 mL is loaded onto the first NAP-25 column.
4. The transcript is eluted from the gel bed using 2.5 mL RNA storage buffer #1. (**Note:** The manufacturer recommends 3.5 mL elution, but this does not purify the RNA sufficiently well.)
5. The eluate is applied to the second NAP-25 column and eluted with 2.5 mL RNA storage buffer #1.
6. Triplicate samples of column-purified transcript are diluted 1:10 into 1.1X PE for A_{260} and A_{280} measurement to estimate concentration.
7. Purity and yield are determined by DE81 chromatography as above. Typically, the yield is 100–150 µg of RNA that is about 95% free of nucleotides after the two NAP-25 columns.
8. At least 40 µg, and preferably 60 µg, of column-purified transcript are reserved for quantification *(15)*. These values assume microcuvets (200 µL) are used for absorbance, phosphate, and hyperchromicity analysis.
9. Using the DE81 estimate of the RNA concentration, the rest of the column-purified transcript is diluted to approx 1 fm/µL in PCR RNA storage buffer for PCR applications or bDNA applications or in RNA storage buffer #2 for bDNA applications only and stored at –80°C.
10. Four 20-µL spots on DE81 are made to validate this dilution and are counted along with the other DE81 filters.
11. The samples are saved for counting together with the final DE81 counts after ultrapurification.

3.6. Formaldehyde Gel Analysis

1. A gel apparatus is prepared by washing with 2% Absolve (Dupont NEN Research Products, Boston, MA), and rinsing thoroughly with DEPC-treated deionized water and drying.
2. A 1.5% agarose gel is prepared with formaldehyde essentially as described *(16)*, except that 1X PE is used as the running buffer.

3. A total of 60 µL denaturation buffer is added to 15 µL of each RNA sample. RNA size markers are treated similarly. After 15 min at 56°C, the samples are quick-cooled in ice water. Samples are run in triplicate (20 µL/lane) on the gel. A lane between distinct RNA samples is skipped to increase accuracy with radioanalytic imager quantification.
4. An overnight run is preferable; however, a 4-h run may be done if the gel is kept cold. In both cases, the gel must be run with vigorous buffer recirculation for accurate sizing.
5. The gel is dried and scanned on a radioanalytic imager.
6. The size of the transcripts can be accurately determined using a least-squares analysis of a plot of M_r in nucleotides of the size markers vs 1/mobility in cm.
7. The percent full-length transcripts is determined as the percentage of the total cpm in the peak fractions in the expected size range.

3.7. Ultrapurification of the HCV RNA: Phenol Extraction and Ethanol Precipitation

The RNA is purified further by phenol extraction and ethanol precipitation before quantification to remove proteinase K and any residual nucleotides.

1. Four phenol-chloroform and two chloroform extractions are done, and the RNA is precipitated three times from 2 M autoclaved ammonium acetate and once from 0.3 M DEPC-treated, autoclaved sodium acetate. The RNA pellet is washed in 75% ethanol after each precipitation.
2. The RNA is dried and resuspended in 100 µL of autoclaved, DEPC-treated water for analysis.

3.8. Estimation of Concentration by A_{260} and of Purity by DE81 Chromatography

1. Three 10-µL aliquots of the RNA are removed and diluted with 200 µL 1X PE for A_{260}. The concentration is estimated using 40 µg/mL/A_{260}.
2. A total of 10 µL of RNA are diluted to 100 µL with autoclaved 1X TE. Four 20-µL aliquots of the RNA are spotted onto DE81 filters, and the purity and recovery estimated. Typically, about 75% of the RNA is recovered, and it is >99% pure.
3. At this time, the DE81 samples from the transcription mix, the column-purified RNA, and the diluted column-purified RNA are recounted with the DE81 filters on the ultrapurified samples. In this way, all the numbers can be compared without correcting for radioactive decay.
4. The cpm/µL of the ultrapurified RNA is calculated.

3.9. Digestion of the RNA Prior to Phosphate Analysis and Hyperchromicity

Complete digestion of the HCV RNA transcripts is necessary for accurate quantification by phosphate analysis and hyperchromicity.

1. RNA (about 25–50 µg in 50 µL) is heated to 100°C for 10 min in DEPC-treated water, quick-cooled on ice, and centrifuged for 10 s.
2. A mixture containing 0.4 U snake venom phosphodiesterase (SVPD) and 2.8 U of calf intestinal phosphatase (CIP) and buffer is prepared in 0.8X One-Phor-All Plus (8 mM magnesium acetate, 8 mM Tris-acetate, pH 7.5, 40 mM potassium acetate) and 3 mM MgCl$_2$. Samples are incubated for 24 h at 32°C.
3. Three DEPC-treated water controls are treated in the same manner for phosphate/hyperchromicity blanks.
4. For hyperchromicity analysis, the four ultrapure (>99%) ribonucleoside triphosphates are subjected (0.5 mM) to the same digestion. A fifth GTP control containing 10 mCi of α-^{32}P-GTP in 0.5 mM unlabeled GTP is used for thin-layer chromatography (TLC) measurement of the completion of dephosphorylation of the rNTP standards.
5. 50 µL of the phosphate standards (NIST-standardized) and the NIST dilutions are incubated for 24 h in the above buffered enzyme mixture. Samples are stored at –20°C until digestion is verified by TLC.

3.10. TLC Analysis of the Extent of Digestion

1. The percent digestion of the RNA samples is determined by chromatography on PEI cellulose plates using 0.8 M ammonium formate, pH 7.0. Undigested ^{32}P-labeled RNA, α-^{32}P-labeled GTP, and ^{32}P-orthophosphate are used as controls.
2. The spots are quantified on a radioanalytic imager. Samples are not further analyzed until >97% conversion of labeled nucleic acid to ^{32}P-orthophosphate is achieved.
3. After verification of complete digestion, 187.5 µL of quench reagent (20 µg/mL proteinase K) are added to all the samples and incubation continued for 10 min at 32°C.

3.11. Phosphate Determination

1. Digests are warmed to 32°C in a dry heat block to decrease sample viscosity.
2. Three 20-µL aliquots of the quenched, digested samples of RNA, nucleotides, and phosphate standards are mixed with 200 µL of fast phosphorus reagent and incubated for 5 min at room temperature.
3. Absorbance is measured at 360 nm on a Hewlett Packard 8451A spectrophotometer. The concentration of phosphate in the unknowns is determined by least squares from the NERL phosphate standard curve.
4. The RNA concentration is determined by dividing the phosphate concentration by the length of the RNA. The length used is that of full-length RNA, not the average size on the gel, since control experiments show that the shorter RNA molecules are breakdown products, not premature termination products. A phosphate assay is considered valid if the average value of the 4, 8, and 16X dilutions of the NIST standard is within 5% of the expected values.
5. The concentration of the digested nucleotide triphosphate standards is determined by dividing by three the value determined by phosphate analysis.

3.12. Hyperchromicity Analysis

1. Three 20-μL aliquots of the quenched, digested samples of RNA and nucleotides are mixed with 200 μL of 1.1X PE, and A_{260} and A_{280} are determined.
2. The extinction coefficients of the nucleoside standards are calculated as the measured A_{260} divided by the concentration (from phosphate analysis).
3. From the DNA sequence, the extinction coefficient of the RNA is calculated as a weighted average of the measured extinction coefficients of the individual nucleosides.
4. The concentration of the RNA is determined by dividing the A_{260} by the product of the RNA extinction coefficient and the length of the RNA. Full-length RNA is used for this calculation.
5. The concentration determined by hyperchromicity must agree within 20% with both the concentration determined by phosphate and that determined by A_{260}.

3.13. Calculation of the Final Concentration of the Column-Purified RNA

1. The concentration of the ultrapurified RNA is calculated in fm/μL from the phosphate analysis.
2. The specific activity of the RNA in cpm/fm is calculated by dividing the cpm/μL from the DE81 analysis of the ultrapurified RNA by the concentration of this RNA in fm/μL determined by phosphate.
3. The RNA cpm/μL of the NAP-25 column-purified and diluted RNA is calculated from the recounted DE81 data (**Subheading 3.8., step 3**) as: Average wash CPM ÷ 20. The ratio, column-purified RNA cpm/diluted RNA, is used to calculate the true dilution factor. From the measured specific activity of the RNA, the true concentration of the diluted, column-purified RNA is determined as fm/μL. Typically, the 1 fm/μL estimate is correct within 10%.

Acknowledgments

We thank Kristina Whitfield for graphics, and Patricia Laurenson and Linda Wuestehube for editorial assistance.

References

1. Simmonds P., Holmes, E. C., Cha, T.-A., Chan, S.-W., McOmish, F., Irvine, B., et al. (1993) Classification of hepatitis C virus into six major genotypes and a series of subtypes by phylogenetic analysis of the NS-5 region. *J. Gen. Virol.* **74,** 2391–2399.
2. Preston, F. E., Jarvis, L. M., Makris, M., Philp, L., Underwood, J. C., Ludlam, C. A., et al. (1995) Heterogeneity of hepatitis C virus genotypes in hemophilia: relationship with chronic liver disease. *Blood* **85,** 1259–1262.
3. Zein, N. N., Rakela, J., Krawitt, E. L., Reddy, R., Tominaga, T., Persing, D. H., et al. (1996) Hepatitis C virus genotypes in the United States: epidemiology, pathogenicity, and response to interferon therapy. *Ann. Intern. Med.* **125,** 634–639.

4. Ohno, T. and Lau, J. Y. N. (1996) The "Gold-Standard," accuracy, and the current concepts: hepatitis C virus genotype and viremia. *Hepatology* **24,** 1312–1315.
5. Bukh, J., Purcell, R. H., and Miller, R. H. (1992) Sequence analysis of the 5' noncoding region of hepatitis C virus. *Proc. Natl. Acad. Sci. USA* **89,** 4942–4946.
6. Hawkins, A., Davidson, F., and Simmnonds, P. (1997) Comparison of plasma virus loads among individuals infected with hepatitis C virus (HCV) genotypes 1, 2, and 3 by Quantiplex HCV RNA assay versions 1 and 1, Roche Monitor assay, and an in-house limiting dilution method. *J. Clin. Microbiol.* **35,** 187–192.
7. Detmer, J., Lagier, R., Flynn, J., Zayati, C., Kolberg, J., Collins, M., et al. (1996) Accurate quantification of HCV RNA from all HCV genotypes using branched DNA (bDNA) technology. *J. Clin. Microbiol.* **34,** 901–907.
8. Lau, J. Y. N., Davis, G. L., Kniffen, J., Qian, K. P., Urdea, M. S., Chan, C. S., et al. (1993) Significance of serum hepatitis C virus RNA levels in chronic hepatitis C. *Lancet* **341,** 1501–1504.
9. Magrin, S., Craxi, A., Fabiano, C., Simonetti, R. G., Fiorentino, G., Marino, L., et al. (1994) Hepatitis C viremia in chronic liver disease: relationship to interferon-alpha or corticosteroid treatment. *Hepatology* **19,** 273–279.
10. Yuki, N., Hayashi, N., Kasahara, A., Hagiwara, H., Takehara, T., Oshita, M., et al. (1995) Pretreatment viral load and response to prolonged interferon-alpha course for chronic hepatitis C. *J. Hepatol.* **22,** 457–463.
11. Toyoda, H., Nakano, S., Kumada, T., Takeda, I., Sugiyama, K., Osada, T., et al. (1996) Comparison of serum hepatitis C virus RNA concentration by branched DNA probe assay with competitive reverse transcription polymerase chain reaction as a predictor of response to interferon-alpha therapy in chronic hepatitis C patients. *J. Med. Virol.* **48,** 354–359.
12. Stuyver, L., Rossau, R., Wyseur, A., Duhamel, M., Vanderborght, B., Van Heuverswyn, H., et al. (1993) Typing of hepatitis C virus isolates and characterization of new subtypes using a line probe assay. *J. Gen. Virol.* **74,** 1093–1102.
13. Stuyver, L., Wyseur, A., Van Arnhem, W., Hernandez, F., and Maertens, G. (1996) Second-generation line probe assay for hepatitis C virus genotyping. *J. Clin. Microbiol.* **34,** 2259–2266.
14. Enomoto, N., Takada, A., Nakao, T., and Date, T. (1990) There are two major types of hepatitis C virus in Japan. *Biochem. Biophys. Res. Commun.* **170,** 1021–1025.
15. Collins, M. L., Zayati, C., Detmer, J. J., Daly, B., Kolberg, J. A., Cha, T. A., et al. (1995) Preparation and characterization of RNA standards for use in quantitative branched DNA hybridization assays. *Anal. Biochem.* **226,** 120–129.
16. Sambrook, J., Fritsch, E. F., and Maniatis, T. (1989) *Molecular Cloning Laboratory Manual,* 2nd ed. Cold Spring Harbor Laboratory, Cold Spring Harbor, NY.

III

DETECTION OF HCV IN LIVER TISSUE

9

Detection of HCV RNA in Formalin-Fixed, Paraffin-Embedded Liver Tissue by RT-PCR

Johnson Y. N. Lau

1. Introduction

Hepatitis C virus (HCV) RNA has been detected in the sera and liver sections of patients with chronic HCV infection using RT-PCR and other sensitive molecular techniques. Since archived formalin-fixed, paraffin embedded tissues from these patients are readily available for retrospective studies, development of an assay for the detection of HCV RNA in these fixed tissues will be useful for studying HCV pathogenesis and the effect of interferon-α therapy.

Attempts to detect HCV RNA from formalin-fixed, paraffin-embedded liver tissue have produced inconsistent results. Shieh et al. were unable to detect HCV RNA from such specimens, whereas Bresters et al. and Sallie et al. reported reliable detection from formalin-fixed tissues *(1–3)*. We have established a protocol for the detection of HCV RNA in this fixed tissue *(4)*. This method was able to detect HCV RNA in liver sections from 98% of the patients referred for the consideration of antiviral therapy.

2. Materials

1. Formalin-fixed, paraffin-embedded liver biopsy specimens from patients with chronic HCV infection to be tested.
2. Formalin-fixed, paraffin-embedded liver biopsy specimens from patients with chronic HCV infection known to be positive for HCV RNA using our assay to be used as positive control.
3. Tissue blocks processed in the same way from patients with non-HCV disease to be used as a negative control.
4. Microtome with an adapter that use disposable blades.
5. Disposable microtome blades.
6. Water bath.

7. Digestion buffer: 100 µg/mL proteinase K, 0.5% SDS, 0.0005 M EDTA, 0.01 M Tris, pH 7.8 (all from Fisher Scientific, Pittsburgh, PA).
8. Other reagents were the same as given in Chapter 4.

3. Methods

1. Five 10-µm thick sections were cut from formalin-fixed, paraffin embedded liver biopsy blocks (length of tissue: 1.0–2.0 cm) and put into a 1.5-mL screw-capped Eppendorf tube. (*see* **Note 1**).
2. RNA was extracted by a modified protocol as described by Shibata et al. and by Jackson et al. *(5,6)*.
3. The tissue was dewaxed in xylene twice (5 min each, 37°C) followed by alcohol three times (5 min each, room temperature) (*see* **Note 2**).
4. The pellet was bought down by centrifugation at 14,000g for 5 min. The resulting pellet was resuspended in 200 µL digestion buffer (*see* **Note 3**).
5. The tube containing the pellet and digestion buffer was then vortexed and briefly centrifuged.
6. Two drops of mineral oil weres then added to prevent evaporation, and digestion was carried out in a water bath (42°C) for 2–5 d (*see* **Note 4**).
7. Following digestion, nucleic acid was extracted by phenol chloroform isoamyl alcohol thrice and precipitated with alcohol in the presence of 20 µg glycogen as carrier. The pellet was washed once with 70% alcohol, dried, and resuspended in 10 µL of diethylpyrocarbonate treated water, or commercially available nuclease-free sterile water.
8. Five microliters of the resulting mixture was used for RT-PCR using the protocol described in Chapter 4 (*see* **Note 5**).

4. Notes

1. A new disposable knife was used for each block to avoid the carryover of HCV between cuttings.
2. Use molecular biology-grade xylene and alcohol. Impurities in these solution may inhibit RT-PCR. Trace amount of xylene may also inhibit RT-PCR, and a thorough washing with alcohol is critical.
3. In the process of optimizing our assay, we discovered that ribonucleoside vanadyl complexes (RVCs) can inhibit PCR *(7)*. A few rounds of phenol-chloroform extraction are required to extract RVCs to avoid inhibition of PCR. We found that RVCs were not necessary and its addition only complicated the assay. Therefore, it was routinely omitted.
4. The period of protease digestion depends on the extent to which the tissue are fixed, e.g., the time of formalin fixation determines the extent of crosslinking, which affects the time required for proteolytic digestion. We routinely observe the tube twice a day and once the tissue sections are completed disintegrated, we will proceed to RNA extraction. This usually takes 2–5 d.
5. We believed that the method of tissue preparation, in particular, the time between the biopsy and the fixation, the freshness of the formalin solution, and the proce-

dure for embedding, may all affect the detection of HCV RNA in these tissue blocks. The size of the biopsy tissue may also affect the detection, i.e., there is a higher chance of detection HCV RNA for a bigger piece of liver tissue. Our Health Center routinely fixed the tissue within 2 min of the biopsy in fresh zinc formalin, and the tissue was embedded within 6–12 h. The biopsy is usually 1.5 cm in length. The detection of HCV RNA in liver sections using this protocol is 90–98% in patients referred for antiviral therapy. Other investigators were able to detect HCV RNA in 70–80% of their patients using our protocol (personal communications).

Acknowledgments

The author was supported by the American Liver Association Hans Popper Liver Scholar Award, the Glaxo Institute of Digestive Health Clinical Investigator Award, and an R01-AI41219 from the National Institute of Health.

References

1. Shieh, Y. S. C., Shim, K. S., Lampertico, P., Balart, L. A., Jeffers, L. J., Thung, S. N., et al. (1991) Detection of hepatitis C virus sequences in liver tissue by the polymerase chain reaction. *Lab. Invest.* **65(4)**, 408–411.
2. Bresters, D., Cuypers, H. T. M., Reesink, H. W., Chamuleau, R. A. F. M., Schipper, M. E. I., Boeser-Nunnink, B. D. M., et al. (1992) Detection of hepatitis C viral RNA sequences in fresh and paraffin-embedded liver biopsy specimens of non-A, non-B hepatitis patients. *J. Hepatol.* **15(3)**, 391–395.
3. Sallie, R., Rayner, A., Portmann, B., Eddleston, A. L. W. F., and Williams, R. (1992) Detection of hepatitis "C" virus in formalin-fixed liver tissue by polymerase chain reaction. *J. Med. Virol.* **37(4)**, 310–314.
4. Diamond, D., Davis, G. L., Qian, K. P., and Lau, J. Y. N. (1994) Detection of hepatitis C virus RNA in liver tissue: effect of interferon-α therapy. *J. Med. Virol.* **42**, 294–298.
5. Shibata, D., Brynes, R. K., Nathwani, S. A., Kwok S., Sninsky, J., and Arnheim, N. (1989) Human immunodeficiency viral DNA is readily found in lymph node biopsies from seropositive individuals: Analysis of fixed tissue using the polymerase chain reaction. *Am. J. Pathol.* **135(4)**, 697–702.
6. Jackson, D. P., Lewis, F. A., Taylor, G. R., Boylston, A. Q., and Quirke, P. (1990) Tissue extraction of DNA and RNA and analysis by the polymerase chain reaction. *J. Clin. Pathol.* **43(6)**, 499–504.
7. Lau, J. Y. N., Qian, K. P., Wu, P. C., and Davis, G. L. (1993): Ribonucleoside vanadyl complexes inhibits polymerase chain reaction. *Nucleic Acids Res.* **21**, 2777.

10

Quantification of HCV RNA in Liver Tissue by bDNA Assay

Peter J. Dailey, Mark L. Collins, Mickey S. Urdea, and Judith C. Wilber

1. Introduction

"Quantitative analysis of liver biopsy specimens is plagued by sampling difficulties and by failure to find a suitable standard of reference."

–*S. Sherlock and J. Dooley (1)*.

With this statement, Sherlock and Dooley have described two of the three major challenges involved in quantitatively measuring any analyte in tissue samples: the distribution of the analyte in the tissue; and the standard of reference, or denominator, with which to make comparisons between tissue samples. The third challenge for quantitative measurement of an analyte in tissue is to ensure reproducible and quantitative recovery of the analyte on extraction from tissue samples. This chapter describes a method that can be used to measure HCV RNA quantitatively in liver biopsy and tissue samples using the bDNA assay. All three of these challenges—distribution, denominator, and recovery—apply to the measurement of HCV RNA in liver biopsies.

The first challenge to be considered is the distribution of HCV RNA in the liver of HCV-infected patients. If quantification of liver biopsy HCV RNA is to be useful, a liver biopsy sample must be representative of the liver as a whole. It has been estimated that a typical needle biopsy contains 1/63,000 of the mass of a normal liver *(2)*. Two groups of investigators have evaluated this issue using the bDNA assay. Idrovo et al. *(3)* have reported good agreement in liver HCV RNA levels in right and left lobe biopsies. Terrault et al. *(4)* demonstrated relatively homogeneous distribution of HCV RNA in liver explants.

The results of these studies support the hypothesis that HCV RNA levels measured in a single liver biopsy are representative of the liver as a whole.

The second challenge to be considered is the appropriate choice of a denominator for expressing HCV RNA quantification results for liver biopsy samples. All quantitative assays express results in terms of both a numerator (e.g., HCV RNA copies) and a denominator (e.g., mL, g). The denominator serves as a reference point, providing a basis for comparison between samples. In the measurement of HCV RNA in serum and plasma, the denominator typically is volume, which is straightforward and easily measured. In tissue samples, the appropriate denominator is less clear. Investigators have used frozen wet weight, amount of extracted RNA, amount of genomic DNA, and amount of an alleged constitutive "housekeeping" mRNA. Each method has advantages and disadvantages. We have used frozen wet weight as a denominator because of its simplicity, and because it allows rational comparison between HCV RNA levels in tissue and serum.

The third challenge—reproducible and quantitative recovery of HCV RNA from liver biopsy specimens—is the focus of this chapter. In order to measure HCV RNA quantitatively in tissue samples, it is essential that HCV RNA be extracted in a reproducible and quantitative manner from the sample. Many investigators have used methods involving acid guanidinium thiocyanate-phenol-chloroform extraction, such as described by Chomczynski and Saachi *(5)*, to extract HCV RNA from liver tissue. However, because of their complexity and multiple steps, including organic extractions, these methods lead to relatively high variability in RNA recovery and reduced yields. We have chosen a simpler, more quantitative and reproducible extraction method that was first described by Cox in 1968 *(6)*. This method involves homogenization of tissue in the chaotropic salt guanidine HCl and 0.3 M sodium acetate, followed by precipitation of RNA with a half volume of ethanol (**Fig. 1**). This extraction method yields excellent differential precipitation of liver tissue RNA and elimination of genomic DNA (**Fig. 2**).

Given its inherent simplicity, this extraction procedure is particularly well suited for HCV RNA quantification using the bDNA assay, and produces consistent, quantitative recovery of HCV RNA (**Fig. 3**). It has been shown that tissue samples can contain inhibitors of RT-PCR *(7)*. In fact, the liver is the site of synthesis of porphyrins, including hemoglobin, known inhibitors of PCR *(8)*. Because of this, PCR-based methods of HCV RNA quantification require complex extraction methods to obtain extremely purified RNA and to remove inhibitors. By contrast, the bDNA assay does not involve enzymatic target amplification and, therefore, is not subject to inhibition. The bDNA assay can therefore accommodate a simpler, more quantitative and reproducible method, such as the Cox procedure, for extraction of RNA from liver samples. In addi-

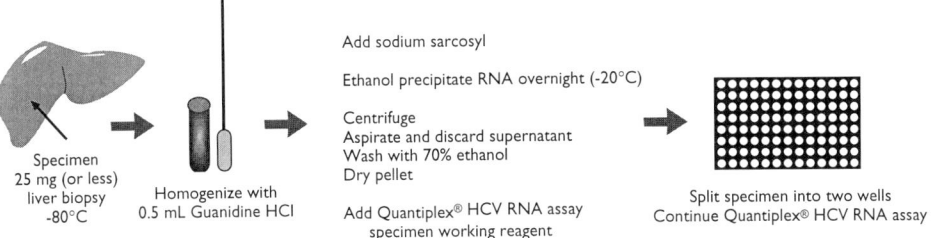

Fig. 1. Overview of the liver biopsy processing protocol for the extraction of HCV RNA from liver tissue for quantification by the bDNA assay.

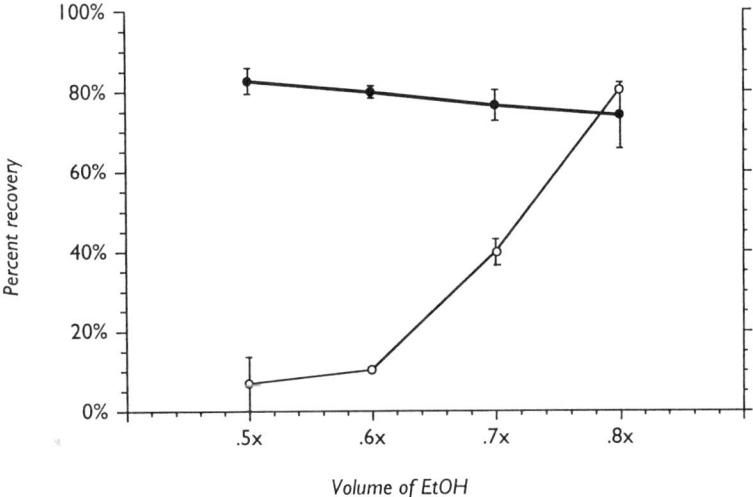

Fig. 2. Selective extraction and precipitation of HCV RNA from liver tissue homogenized in guanidine HCl. ^{32}P-labeled HCV RNA (●) was added to homogenized liver tissue, and the precipitation of RNA was evaluated after addition of different volumes of ethanol. In a separate experiment, ^{32}P-labeled calf thymus DNA (○) was added to liver tissue and its recovery evaluated. Note that 0.5× volume of ethanol yields high recovery of HCV RNA, with nearly complete removal of DNA.

tion, because extremely purified RNA is not required for the bDNA assay, the extracted RNA can remain in an environment inhibitory to RNases throughout the procedure.

The advantage of using the bDNA assay for HCV RNA quantification in liver biopsy specimens was demonstrated in a recent comparison study by Di Bisceglie et al. *(9)*. Although RT-PCR assays can have a greater analytical sensitivity than the bDNA assay, in this study the bDNA assay had a greater

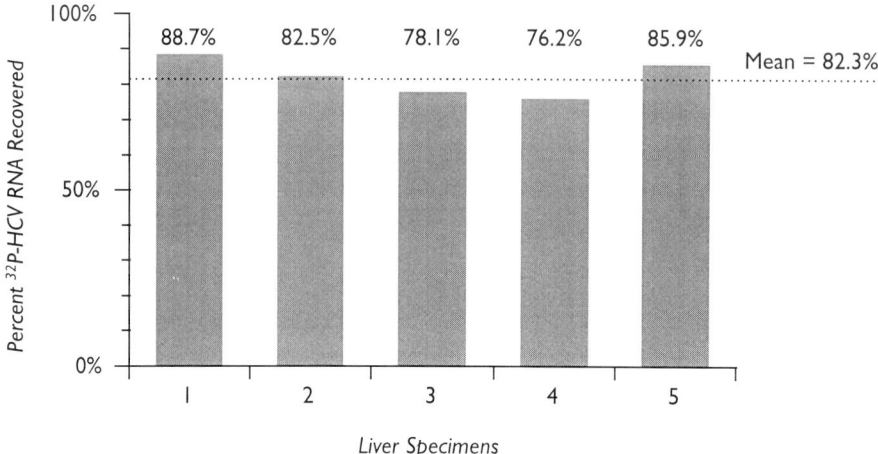

Fig. 3. Efficiency of HCV RNA recovery from liver tissue. ^{32}P-labeled HCV RNA was added to five liver tissue samples and recovered using the protocol described in this chapter.

clinical sensitivity for detection and quantification of HCV RNA in liver tissue. As shown in **Table 1**, the study by Di Bisceglie et al. compared different methods for detecting HCV markers in liver biopsy specimens from chronically infected patients. Liver specimens from 11 HCV seropositive patients were tested for HCV RNA by bDNA assay, RT-PCR, and Northern blot. In addition, HCV antigen in liver tissue was tested by immunofluorescence. Note that the bDNA assay measured HCV RNA in liver specimens from all 11 patients, whereas RT-PCR detected HCV RNA in only 8. The specimens in which RT-PCR failed to detect HCV RNA were from patients with the lowest levels of HCV replication, as measured by HCV RNA levels in liver and serum by bDNA assay. In two out of three of these patients, the presence of HCV also was confirmed by detection of HCV RNA by RT-PCR in serum and/or by HCV antigen staining in liver tissue. The most likely explanation for the higher clinical sensitivity of the bDNA assay is the presence of inhibitors in the tissue samples, which masked the low levels of HCV RNA in these specimens from detection by RTPCR.

Another advantage of the method described in this chapter is that it makes possible the simultaneous evaluation of both serum and liver HCV RNA levels *(10)*. For example, **Fig. 4A–D** shows the profile of HCV RNA levels in liver and serum of four HCV-infected chimpanzees. These animals were part of a preclinical trial of the treatment efficacy of an antisense oligonucleotide in reducing viral load. The measurement of liver HCV RNA for this preclinical trial was performed using the extraction procedure and bDNA assay described

Table 1
HCV Detection and Quantification in Clinical Specimens[a]

Patient	Liver biopsy				Serum	
	bDNA[b] MEq/g	RT-PCR	Northern	HCV Ag	bDNA[b] MEq/mL	RT-PCR
A	520	–	–	+	<2	+
B	680	–	–	–	<2	+
C	710	–	–	–	<2	–
D	1700	+++	+	+	2	+
E	8300	+++	–	+	0.6	+
F	8400	++++	+	+	2.6	+
G	13,000	+++	–	+	15	+
H	18,000	++++	+	+	31	+
I	19,000	+++++	+	nd[c]	2.4	+
J	62,000	++++	+	+	15	+
K	310,000	++++	+	+	3.2	+

[a]See Di Bisceglie et al. *(9)*.
[b]HCV RNA results expressed as megaequivalents (MEq) per mL, where 1 MEq is defined as the amount of HCV RNA in a specimen that generates a level of light emission equivalent to that generated by 10^6 copies of HCV RNA standard *(11)*.
[c]nd, not done.

here. The close correlation of the HCV RNA levels measured in cranial and caudal biopsies is shown in **Fig. 4E**.

Many questions remain regarding the pathogenesis and treatment of HCV-associated liver disease. Within the last few years, quantitative assays for the measurement of HCV RNA in serum have been developed and used in the study of HCV-related disease. It is our hope that the availability of a simple method to quantify HCV RNA levels in liver biopsies will prove useful in studies evaluating new therapeutic agents and regimens, and facilitate a better understanding of the pathogenesis of HCV liver disease.

2. Materials
2.1. Solutions

1. 3 *M* Sodium acetate: Dissolve 40.81 g of sodium acetate · $3H_2O$ in 80 mL of distilled water. Adjust the pH to 5.2 with glacial acetic acid. Adjust the volume to 100 mL with distilled water. Sterilize by autoclaving and aliquot. Store at room temperature.
2. 8 *M* Guanidine-HCl homogenization solution: Mix 280 mL of 8 *M* guanidine-HCl (Sequanal Grade, Pierce Chemical Co., Rockford IL, #24115 G) with 20 mL of 3 *M* sodium acetate (final concentration is 0.2 *M* sodium acetate).

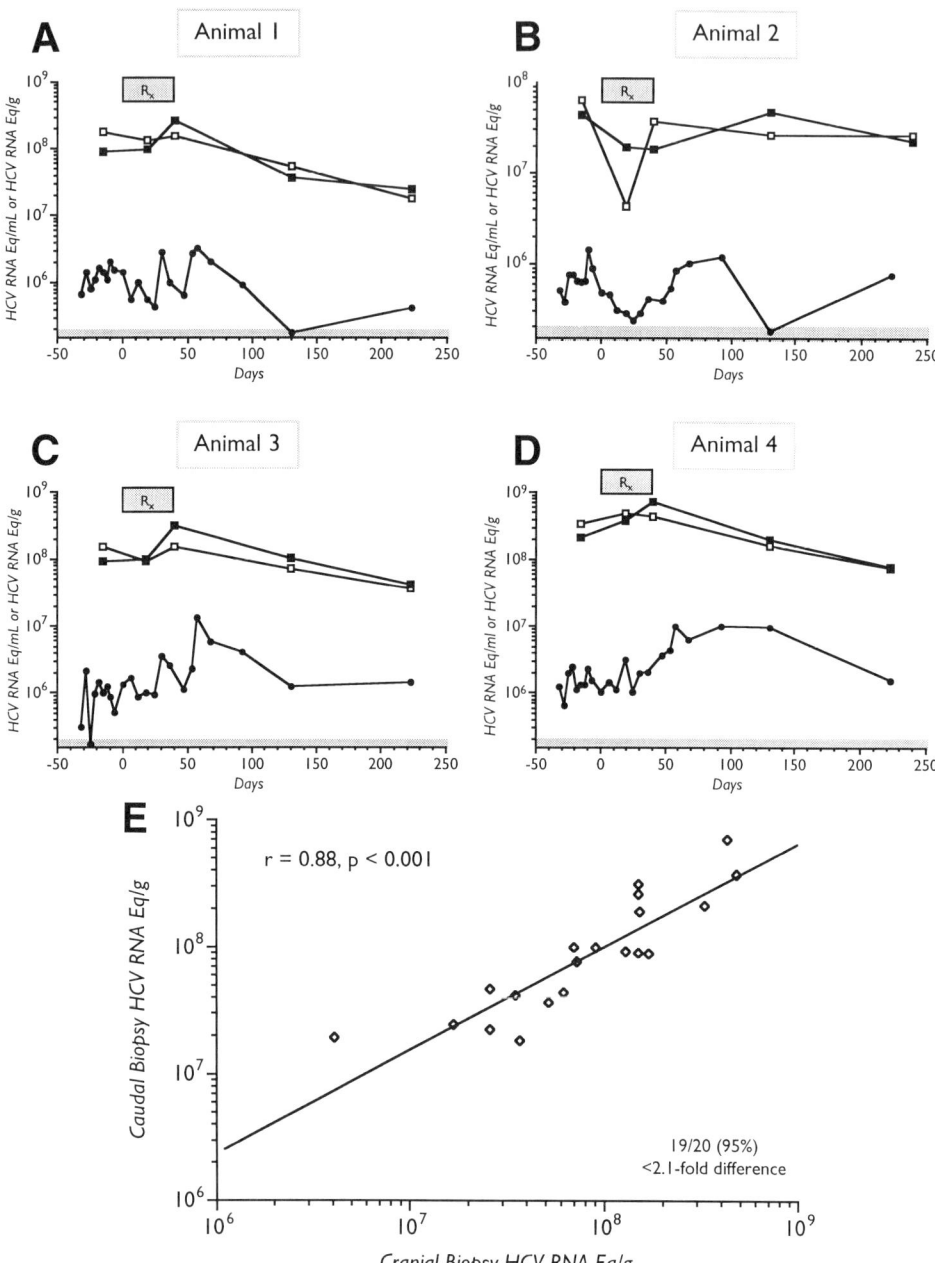

Fig. 4. Effects of an experimental antisense oligonucleotide therapy on HCV RNA levels in serum (●) and paired liver biopsies of chimpanzees. Note in **A–D** the high correlation of HCV RNA levels from liver biopsies obtained simultaneously by caudal (□) and cranial routes (■). Regression analysis of this high correlation is shown in **E**.

Mix very well (so it will not precipitate) and store at 2–8°C (refrigerator temperature).
3. 10 mg/mL Poly [A]: Add Poly [A] (polyadenylic acid [5'], potassium salt, Sigma Chemical Co., St. Louis, MO #P-9403) to distilled water, mix well, and aliquot in 1-mL vol. Store at −18 to −22°C.
4. 10% Sarcosyl: Add *N*-Lauroyl-sarcosine (sodium salt [Sarcosyl], Sigma Chemical Co., #L-5125) to distilled water. Store at room temperature.
5. 100% Ethanol, Gold Shield. Store at −18 to −22°C.
6. 70% Ethanol: Add distilled water to 100% Gold Shield ethanol. Store at −18 to −22°C.

2.2. Equipment

1. Disposable pellet pestle mixer and matched (important) polypropylene 1.5-mL microtubes (manufactured by Kontes, Inc., Owens, IL, #K749520-0000; also available through Fisher Scientific and VWR). These pestles are appropriate for most needle biopsy specimens. Both the pellet pestle mixer and microtubes may be autoclaved. **Critical parameter: Abrasion of the plastic pestle before use with coarse sandpaper assists in rapid homogenization of samples.**
2. Cordless motor for reusable and disposable pellet pestle mixers (Kontes, Inc.; distributed by Fisher Scientific, #K749540-0000).
3. Sterile disposable tissue grinder (Sage Products Inc., Crystal Lake, IL, #3505-small, #3500-large or through Baxter S/P). These are useful for larger specimens (i.e., >25 mg).
4. 2-mL microcentrifuge tubes: **Critical parameter: For ethanol precipitation of tissue homogenized in Guanidine-HCl homogenization solution, it is absolutely necessary to use a larger volume microcentrifuge tube (2.0 mL) with a screw cap and an O-ring (e.g., Sarstedt #72.693, Newton, NC).**
5. A microcentrifuge, which is able to accommodate the large 2.0-mL microcentrifuge tubes (*See* **item 4**).
6. Water bath or heat block set at 53 ± 1°C.
7. Large orifice (micropipet) tips, 1–200 µL (USA/Scientific Plastics, Ocala, FL, #1011-8416); 100–1000 mL (USA/Scientific Plastics, Ocala, FL, #1011-9510).
8. Rotary evaporation device (e.g., Speed-Vac).

2.3. Tissues for Study

Liver biopsy specimens weighing 5 mg or greater are recommended, although HCV RNA has been successfully detected and quantified from smaller specimens. Specimens should be frozen at −60°C or colder as soon as possible after collection and stored frozen until processing. The effects of delay in freezing on HCV RNA recovery have not been completely studied. **Critical parameters: It is important to freeze the biopsy specimen without placing it in any type of preservative or diluent, such as formalin, saline, or isopentane. Also, all**

frozen samples should be diligently maintained at –60°C or lower and not subjected to freeze-thaw conditions. The weight of the specimen should be determined as follows:

1. Select the appropriate tissue grinder. For small specimens (<25 mg), including most needle biopsies, use the pellet pestle mixers and matched microcentrifuge tubes. For larger specimens, use the sterile disposable tissue grinders from Sage Products, Inc. Specimens up to 1 g can be homogenized in the small grinder, and larger specimens in the large grinder.
2. Determine the weight of the tube for grinding using a pan balance accurate to 1 mg (for example, Mettler PM460 Delta Range, Mettler Instruments Corp., Hightstown, NJ).
3. Place the frozen tissue (–60°C or colder) in the tube, and keep on dry ice (at –60°C or colder) before and after weighing. **Critical parameter: Do not allow sample to thaw.**
4. Determine the combined weight of tube and tissue, and calculate the weight of tissue.

3. Methods

3.1. Homogenization of Liver Tissue and Isolation of RNA

Precaution: Homogenization of liver tissue should be performed in a Certified Biological Safety Cabinet, since it is likely to produce aerosols.

1. **Quickly**, add cold guanidine-HCl homogenization solution to the frozen tissue, and homogenize as rapidly as possible with the pellet pestle mixer using the cordless motor (for needle biopsies) or the larger homogenizers from Sage Products (for larger samples, i.e., >25 mg). This step may take several minutes. Keep the homogenized specimen on wet ice. Add the minimum amount of guanidine-HCl homogenization solution that is sufficient to homogenize the specimen. For most needle biopsy specimens (<25 mg), 0.250 mL is sufficient for initial homogenization. After thorough and complete homogenization in this small volume, add an additional 0.250 mL, making a total final volume of 0.5 mL/specimen; homogenize again with the pellet pestle mixer. For larger liver tissue specimens (>25 mg), add proportionally more guanidine-HCl homogenization solution so that the final volume is 0.5 mL/25 mg of tissue. Remove 0.5 mL for further processing and analysis. **Critical parameters: Be sure to homogenize samples thoroughly. Keep homogenized samples on wet ice or in the refrigerator (2–8°C).**
2. To each tube containing 0.5 mL of guanidine-HCl homogenization solution, add 0.025 mL of 10% Sarkosyl (final concentration: 0.5%), vortex gently, and hold for 5 min at 2–8°C.
3. Centrifuge the specimen to sediment particulates. Spin for 1 min at 2–8°C in a microcentrifuge at approx 12,000g.

4. Remove 0.5 mL of the supernatant of the homogenized liver tissue specimen and place in the large-volume (2.0-mL) tubes from Sarstedt. Use of "large orifice" pipet tips (200–1000 mL size) may be helpful in transferring the sample. **Critical parameter: It is essential to use these large-volume (2.0-mL) tubes so that there is adequate space for mixing.**
5. To each tube add 0.010 mL of 10 mg/mL poly [A]. Vortex.
6. Add 0.25 mL of 100% EtOH to each tube, and mix very thoroughly. **Critical parameter: Look carefully at each tube to ensure thorough mixing of EtOH and guanidine-HCl homogenization solutions. These solutions have very different densities and must be mixed well. It is helpful to invert the tube several times in addition to vortexing.**
7. Hold at –18 to –22°C overnight by placing in a freezer (approx 12–18 h). This step **cannot** be performed at lower temperatures.
8. On the following day, centrifuge tubes in a microcentrifuge (10,000–12,000g) for 20 min at 2–8°C, and then carefully aspirate and discard the supernatant without disturbing the pellet (important). Do not aspirate near or disturb the RNA pellet at the bottom of the tube. **Critical parameter: Use large orifice pipet tips (1–200 mL size) on the aspiration device when removing the supernatant. The supernatant contains genomic DNA and it is important to aspirate it carefully and completely.**
9. Add 0.5 mL of cold (2–8°C) 70% EtOH to each tube. Vortex to mix, and centrifuge again for 20 min at 2–8°C. Remember to keep on ice during manipulations.
10. Aspirate the supernatant, and dry down the pellet with a Speed-Vac rotary vacuum device or equivalent. Use the rotary evaporator at room temperature until visible liquid is removed; do not evaporate to complete dryness.

3.2. Quantiplex® HCV-RNA Assay

The procedure outlined in the product insert should be followed for quantification of HCV RNA using the Quantiplex HCV-RNA assay. Considerations specific to quantification of HCV RNA from liver biopsy specimens are detailed in the following steps:

1. Add 0.330 mL of HCV Specimen Working Reagent (from the Quantiplex HCV-RNA Assay) to each tube followed by 0.110 mL of distilled water. Vortex vigorously for 10 s and incubate in a 53°C heat block or water bath for a total of 20 min. Vortex after 10 min of incubation and at the end of 20 min of incubation. The RNA pellet should be solubilized by this treatment. **Critical parameter: Always add the HCV Specimen Working Reagent before the distilled water.**
2. Quickly spin the tube to bring all fluid to the bottom of the microcentrifuge tube and carefully pipet 0.200 mL/well into duplicate Quantiplex® HCV-RNA wells in a standard HCV RNA assay run, including standards, controls, and serum specimens (*see* Chapter 6).
3. Calculate the results in HCV Eq/g based on the weight of tissue processed. The Chiron luminometer automatically calculates the HCV Eq/mL from the relative

light units produced from the average of duplicate testing of 50 μL of serum. When a tissue specimen is used, the result must be adjusted. First, the number calculated by the Chiron luminometer must be adjusted to give the HCV Eq per specimen as opposed to mL (divide by 20), and then normalized to Eq/g based on milligram of tissue used (multiply by 1000 mg/# mg of tissue specimen processed). Finally, the result should be multiplied by two to account for the fact that the specimen was split between two wells. The "result" reported by the Chiron luminometer in "Eq/mL" then is multiplied by 100 and divided by the number of milligrams of the liver biopsy specimen:

$$\frac{\text{Liver tissue result (Eq/mL)} \times 100}{\text{\# mg specimen}} = \text{Eq/g} \qquad (1)$$

4. Results below the assay quantification limit should be reported as "not quantified."
5. To control for the processing of liver biopsy samples, it is recommended that you run HCV-positive and HCV-negative liver tissue samples.

4. Notes

1. This procedure is a modification of the procedure described by Cox *(6)* and involves homogenization of the liver tissue specimen in a chaotropic salt, guanidine hydrochloride, followed by differential precipitation of RNA (as opposed to DNA) with ethanol. The emphasis is on recovery of RNA, not purity.
2. Liver tissue samples should be stored frozen at –60°C or lower. Samples should not be allowed to thaw or partially thaw before homogenization.
3. Before testing important samples with this method, it is recommended that you practice with liver tissue specimens (if available), especially the homogenization and precipitation steps.
4. For maximum recovery of HCV RNA, homogenize **frozen** tissue as rapidly and completely as possible into the guanidine-HCl homogenization solution.
5. The most common problem involves not carefully aspirating all the genomic DNA from the homogenized specimen after the first centrifugation following ethanol precipitation. If all the genomic DNA is not removed at this step, it can cause a viscous white precipitate when the HCV specimen working reagent is added in the last step.
6. Do not hold frozen samples on wet ice while waiting to homogenize them. Keep samples frozen on dry ice. If allowed to thaw before homogenization, degradation of RNA is probable.
7. Remember that the guanidine-HCl homogenization solution also contains sodium acetate. Without the sodium acetate, RNA will not be precipitated.
8. When precipitating RNA from homogenized samples with a half-volume of ethanol, be sure to mix well. Ethanol and the guanidine-HCl homogenization solutions have very different densities and need to be vortexed thoroughly. It helps to invert the tube several times in addition to vortexing.
9. **Homogenize thoroughly and rapidly!**

References

1. Sherlock, S. and Dooley, J. (1993) *Diseases of the Liver and Biliary System,* 9th ed., Blackwell Scientific Publications, London.
2. Feldmann, G. (1995) Critical analysis of the methods used to morphologically quantify hepatic fibrosis. *J. Hepatol.* **22 (Suppl. 2),** 49–54.
3. Idrovo, V., Dailey, P. J., Jeffers, L. J., Coelho-Little, E., Bartholomew, M., and Alvarez, L. (1996) Hepatitis C virus RNA quantification in right and left lobes of the liver in patients with chronic hepatitis C. *J. Viral Hepatitis* **3,** 239–246.
4. Terrault, N. A., Dailey, P. J., Ferrell, L., Collins, M. L., Wilber, J. C., Urdea, M. S., et al. (1997) Hepatitis C virus: quantitation and distribution in liver. *J. Med. Virol.* **51,** 217–224.
5. Chomcyznski, P. A. and Sacchi, N. (1987) Single-step method of RNA isolation by acid guanidinium thiocyanate-phenol-chloroform extraction. *Anal. Biochem.* **162,** 156–159.
6. Cox, R. A. (1968) The use of guanidinium chloride in the isolation of nucleic acids. *Methods Enzymol.* **12B,** 120–129.
7. Mathy, N. L., Lee, R. P., and Walker, J. (1996) Removal of RT-PCR inhibitors from RNA extracts of tissues. *BioTechniques* **21,** 770–774.
8. Higuchi, R. (1989) Simple and rapid preparation of samples for PCR, in *PCR Technology: Principles and Applications for DNA Amplification* (Erlich, H. A., ed.), Stockton, New York, pp. 31–38.
9. Di Bisceglie, A. M., Chung, Y.-W., Dailey, P. J., Shakil, A. O., Krawczynski, K., and Hoofnagle, J. H. (1994) Hepatitis C viral (HCV) markers in serum and liver of chronically infected patients. *Hepatology* **20,** 236A.
10. Coelho-Little, E., Jeffers, L. J., Bartholomew, M., Reddy, K. R., Schiff, E. R., and Dailey, P. J. (1995) Correlation of HCV-RNA levels in serum and liver of patients with chronic hepatitis C. *J. Hepatol.* **22,** 508.
11. Collins, M. L., Zayati, C., Detmer, J. J., Daly, B., Kolberg, J. A., Cha, T. A., et al. (1995) Preparation and characterization of RNA standards for use in quantitative branched DNA hybridization assays. *Anal. Biochem.* **226,** 120–129.

IV

HCV Genotypes

11

Hepatitis C Virus

Types, Subtypes, and Beyond

Donald B. Smith and Peter Simmonds

1. Introduction

Non-A, non-B hepatitis was recognized as a frequent consequence of blood transfusion for many years before the agent responsible, hepatitis C virus (HCV), was first cloned and sequenced in 1989. Very quickly it became apparent that viruses from different parts of the world were distinct, and after a frenzy of sequence analysis, a general picture has now emerged *(1)*. Virus sequences can be divided into major types (identified by numbers) with nucleotide identities of <70% over complete genome sequences. Each type can be subdivided into subtypes (identified by letters) with identities of between 70 and 80%. Complete genome sequences are now available for all six HCV types and for several different subtypes of type 1 (a, b, and c), 2 (a, b, and c) and 3 (a, b, and "10a"). Very similar sequence relationships are obtained by analysis of subgenomic fragments, such as individual genes encoding structural or nonstructural proteins or a region as short as 222 nt of NS5B. On the basis of such comparisons, it is possible to differentiate consistently among six major genotypes (**Fig. 1**), and to an increasing number of subtypes (**Fig. 2**), now exceeding 10 for types 1, 2, 3, 4, and 6, but with only two known for type 5. Some isolates from southeast Asia have a controversial placement in this system, since they are less divergent from each other than virus types, but more divergent than subtypes. However, phylogenetic and serological evidence suggests that they represent divergent subtypes of types 3 and 6 *(2,3)*.

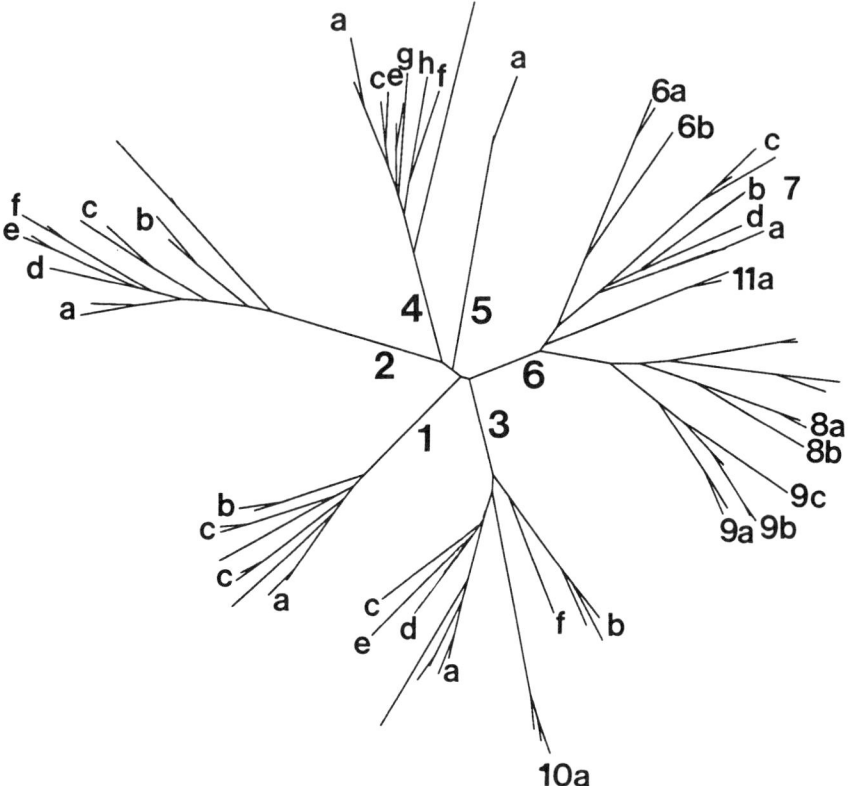

Fig. 1. Phylogenetic tree of HCV NS5B sequences. Nucleotide sequences for positions 7975–8196 (numbered from the polyprotein AUG initiation codon) of NS5B were analyzed using the program Phylip as described previously *(76)*. Major branches are labeled with the type number, and minor branches with letters indicating the subtype. The variant "10a" can be considered as a subtype of type 3, and the variants "7a", "7b", "8a," and so forth, as subtypes of type 6 *(2,3)*.

2. Origin of Virus Genotypes

Reconstructing the evolutionary history of HCV is necessarily an indirect process, since no samples are available that are older than about 25 years. Nevertheless, several lines of evidence suggest that HCV types and subtypes are at least several hundred years old, and possibly much older. In parts of the world such as central and eastern Africa, the Indian subcontinent and southeast Asia only one HCV type is found, but this is represented by numerous subtypes, a pattern consistent with long-standing endemic infection. In other parts of the world, one or more virus types are present, but each is only represented

Hepatitis C Virus Types

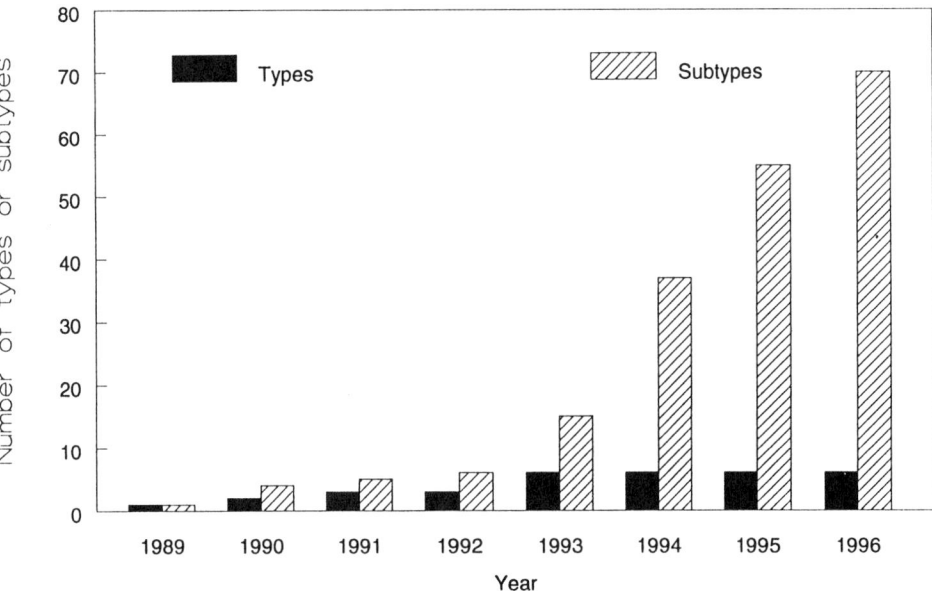

Fig. 2. The discovery of HCV types and subtypes. The total number of HCV types (solid line) and subtypes (broken line) is indicated by year.

by a few subtypes, a pattern suggestive of recent transmission. The rate of evolution of HCV has been estimated from the rate of divergence observed among a cohort of individuals infected 17 yr previously from a common source of anti-D immunoglobulin (4). Using this rate (1.1 or 1.7×10^{-3}/site/yr for synonymous sites in NS5B and E1 respectively), the divergence of different isolates of subtype 1b is equivalent to about 70 yr of divergence, whereas the common ancestor of subtypes 1a and 1b can be dated to more than 300 yr ago. The time of origin of virus types is more difficult to estimate because of increasing saturation of substitutions, but is likely to be more than 500–2000 yr ago. In this context, it is of interest that variants of GBV-A that differ from each other as much as HCV types do from each other are confined to different monkey species (5,5a), suggesting that long periods of isolation are compatible with limited sequence divergence.

3. Clinical Differences Between Virus Genotypes

Characterization of HCV genotypes would be a trivial exercise were there not evidence for significant biological and clinical differences between them. Virus genotype has been found to be a predictor of response to interferon treatment in 37 out of 40 published studies. A poor response is observed in individuals infected with genotypes 1 or 4, and the poor response of type 1 has been associated with slower kinetics of reduction in virus RNA levels in comparison to type 2 infection *(6)*, but no satisfactory explanation for this difference has yet been discovered. Initial reports suggested that levels of virus RNA were higher in individuals infected with type 1 virus and that virus levels were independently correlated with a lack of response to interferon. However, recent work suggests that the differences observed in virus RNA levels between genotypes were owing to the reduced efficiency of detection of types 2 and 3 because of polymorphisms in the regions targeted by the branched DNA 1.0 assay *(7)* or by the primers used in competitive PCR assays *(8,9)*. No significant difference in levels of virus RNA is observed between different genotypes once this is corrected for, or if assays are used that quantify all genotypes with the same efficiency *(9–11)*. Therefore, the differing sensitivities of HCV types to interferon treatment appear to be unrelated to the level of virus replication and may instead reflect intrinsic differences between virus types.

Evidence for differences in the severity of disease produced by different virus genotypes is less clear cut. Some studies have found that serum levels of alanine aminotransferase are higher in individuals infected with type 1 or type 3, or have observed more severe liver histology associated with infection by type 1 virus. However, an equal number of studies have found no significant difference in ALT levels or liver histology between genotypes. Similarly, there is evidence that type 1b virus can superinfect individuals already infected with other genotypes *(12)*, but there is contrary evidence from hemophiliacs exposed to multiple infections, suggesting that all genotypes have similar infectivity *(13)*. A more consistent finding is that liver transplantation into recipients infected with genotype 1a or 1b results in more severe graft disease than in recipients infected with other genotypes *(14,15)*. Infection with type 1b has also been associated with an increased incidence of hepatocellular carcinoma in some *(16–19)*, but not all studies *(20)*. Some of these discrepancies may be owing to biases in the populations infected by different genotypes. Among European and North American patients, individuals infected with type 3a are on average younger, have a shorter duration of infection, and are more likely to have iv drug use as a risk factor than those infected with other genotypes *(11,21–25)*. Multivariate analysis of large cohorts of patients is therefore required to separate out the different effects of patient and virological variables on clinical and therapeutic outcomes.

To date there is no convincing evidence for clinical or virological differences between virus subtypes. Although there are several reports of a reduced responsiveness to interferon for subtype 1b in comparison to subtypes 2a and 2b, these studies were conducted on populations where subtype 1a is rare, and more recent work suggests that types 1a and 1b have similar resistance to treatment *(26)*. There is one report that subtype 2c is associated with a poor response to interferon in contrast to the relatively high response rate observed for types 2a and 2b *(27)*, but larger studies are required to confirm this possibility.

4. Serological Differences

Differences between HCV genotypes that are less equivocal are in the serological responses that they induce following infection. All current commercial serological screening assays for HCV infection utilize proteins or peptide sequences derived from three or four different regions of type 1 viruses. Although there is broad crossreactivity between different genotypes for the c22 (core) and c33 (NS3) antigens, serological responses to c100 (and to 5-1-1, a subregion of c100) are weaker in individuals infected with viruses other than type 1 *(21,28–31)*. As a result, samples from individuals infected with genotypes other than type 1 have lower average scores and are more likely to be scored as indeterminate on confirmatory immunoblot tests *(32)*. Decreased serological reactivity to the individual type 1 derived antigens can also be expected to lower the sensitivity of initial screening by ELISA for infection by genotypes other than type 1. For types 2 and 3, serological responses are 75% weaker than for type 1 *(33)*, but additional testing against homologous antigens is necessary in order to exclude the possibility that this reflects reduced immunogenicity of these virus types.

Serological differences between HCV types can be expected to influence the efficacy of an eventual vaccine against HCV infection, since a similar degree of variation produces the different serotypes of poliovirus and dengue. There is evidence that infection with one virus genotype does not protect against reinfection with a different genotype *(34,35)*, whereas experimental challenge of vaccinated chimpanzees was less effective in animals challenged with a heterologous variant of the same subtype *(35a)*. Protection can be expected to be even less efficacious for different subtypes and types, although cross-reactions have been demonstrated in vitro between antibodies elicited by different genotypes that prevent virus binding to cells *(36)*.

5. Typing Assays

Virus genotype can be determined from a clinical sample in a variety of ways. The most direct and accurate method is to sequence the virus genome in a region that is sufficiently divergent to distinguish between virus types and subtypes. Suitable regions for which large reference databases are available include core, E1, NS4B, and NS5B. More rapid, but indirect methods include sequencing with a single dideoxynucleotide *(37)*, or the analysis of fragments amplified by PCR for the presence of type-specific sequence polymorphisms either by hybridization or by RFLP analysis. Most attention has focused on the 5'-noncoding region, since it is highly conserved, but contains type-specific polymorphisms *(8)* that can be detected by hybridization to oligonucleotide probes *(38–40)* or by RFLP analysis of PCR fragments *(28,41,42)*. However, neither of these 5'-NCR based assays are completely accurate in comparison to typing by sequence analysis *(8,40,43)*, and this problem has been compounded by the discovery of subtypes of type 6 that have 5'-NCR sequences similar or identical to those of type 1 viruses *(44)*. In order to recognize these variants, modified assays have been developed that detect type-specific polymorphisms in the core gene *(45,46)*, but the simplicity of the original formats has been lost. A different kind of typing assay involves PCR amplification with type-specific primers specific for the core *(47–49)* or NS5 *(50)* genes. These assays are currently limited to three of the six known HCV types, and the accuracy of the core-based system is relatively low, especially in overestimating the number of mixed infections *(43)*.

A problem shared by all indirect assays is that of distinguishing between the burgeoning number of different subtypes of the same virus type (**Fig. 1**). Although 5'-NCR polymorphisms are correlated with some virus subtypes, the correlations are neither complete nor exclusive *(8)*, whereas subtypes other than 1a, 1b, 2a, 2b, 2c, and 3a are not likely to be amplified by the subtype-specific amplification primers *(51,52)*.

An alternative approach to typing exploits the existence of type-specific differences in antigenicity for core (*[53]* types 1 and 2) or NS4 (*[54]* types 1, 2, and 3), (*[55]* types 1,2), (*[56]* types 1, 2, 3, 4, 5, and 6), or both regions (*[57]* types 1, 2, and 3). Serological assays have the advantage of being relatively simple and inexpensive, but a proportion of individuals do not have type-specific antibodies or are not immunoreactive with NS4, particularly if they are immunocompromised or recently infected, and in these cases virus genotype cannot be deduced. In addition, serological reactivities observed may derive from previous rather than the current infection. Antigenic differences between virus subtypes are less extreme, so serological discrimination between different subtypes is not yet possible.

6. Variation Within Virus Subtypes

Sequences of the same virus subtype from different individuals differ by up to 10% over the complete genome, but it remains to be proven that this variation is of any consequence. Comparison of NS5A sequences before interferon treatment has yielded a correlation between divergence from the consensus amino acid sequence and increasing responsiveness *(58)*, but this has not been confirmed in another study of the same genotype (1b) *(58a)*. Virus antigenic variation does not seem to be responsible for the minority of instances where HCV-infected individuals remain seronegative, and instead this may reflect a lack of recognition by the immune system *(59)*.

7. Variation Within the Infected Host

Comparison of virus sequences from an infected host at different time-points reveals that most substitutions are synonymous (do not affect the amino acid sequence) with the ratio of nonsynonymous to synonymous substitutions in longitudinal studies ranging between 0.18 and 0.5. The most variable region is at the extreme NH_2 terminus of the E2 glycoprotein *(60,61)*, and this hypervariable region (HVR) is also unusual in that for comparisons between different subtype 1b variants, the ratio of nonsynonymous to synonymous distances is almost 1, whereas in other regions of the genome, the ratio is <0.2 *(61a)*. This has been interpreted as the consequence of selection by neutralising antibodies for amino acid replacement, and this is supported by the reduced HVR variability observed in a patient with agammaglobulinemia *(62)*. However, homogeneity of the HVR has also been observed in an experimentally infected chimpanzee *(63)* and in some patients with normal immune function *(64)*, whereas increased variability has been reported in patients coinfected with HIV *(65)*. Variation of the HVR might therefore instead represent a relative lack of selection against amino acid replacement. Evidence for tissue-specific populations of HCV is confusing; one study found different HVR variants in serum and in cancerous and noncancerous portions of the liver *(66)*, but another study found no evidence for different populations between serum and liver *(67)*.

There are several reports that heterogeneity of the virus population within an infected individual in the HVR is correlated with a lack of responsiveness to interferon treatment *(64,68–72)*. However, this correlation has not always been observed *(73)*, and in some studies, HVR heterogeneity was correlated with virus genotype and virus RNA level *(72)*, or with the extent of liver disease or ALT flare-ups *(69,74,75)*. These correlations might explain the association between HVR heterogeneity and a lack of response to interferon, since virus type, viremia, and the extent of liver disease are independent predictors of response in many studies.

Replication of HCV, like most other RNA viruses, is dependent on a virus-encoded RNA-dependent RNA polymerase that is thought to lack a proofreading activity, and so to have a high inherent rate of nucleotide misincorporation. A consequence of this is that virus populations would be expected to contain numerous mutants that deviate from the consensus sequence by a small number of substitutions. However, the significance of such "quasispecies" in the natural history of HCV has yet to be demonstrated.

8. Conclusions

The extent and significance of variation of HCV are beginning to be clarified. Virus variants can be classified into types and subtypes, and several varieties of typing assays are now available that can reliably distinguish between virus types, and to a lesser extent, between virus subtypes. There is strong evidence for serological differences between virus genotypes, and these have implications for the screening of blood donors and patients, and may affect the efficacy of vaccines against HCV infection. There is no consistent difference in the level of viremia in individuals infected by different virus genotypes once differences in the detection efficiency of different assays have been corrected for. One important difference between virus types is in their responsiveness to interferon treatment, but the basis for this is not yet clear. As yet there is no good evidence for significant virological or clinical differences between virus subtypes. Within the infected host, most variation occurs in a hypervariable region at the NH_2-terminus of the E2 protein, and the extent of heterogeneity in this region may correlate with responsiveness to interferon treatment, although this may be an indirect association. Variation occurring elsewhere in the virus genome is of unknown significance.

References

1. Simmonds, P., Alberti, A., Alter, H. J., Bonino, F., Bradley, D. W., Brechot, C., et al. (1994) A proposed system for the nomenclature of hepatitis C viral genotypes. *Hepatology* **19,** 1321–1324.
2. Mizokami, M., Gojobori, T., Ohba, K. I., Ikeo, K., Ge, X. M., Ohno, T., et al. (1996) Hepatitis C virus types 7, 8 and 9 should be classified as type 6 subtypes. *J. Hepatol.* **24,** 622–624.
3. Simmonds, P., Mellor, J., Holmes, E. C., Tamprasert, S., Sakuldamrongpanich, T., Nuchaprayoon, C., et al. (1996) Evolutionary analysis of variants of hepatitis C virus found in South East Asia: Comparison with classifications based upon sequence similarity. *J. Gen. Virol.* **77,** 3013–3024.
4. Smith, D. B., Pathirana, S., Davidson, F., Lawlor, E., Power, J., Yap, P. L., et al. (1997) The origin of hepatitis C virus genotypes. *J. Gen. Virol.* **78,** 321–328.
5. Leary, T. P., Desai, S. M., Yamaguchi, J., Chalmers, M. L., Schlauder, G. G., Dawson, G. J., et al. (1996) Species-specific variants of GB virus A in captive monkeys. *J. Virol.* **70,** 9028–9030.
5a. Butch, J. and Apgar, C. L. (1997) Five new or recently discovered (GBV-A) virus species are indigenous to New World monkeys and may constitute a separate genus of the *Flaviviridae*. *Virology* **229,** 429–436.
6. Kohara, M., Tanaka, T., Tsukiyamakohara, K., Tanaka, S., Mizokami, M., Lau, J. Y. N., et al. (1995) Hepatitis C virus genotypes 1 and 2 respond to interferon-α with different virologic kinetics. *J. Infect. Dis.* **172,** 934–938.
7. Detmer, J., Lagier, R., Flynn, J., Zayati, C., Kolberg, J., Collins, M., et al. (1996) Accurate quantification of hepatitis C virus (HCV) RNA from all HCV genotypes by using branched-DNA technology. *J. Clin. Microbiol.* **34,** 901–907.
8. Smith, D. B., Mellor, J., Jarvis, L. M., Davidson, F., Kolberg, J., Urdea, M., et al. (1995) Variation of the hepatitis C virus 5' non-coding region: implications for secondary structure, virus detection and typing. *J. Gen. Virol.* **76,** 1749–1761.

9. Hawkins, A., Davidson, F., and Simmonds, P. (1997) Comparison of plasma virus load amongst individuals infected with hepatitis C virus genotypes 1, 2 and 3 using Quantiplex HCV RNA Assay version 1 and 2, Roche Monitor and an in-house limiting dilution method. *J. Clin. Microbiol.* **35,** 187–192.
10. Smith, D. B., Davidson, F., Yap, P. L., Brown, H., Kolberg, J., Detmer, J., et al. (1996) Levels of hepatitis C virus in blood donors infected with different viral genotypes. *J. Infect. Dis.* **173,** 727–730.
11. Lau, J. Y. N., Davis, G. L., Prescott, L. E., Maertens, G., Lindsay, K. L., Qian, K. P., et al. (1996) Distribution of hepatitis C virus genotypes determined by line probe assay in patients with chronic hepatitis C seen at tertiary referral centers in the United States. *Ann. Intern. Med.* **124,** 868.
12. Laskus, T., Wang, L. F., Rakela, J., Vargas, H., Pinna, A. D., Tsamandas, A. C., et al. (1996) Dynamic behavior of hepatitis C virus in chronically infected patients receiving liver graft from infected donors. *Virology* **220,** 171–176.
13. Jarvis, L. M., Ludlam, C. A., Ellender, J. A., Nemes, L., Field, S. P., Song, E., et al. (1996) Investigation of the relative infectivity and pathogenicity of different hepatitis C virus genotypes in hemophiliacs. *Blood* **87,** 3007–3011.
14. Cane, E. J., Portmann, B. C., Naoumov, N. V., Smith, H. M., Underhill, J. A., Donaldson, P. T., et al. (1996) Long-term outcome of hepatitis C infection after liver transplantation. *N. Engl. J. Med.* **334,** 815–820.
15. Feray, C., Gigou, M., Samuel, D., Paradis, V., Mishiro, S., et al. (1995) Influence of the genotypes of hepatitis C virus on the severity of recurrent liver disease after liver transplantation. *Gastroenterology* **108,** 1088–1096.
16. Tanaka, K., Ikematsu, H., Hirohata, T., and Kashiwagi, S. (1996) Hepatitis C virus infection and risk of hepatocellular carcinoma among Japanese: Possible role of type 1b (II) infection. *J. Natl. Cancer Inst.* **88,** 742–746.
17. Yamauchi, M., Nakahara, M., Nakajima, H., Sakamoto, K., Hirakawa, J., and Toda, G. (1994) Different prevalence of hepatocellular carcinoma between patients with liver cirrhosis due to genotype II and III of hepatitis C virus. *Int. Hepatol. Commun.* **2,** 328–332.
18. Chen, C. H., Sheu, J. C., Wang, J. T., Huang, G. T., Yang, P. M., Lee, H. S., et al. (1994) Genotypes of hepatitis C virus in chronic liver disease in Taiwan. *J. Med. Virol.* **44,** 234–236.
19. Lee, D. S., Sung, Y. C., and Whang, Y. S. (1996) Distribution of HCV genotypes among blood donors, patients with chronic liver disease, hepatocellular carcinoma, and patients on maintenance hemodialysis in Korea. *J. Med. Virol.* **49,** 55–60.
20. Yotsuyanagi, H., Koike, K., Yasuda, K., Moriya, K., Hino, K., Kurokawa, K., et al. (1995) Hepatitis C virus genotypes and development of hepatocellular carcinoma. *Cancer* **76,** 1352–1355.
21. McOmish, F., Chan, S.-W., Dow, B. C., Gillon, J., Frame, W. D., Crawford, R. J., et al. (1993) Detection of three types of hepatitis C virus in blood donors: Investigation of type-specific differences in serological reactivity and rate of alanine aminotransferase abnormalities. *Transfusion* **33,** 7–13.

22. Tisminetzky, S. G., Gerotto, M., Pontisso, P., Chemello, L., Ruvoletto, M. G., Baralle, F., et al. (1994) Genotypes of hepatitis C virus in Italian patients with chronic hepatitis C. *Int. Hepatol. Commun.* **2**, 105–112.
23. Nousbaum, J. B., Pol, S., Nalpas, B., Landais, P., Berthelot, P., Brechot, C., et al. (1995) Hepatitis C virus type 1b (II) infection in France and Italy. *Ann. Intern. Med.* **122**, 161.
24. Pawlotsky, J. M., Tsakiris, L., Roudotthoraval, F., Pellet, C., Stuyver, L., Duval, J., et al. (1995) Relationship between hepatitis C virus genotypes and sources of infection in patients with chronic hepatitis C. *J. Infect. Dis.* **171**, 1607–1610.
25. Simmonds, P., Mellor, J., Craxi, A., Sancheztapias, J. M., Alberti, A., Prieto, J., et al. (1996) Epidemiological, clinical and therapeutic associations of hepatitis C types in western European patients. *J. Hepatol.* **24**, 517–524.
26. Bell, H., Hellum, K., Harthug, S., Maeland, A., Ritland, S., Myrvang, B., et al. (1997) Genotype, viral load and age as independent predictors of treatment outcome of interferon-alpha 2a treatment in patients with chronic hepatitis C. *Scand. J. Infect. Dis.* **29**, 17–22.
27. Okamoto, H., Crovatto, M., Pozzato, G., Feray, C., Brechot, C., and Mishiro, S. (1995) Molecular and clinical characteristics of the hepatitis C virus genotype "2c" found in Italians in Italy and France. *Int. Hepatol. Commun.* **3**, 161–165.
28. McOmish, F., Yap, P. L., Dow, B. C., Follett, E. A. C., Seed, C., Keller, A. J., et al. (1994) Geographical distribution of hepatitis C virus genotypes in blood donors—an international collaborative survey. *J. Clin. Microbiol.* **32**, 884–892.
29. Zein, N. N., Rakela, J., and Persing, D. H. (1995) Genotype-dependent serologic reactivities in patients infected with hepatitis C virus in the United States. *Mayo Clin. Proc.* **70**, 449–452.
30. Tsuji, H., Shimomura, H., Wato, M., Kondo, J., and Tsuji, T. (1995) Virological and serological characterization of asymptomatic blood donors positive for anti-hepatitis C virus antibody. *Acta Med. Okayama* **49**, 137–144.
31. Matsubara, T., Sumazaki, R., Shin, K., Nagai, Y., and Takita, H. (1996) Genotyping of hepatitis C virus: Coinfection by multiple genotypes detected in children with chronic posttransfusion hepatitis C. *J. Pediat. Gastroenterol. Nutr.* **22**, 79–84.
32. Dow, B. C., Buchanan, I., Munro, H., Follett, E. A. C., Davidson, F., Prescott, L. E., et al. (1996) Relevance of RIBA-3 supplementary test to HCV PCR positivity and genotypes for HCV confirmation of blood donors. *J. Med. Virol.* **49**, 132–136.
33. Dhaliwal, S. K., Prescott, L. E., Dow, B. C., Davidson, F., Brown, H., Yap, P. L., et al. (1996) Influence of viraemia and genotype upon serological reactivity in screening assays for antibody to hepatitis C virus. *J. Med. Virol.* **48**, 184–190.
34. Jarvis, L. M., Watson, H. G., McOmish, F., Peutherer, J. F., Ludlam, C. A., and Simmonds, P. (1994) Frequent reinfection and reactivation of hepatitis C virus genotypes in multitransfused hemophiliacs. *J. Infect. Dis.* **170**, 1018–1022.
35. Lai, M. E., Mazzoleni, A. P., Argiolu, F., De Virgilis, S., Balestriesi, A., Purcell, R. H., et al. (1994) Hepatitis C virus in multiple episodes of acute hepatitis in polytransfused thalassaemic children. *Lancet* **343**, 388–390.

35a. Houghton, M., Choo, Q.-L., Kuo, G., Chien, D., Weiner, A., Selby, M., et al. (1996) HCV vaccine: interim report. *IX Triennial International Symposium on Viral Hepatitis and Liver Disease*, Rome, Italy. Abstract 50.
36. Rosa, D., Campagnoli, S., Moretto, C., Guenzi, E., Cousens, L., Chin, M., et al. (1996) A quantitative test to estimate neutralizing antibodies to the hepatitis C virus: Cytofluorimetric assessment of envelope glycoprotein 2 binding to target cells. *Proc. Natl. Acad. Sci. USA* **93**, 1759–1763.
37. Fox, S. A., Lareu, R. R., and Swanson, N. R. (1995) Rapid genotyping of hepatitis C virus isolates by dideoxy fingerprinting. *J. Virol. Methods* **53**, 1–9.
38. Stuyver, L., Rossau, R., Wyseur, A., Duhamel, M., Vanderborght, B., Van Heuverswyn, H., et al. (1993) Typing of hepatitis C virus isolates and characterization of new subtypes using a line probe assay. *J. Gen. Virol.* **74**, 1093–1102.
39. Tisminetzky, S., Gerotto, M., Pontisso, P., Chemello, L., Prescott, L. E., Rose, K. A., et al. (1995) Comparison of genotyping and serotyping methods for the identification of hepatitis C virus types. *J. Virol. Methods* **55**, 303–307.
40. Stuyver, L., Wyseur, A., Vanarnhem, W., Hernandez, F., and Maertens, G. (1996) Second-generation line probe assay for hepatitis C virus genotyping. *J. Clin. Microbiol.* **34**, 2259–2266.
41. Nakao, T., Enomoto, N., Takada, N., Takada, A., and Date, T. (1991) Typing of hepatitis C virus (HCV) genomes by restriction fragment length polymorphisms. *J. Gen. Virol.* **72**, 2105–2112.
42. Davidson, F., Simmonds, P., Ferguson, J. C., Jarvis, L. M., Dow, B. C., Follett, E. A. C., et al. (1995) Survey of major genotypes and subtypes of hepatitis C virus using restriction fragment length polymorphism of sequences amplified from the 5'non-coding region. *J. Gen Virol.* **76**, 1197–1204.
43. Lau, J. Y. N., Mizokami, M., Kolberg, J. A., Davis, G. L., Prescott, L. E., Ohno, T., et al. (1995) Application of six hepatitis C virus genotyping systems to sera from chronic hepatitis C patients in the United States. *J. Infect. Dis.* **171**, 281–289.
44. Tokita, H., Okamoto, H., Tsuda, F., Song, P., Nakata, S., Chosa, T., et al. (1994) Hepatitis C virus variants from Vietnam are classifiable into the seventh, eighth, and ninth major genetic groups. *Proc. Natl. Acad. Sci. USA* **91**, 11,022–11,026.
45. Stuyver, L., Wyseur, A., Vanarnhem, W., Lunel, F., Laurentpuig, P., Pawlotsky, J. M., et al. (1995) Hepatitis C virus genotyping by means of 5'-UR/core line probe assays and molecular analysis of untypeable samples. *Virus Res.* **38**, 137–157.
46. Mellor, J., Walsh, E. A., Prescott, L. E., Jarvis, L. M., Davidson, F., Yap, P. L., et al. (1996) Survey of type 6 group variants of hepatitis C virus in southeast Asia by using a core-based genotyping assay. *J. Clin. Microbiol.* **34**, 417–423.
47. Okamoto, H., Sugiyama, Y., Okada, S., Kurai, K., Akahane, Y., Sugai, Y., et al. (1992) Typing hepatitis C virus by polymerase chain reaction with type-specific primers: application to clinical surveys and tracing infectious sources. *J. Gen. Virol.* **73**, 673–679.
48. Okamoto, H., Tokita, H., Sakamoto, M., Horikita, M., Kojima, M., Iizuka, H., et al. (1993) Characterization of the genomic sequence of type V (or 3a) hepatitis C virus isolates and PCR primers for specific detection. *J. Gen. Virol.* **74**, 2385–2390.

49. Widell, A., Shev, S., Mansson, S., Zhang, Y. Y., Foberg, U., Norkrans, G., et al. (1994) Genotyping of hepatitis C virus isolates by a modified polymerase chain reaction assay using type specific primers: epidemiological applications. *J. Med. Virol.* **44,** 272–279.
50. Hashimoto, M., Chayama, K., Tubota, A., Kobayashi, M., Saitou, S., Arase, Y., et al. (1996) Typing six major hepatitis C virus genotypes by polymerase chain reaction using primers derived from nucleotide sequences of the NS5 region. *Int. Hepatol. Commun.* **4,** 263–267.
51. Giannini, C., Thiers, V., Nousbaum, J. B., Stuyver, L., Maertens, G., and Brechot, C. (1995) Comparative analysis of two assays for genotyping hepatitis C virus based on genotype-specific primers or probes. *J. Hepatol.* **23,** 246–253.
52. Kleter, G. E. M., Van Doorn, L. J., Stuyver, L., Maertens, G., Brouwer, J. T., Schalm, S. W., et al. (1995) Rapid genotyping of hepatitis C virus RNA-isolates obtained from patients residing in western Europe. *J. Med. Virol.* **47,** 35–42.
53. Machida, A., Ohnuma, H., Tsuda, F., Munekata, E., Tanaka, T., Akahane, Y., et al. (1992) Two distinct subtypes of hepatitis C virus defined by antibodies directed to the putative core protein. *Hepatology* **16,** 886–891.
54. Simmonds, P., Rose, K. A., Graham, S., Chan, S. W., McOmish, F., Dow, B. C., et al. (1993) Mapping of serotype-specific, immunodominant epitopes in the NS-4 region of hepatitis C virus (HCV)—use of type-specific peptides to serologically differentiate infections with HCV type 1, type 2, and type 3. *J. Clin. Microbiol.* **31,** 1493–1503.
55. Tanaka, T., Tsukiyamakohara, K., Yamaguchi, K., Yagi, S., Tanaka, S., Hasegawa, A., et al. (1994) Significance of specific antibody assay for genotyping of hepatitis C virus. *Hepatology* **19,** 1347–1353.
56. Bhattacherjee, V., Prescott, L. E., Pike, I., Rodgers, B., Bell, H., Elzayadi, A. R., et al. (1995) Use of NS-4 peptides to identify type-specific antibody to hepatitis C virus genotypes 1, 2, 3, 4, 5 and 6. *J. Gen. Virol.* **76,** 1737–1748.
57. Dixit, V., Quan, S., Martin, P., Larson, D., Brezina, M., Dinello, R., et al. (1995) Evaluation of a novel serotyping system for hepatitis C virus: strong correlation with standard genotyping methodologies. *J. Clin. Microbiol.* **33,** 2978–2983.
58. Enomoto, N., Sakuma, I., Asahina, Y., Kurosaki, M., Murakami, T., Yamamoto, C., et al. (1996) Mutations in the nonstructural protein 5A gene and response to interferon in patients with chronic hepatitis C virus 1b infection. *N. Engl. J. Med.* **334,** 77–81.
58a. Khorsi, H., Castelain, S., Wyseur, A., Izopet, J., Canva, V., Rombout, A., et al. (1997) Mutations of hepatitis C virus 1b NS5A 2209–2248 amino acid sequence do not predict the response to recombinant interferon-alfa therapy in French patients. *J. Hepatol.* **27,** 72–77.
59. Kao, J. H., Chen, P. J., Yang, P. M., Lai, M. Y., Wang, T. H., and Chen, D. S. (1996) Absence of extensive genetic heterogeneity of hepatitis C virus in antibody-negative chronic hepatitis C. *J. Med. Virol.* **49,** 87–90.
60. Ogata, N., Alter, H. J., Miller, R. H., and Purcell, R. H. (1991) Nucleotide sequence and mutation rate of the H strain of hepatitis C virus. *Proc. Natl. Acad. Sci. USA* **88,** 3392–3396.

61. Okamoto, H., Kojima, M., Okada, S-I., Yoshizawa, H., Iizuka, H., Tanaka, T., et al. (1992) Genetic drift of hepatitis C virus during an 8.2 year infection in a chimpanzee: variability and stability. *Virology* **190**, 894–899.
61a. Smith, D. B. and Simmonds, P. (1997) Characteristics of nucleotide substitution in the hepatitis C virus genome: constraints on sequence change in coding regions at both ends of the genome. *J. Mol. Evol.* **45**, 238–246.
62. Kumar, U., Monjardino, J., and Thomas, H. C. (1994) Hypervariable region of hepatitis C virus envelope glycoprotein (e2 NS1) in an agammaglobulinemic patient. *Gastroenterology* **106**, 1072–1075.
63. Van Doorn, L. J., Capriles, I., Maertens, G., Deleys, R., Murray, K., Kos, T., et al. (1995) Sequence evolution of the hypervariable region in the putative envelope region e2/NS1 of hepatitis C virus is correlated with specific humoral immune responses. *J. Virol.* **69**, 773–778.
64. Okada, S., Akahane, Y., Suzuki, H., Okamoto, H., and Mishiro, S. (1992) The degree of variability in the amino terminal region of the e2/NS1 protein of hepatitis-c virus correlates with responsiveness to interferon therapy in viremic patients. *Hepatology* **16**, 619–624.
65. Sherman, K. E., Andreatta, C., Obrien, J., Gutierrez, A., and Harris, R. (1996) Hepatitis C in human immunodeficiency virus-coinfected patients: Increased variability in the hypervariable envelope coding domain. *Hepatology* **23**, 688–694.
66. Paterlini, P., Driss, F., Nalpas, B., Pisi, E., Franco, D., Berthelot, P., et al. (1993) Persistence of hepatitis-b and hepatitis C viral genomes in primary liver cancers from HBsag-negative patients—a study of a low-endemic area. *Hepatology* **17**, 20–29.
67. Sakamoto, N., Enomoto, N., Kurosaki, M., Asahina, Y., Maekawa, S., Koizumi, K., et al. (1995) Comparison of the hypervariable region of hepatitis C virus genomes in plasma and liver. *J. Med. Virol.* **46**, 7–11.
68. Kanazawa, Y., Hayashi, N., Mita, E., Li, T. C., Hagiwara, H., Kasahara, A., et al. (1994) Influence of viral quasispecies on effectiveness of interferon therapy in chronic hepatitis C patients. *Hepatology* **20**, 1121–1130.
69. Koizumi, K., Enomoto, N., Kurosaki, M., Murakami, T., Izumi, N., Marumo, F., et al. (1995) Diversity of quasispecies in various disease stages of chronic hepatitis C virus infection and its significance in interferon treatment. *Hepatology* **22**, 30–35.
70. Moribe, T., Hayashi, N., Kanazawa, Y., Mita, E., Fusamoto, H., Negi, M., et al. (1995) Hepatitis C viral complexity detected by single-strand conformation polymorphism and response to interferon therapy. *Gastroenterology* **108**, 789–795.
71. Yeh, B. I., Han, K. H., Oh, S. H., Kim, H. S., Hong, S. H., and Kim, Y. S. (1996) Nucleotide sequence variation in the hypervariable region of the hepatitis C virus in the sera of chronic hepatitis C patients undergoing controlled interferon-alpha therapy. *J. Med. Virol.* **49**, 95–102.
72. Gonzalez-Peralta, R. P., She, J. Y., Davis, G. L., Ohno, T., Mizokami, M., and Lau, J. Y. N. (1996) Clinical implications of viral quasispecies heterogeneity in chronic hepatitis C. *J. Med. Virol.* **49**, 242–247.

73. Nakazawa, T., Kato, N., Ohkoshi, S., Shibuya, A., and Shimotohno, K. (1994) Characterization of the 5' noncoding and structural region of the hepatitis C virus genome from patients with non-A, non-B hepatitis responding differently to interferon treatment. *J. Hepatol.* **20,** 623–629.
74. Kurosaki, M., Enomoto, N., Marumo, F., and Sato, C. (1993) Rapid sequence variation of the hypervariable region of hepatitis C virus during the course of chronic infection. *Hepatology* **18,** 1293–1299.
75. Kao, J. H., Chen, P. J., Lai, M. Y., Wang, T. H., and Chen, D. S. (1995) Quasispecies of hepatitis C virus and genetic drift of the hypervariable region in chronic type c hepatitis. *J. Infect. Dis.* **172,** 261–264.
76. Mellor, J., Holmes, E. C., Jarvis, L. M., Yap, P. L., Simmonds, P., and International Collaborators (1995) Investigation of the pattern of hepatitis C virus sequence diversity in different geographical regions: implications for virus classification. *J. Gen. Virol.* **76,** 2493–2507.

12

Molecular Evolutionary Analysis

Its Application in the Study of Hepatitis C Virus

Masashi Mizokami and Johnson Y. N. Lau

1. Introduction

The recent development of high-power personal computer hardware and software has allowed investigators to prepare phylogenetic trees without understanding of the fundamental principles of molecular evolution. Unfortunately, inexperienced investigators are also prone to draw inappropriate or wrong conclusions from this type of analysis. In particular, extreme caution should be taken when phylogenetic trees are applied to clinical settings.

This chapter shall briefly described the principles behind one of the methods frequently used to estimate the number of nucleotide substitutions, which is used to estimate molecular evolution. It will also describe some of the common tools used to construct phylogenetic trees and the estimation of divergence time.

2. Estimation of Nucleotide Substitution

Phylogenetic trees are determined based on the number of nucleotide substitutions that occur in the gene sequences being analyzed *(1,2)*. Therefore, accurate estimation of the number of nucleotide substitutions is the single most important factor in the construction of a reliable phylogenetic tree.

Let us address the issue of multiple substitutions. There are only four types of nucleotides: adenine (A), thymine (T), guanine (G), and cytosine (C). Therefore, for gene sequences with multiple variation at a specific site, the number of substitutions will not be obvious from a simple comparison of the nucleotide sequences. For example, if sequences A and B have the same nucleotide G in a particular position, it is possible that there was no change during evolution, or change occured for a few rounds, but at the time of the assessment, it was the same (i.e., G). If the nucleotides in a particular position are different (e.g., A and T in two different sequences), it is possible that the sequence has undergone multiple substitutions, but at the time of assessment (e.g., G→C→T, G→A→C→T, and so on), that position has a nucleotide T. Therefore, estimating the number of nucleotide substitutions with appropriate adjustments to account for the possibilities of multiple substitutions in the gene sequences has to be addressed before one can construct an accurate phylogenetic relationship.

The same nucleotide in the position assessed	Different nucleotide in the position assessed
Seq AAT<u>G</u>CT Seq BAT<u>G</u>CT	Seq AAT<u>G</u>CT Seq BAT<u>G</u>CT
Possibilities: G–no change G → A → G G → A → C → G and so on	Possibilities: G → T G → C → T G → A → C → T and so on

Theoretically, a real-time follow-up of the changes in sequences is the best approach, but it is obvious that this is impossible from a technical standpoint. Therefore, a number of mathematical models, which are based on the pattern of variations in a particular position, were developed. At present, the following three methods are widely used by experienced investigators in this field to estimate the number of nucleotide substitutions:

1. One-parameter method
2. Two-parameter method
3. Six-parameter method

2.1. One-Parameter Method (Table 1)

As shown in **Table 1**, the one-parameter method is based on the hypothesis that the rate of nucleotide substitutions per site per year is equivalent among various nucleotides. The probability of nucleotide substitution is designated as α. If α is constant throughout the study period, the mean number of nucleotide substitutions K (genetic distance) for the divergence of two sequences with the same starting sequence is calculated with the following equation:

$$K = 2 \times (\text{evolutionary rate}) \times (\text{time}) = 2 \times \lambda \times t \tag{1}$$

It follows that the probability of nucleotide substitution at a specific site of sequence A over 1 yr is 3α, i.e., $\lambda = 3\alpha$, and the probability that no substitution occurs is $1-3\alpha$.

Table 1
The Models of the Nucleotide Substitutions

	Nucleotide before substitution	Nucleotide after substitution			
		A	T	C	G
1-Parameter method	A	—	α	α	α
	T	α	—	α	α
	C	α	α	—	α
	G	α	α	α	—
2-Parameter method	A	—	β	β	α
	T	β	—	α	β
	C	β	α	—	β
	G	α	β	β	—
6-Parameter method	A	—	α^1	α	α
	T	β^1	—	α	α
	C	β	β	—	α^2
	G	β	β	β^2	—

Let us consider the issue that a sequence is going to diverge but the same nucleotide is found in the same site in two different sequences t years afterward. Assume that the probability of a certain nucleotide is $I(t)$, and the probability of that site having other nucleotide is $1 - I(t)$. Let us make the probability of the same site having a certain nucleotide $I(t + 1)$. For two sequences to have the same nucleotide in a particular position at a given time, either both sequences have no change in that site, or both sequences had substitution and they end up with the same nucleotide at the time of assessment. For the sake of assessment, assume that we are looking at the 1-yr interval. For the first possibility that both nucleotides in the same site in both sequences are not changed in the 1-yr interval, the probability that no substitution will occur is $1 - 3\alpha$ *(see above)*, the probability that both sequences that were assessed one year later to have both nucleotides conserved at the same site is $(1 - 3\alpha)^2$. For the second possibility that both nucleotides were changed but they end up having the same nucleotide in the same position 1 yr later, the probability will be $(3\alpha)^2$.

Now, let us consider the situation that the nucleotides in a certain site from two gene sequences are different in year t and are the same in year $t + 1$. There are two possibilities to account for this possible event. First, the nucleotide at that site for one sequence is substituted with the same nucleotide as the other sequence and the other sequence has not changed, which will give rise to the probability of $2\alpha(1 - 3\alpha)$. Alternatively, both nucleotides in the same site from both sequences have changed but they end up having the same nucleotide in 1 yr, with the probability being $2\alpha^2$.

From the above discussion, the relationship between I(t + 1) and I(t) is given by the following equation:

$$I(t+1) = [(1-3\alpha)^2 + 3\alpha^2]I(t) + [\alpha(1-3\alpha) + 2\alpha^2][1-I(t)] \quad (2)$$

Since the value of α is usually very small, the factor α^2 can be ignored. The equation can then be simplified as

$$I(t+1) = (1-6\alpha)I(t) + 2\alpha[1-I(t)] \quad (3),$$

which can be further simplified into

$$I(t+1) = I(t) - 8\alpha(t) + 2\alpha \quad (4)$$

Therefore, the difference between I(t+1) and I(t) can be estimated as

$$I(t+1) - I(t) = 2\alpha - 8\alpha I(t) \quad (5)$$

which can be translated into

$$I(t+1) - I(t) = 8\alpha[(1/4) - I(t)] \quad (6)$$

The increment in I(t) from year t to year t + 1 is a dynamic change depending on α and I(t). If the equation is expressed in the differential form, the following differential equation is obtained.

$$dI(t)/dt = 8\alpha[1/4 - I(t)] \quad (7)$$

$$\text{or, } I(t) = 1/4 + Ce^{-8\alpha t} \quad (8)$$

where C is a constant.

When this is solved based on the initial condition I(0)=1, C is estimated to be 3/4. Therefore, the following equation is obtained:

$$I(t) = 1/4 + (3/4)e^{-8\alpha t} \quad (9)$$

As the mean number of substitutions per site in year t is

$$K = 2 \times I(t) = 2 \times 3\alpha t \quad (10)$$

when I(t) is substituted into this equation, the following equation is obtained:

$$K = -(3/4)\ln[4/3 I(t) - 1/3] \quad (11)$$

$$K = -(3/4)\ln\{1 - (4/3)[1 - I(T)]\} \quad (12)$$

$$K = -(3/4)\ln\{1 - (4/3)p\} \quad (13)$$

where p = 1 – I(t).

Thus, the percentage of sites with different nucleotides in two homologous nucleotide sequences after t years can be calculated.

This is the method originally described by Jukes and Cantor *(3)*. Since this is a relatively simple model, this is the most widely used method to estimate the number of nucleotide substitution.

2.2. Two-Parameter Method (Table 1)

Nucleotides A and G are purines with a similar molecular weight, whereas C and T are pyrimidines. Nucleotide substitutions between the two purines or the two pyrimidines are known as transitions, but those between purines and pyrimidines are called transversions. Transitions between nucleotides with a similar molecular structure are more likely to occur than transversions between nucleotides with different molecular structures. To account for this, Kimura proposed the two-parameter model for estimating nucleotide substitution rate taking into consideration the different rates of transition and transversion *(4)*.

First, let us define the rate of nucleotide substitution for transitions as α, and that for transversions as β **(Table 1)**. When two homologous sequences are compared, P is the proportion of nucleotides which are different resulting from transition (i.e., the proportion of sites with two different sequences were either A and G, or C and T) and Q is the proportion of different nucleotides resulting from transversion. After t years, the differential change of $P(t)$ and $Q(t)$ can be expressed by the following equations:

$$dP(t)/dt = 2\alpha - 4(\alpha + \beta)P(t) - 2(\alpha - \beta)Q(t) \tag{14}$$

$$dQ(t)/dt = 4\beta - 8\beta Q(t) \tag{15}$$

When solved with the initial condition of $P(0) = Q(0) = 0$:

$$P(t) = 1/4 - (1/2)e^{-4(\alpha + \beta)t} + (1/4)e^{-8\beta t} \tag{16}$$

$$Q(t) = 1/2 - (1/2)e^{-8\beta t} \tag{17}$$

Now, let us consider nucleotide A changes to another nucleotide, it changes to G at a rate of α and to C or T at a rate of β. Accordingly, the mean number of nucleotide sequences changes per year, i.e., the speed of substitution, is expressed as $k = \alpha + 2\beta$.

Hence, the total number of nucleotide substitutions per site at t years for two sequences assessed at that time is $K = 2kt = 2\alpha t + 4\beta t$.

Resolving the two equations on $P(t)$ and $Q(t)$ above will give:

$$8\beta t = -\ln[1 - 2Q(t)] \tag{18}$$

$$4\alpha t = -\ln[1 - 2P(t) - Q(t)] + (1/2)\ln[1 - 2Q(t)] \tag{19}$$

Substituting these to the equation expressing K will give the following equations:

$$K = 2\alpha t + 4\beta t \tag{20}$$

$$K = -(1/2)\ln[1 - 2P(t) - Q(t)] - (1/4)\ln[1 - 2Q(t)] \tag{21}$$

$$K = -(1/2)\ln[1 - 2P(t) - Q(t)][1 - 2Q(t)] \tag{22}$$

In above equations, if one assumes that the rates of transition and transversion are the same, i.e., $\alpha = \beta$, then $P = 1/2Q$. If $P = 1/2Q$ is substituted in the last equation:

$$K = -(3/4)\ln\{[1 - (4/3)(P(t) + Q(t)]\} \tag{23}$$

Since $P(t) + Q(t)$ is equivalent to the proportion of all sites with different nucleotides in the two DNA sequences compared, the equation will resolve back to the simple formula given by the one-parameter method.

2.3. Six-Parameter Method (Table 1)

The six-parameter method takes a step further. This method determines the rate of substitution assuming the rate of change from each of the four nucleotides is different, except when nucleotides A or T (with two bonds) were changed to C or G (with three bonds) and vice versa *(5)*. It is called the six-parameter method because the rates of change for each nucleotide are designated as α, $\alpha 1$, $\alpha 2$, β, $\beta 1$, and $\beta 2$.

The formula from the substitution matrix model shown in **Table 1** is depicted below:

$$K = -pq\ln(B/pq) - 2(qAqT/p)\ln[p(F12 - B1 + 3E12/B1)/(3qAqT)]$$
$$- 2(qCqG/q)\ln[q(F34 - B1 + 3E34/B1)/(3qCqG)] \tag{24}$$

where qA, qT, qC, and qG are the mean content rates for A, T, C, and G, for a specific site, respectively, in the two nucleotide sequences being compared. Note that

$$p = qA + qT \tag{25}$$

$$q = qC + qG \tag{26}$$

$$B1 = pq - (xAC + xAG + xTC + xTC + xTG) \tag{27}$$

$$E12 = (qAq - xAC - xAG)(qTq - xTC - xTG) \tag{28}$$

$$E34 = (qCq - xAC - xTC)(qGp - xAC - xTC)(qGp - xAG - xTG) \tag{29}$$

$$F12 = xAA + xTT - xAT - p2 + 3qAqT \tag{30}$$

$$F34 = xCC + xGG - xCG - q2 + 3qCqG \tag{31}$$

$2xij$ (i is not equal to j) is the proportion of sites with different nucleotides at j than those in the two sequences being compared, and xij shows the proportion of sites with the same nucleotide (i,j = A,T,C,G).

A detailed explanation of this method is beyond the scope of this chapter. These equations were given to highlight the complex mathematics involved in these estimations and the caution needed to interpret these data as discussed **Subheading 2.4.** For details of the derivation of these equations, please refer to **ref. 5**.

2.4. Rational Use of These Methods

These methods of estimating nucleotide substitutions must be used with caution, and each method has its set of advantages and disadvantages.

For example, the one-parameter method is simple, but the estimated value becomes too low when the estimated number of nucleotide substitutions is 1.0 or more per site. The two-parameter method is useful in situations where the rate of nucleotide substitutions by transition and transversion is very different, e.g., mitochondrial genes of humans and monkeys. However, when the rates of transition and transversion are approximately the same, the results obtained are almost identical to that estimated by the one-parameter method. In this case, there is no reason to use the more complicated two-parameter method, and one-parameter is preferred.

The six-parameter method has the advantage that it is based on the frequency of appearance of each nucleotide in a large number of sequences. Therefore, when the nucleotide sequence used for comparison is short, the anti-logarithm portion of logarithmic functions may become negative and further calculation is impossible. On the other hand, as more parameters are considered by this method, the estimates are likely to be the most accurate.

3. Methods of Constructing Phylogenetic Trees

Phylogenetic trees are constructed based on the number of nucleotide substitutions estimated by the methods described previously. A few techniques are available to construct phylogenetic trees, the most commonly used techniques being the unweighed pair grouping method with arithmatic mean (UPGMA) method *(6)*, the neighbor joining (NJ) method, and the maximum likelihood (ML) method *(8)*.

The UPG method is based on the assumption that the rate of nucleotide substitution per site per year is constant. When the rate of nucleotide evolution is not constant, the NJ method is the technique of choice. The ML method is completely different from the other two. This method establishes a hypothesis for each factor from the nucleotide substitution data, and constructs a phylogenetic tree based on each hypothesis. The validity of these hypotheses is proven by estimating the structure of the phylogenetic tree prepared statistically. The likelihood of the data obtained is a coefficient of the unknown parameters and the parameters are estimated so that this likelihood reaches a maximum.

From the above description, one should realize that each method is based on a different set of assumptions. Therefore, one should try to understand the biological basis involved before deciding which is the appropriate method for determining molecular evolution. For example, the UPG method provides phylogenetic trees for situations that have a constant rate of evolution (number of nucleotide substitutions/site/year). However, even when the rate of evolution is almost constant over time, this method cannot be used if the rate of evolution is extremely high and the time span between the isolation of the sequences studied is long. This is because phylogenetic trees prepared by the UPG method consist of branches branching from the initial points, and the distance from the initial point to the terminal points for all branches are equal in length, indicating the same evolutionary distance for all branches. However, if the sequences obtained differ by a long span and the rate of evolution is high, the difference in evolution distance will not be accounted for by this construction, even if the rate of evolution is constant. This is of importance to this chapter since RNA viruses, including HCV, have a high rate of molecular evolution, which averages 10^6 times that of host DNA (e.g., human DNA). It means that the evolution of these viruses in 1 yr is the same as the evolution of humans in one million years. With such high rate of evolution, the NJ method is more suitable for constructing phylogenetic trees for viral genes, including HCV genes. However, the NJ method creates phylogenetic trees with no indication of the root of the tree, i.e. the origin of evolution is not determined. Therefore, most investigators studying RNA virus evolution construct a phylogenetic tree with roots based on the UPG method to determine the root (i.e., showing the route of the evolution), and then construct another phylogenetic tree by the NJ method to determine the evolutionary relationship.

The ML method can provide accurate models if the investigators know the validity of the hypotheses. However, this method has the disadvantage of having to do a very significant amount of calculation to construct phylogenetic trees until the likelihood of the tree in representing the phylogenetic relationship reaches a maximum. For example, a total of 3,628,800 separate trees are required for the analysis of 10 sequences. Therefore, handling of large number of sequences is beyond the capability of most of the personal computers. The recent rapid development of computer technology may make the utilization of these tools using personal computers easier in the near future.

4. Molecular Phylogenetic Trees of HCV

Figure 1 shows the phylogenetic trees of HCV constructed by the three methods discussed in **Subheading 3. Figure 1A** showed a phylogenetic tree constructed by the UPG method, **Fig. 1B** the NJ method, and **Fig. 1C** the ML method. Note that in these three phylogenetic trees, the pattern of divergence differs. However, all isolates are clustered into the same types and subtypes based on each of three methods, supporting the validity of the classification of HCV based on molecular evolutionary analysis.

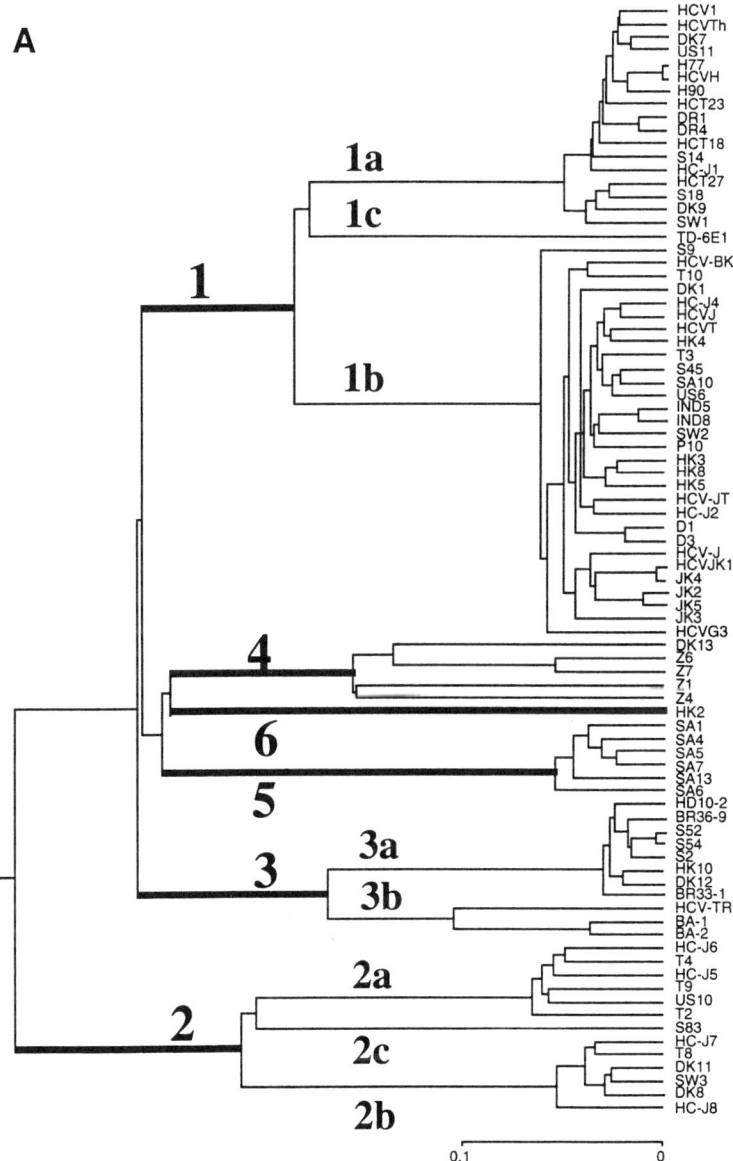

Fig. 1. Phylogenetic tree for HCV isolates as constructed by (**A**) UPGMA, (**B**) NJ, and (**C**) ML methods. Note that all HCV isolates clustered together into the same branch with all three methods. Also note that HCV isolates can be classified into six major types (given as 1, 2, 3, 4, 5, and 6) and a series of subtypes (given as a, b, and so forth).

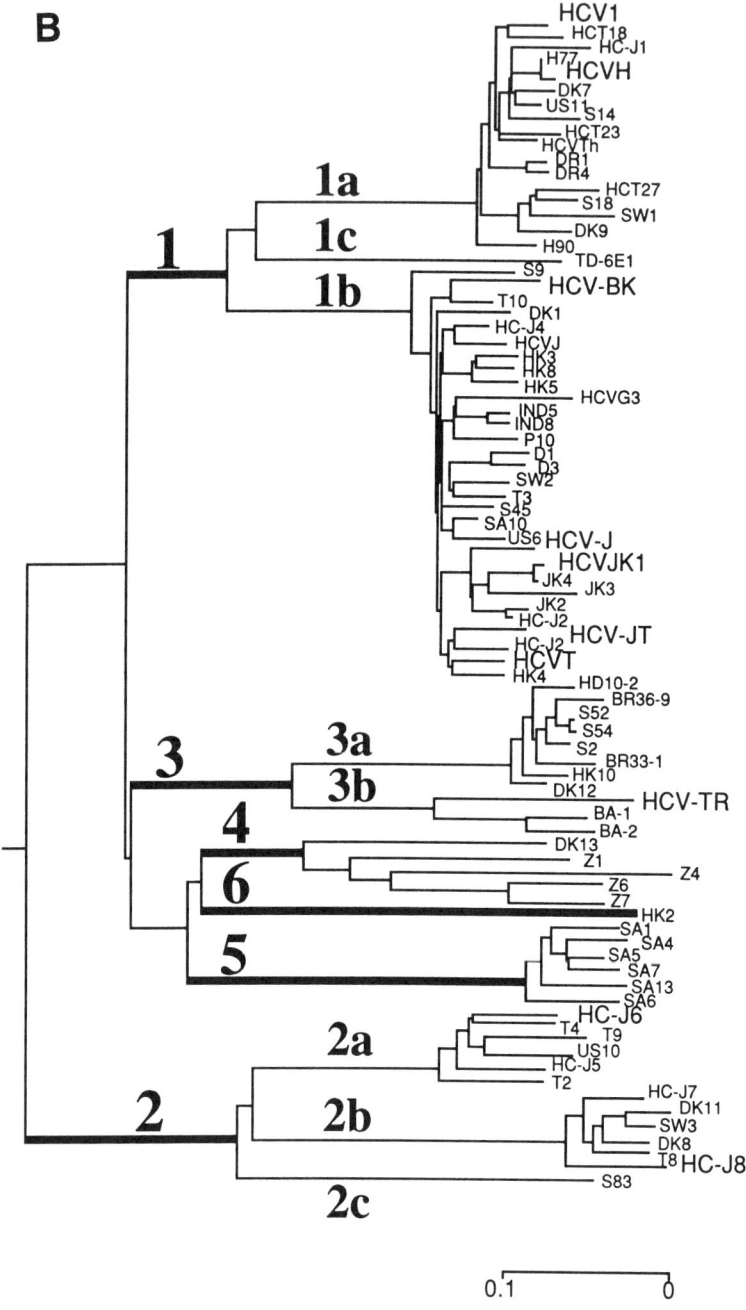

Fig. 1 (**B**)

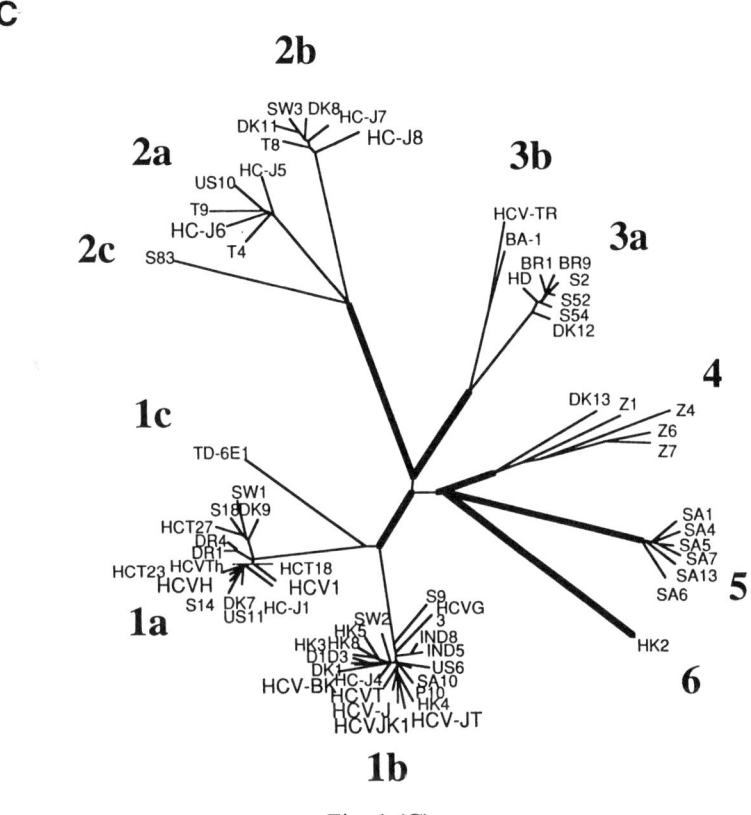

Fig. 1 (**C**)

References

1. Nei, M. (1987) *Molecular Evolutionary Genetics.* Columbia University Press, New York.
2. Kimura, M. (1993) *The Neutral Theory of Molecular Evolution.* Cambridge University Press, Cambridge.
3. Jukes, T. H. and Cantor, C. R. (1969) Evolution of protein molecules, in *Mammalian Protein Metabolism* (Munro, H. N., ed.), Academic, New York, pp. 21–132.
4. Kimura, M. (1980) A simple method for estimating evolutionary rate of base substitutions through comparative studies of nucleotide sequences. *J. Mol. Evol.* **16,** 111–120.
5. Gojobori, T., Ishii, K., and Nei, M. (1982) Estimation of average number of nucleotide substitutions when the rate of substitutions varies with nucleotide. *J. Mol. Evol.* **18,** 414–423.

6. Nei, M. (1975) *Molecular Population Genetics and Evolution.* North-Holland, Amsterdam.
7. Saitou, N. and Nei, M. (1987) The neighbor-joining method: a new method for reconstructing phylogenetic trees. *Mol. Biol. Evol.* **3,** 418–426.
8. Felsenstein, J. (1981) Evolutionary trees from DNA sequences: a maximum likelihood approach. *J. Mol. Evol.* **17,** 368–376.

13

Genotyping by Type-Specific Primers That Can Type HCV Types 1–6

Tomoyoshi Ohno and Masashi Mizokami

1. Introduction

Hepatitis C virus (HCV) was identified as a major causative agent of non-A, non-B hepatitis *(1)*. Numerous complete or partial nucleotide sequences of HCV isolates have been reported worldwide, and comparison of these sequences revealed their marked genetic heterogeneity nature, suggesting the existence of HCV genotypes.

On the basis of sequence variation in both the coding and noncoding regions, several classifications have been proposed, leading to confusion in the nomenclature of HCV genotypes. However, in the currently proposed nomenclature for HCV genotyping, HCV can be classified into at least six major genotypes based on phylogenetic analyses of the 5'-untranslated region, core, E1, and NS5 regions *(2)*.

Recent studies have pointed out that different HCV genotypes are associated with different profiles of pathogenicity, infectivity, and response to antiviral therapy. The establishment of a simple and precise genotyping system for HCV is essential to address these issues. There are several genotyping systems for HCV; one is based on PCR with genotype-specific primers, and some are by restriction fragment length polymorphism (RFLP). Both systems have been developed by focusing on genotype-specific sequences; therefore, the more the number of HCV isolates employed in designing a genotyping system, the higher would be the specificity of the system designed. To develop a typing system using PCR, the region used is necessary to be in part variable and in part conservative. Therefore, we focused on HCV core region, although you could use whichever region you wanted. Our genotype-specifc primers are designed on the basis of 91 HCV sequences, 90 of which were reported to be classified into genotype 1a, 1b, 1d, 2a, 2b, 3a, 3b, 4, or 5a in a previous study *(3)*, and the remaining one of which was isolated as genotype 6a.

1. Reverse Transcription

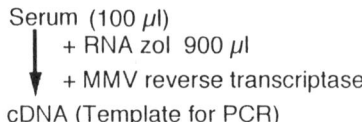

2. PCR

1st PCR ; primer pair of S2 and A2

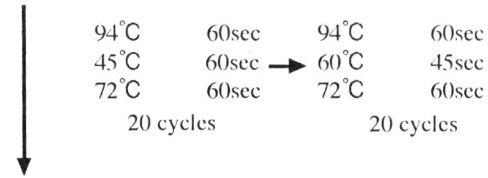

Genotyping PCR; Mix 1 & Mix 2 (TABLE 1 and FIGURE 2)

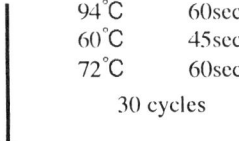

3. Electrophoresis on separate gels

Fig. 1. A simplified flowchart that describes this protocol.

In this chapter, a new genotyping system that allows for the determination of HCV genotypes 1a, 1b, 2a, 2b, 3a, 3b, 4, 5a, and 6a is described *(4)*.

2. Materials

1. Clinical samples.
2. RNAzol B (Cinna/Biotecx Laboratories, Friendswood, TX).
3. M-MLV-RT (Gibco-BRL, Gaithersburg, MD).
4. RNasin (TOYOBO, Osaka, Japan).
5. RT buffer: 50 mM Tris-HCl, pH 8.3, 75 mM KCl, 3 mM MgCl$_2$, and 10 mM DDT.
6. Thermal cycler (Perkin-Elmer Cetus, Norwalk, CT).
7. *Taq* polymerase and reaction buffer (Promega, Madison WI).
8. PCR buffer: 10 mM Tris-HCl, pH 9.0, 50 mM KCl, 1.5 mM MgCl$_2$, 0.01% gelatin, and 0.1% Triton X-100.
9. Seakem agarose (FMC BioProducts, Rockland, ME).
10. UV chamber (*see* **Note 1**).

3. Methods

Figure 1 shows a flowchart summary of our protocol for typing HCV samples.

3.1. RNA Extraction

1. Extract RNA from 100 µL of serum with guanidinium salt, phenol and chloroform (RNAzol B, Cinna/Biotecx Laboratories) using the manufacturer's protocol.
2. Precipitate the extracted RNA with isopropanol and wash with ethanol.
3. Dissolve the RNA pellet in diethylpyrocarbonate-treated distilled water containing 100 U of human placental ribonuclease inhibitor (RNasin, TOYOBO, Osaka, Japan).

3.2. Reverse Transcription

1. Synthesize the first-strand cDNA from RNA samples at 37°C for 60 min with 200 U of Moloney murine leukemia virus reverse transcriptase (M-MLV-RT, Gibco-BRL) in a 20 µL mixture containing 1X RT buffer and 600 µM dNTP (Promega).
2. Terminate reactions by heating at 95°C for 10 min, and then chill the mixtures on ice.

3.3. Polymerase Chain Reaction (PCR)

1. For amplification by PCR, prepare a 50-µL mixture containing 1X PCR buffer, 2 µL of the cDNA, 1.25 U of *Taq* DNA polymerase (Promega), and primers. Amplify 2 µL of the cDNA for 40 cycles with the following parameters: a preliminary 20 cycles of amplification with 94°C for 1 min (denaturation), 45°C for 1 min (annealing), and 72°C for 1 min (extension), followed by 20 additional cycles at 94°C for 1 min, 60°C for 1 min, and 72°C for 1 min.
2. For the second-round PCR, amplify 1 µL of the first-round PCR product for another 30 cycles; each cycle consists of 94°C for 1 min, 62°C for 45 s, and 72°C for 1 min (*see* **Note 2**).
3. Use primers S2 and A2 for the first-round PCR. In PCR of genotyping HCV, prepare two different primer mixtures, one containing S7, S2a, G1b, G2a, G2b, and G3b primers (Mix-1), and another including S7, G1a, G3a, G4, G5a, and G6a primers (Mix-2) (**Table 1**). Perform two second-round PCRs for each sample, one with primers Mix-1 and the other with Mix-2 (**Table 1**) (*see* **Note 3**).

3.4. Gel Electrophoresis

1. Electrophorese 8 µL of the second-round PCR products on a 2% agarose gel, stain with ethidium bromide, and evaluate under UV light.
2. Determine the HCV genotype in each sample by identifying the genotype-specific cDNA bands, as exemplified in **Fig. 2** (*see* **Note 4**).

4. Notes

1. PCR experiments are susceptible to contaminations. In addition to all the unusual precautions to avoid PCR contaminations, all pipets and racks were placed under UV light before use.

Table 1
Primers for PCR, Sequencing, and Genotyping[a]

Primer	Sequence (5'–3')	Nucleotide position
1st-round PCR		
S2	GGGAGGTCTCGTAGACCGTGCACCATG	–24–3
A2	GAG(AC)GG(GT)AT(AG)TACCCCATGAG(AG)TCGGC	417–391
2nd-round PCR for typing HCV		
Mix 1		
S7	AGACCGTGCACCATGAGCAC	–12–8
S2a	AACACTAACCGTCGCCCACAA	40–60
G1b	CCTGCCCTCGGGTTGGCTA(AG)	222–203
G2a	CACGTGGCTGGGATCGCTCC	178–159
G2b	GGCCCCAATTAGGACGAGAC	325–306
G3b	CGCTCGGAAGTCTTACGTAC	164–145
Mix 2		
S7	AGACCGTGCACCATGAGCAC	–12–8
G1a	GGATAGGCTGACGTCTACCT	196–177
G3a	GCCCAGGACCGGCCTTCGCT	220–211
G4	CCCGGGAACTTAACGTCCAT	87–58
G5a	GAACCTCGGGGGGAGAGCAA	308–289
G6a	GGTCATTGGGGCCCCAATGT	334–315

[a]Pairs of nucleotides inside parentheses are degenerate nucleotides. Notations 1a–6a are according to the nomenclature proposed by Simmonds et al. *(2)*. Numbering is from the start of the main open reading frame. The expected size of the genotype-spcific band amplified by typing PCR is as follows: genotype 1a 208 bp in size, genotype 1b 234 bp, genotype 2a 139 bp, and 190 bp (both bands are specific; if it happens, the 190 bp-band might be amplified in type 4 samples), genotype 2b 337 bp, genotype 3a 232 bp, genotype 3b 176 bp, genotype 4 99 bp, genotype 5a 320 bp, and genotype 6a 336 bp (**Fig. 2**).

2. The concentration of $MgCl_2$ affects the specificity of primer annealing. The same holds true for the primer and template of PCR even if all of genotype-specifc primers are completely specific. The PCR conditions described here were the optimal based on a series of experiments to optimize the conditions.
3. The system presented here uses genotype-specific primers designed on the basis of nucleotide sequences of the 91 HCV isolates. When more HCV sequences become available, the primers may need to have minor modifications.
4. In those case with difficulties in assigning HCV genotypes, it is necessary to both compare to genotyping results with other systems and also to determine the nucleotide sequence. This approach will provide information needed for further improvement of this system and in identifying new HCV genotypes.

【Mix-1】

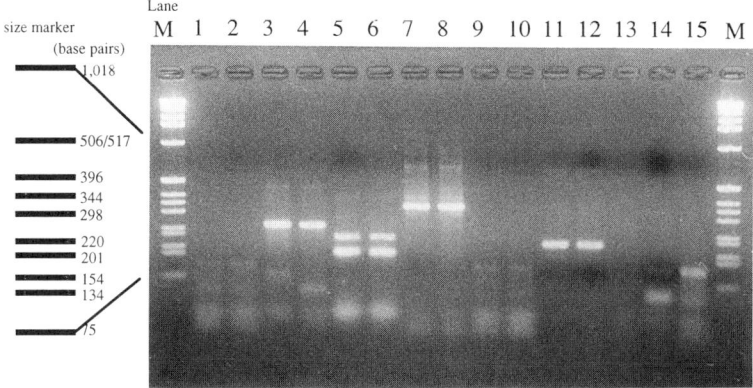

【Mix-2】

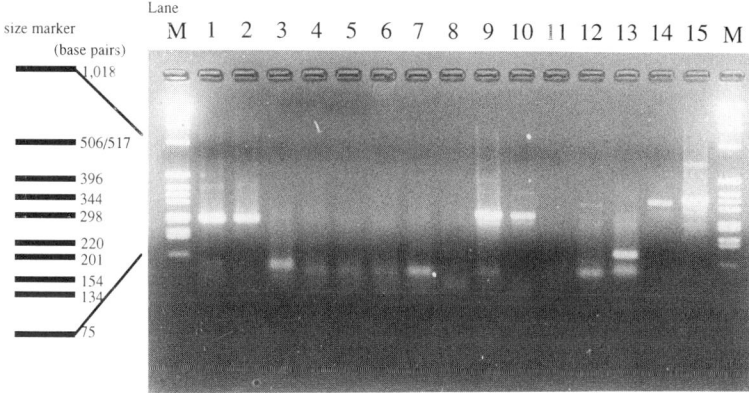

Fig. 2. Typical electrophoresis pattern of PCR products from different HCV genotypes using our new typing system. All samples were analyzed twice by PCR with either Mix-1 or Mix 2. Mix 1 will allow for the specific detection of PCR products for HCV genotypes 1b, 2a, 2b, and 3b. Mix 2 will allow for the specific detection of HCV genotypes 1a, 3a, 4, 5a, and 6a. The detection of genotype-specific products in Mix 1 and Mix 2 was designed so that the difference in the size of PCR products can be evaluated on gel easily. In the analysis of results, one should look for the strong specific bands seen on either gels. Faint nonspecific bands may be generated through weak priming, but they are usually very weak when the reaction conditions that we have optimized are used. The size of the HCV genotype-specific products are given in the footnote of **Table 1**. For example, in lanes 1 and 2, no specific product is detected in Mix 1 (upper panel), but a specific band of 209 bp is seen. (Note that the molecular-marker scale is enlarged and the PCR product band corresponds to the size of between 201 and 220.) Similarly, HCV genotype 1b samples only showed two bands of 234 bp in Mix 1 (lanes 3, 4); genotype 2a showed two bands (139 and 190 bp) in Mix 1 (with two different sense primers, lanes 5 and 6; genotype 2b showed a specific band of 337 bp in Mix 1 (lanes 7 and 8). Similar interpretation applied to genotype 3a (lanes 9 and 10; 232 bp in Mix 2), genotype 3b (lanes 11 and 12; 176 bp in Mix 1); genotype 4 (lane 13; 99 bp in Mix 2, a faint nonspecific band was also seen in this case); genotype 5a (lane 14; expected size of 320 bp in Mix 2); and genotype 6a (lane 15, 336 bp in Mix 2).

References

1. Choo, Q. L., Kuo, G., Weiner, A. J., Overby, L. R., Bradley, D. W., et al. (1989) Isolation of a cDNA clone derived from a blood-borne non-A, non-B viral hepatitis genome. *Science* **244,** 359–362.
2. Simmonds, P., Alberti, A., Alter, H. J., Bonino, F., Bradley, D. W., Brecho, T. C., et al. (1994) A proposed system for the nomenclature of hepatitis C viral genotypes. *Hepatology* **19,** 1321–1324.
3. Ohba, K., Mizokami, M., Ohno, T., Suzuki, K., Orito, E., Ina, Y., et al. (1995) Classification of hepatitis C virus into major types and subtypes based on molecular phylogenetic tree analysis. *Virus Res.* **36,** 201–214.
4. Ohno, T., Mizokami, M., Wu, R. R., Saleh, M. G., Ohba, K.-I., Orito, E., et al. (1997) New hepatitis C virus (HCV) genotyping system that allows for identification of HCV genotypes 1a, 1b, 2a, 2b, 3a, 3b, 4 5a, and 6a. *J. Clin. Microbiol.* **35,** 201–207.

14

Genotyping Hepatitis C Virus by Type-Specific Primers for PCR Based on NS5 Region

Kazuaki Chayama

1. Introduction

Hepatitis C virus (HCV), a flavi-like virus with a positive-sense, single-stranded genome RNA *(1–3)*, shows considerable variation in nucleotide sequences. These variations fall into a series of specific patterns and are the basis for classification of HCV into different types and genotypes *(4–9)*. Typing of HCV is of special interest because it has been suggested that different types or genotypes may cause different disease severities and show different sensitivity to interferon treatment *(10–12)*. The number of types and genotypes of HCV continue to increase with the description of new sequences particularly from southeast Asian countries *(13–16)*. More than 34 genotypes have been reported so far, and there is no doubt that the number will increase in the future with identification of new genotypes. Although there are several methods for determining the genotypes of HCV *(5, 17–19)*, it is impossible to determine all these genotypes by one method. However, the prevalence of HCV genotypes has been well studied in some countries, including Japan and the United States *(20–23)*. Detection of genotypes by polymerase chain reaction (PCR) using type-specific primers or probes is useful in this area where only a limited number of genotypes are known to exist. In this chapter, I describe a simple one-step PCR method to detect six major HCV genotypes (1a, 1b, 2a, 2b, 3a, and 3b) using genotype-specific primers based on the nucleotide sequences of the NS5 region.

2. Materials

1. Guanidine thiocyanate buffer: 4.2 M guanidine thiocyanate, 100 mM Tris-HCl, pH 7.5, 0.6% lauryl sarosine sodium salt.
2. Glycogen (20 g/L) in diluted water.

3. Dithiothreitol (DTT).
4. Phenol and chloroform.
5. RNase inhibitor (100 U/μL in 1 mM DTT, Takara Syuzo, Otsu, Japan).
6. Random primer (Takara Syuzo).
7. Reverse transcriptase (Gibco-BRL, Rockville, MD).
8. 5X reverse transcripitase buffer: 250 mM Tris-HCl, pH 8.3, 375 mM KCl, 15 mM MgCl$_2$.
9. Taq DNA polymerase (Promega, Madison, WI).
10. 10X PCR buffer: 10 mM Tris-HCl, pH 9.0, 50 mM KCl, 0.1% Triton X-100.
11. SeaKem GTG agarose (FMC BioProducts, Rockland, ME).
12. TAE buffer: 40 mM Tris-acetate, pH 8.0, 1 mM EDTA.
13. Primers:
    5'-CAGTCACTGAGAGCGACATCCGTACG-3' (for 1a)
    5'-AGGCCACTGCGGCCTGTCGAGCTGCGAA-3' (for 1b)
    5'-TATGTTCAACAGCAAGGGCCAGA-3' (for 2a)
    5'-GGCTTGTTCCCTGCCTCAAGAGGCCA-3' (for 2b)
    5'-CTCGGACCCTGACTTTCT-3' (for 3a)
    5'-CCGCGCTAGCGGCGTCTTGC-3' (for 3b)
    5'-CCTGGTCATAGCCTCCGTGAA-3' (antisense primer for all genotypes).
    Primers are purified by HPLC or column chromatography. All primers should be dissolved in distilled water at 0.1 mg/mL.
14. 1.5 mL silicon-coated polypropyrene sampling tubes.
15. Thermocycyler: e.g., Perkin-Elmer DNA thermal cycler 9600.

3. Methods

1. To a 1.5 mL sampling tube, add 100 μL of test serum sample, or negative (serum of a healthy individual) or positive control (positive serum for genotyping PCR), 4 μL of 2-mercaptoethanol, and 425 μL guanidine thiocyanate buffer (4.2 M guanidine thiocyanate, 100 mM Tris-HCl, pH 7.5, 0.6% N-lauryl sarcosine sodium salt). Guanidine buffer can be stored for several month, but fresh 2-mercaptoethanol should be added before use. Mix gently for 30 min at room temperature on a rotator or by hand. Extract RNA by adding 500 μL phenol/chloroform (1/1). Spin the mixture at 13,000 rpm (15,000g) for 5 min in a microcentrifuge at room temperature. Move supernatant to a next tube. Repeat this process three times, then add 500 μL chloroform. Move supernatant to a next tube. Precipitate RNA by adding 1/10 vol of 3 M sodium acetate and 2.5 volume of absolute ethanol with one microgram glycogen as a carrier. After cooling to –80°C for 5 min or –20°C for 20 min, centrifuge at 4°C for 30 min at 13,000 rpm (15,000g). Rinse the RNA pellet once with 1 mL of 70% ethanol and once with 1 mL of 100% ethanol. Dry the pellets by gentle suction. Dissolve the RNA pellet in 9 μL of RNase inhibitor (1 U/μL in 1 mM DTT). Care should be taken when diluting RNase inhibitor, since irreversible inactivation of this reagent may occur when diluted in the absence of more than 1 mM DTT. Alternatively, RNA extraction kits from commercial sources may be used,

although some of these are inappropriate for subsequent reverse transcription and PCR (see **Note 1**).
2. Reverse-transcribe RNA with random hexamer and reverse transcriptase. For this purpose, mix all necessary reagents according to the instructions of each reverse transcriptase. The following is an example using MMLV reverse transcriptase (Gibco-BRL).

Component	Amount (µL)
5X reverse transcriptase buffer	4
100 mM DTT	2
RNase inhibitor (100 U/L)	0.2
10 mM dNTP	2
Random primer (0.5 OD/25 L)	2
M-MLV reverse transcriptase (200 U/L)	1
Total	11.2

Prepare 1.2 times larger amount of a master mix than calculated for reverse transcription reaction for test samples and negative controls. Add 11.2 µL master mix to test sample and control (total volume 20.2 µL). Incubate for 30–60 min at 42 or 37°C depending on the preferred temperature of each reverse transcriptase. We have tested many commercial reverse transcriptases and almost all of them work well when used according to the instructions provided by each manufacturer. It should be cautioned that a particular reverse transcriptase does not work with buffers prepared for different reverse transcriptases.
3. Prepare a master mix solution of genotyping PCR sufficient for the number of test samples and negative controls. Do not add primers to this master mix.

Component	Amount (µL)
10X PCR	2.5
10 mM dNTP	0.5
25 mM MgCl$_2$	1.5
distilled water	q.s.
cDNA solution	1–5
Taq DNA polymerase (5 U/L)	0.13
Total	18.13

*Quantity sufficient to prepare a total volume of 18 µL.

We recommend preparing a master mix volume 1.2 times larger than required. In 0.5 mL microcentrifuge tubes, mix all necessary solutions, except the seven primers. Overlay the solution with mineral oil and preheat the tubes to 70°C.
4. Add 7 µL of the remaining seven primer mixtures (1 µL for each of the seven primers) through the thin layer of mineral oil (see **Note 2**). Alternatively, Taq Start (Clontech) can be used instead of manual hot starting. AmpliWax (Perkin-Elmer) can also be used, but in the latter instance, the total volume of PCR mixture should be increased to 50–100 µL to allow the upper layer solution to go down through the wax layer.

168

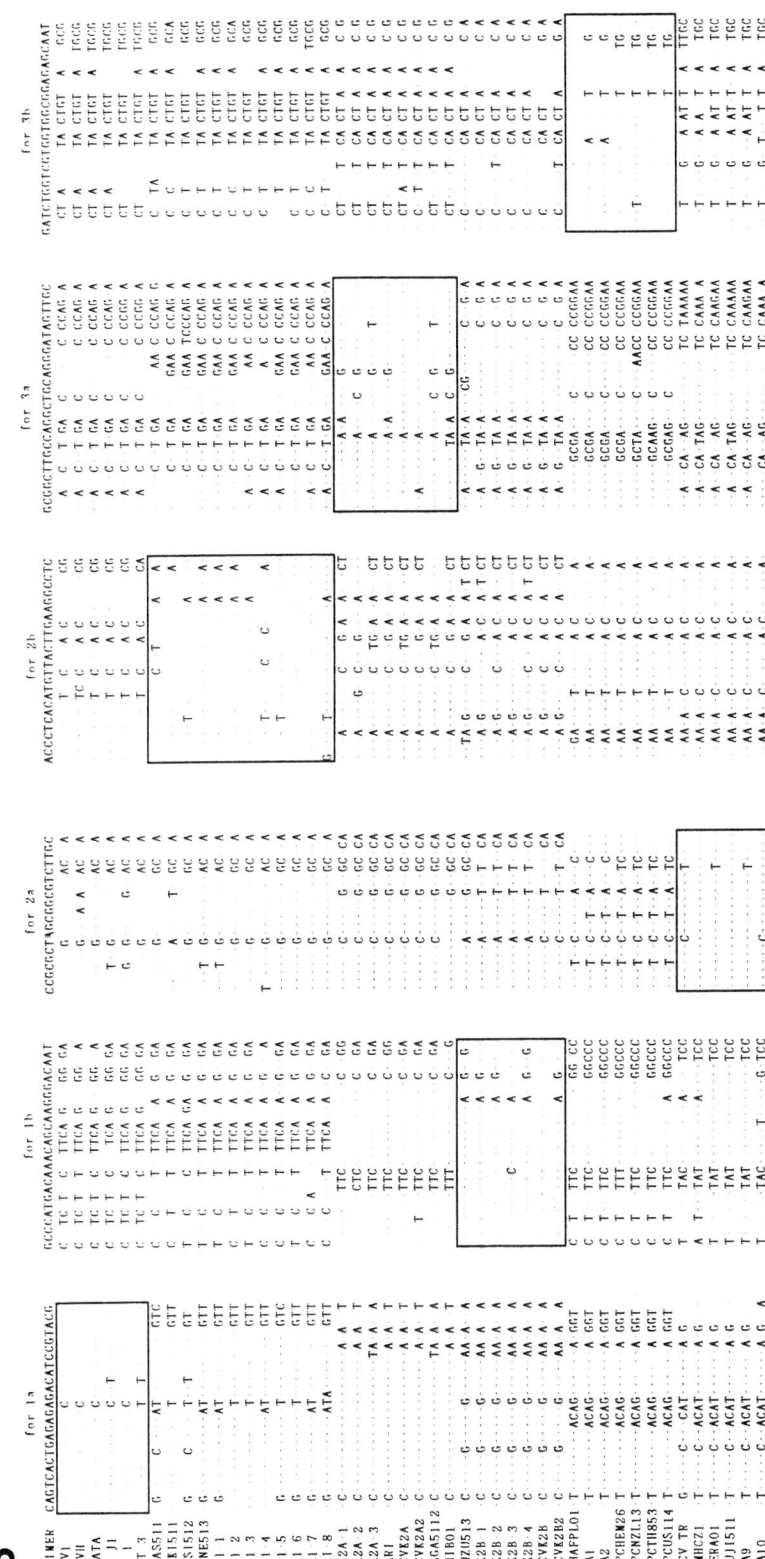

Fig. 1. (A) and (B) Examples of primer designs. Primers should be situated where characteristic features of the nucleotide sequence of each genotype allow only genotype-specific primer annealing. Nucleotide sequences of the primers are on the top of each row, and aligned nucleotide sequences of each genotypes are shown. Nucleotide sequences of target genotypes are shown in boxes.

5. Run PCR reaction as follows, 10 cycles of amplifications at 94°C for 1 min, 61°C for 1 min, 72°C for 1 min, followed by 30 cycles of amplification at 90°C for 0.5 min, 59°C for 1 min, 72°C for 1 min, and final extension at 72°C for 7 min (*see* **Note 3**).
6. Mix 10 µL of the PCR products with bromo-phenol-blue/glycerol solution and run on 3% agarose gel in TAE buffer (40 mM Tris-acetate, pH 8.0, 1 mM EDTA) (*see* **Notes 4–6**).

4. Notes

1. RNA extraction should be done very carefully. Since this method employs only a single-step PCR, obtain as much as good quality RNA and cDNA as is necessary for satisfactory results.
2. This method can be expanded to detect other genotypes present in the area of interest. Primer design is essential for the detection of genotypes by PCR. Each selected primer should be situated on a domain of the target genotype where characteristic sequence features would allow only genotype-specific primer annealing. Furthermore, the 3' end of each primer is positioned on the first or second letter of the codon because mutations at the third letter of the codon, are frequently observed (**Fig. 1**). Each primer should also be positioned on a different domain, so that one can determine the genotype by simply comparing the size of the amplified DNA fragments (**Fig. 2**). One may design primers for another genotype based on similar considerations. However, whether the designed primers work well or not should be confirmed using plasmids or phage clones of known genotypes (**Fig. 3**).
3. The above 40-cycle PCR has a good sensitivity sufficient to detect the genotype of samples containing approx 1000 molecules of single-stranded M13 phage DNA of each genotype.
4. Some samples may show negative results, although they contain a sufficient quantity of HCV RNA. This may be owing to a mismatch of the primer at its 3'-end that happens to present on the target sequence. One may determine the genotype of such samples using different sets of primers. However, only one nucleotide substitution does not prevent detection, since extension of such primer actually occurs because of a lack of proofreading activity of *Taq* DNA polymerase. In our laboratory, the detection rate of the six major genotypes is usually more than 90% when the primer set described in this chapter is used.
5. Three to four percent agarose gel can be used to determine genotypes. Agarose gels designed to separate low-mol-wt DNA fragment (e.g., Nusieve GTG agarose, FMC BioProducts, ME or similar products) can be added to allow easy preparation of high concentration gels.
6. In addition to the problem of detecting small amounts of DNA, care should be taken to prevent contamination during PCR. The contamination prevention measures recommended by Kwok and Higuchi *(24)* should be strictly applied.

Type-Specific Primers

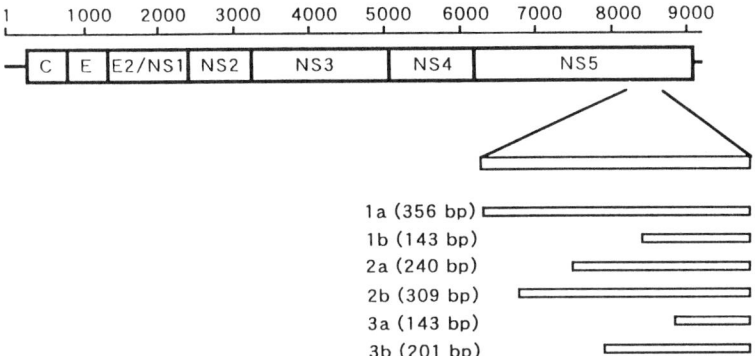

Fig. 2. Schematic representation of DNA fragments amplified by genotyping PCR. Nucleotide sequence numbers of HCV are shown at the top. Expected sizes of DNA fragments are shown on the bottom.

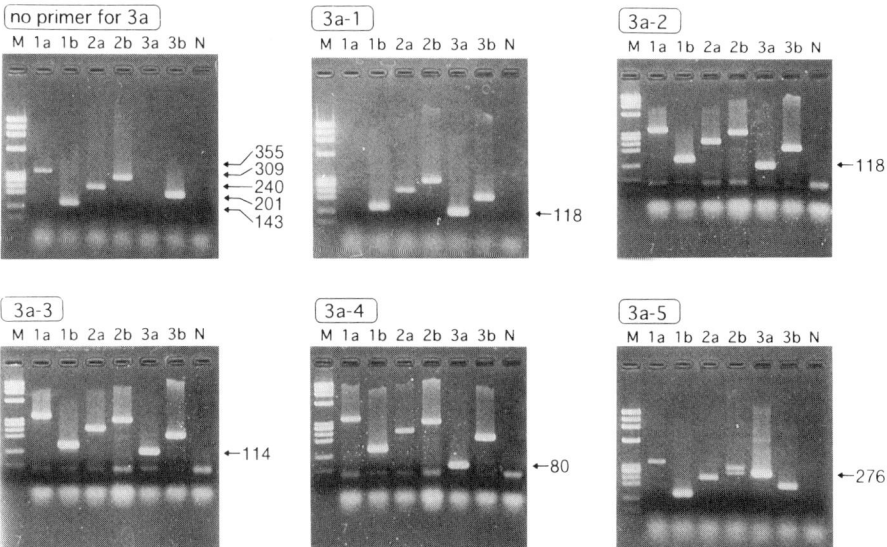

Fig. 3. Examples of tests where designed primers work appropriately as a mixed primer in genotyping PCR *(21)*. About 1000 molecules of M13 clones of each genotype were used as template (1a–3b in each lane). *M*; molecular wt size marker φX174 DNA digested with *Hae*III, N: negative control. "no primer for 3a," PCR without any primer for genotype 3a, 3a-1–3a-5, tests for five primers for genotype 3a. Note that no band can be seen in lane 1a in 3a-1 and doublet band in lane 2b in 3a-5. These combinations of primers should be avoided. Expected sizes of genotypes 1a, 1b, 2a, 2b and 3b are shown on the right in "no primer for 3a," and those of 3a are shown in 3a-1–3a-5.

References

1. Choo, Q.-L., Kuo, G., Weiner, A. J., et al. (1989). Isolation of a cDNA clone from a blood borne non-A, non-B hepatitis genome. *Science* **244,** 359–362.
2. Inchauspe, G., Zebedee, S., Lee, D. H., et al. (1991) Genomic structure of the human prototype strain H of hepatitis C virus: comparison with American and Japanese isolates. *Proc. Natl. Acad. Sci. USA* **88,** 10,292–10,296.
3. Kato, N., Hijikata, M., Ootsuyama, Y., et al. (1990). Molecular cloning of the human hepatitis C virus genome from Japanese patients with non-A, non-B hepatitis. *Proc. Natl. Acad. Sci. USA* **87,** 9524–9528.
4. Enomoto, N., Takada, A., Nakao, T., and Date, T. (1990) There are two major types of hepatitis C virus in Japan. *Biochem. Biophys. Res. Commun.* **170,** 1021–1025.
5. Chayama, K., Tsubota, A., Arase, Y., et al. (1993) Genotypic subtyping of hepatitis C virus. J. Gastroenterol. *Hepatology* **8,** 150–156.
6. Mori, S., Kato, N., Yagyu, A., et al. (1992) A new type of hepatitis C virus in patients in Thailand. *Bichem. Biophys. Res. Commun.* **183,** 334–342.
7. Cha, T. A., Beall, E., Irvine, B., et al. (1992) At least five related, but distinct hepatitis C viral genotype exist. *Proc. Natl. Acad. Sci. USA* **89,** 7144–7148.
8. Bukh, J., Purcell, R., and Miller, R. H. (1993) At least 12 genotypes of hepatitis C virus predicted by sequence analysis of the putative E1 gene of isolates collected worldwide. *Proc. Natl. Acad. Sci. USA* **90,** 8234–8238.
9. Simmonds, P., Holmes, E., Cha, T., et al. (1993) Classification of hepatitis C virus into six major genotypes and a series of subtypes by phylogenetic analysis of the NS-5 region. *J. Gen.Virol.* **74,** 2391–2399.
10. Tsubota, A., Chayama, K., Ikeda, K., et al. (1994) Factors predictive of response to interferon-alpha therapy in hepatitis C virus infection. *Hepatology* **19,** 1088–1094.
11. Kohara, M., Tanaka, T., Tsukiyama-Kohara, K., et al. (1996) Hepatitis C virus genotypes 1 and 2 respond to interferon-alpha with different virologic kinetics. *J. Infect. Dis.* **172,** 934–938.
12. Chayama, K., Tsubota, A., Arase, Y., et al. (1995) Genotype, slow decrease in virus titer during interferon treatment and high degree of sequence variability of hypervariable region are indicative of poor response to interferon treatment in patients with chronic hepatitis type C. *J. Hepatol.* **23,** 648–653.
13. Tokita, H., Shrestha, S. M., Okamoto, H., et al. (1994) Hepatitis C virus variants from Nepal with novel genotypes and their classification into the third major group. *J. Gen. Virol.* **75,** 931–936.
14. Tokita, H., Okamoto, H., Tsuda, F., et al. (1994) Hepatitis C virus variants from Vietnam are classifiable into the seventh, eighth, and ninth major genetic groups. *Proc. Natl. Acad. Sci. USA* **91,** 11,022–11,026.
15. Tokita, H., Okamoto, H., Tsuda, F., et al. (1995) Hepatitis C virus variants from Thailand classifiable into five novel genotypes in the sixth (6b), seventh (7c,7d) and ninth (9b,9c) major genetic groups. *J. Gen. Virol.* **76,** 2329–2335.
16. Tokita, H., Okamoto, H., Iizuka, H., et al. (1996) Hepatitis C virus variants from Jakarta, Indonesia classifiable into novel genotype in the second (2e and 2f), tenth (10a) and eleventh (11a) genetic groups. *J. Gen. Virol.* **77,** 293,301.

17. Okamoto, H., Sugiyama, Y., Okada, S., et al. (1992) Typing hepatitis C virus by polymerase chain reaction with type-specific primers: application to clinical surveys and tracing infectious sources. *J. Gen. Virol.* **73,** 673–679.
18. Okamoto, H., Tokita, H., Sakamoto, M., et al. (1993) Characterization of the genomic sequence of type V (or 3a) hepatitis C virus isolates and PCR primers for specific detection. *J. Gen. Virol.* **74,** 2385–2390.
19. Nakao, T., Enomoto, N., Takada, N., et al. (1991) Typing of hepatitis C virus genomes by restriction fragment length polymorphism. *J. Gen. Virol.* **72,** 2105–2112.
20. Stuyver, L., Rossau, R., Wyseur, A., et al. (1993) Typing of hepatitis C virus isolates and characterization of new subtypes using a line probe assay. *J. Gen. Virol.* **74,** 1093–1102.
21. Hashimoto, M., Chayama, K., Tsubota, A., et al. (1996) Typing six major hepatitis C virus genotypes by polymerase chain reaction using primers derived from nucleotide sequences of the NS5 region. *Intern. Hepatol. Commun.* **4,** 263–267.
22. Pontisso, P., Ruvoletto, M. G., Nicoletti, M., et al. (1995) Distribution of three major hepatitis C virus genotypes in Italy. A multicentre study of 495 patients with chronic hepatitis C. *J. Viral. Hepatol.* **2,** 33–38.
23. Lau, J. Y. N., Davis, G. L., Prescott, L. E., et al. (1996) Distribution of hepatitis C virus genotypes determined by line probe assay in patients with chronic hepatitis C seen at tertiary referral centers in the United States. Hepatitis Interventional Therapy Group. *Ann. Intern. Med.* **124,** 868–876.
24. Kwok, S. and Higuchi, R. (1989) Avoiding false positives with PCR. *Nature* **339,** 237,238.

15

Determination of HCV Genotypes by RFLP

Fiona Davidson and Peter Simmonds

1. Introduction

Several different methods have been developed for the typing of HCV variants: direct sequence analysis, slot-blot hybridization analysis of reverse transcriptase-polymerase chain reaction (RT-PCR) products using cDNA probes specific to each HCV genotype and PCR amplification using type-specific primers that are designed to match only virus sequences of a defined HCV type and will fail to amplify sequences of other types. An alternative method is the nonselective amplification of virus cDNA using conserved primers followed by restriction fragment length polymorphisms (RFLP). The coding regions of the HCV genome are highly variable, so reliable amplification of different HCV genotypes with the same set of primers is difficult. For this reason, typing methods based on analysis of amplified DNA are more reliable if carried out in the highly conserved 5' noncoding region (5' NCR). Different typing assays are discussed in Chapters 14, 16, and 17. The RFLP assay method described in the following section has been developed to enable the detection HCV genotypes 1–6 *(1)*. The advantages that this particular method offers are that it is relatively easy to carry out, the apparatus required is generally available in most laboratories or is inexpensive to buy and a large number of samples can be genotyped at the same time as those being tested by PCR in the laboratory. The major problem associated with the technique is the possible misidentification of novel subtypes of HCV type 6 as type 1 variants *(2)*. In addition, it is not possible to identify HCV subtypes without carrying out a further set of restriction digests *(3)*.

2. Materials

1. Microcentrifuge tubes, 0.5 and 1.5 mL (Alpha Laboratories Limited, Eastleigh, Hants, UK).

2. Ultraflux tubes, 0.2 mL (Scotlab Limited, Coatbridge, Strathclyde, Scotland).
3. Pastettes, 1 mL (Alpha Laboratories Limited).
4. Phenol, water-saturated (Rathburn Chemicals Ltd., Walkerburn, Scotland).
5. Chloroform (Merck Ltd., Poole, Dorset, UK).
6. Ethanol, (Rathburn Chemicals Ltd.).
7. TNE solution: 4 M sodium chloride, final concentration 0.11 M, 1 M Tris (hydroxymethyl)-methylamine, pH 8.0, final concentration 55 mM (Merck Ltd.), 0.2 M EDTA, pH 8.0, final concentration 1.1 M, 10% SDS, final concentration 0.55% (Sigma-Aldrich Company Ltd., Poole, Dorset, UK).
8. Di-ethylpyrocarbonate (DEPC)-treated water (DEPC supplied by Sigma-Aldrich Co. Ltd.). Add 500 µL DEPC to 1 L of water, and leave to stand at room temperature for 2 h before autoclaving.
9. Sodium acetate: Make a stock solution of 3 M sodium acetate (Sigma-Aldrich Co. Ltd.).
10. Isoamylalcohol (Merck Ltd.).
11. Proteinase K (Boehringer Mannheim UK Ltd., UK). Make a stock of 10 mg/mL and store frozen at $-20°C$ in 1 mL aliquots. Thaw the aliquot immediately prior to use and do not refreeze.
12. 10X RT buffer: 500 mM Tris-HCl, pH 8.0, 50 mM magnesium chloride, 50 mM DTT, 500 mM potassium chloride, 0.5 mg/mL bovine serum albumin (BSA).
13. RT (Promega UK Ltd., Southampton, UK).
14. RNasin (Promega UK Ltd.).
15. Polyadenylic acid (Poly A): Make a stock solution of 2 mg/mL and store frozen at $-20°C$ (Boehringer Mannheim UK Ltd.).
16. 10X *Taq* polymerase buffer (containing magnesium) (Promega UK Ltd.).
17. *Taq* polymerase (Promega UK Ltd.).
18. Nucleoside triphosphates: 3-mM and 4-mM stock solutions should be made containing each of dATP, dGTP, dTTP, and dCTP, and frozen in aliquots of 100 µL (Boehringer Mannheim UK Ltd.).
19. 5' NCR oligonucleotide primers (Oswell DNA Service, Southampton, UK). These should be diluted to give a stock of 100 M.
    (939) Outer sense 5'-CTGTGAGGAACTACTGTCTT- 3'
    (209) Outer antisense 5'-ATACTCGAGGTGCACGGTCTACGAGACCT- 3'
    (940) Inner sense 5'-TTCACGCAGAAAGCGTCTAG- 3'
    (211) Inner antisense 5'-CACTCTCGAGCACCCTATCAGGCAGT- 3'
20. Mol-wt markers: DNA mol-wt marker VIII (Boehringer Mannheim, UK Ltd.).
21. Liquid paraffin (Thornton and Ross, Huddersfield, UK).
22. Pipet tips (Alpha Laboratories).
23. Dimethylsulfoxide DMSO (Sigma-Aldrich Co. Ltd.).
24. 10X TBE buffer: 1.3 M Tris base, 0.68 M boric acid, 0.025 M EDTA, pH 8.5.
25. Agarose (Flowgen Instruments Ltd., Sittingbourne, Kent, UK).
26. Metaphor agarose (Flowgen Instruments Ltd.).
27. Ethidium bromide (Sigma-Aldrich Co. Ltd.).
28. Restriction enzymes: *Hae*III, *Rsa*I, *Hinf*I, *Mva*I (Boehringer Mannheim UK Ltd.).
29. Tegador (Mackay & Lynn, Edinburgh, Scotland).

3. Methods

3.1. Extraction of Viral RNA from Plasma

1. Prepare a solution of extraction buffer. 9 vol TNE buffer: 1 vol proteinase K (10 mg/mL), and 20 µL/mL Poly A (2 mg/mL). For 12 tubes, this is 4.5 mL TNE buffer, 500 µL proteinase K, and 100 µL Poly A.
2. Preincubate the solution for 10 min at 37°C.
3. Dispense 400 µL of extraction buffer into a 0.5 mL Eppendorf tube and add 100 µL of plasma.
4. Incubate for 1.5–2 h at 37°C, in a waterbath.
5. Spin tubes briefly to bring down condensation from the lids.
6. Add 450 µL phenol to each tube. Vortimix for 5 min.
7. Centrifuge at 15,000 rpm (15,000g) for 5 min to separate the phases.
8. Transfer aqueous (top) layer using a gilson pipetteman to a fresh tube containing 450 µL chloroform/isoamyl alcohol (50:1) (make up fresh for each extraction set). Vortimix for 5 min.
9. Centrifuge at 15,000 rpm (15,000g) for 5 min.
10. Place 40 µL 3 M sodium acetate, pH 5.2, in a 0.5-mL Eppendorf tube. Transfer 400 µL of aqueous (top) layer using a gilson pipetman.
11. Add 600 µL of 100% ethanol (kept at –20°C) to each tube, and mix by inverting the tub (do not vortimix).
12. Precipitate nucleic acids overnight at –20°C.
13. Prepare the nucleic acid by centrifugation of the tubes at 15,000 rpm (15,000g) at 4°C for 10 min.
14. Discard the supernatant, and wash the pellet with 600 µL 80% ethanol. Centrifuge again for 5 min at 15,000 rpm (15,000g) to prevent loss of pellet.
15. Remove supernatant and dry pellet at 42°C then dissolve in 25 µL of DEPC-treated H_2O. (It is best to carry out the RT reaction immediately after preparing the nucleic acid, since freezing and thawing can result in a loss in sensitivity.) Five milliliters of this product are then used in the RT reaction.

3.2. Reverse Transcriptase Reaction

1. Reverse transcription is performed by specific viral primer-initiated cDNA synthesis. cDNA synthesis is carried out by adding 5 µL of the extracted RNA to 15 µL of reaction mix composed of 1 µL outer antisense primer (209), 2 µL 10X reverse transcription buffer, 3 µL 4 mM dNTPs, 3 µL DMSO, 4.5 µL DEPC dH_2O, 10 U of reverse transcriptase; 10 U of RNasin (the volume of DEPC dH_2O may have to be ajusted to give a total volume of 15 µL of reaction mix to be added to the 5 µL of nucleic acid). It is easiest to make up a reaction mix for the total number of samples to be tested then aliquot the appropriate volume into each tube.
2. The mix is then incubated at 42°C for 30 min. (It is best to carry out the PCR reaction immediately after the reverse transcription step, since freezing and thawing may cause a loss in sensitivity.)

3.3. PCR Amplification

1. For the amplification of HCV, a modified hot-start nested PCR method is employed. Prepare PCR mix containing, 1X Promega *Taq* buffer (1:10 dilution), 3.3 µM each of dGTP, dATP, dCTP, and dTTP (a 1:100 dilution of the 3 mM stock), 0.5 µM of each of the outer primers (209 and 939) (1:200 dilution of stock); and 20 U/mL *Taq* polymerase. Forty-five microliters of mix should be aliquoted into the Ultraflux PCR tubes, and two drops of liquid paraffin layered on top.
2. These are then placed in the PCR machine and heated to 80°C for 2 min. This temperature is maintained while 5 µL of cDNA from the RT reaction is added to each tube.
3. The tubes are then closed, and the PCR reaction steps immediately started without allowing the temperature of the tubes to drop below 80°C.
4. Twenty-five rounds of amplification are carried out consisting of 18 s at 94°C, 21 s at 50°C, and 90 s at 72°C. This is followed by a final cycle of 7 min at 72°C.
5. One microliter of this first-round amplification product is then transferred to a new Ultraflux tube and 19 µL of PCR mix (as described in **step 1**), but containing inner primers 211 and 940 added and mixed by pipeting. A further 25 cycles of amplification are carried out using the same times and temperatures as for the first-round reaction. (The remaining 19 µL of first-round PCR product can be stored at –20°C.)

3.4. Visualization of Amplified Product

1. The amplified PCR product is visualized by running the second-round amplification product on a 2% agarose gel stained with ethidium bromide. To prepare a gel, dissolve 6 g of agarose in 300 mL 1X TBE buffer, and heat until dissolved (this can be carried out in a microwave oven). The gel should then be allowed to cool to approx 50°C and 10 µL of ethidium bromide (0.5 µg/µL) should be added, and the gel should be poured onto a preleveled electrophoresis plate and allowed to set for about 30 min, at room temperature. The secondary PCR product (20 µL) is loaded into the wells of the gel along with mol-wt marker.
2. The electrophoresis is carried out at 150 V for 20 min. The positive PCR products identified as a discrete band of 251 bp in size and are visualised by UV light.

3.5. HCV Genotyping

1. Following identification of a positive sample, the corresponding first-round PCR product should be retrieved. A second-round PCR should be carried out as described in **Subheading 3.3., step 5**. with the modification that the total reaction volume should be 50 µL for each sample to be genotyped.
2. On completion of the PCR, the 50-µL volume should be split into two separate 0.5-mL Eppendorf tubes each containing 25 µL. The whole sample is then digested using a combination of two sets of different enzymes in a final reaction volume of 30 µL.
3. Again it is easiest to prepare a reaction mix for the total number of samples and then aliquot the appropriate volume into each tube. For each sample, one digestion

Fig. 1
Cleavage with *Hae*III/*Rsa*I

HCV Genotype

a	44		58			114/5		9	26
b		102				114/5		9	26
c	44	12	46		58		56	9	26
d	44	12	46			114		9	26
e	56		46			114		9	26
f	33		69			114		9	26
g	33	23	46			114		9	26
h	44	12	46			117		9	26

[a]Predicted association of different cleavage patterns of the 5'-NCR with sequences of HCV types 1–6. Location of cleavage sites indicated by vertical lines in the left-hand box. The position of 1- or 2-bp insertions found in some 5'-NCR sequences by cross-hatching. Expected size of fragments shown in basepairs.

set is carried out using a mix of 3 µL of restriction enzyme buffer (1.5 µL of buffer M + 1.5 µL buffer L supplied by Boehringer Mannheim), 1 µL of *Hae*III enzyme (10 U/µL), 1 µL *Rsa*I enzyme (10 U/µL). (Restriction enzymes should be stored at –20°C at all times, and the reaction mix held on ice and used immediately once prepared). Five microliters of this mix are then added to one aliquot of the 25 µL sample to be genotyped. For the second digestion set, prepare a mix of 3 µL of restriction enzyme buffer (3.0 µL of buffer H), 1 µL *Mva*I (10 U/µL); 1 µL *Hinf*I (10 U/µL). Add 5 µL of this mix to the second aliquot of amplified PCR product.

4. Incubate the tubes at 37°C for a minimum of 2 h (an overnight incubation can be carried out).

3.6. Identification of Genotypes

1. Prepare a 4% Metaphor agarose gel by dissolving 12 g of Metaphor agarose in 300 mL of 1X TBE, and add ethidium bromide and prepare gel as described in **Subheading 3.4., step 1**.
2. Load the whole 30 µL digested sample onto the gel along with mol-wt markers and electrophorese for 1 h at 150 V. It is difficult to obtain a marker with an appropriate range of sizes. However, once the patterns have been identified, these can then be used as internal markers.

4. Notes

1. The predicted fragment sizes corresponding to the different genotypes is shown in **Figs. 1** and **2**. The pattern of bands obtained on running the cleaved products on a metaphor gel are shown in **Fig. 3A,B**. It is sometimes difficult to visualize

Fig. 2
Cleavage with Mval/HinfI

A	53	63	41	94
B	53	63	44	94
C	53	56	142/3	
D	53	198		

[a]Predicted association of different cleavage patterns of the 5'-NCR with sequences of HCV types 1–6. Location of cleavage sites indicated by vertical lines in the left-hand box. The position of 1- or 2-bp insertions found in some 5'-NCR sequences by cross-hatching. Expected size of fragments shown in basepairs.

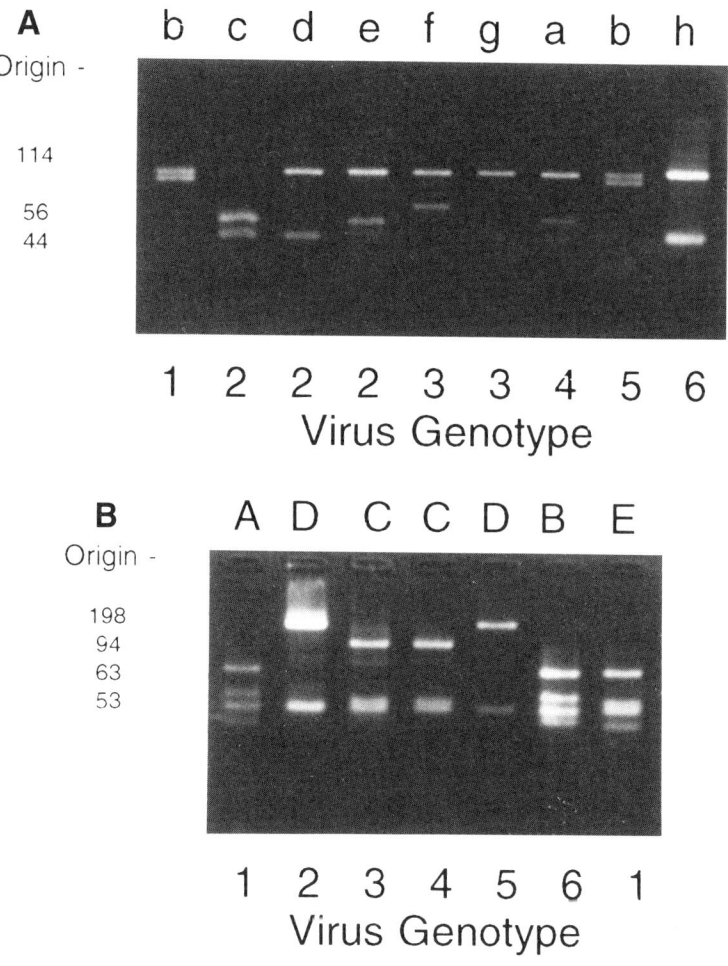

Fig. 3. Restriction patterns obtained by restriction endonuclease digestion of RT-PCR amplified 5'-NCR sequences with **(A)** HaeIII/RsaI and **(B)** MvaI/HinfI: letters correspond to patterns classified in **Figs. 1** and **2**.

the smaller fragments (i.e., the 26- and 9-bp fragments). However, the identification of all six genotypes can be made reliably from the combination of both restriction digests.

HCV genotype	HaeIII/RsaI pattern	MvaI/HinfI pattern
1	a or b	A
2	c, d, or e	D
3	f or g	C
4	a or b	C
5	b	D
6	h	B

2. The pattern corresponding to HCV type 6 is probably the most difficult to identify, since it relies on the identification of a 3-bp size difference to distinguish pattern h (for type 6) from pattern d (for type 2). However, the MvaI/HinfI digest would clarify the genotype determination.

References

1. McOmish, F., Yap, P. L., Down, B. C., Follett, E. A. C., Seed, C., Keller, A. J., et al. (1994) Geographical distribution of hepatitis C virus genotypes in blood donors: an international collaborative survey. *J. Clin. Microbiol.* **32,** 884–892.
2. Mellor, J., Walsh, E. A., Prescott, L., Jarvis, L. M., Davidson, F., Yap, P. L., et al. (1996) Survey of type 6 group variants of hepatitis C virus in Southeast Asia by using a core-based genotyping assay. *J. Clin. Microbiol.* **34(2),** 417–423.
3. Davidson, F., Simmonds, P., Ferguson, J. C., Jarvis, L. M., Dow, B. C., et al. (1995) Survey of major genotypes and subtypes of hepatitis C virus using RFLP of sequences amplified from the 5' non-coding region. *J. Gen. Virol.* **76,** 1197–1204.
4. Smith, D. B., Mellor, J., Jarvis, L. M., Davidson, F., Kolberg, J., Urdea, M., et al. (1995) Variation of the hepatitis C virus 5' non-coding region: implications for secondary structure, virus detection and typing. *J. Gen. Virol.* **76,** 1749–1761.

16

HCV Genotyping by the Line Probe Assay INNO-LiPA HCV II

Geert Maertens and Lieven Stuyver

1. Introduction

Hepatitis C viruses (HCVs) constitute a highly variable genus within the Flaviviridae, with closest homology to the hepatitis G and GB viruses, and Pestiviruses. The positive-stranded RNA genome encodes a polyprotein which is co- and posttranslationally cleaved into at least nine proteins: Core, E1, and E2 (the structural proteins) and NS2, NS3, NS4A, NS4B, NS5A, and NS5B (the nonstructural [NS] proteins). A theoretical protein of 7 kDa (tp7) may be processed from the carboxy terminal E2 region *(1)*.

The NS5B region encodes an RNA-dependent RNA polymerase that lacks proofreading activity. Consequently, many different, but closely related variants are generated within the infected patient. Since as many as 2.4×10^{13} genomes may be produced/year, ample opportunity exists for variant genomes incorporating advantageous mutations to emerge. Such mutants always appear spontaneously, but their fitness highly depends on the host's immune response or on the therapy received. The accumulation of such minor differences over time cause isolates to drift phylogenetically. Over time (hundreds to thousands of years), these processes gave rise to multiple genotypes. Currently, 11 types, including over 90 subtypes, have been identified *(1)*.

1.1. Clinical Importance of HCV Genotypes

Evidence has now accumulated from a large number of studies teaching that HCV genotype is correlated with response to interferon alpha (IFN-α) therapy *(2)*. Percentages of long-term response have been calculated for some of the most prevalent HCV genotypes in several studies *(3–6)*, with the exception of genotype 4 for which only preliminary data are available *(7)*. Subtype 1b and type 4-infected patients respond poorly (<8%) to IFN-α, subtype 1a shows a markedly better response rate as compared with subtype 1b (15–20%), but complete responses are seen in over 30% of patients infected with subtypes 2 or 3a. Subtype 2c infections are sometimes referred to as having a poor response to IFN-α *(8)*, but this has only been documented in one small study of eight subtype 2c infected patients *(9)*. Larger studies are needed to investigate whether clinical differences exist between type 2 subtypes.

Recently, results from the first IFN-α/Ribavirin combination trials *(10)* indicated increased responses for all HCV genotypes to combination treatment as compared with IFN- monotherapy, with similar relative differences maintained between HCV genotypes. Multiple variables often seem to be associated with response to IFN therapy after univariate analysis, but from studies that included multivariate analyses, the predictive value of HCV genotype was independent from either viremia level, age, etiology, duration of disease, or histology *(3–6)*.

As concluded from the studies at King's College (London), subtype 1b infections show a fast recurrence and progression toward chronic active hepatitis and cirrhosis in the liver graft. Also, type 4 infections seem to be associated with severe recurrence, but this observation could not yet be demonstrated statistically *(11,12)*. As stated by Féray et al. *(13)*, an intrinsic property of subtype 1b is involved in the severe pathogenicity after transplantation. Both the incidence and severity of recurrence were similarly reduced for subtypes 1a and 2a as compared to subtype 1b infections *(14)*. In addition to specific genotypes, mixed infections also seem to be associated with unfavorable outcome of disease. As a first approach, HCV genotyping may allow confirmation of the suspicion of patient-to-patient transmission, especially when multiple cases are involved, as demonstrated for a subtype 1a infection in New South Wales by Chant and coworkers *(15)*. Furthermore, genotype 2 infection is associated with type II cryoglobulinemia, especially in cases with apparently benign liver disease or cases with autoantibodies *(16)*.

These data confirm the existence of major clinical differences between HCV subtypes and emphasize the need for sophisticated subtyping methods. Subtyping will be required not only for the initiation and monitoring of therapy, but also for the choice of vaccine and further follow-up of vaccinees.

1.2. Analysis of HCV Isolates

HCV diversity can be studied according to three different approaches. The quasispecies nature of a given isolate is investigated by analysis of the E2 hypervariable region I. Such analysis is performed by sequence determination of multiple clones of an RT-PCR fragment obtained from the E2 HVR I or by single-stranded conformation polymorphism (SSCP) analysis of such a PCR fragment. The extend of quasispecies diversity seems to be associated with response to IFN treatment *(17)* and with severity of liver disease *(18)*. The technique is also useful to investigate the relatedness of HCV isolates, e.g., in hospital infections *(19)*, but cannot be employed to determine the HCV genotype because of the high variability in this region of the HCV genome. A second approach is the thorough study of HCV isolates with the purpose of their classification into genotypes. To this end, isolates are first screened by routine genotyping systems (*see* **Subheading 1.3.**), and isolates showing aberrant results are submitted to sequence determination and phylogenetic analysis. According to international guidelines *(20)*, at least two regions of the genome have to be analyzed before assignment of the subtype name. Such analysis of the C/E1 region of >579 bp and an NS5B region of >329 bp allows classification of >99.8% of isolates studied so far *(21,22)*. For the rapid genotype determination in a routine clinical laboratory (third approach), other more user-friendly techniques are required.

1.3. Routine Genotyping of HCV Isolates

Since routine sequence analysis of larger genomic regions is extremely laborious, many laboratories have developed more rapid genotyping methodologies. Crucial to the development of genotyping assays is the choice of the genomic region to be analyzed. First of all, the region must contain subtype- and type-specific motifs, which faithfully represent the diversity of the entire genome. Secondly sufficient conservation within the subtype is essential for the development of sensitive and specific primers or probes, but sufficient variability is needed to allow discrimination between subtypes. Furthermore, variability of the region to be analyzed should be sufficiently low to allow PCR amplification of all HCV genotypes.

The 5'-NCR is highly conserved, yet contains multiple genotype-specific motifs distributed over seven small variable regions, the analysis of which allows discrimination of over a hundred different genotype-specific sequences *(23)*. The sequence motifs are highly conserved within the genotype; therefore, genotyping in the 5'-NCR is very sensitive and specific. Furthermore, the region is routinely amplified for the detection of HCV RNA, and thus, the same amplicon can be conveniently analyzed in a genotyping assay. On the other hand, the low variability of this region does not always allow discrimination of all genotypes. The Core and NS5B regions are mildly conserved. These regions offer more possibilities for differentiation between different subtypes, yet their high degree of variability renders the respective methods less sensitive, especially if only 1 probe/subtype is used. Current methods for routine subtyping employ different ways of analyzing PCR fragments. Methodologies include type-specific amplification of the Core or NS5B regions, or analysis of 5'-NCR, core, or NS5B fragments by hybridization to type-specific probes (line probe assay [LiPA*]), or by RFLP.

1.4. The Line Probe Assay (LiPA)

A particular kind of reverse hybridization assays, called LiPA, were developed at Innogenetics, which allow an easy and fast determination of multiple genetic variations, as has been documented for HCV genotyping *(24)*. New assays have recently been developed for HLA class I A, B, and C typing, HIV reverse transcriptase drug resistance *(25)*, and for determination of HBV genotypes *(26)* and precore mutants.

1.5. Test Principle

The INNO-LiPA HCV II employs the distinction of 5'-NCR polymorphisms specific for the different HCV genotypes. In the prototype assay *(24)*, probes of 16 nucleotides were tailed with a poly(T)-tail by terminal deoxynucleotidyl transferase and attached to nitrocellulose membranes (*see* **Note 1**; *27*). Biotin-labeled PCR products are reversely hybridized to the probes on the strip (**Fig. 1**). The biotin group can be incorporated by addition of biotinylated dUTP or a 5'-biotinylated primer during PCR. Usually, nested PCR with biotinylated primers is performed on fragments previously generated for the purpose of HCV RNA detection. Alternatively, biotin compounds can be incorporated during HCV RNA detection. Biotinylated amplicons can be readily transferred to the LiPA procedure. The labeled PCR product obtained from the 5'-NCR will only hybridize to a probe (or line) perfectly matching the sequence of the isolate, allowing stringent discrimination at the subtype level. Such a high specificity can be obtained by using very stringent hybridization conditions ($50 \pm 0.5°C$). Consequently, a 100% correlation with 5'-NCR sequences could be demonstrated (*see* **Note 2**; *28–31*). After an isothermal stringent wash, the presence of probe/amplicon–biotin hybrids is revealed by an alkaline phosphatase-labeled streptavidin conjugate. The captured enzyme converts NBT and BCIP into a purple color, which uncovers the sequence of part of the 5'-NCR of the isolate studied (**Fig. 1**).

A first-generation kit (INNO-LiPA™ HCV, Innogenetics, Gent, Belgium) already discriminated genotypes 1a, 1b, 2a, 2b, 3a, 3b, 4, and 5a. A second-generation test (INNO-LiPA™ HCV II, Innogenetics, Gent, Belgium) is now available, which allows better discrimination of types 1–6 and subtypes 1a, 1b, 2a/c, 2b, 2d, 2i, 3a–c, 4a–h, 5a, 6a, and 10a. Some cases have been detected which displayed aberrant LiPA reactivity patterns. In the majority of such cases, typing is possible, but no subtype can be deduced. After sequencing of the NS5B and core/E1 regions, such aberrant LiPA II reactivity patterns could be linked to new subtypes *(23,32,33)*. Although the use of the 5'-NCR allows

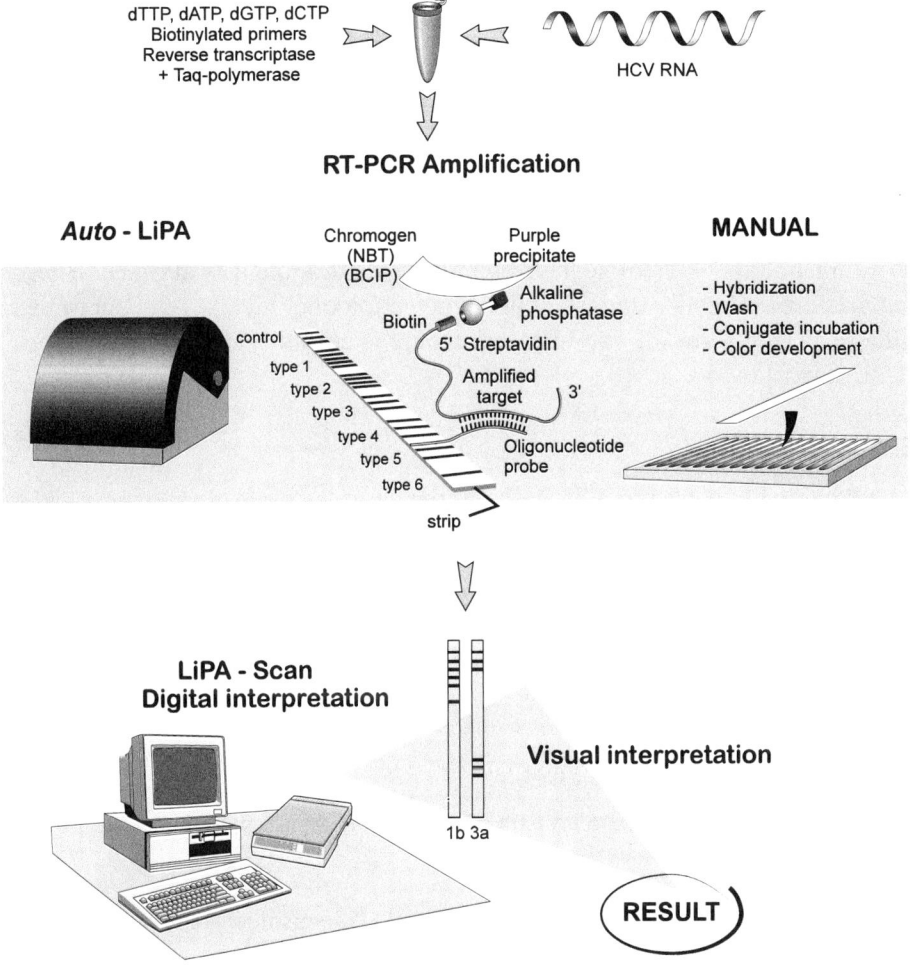

Fig. 1. INNO-LiPA HCV II.

highly specific and sensitive genotyping, the lack of sequence polymorphisms for certain subtypes constitutes the major limitation of assays employing 5'-NCR sequence variability (*see* **Note 3**; *32–34*). On the other hand, methods employing core region polymorphisms perform less specifically because of the high degree of heterogeneity (*see* **Note 4**; *35–39*). Although reverse hybridization technology allows targeting of any desired polymorphism, RFLP analysis will always remains dependent on the availability of endonuclease restriction sites coinciding with the genotype-specific polymorphism (*see* **Note 5**; *40*). Serotyping techniques do not allow determination of subtypes and show problems of specificity at the typing level *(39–43)* (*see* **Note 6**). Thus far, 58 different LiPA II patterns have been encountered, all of which are characteristic for a given genotype. The principle of reverse hybridization allows simultaneous testing of multiple probes on a single test strip. With some isolates, up to 60% of the 5'-NCR sequences can be deduced from a single hybridization. Although mixed infections can only be detected by direct sequencing or RFLP analysis when the minor genotype is present in at least 20% of sequences, INNO-LiPA can detect a minor genotype as soon as a threshold of ~1% of sequences in the PCR fragment is attained. These features are especially important in the detection of clinically relevant mixed infections (*see* **Note 7**). The LiPA procedure is currently used in many laboratories worldwide.

2. Materials

1. We recently published a detailed description of the genotype-specific 5'-NCR motifs targeted by the INNO-LiPA HCV II probes *(23)*. The following reagents are provided with the kit.
   a. 20 INNO-LiPA HCV II strips marked with a black line.
   b. Ready-for-use denaturation solution.
   c. Ready-for-use hybridization solution (SSC/0.1% SDS).
   d. Stringent wash solution (SSC/0.1% SDS).
   e. Concentrated conjugate (to be diluted 1:100 in conjugate diluent before use).
   f. Conjugate diluent.
   g. Concentrated BCIP/NBT substrate solution (5-bromo-4-chloro-3-indolyl phosphate and nitro blue tetrazolium in dimethylformamide, to be diluted 1:100 in substrate buffer before use).
   h. Substrate buffer.
   i. Concentrated rinse solution (to be diluted 1:5 in distilled water before use).
   j. Three incubation trays containing eight troughs each.
   k. One plastic transparent reading chart for identification of positive lines.
2. Water bath with shaking platform (80 rpm with inclined lid, and temperature adjustable to $50 \pm 0.5°C$).
3. An orbital or longitudinal shaker or rocker (*see* **Note 8**).
4. Aspiration device.
5. Calibrated thermometer.
6. Distilled or deionized water.
7. Precision pipets (with disposable tip) capable of delivering 10, 20–200, and 200–1000 µL. To avoid contamination, the use of cotton-plugged (aerosol-resistant) tips is advisable if the same sample is intended to be used for HCV RNA determination.
8. Tweezers for manipulation of the strips
9. Graduated cylinders; 10, 25, 50, and 100 mL.

HCV Genotyping

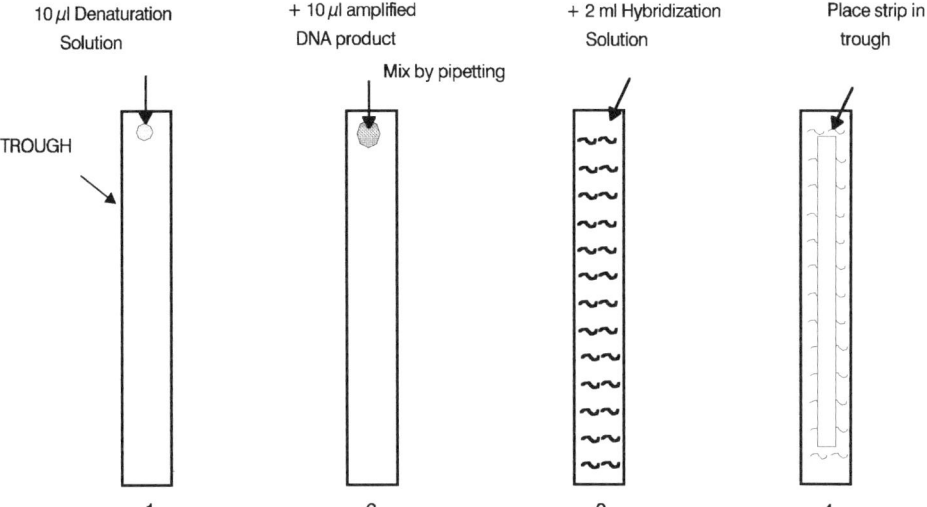

Fig. 2. Addition of the HCV 5' NCR amplicon.

3. Methods
3.1. Manual Procedure

1. Heat a shaking water bath to 50 ± 0.5°C. Check temperature using a calibrated thermometer, and adjust the temperature if necessary. Prewarm the hybridization solution in a water bath of at least 37°C, and do not exceed the hybridization temperature (50°C). Mix before use to dissolve any crystals.
2. Remove the required number of INNO-LiPA HCV II strips from their container using a pair of tweezers, taking a positive (positive PCR sample from a previous run) and negative (no DNA added) control strip into account. Provide each strip with an identification number above the marker line.
3. Take the required number of test troughs, and place them in the tray.
4. Add 10 µL of denaturation solution into the upper corner of each trough. It is important to close the vial immediately after use (**Fig. 2**, step 1).
5. Add 10 µL amplified product to the denaturation solution, and carefully mix by pipeting up and down (**Fig. 2**, step 2). A sufficient amount of HCV cDNA is required to obtain unequivocally interpretable strips (*see* **Note 9**). Always use cotton-plugged pipet tips. Allow denaturation to proceed for 5 min at room temperature.
6. Mix the prewarmed ready-for-use hybridization solution and gently add 2 mL to the denatured amplified product into each trough. Mix by gently shaking (**Fig. 2**, step 3). Take care not to contaminate neighboring troughs during pipeting.
7. Immediately place the strip, marker line up, into the trough as shown in **Fig. 2**, step 4. The strips should be completely submerged in the solution. It is advisable to wear disposable gloves and to use a pair of tweezers.

8. Place the tray into the water bath, which has been heated to 50 ± 0.5°C. Start shaker, close lid, and incubate for 60 min (*see* **Note 8**).
9. After hybridization, remove the tray from the water bath.
10. Hold the tray slightly inclined, and aspirate the liquid from the trough with a pipet, preferably attached to a vacuum aspirator. Add 2 mL prewarmed ready-for-use stringent wash solution into each trough, and rinse by rocking the tray briefly (10–20 s) at room temperature. Aspirate the solution from each trough.
11. Repeat **step 10** once.
12. Incubate each strip with 2 mL prewarmed ready-for-use stringent wash solution in the shaking water bath at 50 ± 0.5°C for 30 min. Close the lid of the water bath.
13. Dilute the concentrated rinse solution and conjugate during the stringent wash.
14. Perform all subseq uent incubations at a room temperature of about 20–30°C on a shaker or rocker (*see* **Note 8**). During the incubations, the liquid and test strips should move back and forth in the troughs to achieve homogeneous staining.
15. Wash the strips twice for 1 min using 2 mL diluted rinse solution.
16. Add 2 mL diluted conjugate to each trough, and shake for 30 min at room temperature.
17. Dilute substrate 10 min prior to the end of the conjugate incubation.
18. Wash each strip twice for 1 min using 2 mL diluted rinse solution.
19. Wash once using 2 mL substrate buffer.
20. Add 2 mL of prepared substrate solution to each trough, and shake for 30 min.
21. Wash strips with 2 mL distilled water by shaking for at least 5 min.
22. Using tweezers, remove the strips from the troughs and place on absorbent paper. Let dry completely before reading the results. Developed strips will retain color if protected from light.

3.2. Automated Procedure Using the Auto-LiPA™ System

The *Auto*-LiPA procedure enables automated processing of up to 30 strips. After addition of the sample, the system allows full walk-away processing and excludes manipulation errors. It allows highly standardized and reliable HCV genotyping and can be combined with automated interpretation by the LiPA-Scan system (**Fig. 1**).

3.3. Interpretation of the LiPA II Strip

3.3.1. Validation

1. Line 1 monitors the addition of reactive conjugate and substrate solution during the detection procedure. This line should always stain positive and should exhibit a similar intensity for each strip included in a given run.
2. The negative control should only have line 1 stained. The positive control and test samples should have lines 1, 2, and isolate-specific lines stained.
3. Color intensities between lines on a single strip may differ from one line to another.

3.3.2. Interpretation

1. For ease of interpretation, the strips and reading chart are lined up using the conjugate control lines.
2. Collect all line numbers that are positive on the INNO-LiPA HCV II strip, and deduce the genotype by using the INNO-LiPA HCV II interpretation chart.

3.3.3. Interpretation by the LiPA-Scan System

Objective interpretation can be obtained by scanning of the LiPA strips, as is currently the case for INNO-LiPA HLA. Conventional scanners, such as Hewlett Packard or Apple One, are compatible with a specific LiPA-Scan software program that is currently under development for HCV genotyping (LiPA-Scan, **Fig. 1**).

4. Notes

1. Probe sequences were previously reported for the prototype assay *(24)*. In the meantime, probes have been significantly improved in the commercial versions of the assay, and multiple probes can be added to a single line to compensate for polymorphisms within types or subtypes. Based on the sequences reported for the prototype assay, theoretical assumptions of sensitivities of the commercial INNO-LiPA tests may be severely underestimated *(27)*.
2. Comparison with sequencing: Genotyping results obtained with the INNO-LIPA HCV kit have been compared with results obtained by direct sequencing of the 5'-NCR of 54 isolates by van Doorn and coworkers, who found a 100% correlation *(28)*. LiPA genotyping has also been compared with RFLP analysis of 5'-NCR PCR fragments obtained from 98 American patients by Mahaney et al. *(29)* who detected a 100% correlation with RFLP for typing, with additional possibilities for subtyping in the LiPA procedure. In 208 Italian and French cases also Giannini and coworkers *(30)* demonstrated a 100% correlation between 5'-NCR sequences and LiPA results, although the polymorphism at position –99 of the 5'-NCR did not always prove to be specifically linked to subtype 1a or 1b sequences detected in the core region (2% of investigated cases). Zeuzem and coworkers *(31)* compared LiPA results with NS5B sequences in German cases. Again a 100% correlation was reported for typing and type 2 subtyping. 5'-NCR sequences exhibited 90% correlation with type 1 subtype sequences of NS5B. A 100% correlation was demonstrated between LiPA typing and classification based on sequencing and phylogenetic analysis of a series of 506 atypical samples and 448 Genbank sequences, with the sole exception of 3 Vietnamese patients *(23)*.
3. The use of the 5'-NCR does not allow discrimination of all subtypes or types. For example, in the region analyzed (nucleotides –263 to –30), the sequence of subtype 2c is identical to that of 2a. Some other recently discovered type 2 subtypes from Africa also have identical sequences, whereas subtype 2d, 2i, and the recently discovered French subtype 2' (isolates FR14, FR15, and FR19) can be discriminated with the second-generation LiPA *(32)*. 5'-NCR motifs, thought to

be unique for type 1 (usually identical to subtype 1b), now also appear to be present in type 7, 8, or 9 subtypes *(33)*. Based on a recent survey by Mellor et al. *(34)*, covering isolates from Thailand, Burma, Hong Kong, Macau, Taiwan, Singapore, and Malaysia, such variants seem to be restricted to Vietnam. Type 7–9 variants have also been detected in Thailand, but most of the latter isolates show 5'-NCR sequences distinct from type 1 *(34)*.

4. Using primers for genotype-specific amplification of the HCV core region *(35)*, up to 30% of European isolates cannot be amplified with any of the subtype-specific primers *(31,36)*. Type 2 isolates, which contained several mismatches in the region of the subtype 2a primer, could not be genotyped with this method. We now understand that this is owing to the low prevalence of subtype 2a in Europe, whereas the more recently discovered subtype 2c is more prevalent *(31,36)*. Nevertheless, nonspecific amplification was reported in at least four studies. For example, genotype 1a sequences were falsely amplified by the subtype 1b primer *(30,37–39)*. In addition to mistyping, such nonspecificity during primer annealing also generated an overestimation of the number of mixed infections. Although it is currently believed that mixed HCV infections appear at a frequency of about 1–3%, mixed infections were frequently reported in 10–30% of cases analyzed by the Okamoto method *(30,39)*. Although the separation of nested PCR reactions into five different tubes can markedly improve specificity, the method becomes considerably more tedious to perform. Given the high number of subtypes characterized today, routine application of this technique has become less appealing. The method is still used in a screening phase for variability research, after which nontypeable samples are analyzed by sequencing and phylogenetic analysis.

5. RFLP: Since restriction fragments are often of relatively small size, radiolabeling may be required. Only sequence polymorphisms that coincidentally generate or destroy a restriction enzyme recognition site can be analyzed by RFLP. None of the described RFLP methods are commercially available; the methods are usually applied in a research environment *(40)*.

6. Comparison with serotyping: Type-specific B-cell epitopes are present in the NS4A and NS4B regions. Single or branched peptides derived from both of these regions can be used for serotyping. Simmonds et al. *(41)* coated multiple-antigen peptides from the NS4A and NS4B regions of types 1, 2, and 3 onto three different microwells. Type-specific responses could be demonstrated, but some crossreactivities were still observed. This method is used in a commercially available kit (HCV Serotyping Assay, Murex Diagnostics, Dartford, UK), and a second generation *(42)* for types 1–6 has been introduced recently. No reports are available yet on the comparison of serotyping results with sequencing. In a study by Martinot et al. *(43)*, who compared serotyping with INNO-LiPA HCV I in 220 patients with chronic hepatitis C, sensitivity of serotyping was 78% and that of genotyping was 98%. Of the serotyping results, 8% showed discordancies with genotyping (note that genotyping by LiPA shows 100% correlation with sequencing *[28]*), a specific serotyping result was obtained in only 72% of cases. For

example, only 81/110 (74%) of subtype 1b isolates were correctly diagnosed as serotype 1 using NS4 antibodies *(43)*. van Doorn et al. *(44)* obtained very similar results in a series of 106 chronically infected patients with an overall concordance of 73%. A difficulty in the analysis of such comparative studies is the impossibility of ruling out the existence of antibodies to previous infections with heterologous HCV genotypes, or of differentiating these from ordinary cross-reactivity. However, anti-NS4 antibodies are usually cleared rapidly after resolving HCV infection *(45)*, and the number of acute-resolving cases of hepatitis C is very low. Combined with the lower sensitivity, overall concordance of NS4 serotyping with genotyping is only 65–75%, with concordances of 50–60% in immunocompromised patients. Tuveri and coworkers recently reported concordances between serotyping and LiPA of only 12/21 (57%) in HIV-negative patients and of 4/19 (21%) in patients coinfected with HIV; some samples were further investigated by sequencing of the core region and confirmed the LiPA results *(39)*.

HCV types 1 and 2 show sufficient degrees of divergence in the core-variable region to be discriminated serologically, but sequences of type 3 and 4 isolates are very similar to type 1 in this region. Type 1 can therefore not be discriminated from type 3 and type 4 in the core region. Dixit et al. *(46)* applied type 1 and 2 core peptides, and types 1–3 NS4 peptides on a serotyping strip (RIBA Serotyping, Chiron, Emeryville, CA). The system was only recently introduced and has not yet been evaluated extensively.

7. Mixed infections: The detection of infection with a mixture of HCV genotypes is currently highly debated. As a consequence of its high sensitivity for capturing minor sequence variants, the LiPA proved to be particularly useful for the detection of mixed infection *(47)*. Tuveri et al. *(39)* studied French hemophiliacs using several genotyping techniques, of which subtype-specific amplification of the Core region detected mixed infection in 8 out of 45 cases. Six of these were 1a + 1b coinfections, of which only one was confirmed by LiPA II and sequencing of the Core region *(39)*. These results, in addition to the majority of type 1 isolates that show regular subtype 1a and 1b patterns, indicate the high specificity of subtype 1a and 1b probes in the LiPA II assay. Nevertheless, some exceptional cases infected with a single subtype 1a or 1b genotype reacted with both subtyping probes *(33)*. Consequently, any probe reactivity must result from specific sequences present in the isolate studied. Some type 1 isolates may therefore exhibit quasispecies variation at position –99, which is used for discrimination of subtype 1a from 1b.

8. Hybridization and stringent wash: Incubation at $50 \pm 0.5°C$ during hybridization and stringent washing are the most critical steps in avoiding false-positive (too low temperatures), or false-negative, or weak signals (resulting from too high temperatures). A shaking water bath with inclined lid allows optimal control of temperature variations. Strict temperature control using a calibrated thermometer is necessary. Always close the lid of the water bath during incubations in order to avoid false-positive signals. A hot-air shaker should not be used either for

hybridization or stringent wash steps. The amplitude of the motion generated by both the shaker in the water bath (hybridization procedure) and the orbital shaker/rocker (color development procedure) is critical for achieving maximum sensitivity and homogeneous staining. The amplitude should be as high as possible, but spilling of liquid over the edges of the troughs needs to be avoided. For hybridization and stringent wash, the troughs are placed on the shaking platform of the water bath. Water level is adjusted between one-third and one-half of the height of the trough. Troughs should not float, and the water should be in direct contact with the troughs. Hybridization and stringent wash incubation steps are performed in a water bath with closed lid, capable of shaking at 80 rpm. All 20–25°C incubation steps should be performed using an orbital shaker (160 rpm) or rocker (50 rpm). Shaking of the hybridization, wash, rinse, conjugate, and substrate solutions over the strips is important to achieve the maximum sensitivity and homogeneous staining. Shaking during incubation of the strips should be performed in such a way that both the liquid and the test strips move back and forth in the trough, without liquid being spilled over the edges. During hybridization and stringent wash incubations, the troughs must be left uncovered in the water bath. Covering the troughs with microplate sealers may cause crosscontamination.

9. Agarose-gel control. Although the combined INNO-LiPA procedure based on *Auto*-LiPA and LiPA-Scan provides highly reliable genotyping, it remains dependent on the quality and quantity of the input HCV cDNA. Standardization of the RT-PCR procedure or the use of commercially available HCV RNA detection kits combined with LiPA permits quick and economical subtyping of the viral genome, as reported by Huber et al. *(48)*. If in-house RT-PCR procedures are used, HCV 5'-NCR amplicons should always be examined by agarose-gel electrophoresis before submission to LiPA analysis. Both the specificity and intensity should can be kept under control by inclusion of this step. EtBr-stained bands with apparent molecular weight of ~325 bp and ~275 bp should be obtained for the 300-bp outer and 250-bp nested PCR fragments (the biotin groups increase the apparent MW), respectively. In the course of 1997, a 275-bp control fragment based on non-HCV sequences has been included in the kit. This control serves both as a marker (migrating close to the position of the nested PCR fragment) and as a cutoff (inclusion of a specific amount of this fragment). Amplicons stained with an intensity equal to or higher than the 275-bp cutoff fragment can be used for further analysis. Although as little as 10 pg of amplicon can be detected by LiPA, proceeding with less material may cause certain lines to be colored very faintly.

Acknowledgment

This work was supported in part by the Flemish Government, Ministry of Economics (Grants FIOV/IWT/91/007.tv1 and ADV/94072/Innogenetics) as part of Eureka Project EU680 "hepatitis C."

References

1. Maertens, G. and Stuyver, L. (1997) Genotypes and Genetic variation of hepatitis C virus, in *Molecular Medicine of Viral Hepatitis* (Zuckerman, A. and Harrison, T., eds.), *Molecular Medical Science Series* (James, K. and Morris A., eds.), John Wiley, Chichester, England, pp. 183–233.
2. Hoofnagle, J. and Di Bisceglie, A. (1997) The treatment of chronic viral hepatitis. *N. Engl. J. Med.* **336**, 347–356.
3. Chemello, L., Bonetti, P., Cavalletto, L.,Talato, F., Donadon, V., Casarin, P., et al. (1995) Randomized trial comparing three different regimens of alpha-2a-interferon in chronic hepatitis C. *Hepatology* **22**, 700–706.
4. Qu, D., Li, J.-S., Vivitski, L., Mechai, S., Berby, F., Tong, S.-P., et al. (1994) Hepatitis C virus genotypes in France: comparison of clinical features of patients infected with HCV type I and type II. *J. Hepatol.* **21**, 70–75.
5. Tsubota, A., Chayama, K., Ikeda, K., Yasuji, A., Koida, I., Saitoh, S., et al. (1994) Factors predictive of response to interferon-alfa therapy in hepatitis C infection. *Hepatology* **19**, 1088–1094.
6. Nousbaum, J.-B., Pol, S., Nalpas, B., Landais, P., Berthelot, P., and Bréchot, C. (1995) Hepatitis C virus type 1b (II) infection in France and Italy. *Ann. Intern. Med.* **122**, 161–168.
7. El-Zayadi, A., Selim, O., El Haddad, S., and Hamdy, H. (1995) Combination treatment of alpha interferon-2b and Ribavirin in chronic hepatitis C genotype 4 patients resistant to interferon therapy [Abstract]. *Hepatology* **22 (Pt. 2)**, 152A.
8. Maggi, F., Vatteroni, M., Fornai, C., Morrica, A., Giorgi, M., Bendinelli, M., et al. (1997) Subtype 2c hepatitis C virus is highly prevalent in Italy and is heterogeneous in the NS5A region. *J. Clin. Microbiol.* **35**, 161–164.
9. Okamoto, H., Crovatto, M., Pozzato, G., Féray, C., Bréchot, C., and Mishiro, S. (1995) Molecular and clinical characteristics of the hepatitis C virus genotype 2c found in Italians in Italy and France. *Int. Hepatol. Commun.* **3**, 161–165.
10. Chemello, L., Cavaletto, L., Bernardinello, E., Guido, M., Pontisso, P., and Alberti, A. (1995) The effect of interferon alfa and ribavirin combination therapy in naive patients with chronic hepatitis C. *J. Hepatol.* **23 (Suppl. 2)**, 8–12.
11. Gane, E., Naoumov, N., Qian, K.-P., Mondelli, M., Maertens, G., Portmann, B., et al. (1996) A longitudinal analysis of hepatitis C virus replication following liver transplantation. *Gastroenterology* **110**, 167–177.
12. Gane, E., Portmann, B., Naoumov, N., Smith, H., Underhill, J., Donaldson, P., et al. (1996) Long-term outcome of hepatitis C infection after liver transplantation. *N. Engl. J. Med.* **334**, 815–820.
13. Féray, C., Gigou, M., Samuel, D., Paradis, V., Mishiro, S., Maertens, G., Reynès, M., et al. (1995) Influence of the genotypes of hepatitis C virus on the severity of recurrent liver disease after liver transplantation. *Gastroenterology* **108**, 1088–1096.
14. Di Martino, V., Féray, C., Saurini, F., Samuel, D., Reynès, M., and Bismuth, H. (1995) Relation between intra-hepatic replication, genotypes and recurrent liver disease due to hepatitis C virus after liver transplantation [Abstract]. *J. Hepatol.* **23 (Suppl. 1)**, 152.

15. Chant, K., Kociuba, K., Munro, R., Crone, S., Kerrdige, R., Quin, J., et al. (1994) Investigation of possible patient-to-patient transmission of hepatitis C in a hospital. *New South Wales Heath Bull.* **5,** 47–51.
16. Zignego, A., Ferri, C., Giannini, C., Monti, M., La Civita, L., Careccia, G., et al. (1996) Hepatitis C virus genotype analysis in patients with type II mixed cryoglobulinemia. *Ann. Intern. Med.* **124,** 31–34.
17. Kanazawa, Y., Hayashi, N., Mita, E., Li, T., Hagiwara, H., Kasahara, A., et al. (1994) Influence of viral quasispecies on effectiveness of interferon therapy in chronic hepatitis C patients. *Hepatology* **20,** 1121–1130.
18. Honda, M., Kaneko, S., Sakai, A., Unoura, M., Murakami, S., and Kobayashi, K. (1994) Degree of hepatitis C virus quasispecies and progression to liver disease. *Hepatology* **20,** 1144–1151.
19. Allander, T., Medin, C., Jacobson, S., Grillner, L., and Persson, M. (1994) Hepatitis C transmission in a hemodialysis unit: molecular evidence for spread of virus among patients not sharing equipment. *J. Med. Virol.* **43,** 514–419.
20. Simmonds, P., Alberti, A., Alter, H., Bonino, F., Bradley, D.W., Bréchot, C., et al. (1994) A proposed system for the nomenclature of hepatitis C virus genotypes. *Hepatology* **19,** 1321–1324.
21. Stuyver, L., van Arnhem, W., Wyseur, A., Hernandez, F., Delaporte, E., and Maertens, G. (1994) Classification of hepatitis C viruses based on phylogenetics analysis of the E1 and NS5B regions and identification of 5 new subtypes. *Proc. Natl. Acad. Sci. USA* **91,** 10,134–10,138.
22. Tokita, H., Okamoto, H., Tsuda, F., Song, P., Nakata, S., Chosa, T., et al. (1994) Hepatitis C virus variants from Vietnam are classifiable into the seventh, eighth, and ninth major genetic groups. *Proc. Natl. Acad. Sci. USA* **91,** 11,022–11,026.
23. Stuyver, L., Wyseur, A., van Arnhem, W., Hernandez, F., and Maertens, G. (1996) A second generation INNO-LiPA for hepatitis C virus genotyping. *J. Clin. Microbiol.* **34 (9),** 2259–2266.
24. Stuyver, L., Rossau, R., Wyseur, A., Duhamel, M., Vanderborght, B., Van Heuverswyn, H., et al. (1993) Typing of hepatitis C virus isolates and characterization of new subtypes using a line probe assay. *J. Gen. Virol.* **74,** 1093–1102.
25. Stuyver, L., Wyseur, A., Rombout, A., Louwagie, J., Scarcez, T., Verhofstede, C., et al. (1997) Line probe assay for rapid detection of drug-selected mutations in the human immunodeficiency virus type 1 reverse transcriptase gene. *Antimicrob. Agents Chemother.* **41,** 284–291.
26. Stuyver, L., Rossau, R., and Maertens, G. (1996) Line probe assays for the detection of HCV and HBV genotypes. *Antiviral Ther.* **1 (Suppl. 3),** 53–57.
27. Smith, D., Mellor, J., Jarvis, L., Davidson, F., Kolberg, J., Urdea, M., et al. (1995) Variation of the hepatitis C virus 5' non-coding region: implications for secondary structure, virus detection and typing. *J. Gen. Virol.* **76,** 1749–1761.
28. van Doorn, L.-J., Kleter, B., Stuyver, L., Maertens, G., Brouwer, J., Schalm, S., et al. (1994) Analysis of hepatitis C virus genotypes by a line probe assay (LiPA) and correlation with antibody profiles. *J. Hepatol.* **12,** 122–129.

29. Mahaney, K., Tedeschi, V., Maertens, G., Di Bisceglie, A., Vergalla, J., Hoofnagle, J., et al. (1994) Genotypic analysis of hepatitis C virus in American patients. *Hepatology* **20**, 1405–1411.
30. Giannini, C., Thiers, V., Nousbaum, J.-B., Stuyver, L., Maertens, G., and Bréchot, C. (1994) Comparative analysis of the hepatitis C virus core PCR and LiPA genotyping assays. *J. Hepatol.* **23**, 246–253.
31. Zeuzem, S., Rüster, B., Lee, J.-H., Stripf, T., and Roth, K. (1995) Evaluation of a reverse hybridization assay for genotyping of hepatitis C virus. *J. Hepatol.* **23**, 654–661.
32. Stuyver, L., Fretz, C., Esquivel, C., Boudifa, A., Jaulmes, D., Azar, N., et al. (1996) HCV genotype analysis in apparently healthy anti-HCV positive Parisian blood donors. *Transfusion* **36**, 552–558.
33. Stuyver, L., Wyseur, A., van Arnhem, W., Lunel, F., Laurent-Puig, P., Pawlotsky J.-M., et al. (1995) Hepatitis C virus genotyping by means of 5'UR/Core line probe assays and molecular analysis of untypeable samples. *Virus Res.* **38**, 137–157.
34. Mellor, J., Holmes, E., Jarvis, L., Yap, P.-L., and Simmonds, P. (1995) Investigation of the pattern of hepatitis C virus sequence diversity in different geographical regions: implications for virus classification. *J. Gen. Virol.* **76**, 2493–2507.
35. Okamoto, H., Sugiyama, Y., Okada, S., Kurai, K., Akahane, Y., Sugai, Y., et al. (1992) Typing of hepatitis C virus by polymerase chain raction with type-specific primers: application to clinical surveys and tracing infectious sources. *J. Gen. Virol.* **73**, 673–679.
36. Cammarota, G., Maggi, F., Vatteroni, M., Da Prato, M., Barsanti, L., Bendinelli, M., et al. (1995) Partial nucleotide sequencing of six subtype 2c hepatitis C viruses detected in Italy. *J. Clin. Microbiol.* **33**, 2781–2784.
37. Kleter, G., van Doorn, L.-J., Stuyver, L., Maertens, G., Brouwer, J., Schalm, S., et al. (1995) Rapid genotyping of hepatitis C virus RNA-isolates obtained from patients residing in Western Europe. *J. Med. Virol.* **47**, 35–42.
38. Andonov, A. and Chaudary, R. (1994) Genotyping of Canadian hepatitis C virus isolates by PCR. *J. Clin. Microbiol.* **32**, 2031–2034.
39. Tuveri, R., Rotschild, C., Pol, S., Reijasse, D., Persico, T., Gazengel, C., et al. (1997) Hepatitis C virus genotypes in French haemophiliacs: kinetics and reappraisal of mixed infections. *J. Med. Virol.* **51**, 36–41.
40. McOmish, F., Yap, P.-L., Dow, B., Follett, E., Seed, C., Keller, A., et al. (1994) Geographical distribution of hepatitis C virus genotypes in blood donors: an international collaborative survey. *J. Clin. Microbiol.* **32**, 884–892.
41. Simmonds, P., Rose, K., Graham, S., Chan, S.-W., McOmish, F., Dow, B., et al. (1993) Mapping of seotype-specific epitopes in the NS4 region of hepatitis C virus (HCV): use of type-specific peptides to serologically differentiate infections with HCV types 1, 2, and 3. *J. Clin. Microbiol.* **31**, 1493–1503.
42. Battacherjee, V., Prescott, L., Pike, I., Rodgers, B., Bell, H., El-Zayadi, A., et al. (1995) Use of NS4 peptides to identify type-specific antibody to hepatitis C virus genotypes 1, 2, 3, 4, 5, and 6. *J. Gen. Virol.* **76**, 1737–1748.

43. Martinot M., Marcellin, P., Pellet, C., Le Breton, V., Darthuy, F., Rémiré, J., et al. (1995) Serological assay to determine HCV genotype: comparison with PCR based HCV genotyping. *Hepatology* **22 (Pt. 4),** 358A.
44. van Doorn, L.-J., Kleter, B., Pike, I., and Quint, W. (1996) Analysis of hepatitis C virus isolates by serotyping and genotyping. *J. Clin. Microbiol.* **34,** 1784–1787.
45. Saracco, G., Abate, M., Baldi, M., Calvo, P., Manzini, P., Brunetto, M., et al. (1994) Hepatitis C virus markers in patients with long-term biochemical and histological remission of chronic hepatitis. *Liver* **14,** 65–70.
46. Dixit, V., Quan, S., Martin, P., Larson, D., Brezina, M., DiNello, R., et al. (1995) Evaluation of a novel serotyping system for hepatitis C virus: strong correlation with standard genotyping methodologies. *J. Clin. Microbiol.* **33,** 2978–2983.
47. Lau, J., Davis, G., Prescott, L., Maertens, G., Lindsay, K., Qian, K., et al. (1996) Distribution of hepatitis C virus genotypes determined by a line probe assay in patients with chronic hepatitis C seen at trertiary referral centers in the united states. *Ann. Intern. Med.* **124,** 868–876.
48. Huber, K., Knapp, M., and Bauer, K. (1995) Subtyping of hepatitis C virus. *Clin. Chem.* **41,** 319,320.

17

Serological Genotyping Using Synthetic Peptides Derived from the NS4 Region

Linda E. Prescott and Peter Simmonds

1. Introduction

The RNA genome of hepatitis C virus (HCV) displays extensive sequence variation, and consequently, the virus is classified into six major genotypes. The severity of disease and response to antiviral treatment are thought to be influenced by both viral and host-related factors, including age of aquisition, duration of infection, circulating virus load, and the genotype of infecting virus. Many investigators have reported that infections with HCV type 1 are associated with an increase in the likelihood of progression to hepatocellular carcinoma *(1–3)*, and with nonresponsiveness to interferon therapy when compared to genotypes 2 or 3 (reviewed in **refs.** *4,5*). This discovery emphasizes the need for genotyping methods in current clinical practice, in providing a predictor of the outcome of treatment, and perhaps helping to target appropriate treatment to the most relevant patient groups.

A number of different methods have been developed to identify the genotype of infecting virus. The majority of these techniques use the polymerase chain reaction (PCR) for the amplification of HCV DNA sequences. Although accurate for HCV genotypes encountered in Western clinical practice, PCR-based genotyping methods are both time-consuming and expensive, and are therefore currently unsuitable for the analysis of high numbers of routine samples in a clinical laboratory. A different, indirect method for HCV genotyping is based on the observation that genetic heterogeneity between genotypes results in the production of type-specific antibodies, which can be detected by an enzyme-linked immunosorbent assay (ELISA). The majority of the serotyping assays designed to date aim to distinguish between genotypes by a direct comparison of antibody reactivity to type-specific antigens on the solid phase. These include NS4 recombinant proteins for the identification of HCV types 1 and 2 *(6)*, and monomeric peptides to core/NS4 for the identification of either 2 *(7)* or 3 *(8)* genotypes, respectively. The assay described in this chapter is a competetive ELISA, which uses NS4 branched peptides to differentiate between all the six major genotypes described. *(9,10)*.

1.1. Development of a Serotyping Assay Based on Branched Peptides

Epitope mapping of the NS4 protein revealed two major antigenic regions (amino acid residues 1691–1708 and 1710–1728) that were highly variable among HCV genotypes 1, 2, and 3, and to which type-specific antibody could be detected *(9)*. Type-specific branched peptides were made corresponding to both these regions and used in an indirect ELISA. As more genotypes were detected, a full range of peptides for all six genotypes were designed and included in the assay (21 peptides in total) *(10)*.

In order to detect type-specific antibody, yet eliminate crossreactivity with heterologous peptides, a competition ELISA was designed. Serum samples are incubated alongside blocking solutions containing heterologous peptides, which absorb cross reactive antibody. A strip of eight wells is used for each sample to be tested (12 samples/microtiter plate), which includes a positive and negative reference well, and six typing wells. Each well is initially coated with all 21 peptides. Prior to the addition of serum to the wells, blocking solutions of heterologous competing peptides (in a 100-fold excess over those used for coating) were added to the appropriate typing wells on the microtiter plate. For example, the HCV-1 typing well will have a competing solution added, which contains peptides for genotypes 2–6, whereas the HCV-2 typing well will have competing peptides for types 1, 3, 4, 5, and 6 added. The result is that the only antibody able to bind to the antigen on the solid phase is that which has not reacted with any of the heterologous peptides in solution. The positive reference well has no competing peptides added, which leaves any NS4 antibody present in the serum free to bind to the solid phase, whereas the negative reference well has competing peptides for all six genotypes added, designed to absorb all antibody whether type-specific or to shared epitopes in NS4. Serum is then added to the wells at a dilution of 1:20, and the plate incubated at 37°C for 1 h. Secondary antibody is added in the form of antihuman IgG horseradish peroxidase (HRP) labeled conjugate, with color development appearing on incubation with o-phenylenediamine (OPD)/hydrogen peroxide substrate. The colormetric reaction is stopped with 8 M sulfuric acid.

1.2. Correlation with Other Assays

The main advantage of serological methods over PCR-based genotyping is the ability to process large numbers of samples in a single working day, although this should not be at the expense of sensitivity and specificity. To investigate the performance of the serotyping assay, a total of 210 samples of known genotype were analyzed (Table 1 taken from **ref. *10***). The sensitivity of the assay was calculated as the percentage of samples analyzed in which NS4 type-specific antibody could be detected. Values range from 100 (type 2b) to 66.7% (type 6). The specificity of the assay was measured as the percentage of typeable samples, in which the serotyping results were concordant with genotyping by RFLP *(11,12)*. Concordance values are generally high, with the overall concordance of the assay in this study being 97.3%. However, concordance may be lower if the patients, such as hemophiliacs who have been multiply exposed to HCV. In such individuals, antibody may be detected to previously circulating genotypes subsequently replaced through reinfection or reactivation of other genotypes *(13)*.

2. Materials
2.1. Preparation

1. Flat-bottomed immunoplates (polystyrene/polypropylene) (NUNC Maxisorp; Gibco-BRL, Paisley, Scotland).
2. Phosphate-buffered saline (PBS) with $MgCl_2$ (Sigma, Dorset, UK).
3. PBST: PBS + 0.05% Tween-20, BDH, Merck Ltd, UK.
4. Bovine serum albumin (BSA) >98%. (Sigma). Store at 2–8°C. Make up 2% solution in PBS.

2.2. ELISA

1. Sample diluent: PBST + 2% BSA. Make up a fresh solution every day.
2. Conjugate: Concentrated antihuman IgG HRP-labeled conjugate (Sigma).
3. Conjugate diluent: 2% BSA in PBST.
4. Substrate: OPD 50 µL/mL + 0.1% hydrogen peroxide (OPD—Dako Ltd, Bucks, UK; H_2O_2—Analar, BDH, Merck Ltd, UK). Store at 2–8°C.
5. Substrate diluent: Citrate phosphate buffer: 20 mL 1 M citric acid (Sigma) + 50 mL 0.5 M Na_2HPO_4. Adjust pH to 4.0 using NaOH, and make up to 250 mL with water. Store at 4°C, maximum 4 wk.
6. "Stop solution": 8 M sulfuric acid.

3. Method
3.1. Preparation

1. Microtiter plates are coated with PBS containing all 21 peptides, each at a concentration of 50 ng/mL. Add 100 µL to each well, and incubate at either 4°C overnight or at 37°C for a minimum of 2 h (*see* **Note 1**).
2. Wash the plates four times with PBST, and block with 125 µL vol of 2% BSA in PBS, for a minimum of 1 h at room temperature (*see* **Note 2**).
3. Wash with PBST and air-dry (*see* **Note 3**).

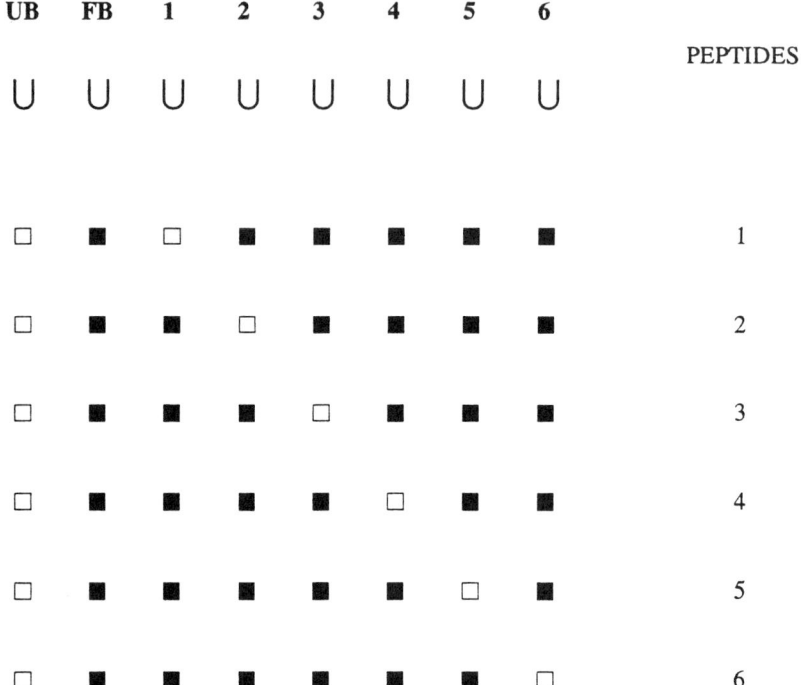

Fig. 1. Basis for HCV serotyping assay. UB; Unblocked well. FB; Fully blocked well. ☐ Peptide absent in competing solution. ■ Peptide added in competing solution.

3.2. ELISA

1. Each sample is incubated in a row of eight wells. Prior to the addition of serum to the wells, blocking solutions of competing peptides (in a 100-fold excess over those used for coating) are added to the immunoplate wells as shown in **Fig. 1**. Each blocking solution consists of 100 µL vol of the appropriate peptides, with the final volume being made up to 2.1 mL with distilled water, if necessary. Blocking solutions are added to their relevant wells in 10 µL vol.
2. Dilute the plasma in 800 µL sample diluent at a concentration of 1:20. Immediately add 100 µL to each of the eight wells, and incubate (covered) at 37°C for 1 h. Do not allow the pipet tip to touch the wells at any time, since blocking solutions may be carried over.
3. Wash the plates four times with PBST.
4. Dilute the concentrated antihuman IgG HRP conjugate in PBST–2% BSA at a concentration of 1:20,000. Add 100 µL to each well, and incubate (covered) for 1 h at 37°C.
5. Wash the plate four times with PBST.
6. Dilute substrate (OPD) in a suitable volume (10 mL needed/plate) of citrate buffer, pH 4.0, at a concentration of 0.5 mg/mL. Immediately prior to use, add

Serological Genotyping 203

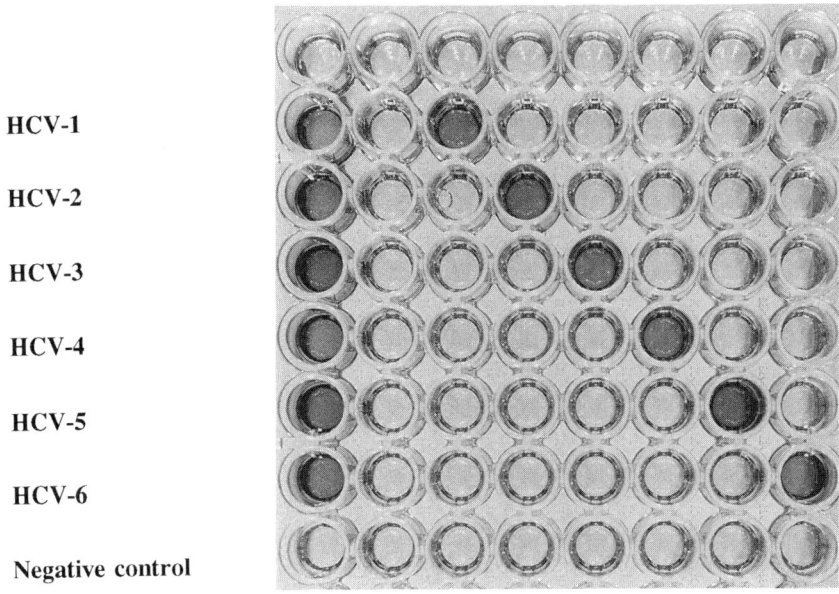

Fig. 2. Positive serotyping results for genotypes 1–6. UB; unblocked well—has no competing peptides added. FB; fully blocked well—has competing peptides for all genotypes added.

hydrogen peroxide at a concentration of 2 μL/mL. Add 100 μL prepared substrate to each well and incubate (covered) for 30 min at 37°C, preferably in the dark (*see* **Note 4**).
7. Add 50 μL 8 *M* sulfuric acid to each well to stop the reaction.
8. Read the plates against a negative control blank at a wavelength of 450 nm, with a reference wavelength of 650 nm.

3.3. Interpretation of Results

Most of the samples can be read clearly by eye, with a high OD reading in the unblocked well (positive control well) and in one or more (in the case of multiple infection) of the six typing wells. The fully blocked well should be negative or a low OD. Weak reactivity can still be recognized by a comparison of OD values, although these samples should be retested with a higher concentration of serum for confirmation. Type-specific reactivity was considered significant when it was more than twice the OD in the negative reference (unblocked) well. Positive results for types 1–6 are shown in **Fig. 2**.

1. Nonreactive samples: Samples that do not contain antibody to NS4 should be negative in all eight wells.
2. Nontype-specific results: If a sample shows the presence of NS4 antibody, but the serotype cannot be distinguished by the assay, then the sample is classed as having a nontype-specific result. There are two ways in which this kind of reactivity can be observed on the microtiter plate:
    a. The unblocked well is positive with all other typing wells negative. In these cases, crossreactivity must be taking place between the NS4 antibody in the sample and one or more of the competing peptides in solution. An example of when this may occur would include a patient infected with an unusual HCV subtype, in which antigenic variation in NS4 has resulted in shared epitopes with those of a different genotype. Sequencing in NS4 would confirm this.
    b. All eight wells show high levels of reactivity. The antibody titer in these samples is extremely high and the 100 fold excess competing peptide solution is not high enough to absorb all nonspecific antibody. Repeat the test using a higher dilution of serum to obtain clear result.

4. Notes

1. Solid NS4 peptides were dissolved in Analar water (BDH) at a concentration of 1 mg/mL, and stored at 4°C. Some peptides would not dissolve immediately, and were helped by either the addition of a small volume of acetic acid (type 3 peptides) or by bubbling ammonia vapor through the suspension. Stock peptide solutions should not be frozen, since as they may come out of solution and be difficult to redissolve. It is not advisable to store stock solutions at 4°C for more than 2 wk.
2. Protein in the form of BSA is used to "block" any remaining binding sites on the plastic microtiter wells. This is important to prevent the binding of nonspecific antibody used later in the assay, leading to misleading results.
3. Plates should be kept at 4°C prior to use. Sealed plates stored in this way can be kept for several months without a significant loss of reactivity.
4. Exposure to light for long periods may reduce the effectiveness of the hydrogen peroxide in this reaction owing to the presence of free radicals.

References

1. Haydon, G. H., Jarvis, L. M., Simmonds, P., and Hayes, P. C. (1995) Association between chronic hepatitis C infection and hepatocellular carcinoma. *Lancet* **345,** 928,929.
2. Takada, A., Tsutsumi, M., Zhang, S. C., Okanoue, T., Matsushima, T., Fujiyama, S., et al. (1996) Relationship between hepatocellular carcinoma and subtypes of hepatitis C virus: A nationwide analysis. *J. Gastroenterol. Hepatol.* **11,** 166–169.
3. Kobayashi, M., Tanaka, E., Sodeyama, T., Urushihara, A., Matsumoto, A., and Kiyosawa, K. (1996) The natural course of chronic hepatitis C: A comparison between patients with genotypes 1 and 2 hepatitis C viruses. *Hepatology* **23,** 695–699.

4. Davis, G. L. (1994) Prediction of response to interferon treatment of chronic hepatitis C. *J. Hepatol.* **21**, 1–3.
5. Dusheiko, G., Schmilovitzweiss, H., Brown, D., McOmish, F., Yap, P. L., Sherlock, S., et al. (1994) Hepatitis C virus genotypes—an investigation of type-specific differences in geographic origin and disease. *Hepatology* **19**, 13–18.
6. Tanaka, T., Tsukiyamakohara, K., Yamaguchi, K., Yagi, S., Tanaka, S., Hasegawa, A., et al. (1994) Significance of specific antibody assay for genotyping of hepatitis C virus. *Hepatology* **19**, 1347–1353.
7. Machida, A., Ohnuma, H., Tsuda, F., Munekata, E., Tanaka, T., Akahane, Y., et al. (1992) Two distinct subtypes of hepatitis C virus defined by antibodies directed to the putative core protein. *Hepatology* **16**, 886–891.
8. Dixit, V., Quan, S., Martin, P., Larson, D., Brezina, M., Dinello, R., et al. (1995) Evaluation of a novel serotyping system for hepatitis C virus: strong correlation with standard genotyping methodologies. *J. Clin. Microbiol.* **33**, 2978–2983.
9. Simmonds, P., Rose, K. A., Graham, S., Chan, S. W., McOmish, F., Dow, B. C., et al. (1993) Mapping of serotype-specific, immunodominant epitopes in the NS-4 region of hepatitis C virus (HCV)—use of type-specific peptides to serologically differentiate infections with HCV type 1, type 2, and type 3. *J. Clin. Microbiol.* **31**, 1493–1503.
10. Bhattacherjee, V., Prescott, L. E., Pike, I., Rodgers, B., Bell, H., Elzayadi, A. R., et al. (1995) Use of NS-4 peptides to identify type-specific antibody to hepatitis C virus genotypes 1, 2, 3, 4, 5 and 6. *J. Gen. Virol.* **76**, 1737–1748.
11. Davidson, F., Simmonds, P., Ferguson, J. C., Jarvis, L. M., Dow, B. C., Follett, E. A. C., et al. (1995) Survey of major genotypes and subtypes of hepatitis C virus using RFLP of sequences amplified from the 5' non-coding region. *J. Gen. Virol.* **76**, 1197–1204.
12. McOmish, F., Yap, P. L., Dow, B. C., Follett, E. A. C., Seed, C., Keller, A. J., et al. (1994) Geographical distribution of hepatitis C virus genotypes in blood donors—an international collaborative survey. *J. Clin. Microbiol.* **32**, 884–892.
13. Prescott, L. E., Berger, A., Pawlotsky, J. M., Conjeevaram, P., Pike, I., and Simmonds, P. (1997) Sequence analysis of hepatitis C virus variants producing discrepant results with two different genotyping assays. *J. Med. Virol.* **53**, 237–244.

18

Determination of HCV Quasispecies by Cloning and Sequencing

Masashi Mizokami and Tomoyoshi Ohno

1. Introduction

Most RNA viruses exists as a heterogeneous mixture of closely related viral genome in the host, which is the result of high error rates in RNA replication and selected by various viral and host factors. The spectrum of this spectrum of related genomes within a host is referred as quasispecies *(1)*. This important biological characteristics of RNA virus is believed to contribute to viral persistence in the presence of host immune system and during treatment with antiviral agents. Hepatitis C virus (HCV), being a single-strand RNA virus, is no exception. In HCV genome, the most heterogeneous regions lie within the envelope 2 region, which are referred to as hypervariable regions (HVRs). The HVRs in HCV are believed to be the result of high nucleotide variation and immune selection pressure *(2)*. Because of its heterogeneity, this is a good region for the study of HCV quasispecies.

Interferon (IFN) therapy has been shown to be effective in the treatment of patients with chronic hepatitis C *(3)*. Approximately 15–30% of patients who received IFN therapy have normalization of their serum ALT levels and the elimination of HCV RNA. The remaining patients had persistent viremia and LAT elevations, or had a relapse shortly after IFN was discontinued *(4,5)*. There is evidence that certain virologic factors are associated with the outcome of IFN therapy, including HCV genotype, viremia level, and the level of heterogeneity of HCV quasispecies *(6,7)*. This chapter describes our technique of studying HCV quasispecies before and after IFN therapy using a combination of cloning and sequencing, with the sequences analyzed by molecular evolutionary analysis *(8,9)*.

2. Materials

1. Serum samples: In the study described, samples were obtained from a Japanese patient with genotype 1b; five time points were studied (A: 1 yr before IFN, B: just before IFN, C: just before IFN, D: at the biochemical relapse time, E: 1 yr after IFN).
2. RNAzol B (Cinna/Biotecx Laboratories, Friendswood, TX).
3. Moloney Murine Leukemia Virus Reverse Transcriptase (M-MLV-RT, Gibco-BRL, Gaithersburg, MD).
4. 1X RT buffer: 50 mM Tris-HCl, pH 8.3, 75 mM KCl, 3 mM MgCl$_2$, and 10 mM DDT.
5. dNTP (Promega, Madison, WI).
6. Placental RNase inhibitor (RNasin, TOYOBO, Osaka, Japan).
7. Thermal cycler (Perkin-Elmer Cetus, Norwalk, CT).
8. *Taq* polymerase and reaction buffer (Promega).
9. 1X PCR buffer (10 mM Tris-HCl, pH 9.0, 50 mM KCl, 1.5 mM MgCl$_2$, 0.01% gelatin, and 0.1% Triton X-100).
10. Seakem agarose (FMC BioProducts, Rockland, ME).
11. Magic Minipreps (Promega).
12. *Bam*HI and *Eco*RI (Takara, Shiga, Japan).
13. pGEM-3zf(+) vector (Applied Biosystems, Foster City, CA).
14. DNA ligation kit (Takara, Shiga, Japan).
15. Competent cell *Escherichia coli*: DH5a (Takara).
16. 373A DNA sequencer (Applied Biosystems).
17. PRISM Ready Reaction Dye Primer Cycle Sequencing Kit (Applied Biosystems).

3. Methods

1. RNA extraction: RNA is extracted from 100 μL of serum with RNAzol B. The extracted RNA was precipitated with isopropanol and washed with ethanol. The RNA pellet is dissolved in diethylpyrocarbonate-treated distilled water containing 100 U of human placental ribonuclease inhibitor (RNasin).
2. Reverse transcription: The first-strand cDNA is synthesized from the extracted RNA at 37°C for 60 min using random hexamer, and with 200 U of M-MLV-RT in a 20-μL mixture containing 1X RT buffer and 600 μM each dNTP. Reaction is terminated by heating at 95°C for 5 min, and mixtures are then chilled on ice.
3. PCR: For PCR, a 50-μL mixture containing 1X PCR buffer, 2 μL of the resulting cDNA, 1.25 U of *Taq* DNA polymerase (Promega), and primers is prepared. The cDNA is amplified for 40 cycles with the following parameters: a preliminary 20 cycles of amplification with 94°C for 1 min (denaturing), 45°C for 1 min (annealing), and 72°C for 1 min (extension), followed by 20 additional cycles at 94°C for 1 min, 60°C for 1 min, and 72°C for 1 min. For the second-round PCR, two μL of the first round PCR product is amplified for another 30 cycles. Each cycle is at 94°C for 1 min, 60°C for 45 s, and 72°C for 1 min. The primers used are as follows (*see* **Note 1**):

    Outer primers 5'-CAG(C/T)T(A/G)CTCCGGATCCCACAAGC-3', and
    5'-ACGTCCGTCTCATT(C/T)(T/G)C(A/C)CCCCA-3'.

HCV Quasispecies

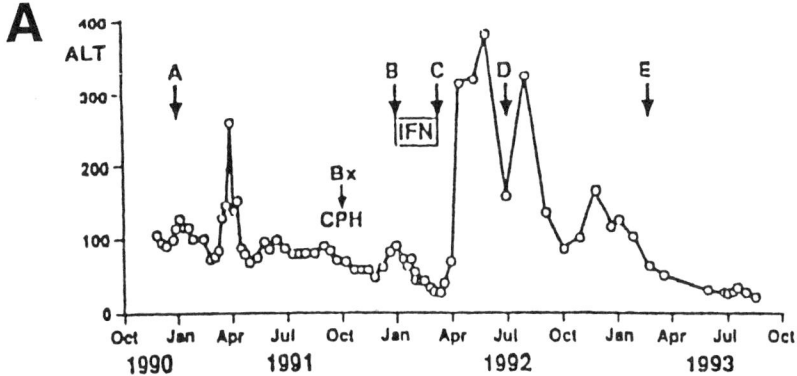

Fig. 1. **(A)** Biochemical profile of the patient and the study time points. *(continued)*

Inner primer 5'-TCTGGATCCTATTCCATGGTGGGGAACTGG-3' (with a *Bam*HI site) and
5'-AATGAATTCTACAACAGGGCT(T/G)GG(A/G)GTGAA-3' (with an *Eco*RI site).

Ligation and transformation: The PCR amplicons are digested with the respective enzymes and gel-purified with Magic MiniprepsTM. The pGEM-3zf(+) vector and purified PCR product are then ligated with T4 ligase at a ratio of 1:1–3 at 16°C for 30 min (as described in the DNA ligation kit). The DNA is then transformed into competent cells, the cells were spread on the LB plate, and colonies with insert are color-selected with X-gal staining (the DNA insert will disrupt the *lacZ* gene and the colonies with the vector with DNA insert should not change X-gal from colorless to blue) (*see* **Note 2**).

4. Sequencing and analysis: To avoid selection bias, at least 10 clones (in the experiment described, at time point A: 11 colonies, B: 47, C: 12, D: 24, and E: 12 clones) are selected and their sequence determined bidirectionally with the dideoxynucleotide chain-termination method using a 373A DNA sequencer. The sequences obtained are maximally aligned, the number of nucleotide substitutions and nucleotide diversity are then estimated by the six-parameter method, and phylogenetic tree is constructed using the neighbor-joining method, as described in Chapter 12 (*see* **Note 3**).

4. Notes

1. PCR experiments are prone to contaminations. The general precautions to avoid PCR contamination must be followed.
2. In ligation, transformation and sequencing, a number of potential problems may occur in every step. Therefore, positive and negative controls should be employed in every step. For details, refer to standard molecular biology textbooks.
3. In the experiments performed and described in this chapter, the quasispecies nature of HCV is obvious as seen in the phylogenetic tree (**Fig. 1**). All clones obtained

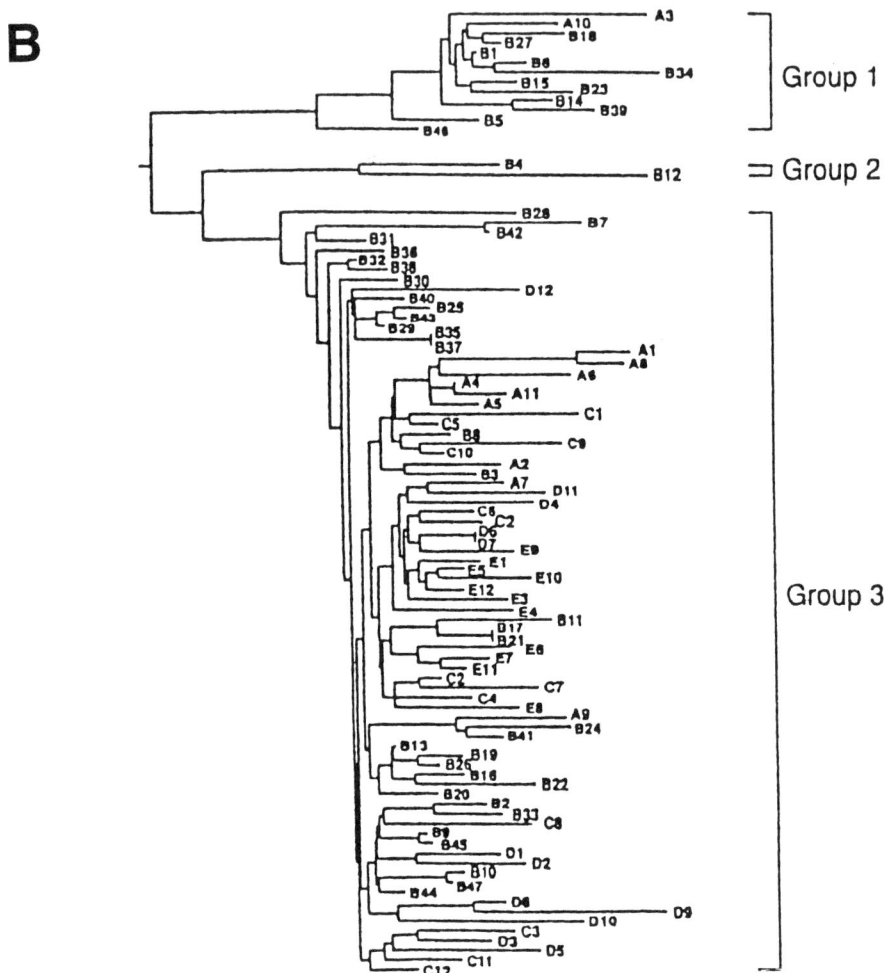

Fig. 1. **(B)** The phylogenetic tree analysis of the clones. Letters represent time points and numbers represent the clone numbers. The clones can be divided into three groups based on evolutionary distances *(9)*.

from the same time-point are referred to by the letter followed by the clone number. Note that IFN therapy drifted the quasispecies equilibrium of HCV.

References

1. Steinhauer, D. A. and Holland, J. J. (1987) Rapid evolution of RNA viruses. *Annu. Rev. Microbiol.* **41,** 409–433.
2. Weiner, A. J., Geysen, H. M., Christopherson, C., Hall, J. E., Mason, T. J., Saracco, G., et al. (1992) Evidence for immune selection of hepatitis C virus

(HCV) putative envelope glycoprotein variants: potential role in chronic HCV infections. *Proc. Natl. Acad. Sci. USA* **89**, 3468–3472.
3. Hoofnagle, J. H., Mullen, K. D., Jones, D. B., Rustig, V., Di Bisceglie, A., Peters, M., et al. (1986) Treatment of chronic non-A, non-B hepatitis with recombinant human alpha interferon. A preliminary report. *N. Engl. J. Med.* **315**, 1575–1578.
4. Davis, G. L., Balart, L. A., Schiff, E. R., Lindsay, K., Bodenheimer, H. C., Perrillo, R. P., et al. (1989) Treatment of chronic hepatitis C with recombinant interferon alfa. A multicenter randomized, controlled trial. Hepatitis Interventional Therapy Group. *N. Engl. J. Med.* **321**, 1501–1506.
5. Hagiwara, H., Hayashi, N., Mita, E., Takehara, T., Kasahara, A., Fusamoto, H., et al. (1993) Quantitative analysis of hepatitis C virus RNA in serum during interferon alpha therapy. *Gastroenterology* **104**, 877–883.
6. Tsubota, A., Chayama, K., Ikeda, K., Yasuji, A., Koida, I., Saitoh, S., et al. (1994) Factors predictive of response to inetrferon-a therapy in hepatitis C virus infection. *Hepatology* **19**, 1088–1094.
7. Kanazawa, Y., Hayashi, N., Mita, E., Li, T., Hagiwara, H., Kasahara, A., et al. (1997) Influence of viral quasispecies on effectiveness of interferon therapy in chronic hepatitis C patients. *Hepatology* **20**, 1121–1130.
8. Mizakami, M., Lau, J. Y. N., Suzuki, K., Nakano, T., and Gojobori, T. (1994) Differential sensitivity of hepatitis C virus quasispecies to interferon-α therapy. *J. Hepatol.* **21**, 884–886.
9. Mizokami, M., Gojobori, T., and Lau, J. Y. N. (1994) Molecular evolutionary virology: its application to hepatitis C virus. *Gastroenterology* **107**, 1181,1182.

19

Detection of Hepatitis C Virus Quasispecies Heterogeneity by Single-Strand Conformational Polymorphism

Regino P. González-Peralta

1. Introduction

Hepatitis C virus (HCV) is believed to replicate via a viral-encoded, RNA-dependent RNA polymerase. This replication strategy has limited fidelity. Thus, HCV is genetically heterogenous. To date, six HCV genotypes and more than 80 viral subtypes have been identified. Further, even within individually infected patients, HCV exists as a highly heterogenous population of closely related genome called quasispecies *(1–3)*. Viral quasispecies have been shown to have important pathobiological implications.

Detection of quasispecies heterogeneity by conventional cloning and sequencing techniques is labor-intensive and expensive. Thus, to study HCV quasispecies, we have developed a rapid and reliable technique based on single-strand conformational polymorphism (SSCP). Three technical requirements for the development of an SSCP assay were anticipated. First, to assure sensitivity and avoid quasispecies selection bias, PCR primers designed from relatively well-conserved regions of the HCV Envelope 2 (E2) gene were used. However, to allow for assessment of heterogeneity, the primers flanked a hypervariable region (HVR1). Second, the "nested" PCR products were <400 bp long, which allows optimal SSCP electrophoresis separation. Third, a predetermined quantity of cDNA was gel-loaded for SSCP analysis. This is important, since patients with high-level HCV viremia would have more amplicon per PCR reaction volume, and would be more likely to have detectable quasispecies. Thus, the quantity, rather than the volume of amplicon DNA was controlled in the SSCP process.

From: *Methods in Molecular Medicine, Vol. 19: Hepatitis C Protocols*
Edited by: J. Y. N. Lau © Humana Press Inc., Totowa, NJ

**Table 1
SSCP Optimization Conditions**

Condition tested	Range tested	Optimal condition
Temperature	4–30°C	25°C
Electrophoresis power	100–400 V	200 V
Gel density	4–20%	12.5%
cDNA loaded	1–200 ng	25 ng

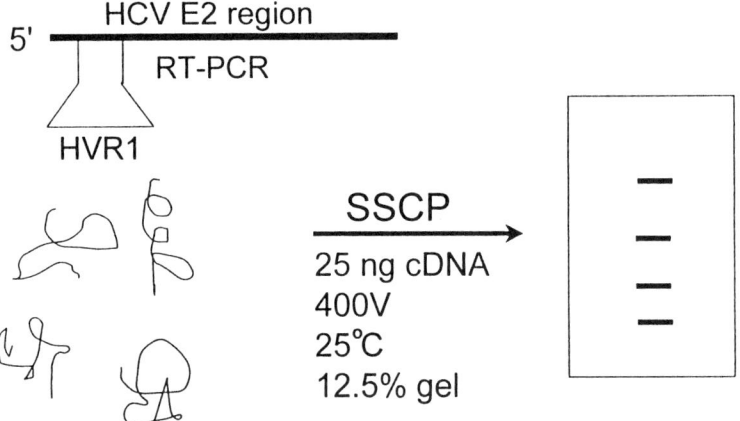

Fig. 1. Outline of SSCP experimental approach.

To ensure reproducibility of results, an automated minigel electrophoresis system (PhastSystem, Pharmacia Biotech, Piscataway, NJ) was used for SSCP analysis. In the development of the assay, the following parameters were systematically studied:

1. Amount of DNA loaded onto the gel/sample (10–200 ng).
2. Gel density (4–20% polyacrylamide).
3. Electrophoresis power (100–400 V).
4. Electrophoresis temperature (4–30°C) (**Table 1**).

Mixing experiments with different ratios of amplicons of known sequence was done to ensure that multiple quasispecies populations in the same PCR product did not interfere with band resolution. This chapter will describe the optimized SSCP method developed in our laboratory, based on the results of this approach *(4)* (**Fig. 1**).

2. Materials

1. Serum samples, collected, spun, and frozen within 4 h of venesection (*see* **Note 1**).
2. RNA extraction solutions (*see* Chapter 4):
   a. Chomczynski solution D: 2 M sodium acetate (NaAc, pH 4.0), 3 M NaAc, pH 6.5).
   b. Glycogen-acetate mix: 0.1 M dithioreitol (DTT), 5 mg/mL bromophenol blue (BPB), water-saturated acid phenol, pH 4.3, 2-mercaptoethanol, nonidet detergent (NP-40), 70 and 100% ethanol, chloroform-isoamyl alcohol, mineral oil (*see* **Notes 2** and **3**).
3. RNA dissolution buffer (prepare fresh on the day of use): Add 10 µL of 1 M Tris-HCl (pH 8.3 at 25°C), 50 µL of 1 M KCl, 5 µL of 100% NP-40, 4 µL of 5 mg/mL BPB, and water to make 1 mL. For 10 reactions, transfer 200 µL to a sterile 500 µL microcentrifuge tube, and add 10 µL of 0.1 M DTT and 2.5 µL of RNase inhibitor. Mix well with flicking; do not vortex, since this results in significant foaming.
4. RT-PCR stock solutions: 1 M Tris-HCl (pH 8.3 at 25°C): mix 157.6 g in 1 L of water and adjust pH. 1 M potassium chloride (KCl): mix 74.6 g in 1 L of water.
5. RT-PCR Enzymes: Moloney murine leukemia virus reverse transcriptase (M-MLV-RT, 200 U/µL, Promega), RNase inhibitor (40 U/µL, Promega), *Thermophilus aquaticus* DNA polymerase (*Taq*, 5 U/µL, Boehringer-Mannheim, Indianapolis, IN).
6. SSCP denaturing solution: 98% formamide, 2% glycerol, 0.05% BPB, and 0.05% xylene cyanol.
7. Silver-staining solutions in deionized water: 20% tricarboxylic acid, 50% ethanol/10% acetic acid (HAC), 10% ethanol/5% HAC, 0.4% silver nitrate, developer (0.13% formaldehyde in 2.5% sodium carbonate), background reducer (sodium thiosulfate: dissolve 1.6 and 3.7 g Tris-HCl in 100 mL deionized water, adjust pH to 5.0–6.0 with glacial HAC), 5% glycerol.
8. Thermal cycler (Perkin-Elmer-Cetus, Norwalk, NJ).
9. Fluorometer (DyNA Quant™ 200, Hoefer-Pharmacia Scientific, San Francisco, CA).
10. Electrophoretic and development unit (Phast system™, Pharmacia Biotech).

3. Methods

3.1. RNA Extraction (see Chapter 4)

1. Add 36 µL of 2-mercaptoethanol and 20 µL of 5 mg/mL BPB to 5 mL of Chomczynski solution D. Vortex and aliquot 450 µL to a labeled sterile 2 mL polypropylene screw-capped tube. To this, add 100 µL of serum (mix by pipetting), 50 µL of NaAc (pH 4.0), 500 µL phenol, and 125 µL of chloroform-isoamyl alcohol solution.
2. Screw caps on tightly and vortex vigorously for 30 min. Change gloves.
3. Place tubes in refrigerated centrifuge. Let stand at 4°C for 15 min, and then spin at 13,000*g* for 15 min.

4. Transfer 400 µL of the aqueous phase (top) to a sterile propylene tube containing 40 µL of glycogen acetate mix, and 1 mL 100% alcohol. Mix well with vortex and precipitate RNA at –20°C overnight.
5. Remove tubes from freezer and spin at 4°C, 13,000g for 45 min. Carefully discard the supernatant, and add 1 mL of 75% ethanol (trying not to disturb the RNA pellet). Do not shake.
6. Spin at 4°C, 13,000g for 10 min. Carefully discard supernatant, and remove excess alcohol by swabbing the sides of the tubes using a sterile cotton-tipped applicator. Do not touch RNA pellet.
7. Add 20 µL of freshly prepared RNA dissolution buffer, and 40 µL of mineral oil. Mix with flicking and dissolve RNA pellet at 37°C for 20 min.
8. Quick-spin to separate aqueous and oil layers.

3.2. RT-PCR Assay (see Notes 4–6)

1. Thaw RT-first-round PCR batch solution (160 µL) at room temperature, and add 8 µL of 0.1 M DTT, 2.5 µL of RNase inhibitor, 1.5 µL of M-MLV-RT, and 1.6 µL of *Taq* DNA polymerase. Mix by flicking (vortex causes foaming), and quick-spin.
2. Transfer 16 µL of RT-PCR buffer (from above) to 500 µL microcentrifuge tubes, and add 4 µL of dissolved RNA from above and 40 µL of mineral oil. Mix with flicking, briefly centrifuge, and place in thermal cycler at 37°C for 45 min (for reverse transcription) followed by 94°C for 4 min (denaturing), and 40 cycles each of 94°C for 1 min (denaturing), 50°C for 1.5 min (annealing), and 72°C for 2 min (extension).
3. Remove from thermal cycler, mix first-round product by flicking, and briefly centrifuge.
4. Thaw second-round "nested" PCR batch solution (500 µL) at room temperature and add 2 µL of *Taq* DNA polymerase. Mix by flicking, briefly centrifuge, and transfer 40 µL to 500 µL centrifuge tubes.
5. To each tube, add 4 µL of first round PCR product and 40 µL of mineral oil. Flick tubes, briefly centrifuge, and place in thermal cycler at 94°C for 4 min (denaturing), followed by 40 cycles each of 94°C for 1 min (denaturing), 52°C for 1.5 min (annealing), and 72°C for 2 min (extension), and a final extension step at 37°C for 5 min.
6. Visualize the expected 196 bp "nested" PCR product under UV illumination after separation in 4% agarose and ethidium bromide staining.
7. Determine DNA concentration of "nested" PCR product using a fluorometer.
8. RT-first-round PCR: Add 100 µL of 1 M Tris-HCl (pH 8.3 at 25°C), 500 µL of 1 M KCl, 25 µL of each of 4 dNTPs (Pharmacia Biotech, 100 mM), 1.6 mL of 25 mM magnesuim chloride ($MgCl_2$, Promega, Madison, WI), 20 µL of 5 mg/mL BPB, 16 pmol each of primers 127 and 128 (*see* **Table 2**), and water to make 10 mL of solution. Mix well with vortex, aliquot into 160 µL (10 reactions), and store at –20°C.
9. Second-round "nested" PCR: Add 100 µL of 1 M Tris-HCl (pH 8.3 at 25°C), 500 µL of 1 M KCl, 20 µL of each of 4 dNTPs, 800 µL of 25 $MgCl_2$ (Promega),

Table 2
PCR Primers Used for Detection of HCV HVR1[a]

Primer	Sense	Numbering	Nucleotide sequence (5'→3')
JL128	+	1298–1320	TGGGATATGATGATGAACTGGTC
JL129	+	1413–1432	GCCTTGCCTACTATTCCATG
REG4	+	1413–1432	GCATAGCGTATTTCTCCATG
JL127	–	1891–1871	AATGAATTCTACAACAGG GCT{TG}GG{AG}GTGAA
JL130	–	1608–1589	TTGATGTGCCAACTGCCATT
REG5	–	1608–1589	TTGATGTGCCAACTGCCGTT

[a]Nucleotide numbering according to Okamoto's system (Okamoto et al., 1991); {} indicates degenerate nucleotides at that position, and *Eco*RI sequence is underlined.

60 pmol each of primers 129 and 130 or REG4 and REG5 (**Table 2**), and water to make 10 mL. Mix well with vortex, aliquot into 500 µL (10 reactions), and store at –20°C.

3.3. SSCP Electrophoresis

1. Add 25 ng of cDNA (on average 1.5–2.5 µL) to microcentrifuge tubes and SSCP denaturing solution to make 4 µL total volume. Mix and place in thermal cycler, and denature at 94°C for 10 min.
2. Place SSCP native buffer strips and 12.5% polyacrylamide precast minigels on electrophoretic apparatus and "pre-run" at 400 V, 25°C for 15 min.
3. Quick-chill denatured cDNA on ice and pipet 4 µL on paraffin paper imprinted with sample wells (using template supplied with Phast system). Quickly load denatured samples on the "prerun" polyacrylamide gels using 4 µL sample applicators (*see* **Note 7**).
4. Electrophorese at 200 V, 25°C for 200 V-ho (approx 30–40 min).
5. Carefully remove gels from electrophoresis apparatus, and place them in the silver-staining development unit. Run developing program: 20% tricarboxylic acid (20°C for 5 min), 50% ethanol/10% HAC (50°C for 2 min), 10% ethanol/5% HAC (50°C for 6 min), 5% glutaraldehyde (50°C for 6 min), 10% ethanol/5% HAC (50°C for 8 min), water (50°C for 4 min), 0.4% silver nitrate (40°C for 10 min), water (30°C for 1 min), developer (30°C for 6 min), background reducer (30°C for 8 min), and 5% glycerol (50°C for 5 min) (*see* **Note 8**).
6. Remove gels from development unit, allow to air-dry overnight, enumerate the number of bands, and photograph (*see* **Note 9** and **Figs. 2** and **3**).

4. Notes

1. The method of serum preparation significantly affects HCV RNA levels. The processing conditions described in the protocol have been shown by our laboratory to preserve HCV RNA best *(5)*.

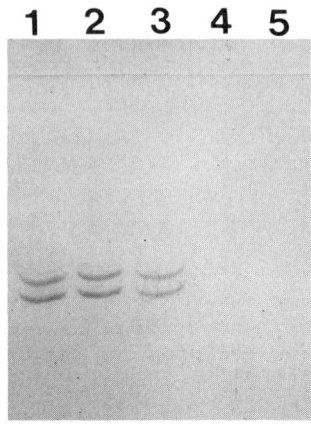

Fig. 2. Detection sensitivity of SSCP analysis using optimal electrophoretic conditions. Amount of amplicon loaded: Lane 1: 10 ng DNA, lane 2: 5 ng DNA, lane 3: 2 ng DNA, lane 4: 1 ng DNA, lane 5: no DNA loaded. Note that double-strand amplicons appear as two discrete bands, each representing single-strand DNA with different conformation.

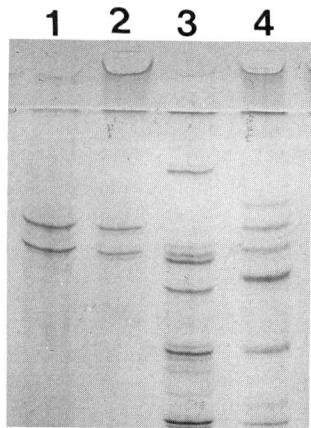

Fig. 3. SSCP analysis of four patients before interferon-α therapy; lanes 1 and 2 are from patients who had a subsequent complete and sustained response, whereas lanes 3 and 4 are from patients who had complete response with relapse or no response to therapy, respectively. Note the decreased HCV quasispecies heterogeneity in patients with a beneficial response to therapy.

2. As was discussed in Chapter 4, to avoid RNA degradation, it is essential to reduce sample contact with RNase. Thus, during all phases of RNA work, it is important to wear gloves and to use either nuclease-free water (commercially available) or water that has been treated with diethylpyrocarbonate (DEPC, mix 1 mL of

DEPC/L of water, incubate at room temperature for 2 h and autoclave the solution). Also, unused glycogen:acetate mix should be discarded and not reused since this solution easily becomes contaminated.
3. To ensure consistent RNA extraction, we routinely use commercially available water-saturated acid phenol (Amresco, Solon, OH).
4. To avoid crosscontamination during the RT-PCR process, we adhere to all of the general measures suggested by Kwok and Higuchi (6), except that different sets of pipets were used for different phases of the work instead of using positive displacement pipets. HVR1-positive and negative serum samples are included with every RT-PCR run.
5. Using degenerate primers for "nested" PCR enhances detection rate, but it necessarily introduces nucleotide variability within the amplified product, which interferes with SSCP analysis. Thus, to increase the detection rate without such primer-induced nucleotide variability, two different sets of "nested" primers from regions flanking the HVR1 region were used, in separate PCR reactions. The overall HVR1 detection rate using the RT-PCR assay described is 75–95%.
6. RT-PCR amplification efficiency is important to avoid unrepresentative sampling of quasispecies populations. Because the viral genomic region studied (HVR1) is heterogenous, it is difficult to demonstrate that all quasispecies populations in a given serum sample are equally detected. Because of this, the PCR primers used were designed from within relatively conserved areas of the HVR1, based on all sequences available in Genebank. Also, HVR1 was amplified in a similar proportion of patients infected with HCV types 1, 2, and 3, suggesting that PCR amplification efficiency was similar, at least with respect to HCV genotypes (7).
7. To avoid premature reannealing of cDNA, denatured samples should be kept on ice and gel-loaded as quickly as possible.
8. During initial experiments, we observed occasional inconsistent development when silver nitrate, developer, and background reducing solutions prepared in the laboratory were used. Such problems have been obviated by using the PhastGel™ Silver kit (Pharmacia).
9. Using the optimal conditions, the sensitivity of the SSCP assay has been consistently determined to be 1 ng/band (**Fig. 2**). Thus, viral quasispecies representing at least 4% of the total HCV population in a given sample are detected.

Acknowledgments

The oligonucleotide primers used were synthesized by the DNA Synthesis Core facilities, ICBR, University of Florida. The author would like to thank Wei-zhen Liu for her excellent technical assistance and Johnson Y. N. Lau, my mentor, for his support and encouragement. RPGP is supported in part by grants from the National Institutes of Health (KO 8AI01486), the Blowitz-Ridgeway Foundation Health Scholar Award, the Children's Miracle Network Research Fund, and the Division of Sponsored Research of the University of Florida (DSR-D-89596).

References

1. Martell, M., Esteban, J. I., Quer, J., Genesca, J., Weiner, A., Esteban, R., et al. (1992) Hepatitis C virus circulates as a population of different but closely related genome: quasispecies nature of HCV genome distribution. *Virology* **66**, 3225–3229.
2. Higashi, Y., Kakumu, S., Yoshioka, K., Wakita, T., Mizokami, M., Ohba, K., et al. (1993) Dynamics of genome change in the E2/NS1 region of hepatitis C virus in vivo. *Virology* **197**, 659–668.
3. Weiner, A. J., Brauer, M. J., Rosenblatt, J., Richman, K. H., Tung, J., Crawford, K., et al. (1991) Variable and hypervariable domains are found in the regions of HCV corresponding to the flavirus envelope and NS1 proteins and the pestivirus envelope glycoprotein. *Virology* **180**, 842–848.
4. González-Peralta, R. P., Qian, K., She, J. Y., Davis, G. L., Ohno, T., Mizokami, M., et al. (1996) Clinical implications of viral quasispecies in chronic hepatitis C. *J. Med. Virol.* **49**, 242–247.
5. Davis, G. L., Lau, J. Y. N., Urdea, M. S., Neuwald, P., Wilber, J. C., Lindsay, K., et al. (1994) Quantitative detection of hepatitis C virus RNA by solid phase branched DNA amplification method: definition and optimal conditions for specimen collection and clinical application in interferon-treated patients. *Hepatology* **19**, 1337–1341.
6. Kwok, S. and Higuchi, R. (1989) Avoiding false positives with PCR. *Nature* **339**, 237,238.
7. González-Peralta, R. P., Liu, W. Z., Davis, G. L., Qian, K., and Lau, J. Y. N. (1997) Modulation of hepatitis C virus quasispecies heterogeneity by interferon- and ribavirin therapy. *J. Viral Hepatitis* **4**, 99–106.

20

Hepatitis C Virus Heteroduplex Tracking Assay

Application to Genotype Determination, Quasispecies Analysis, and Molecular Evolution Studies

Amy J. Weiner, Piero L. Calvo, Joe Kansopon, David Gretch, Ferruccio Bonino, Maurizia Brunetto, and Michael Houghton

1. Introduction

The heteroduplex tracking assay (HTA) is a tool that can be used for determining genotype, quasispecies analysis, molecular evolution, and epidemiological studies *(1–7)*. By hybridizing a labeled, single-stranded DNA probe to colinear, reverse transcriptase (RT) PCR products from a sample of interest, the probe will either form a homoduplex with identical molecules or a heteroduplex with nonidentical sequences. The hybridization products are separated on MDE or polyacrylamide gels and visualized. Delwart et al., the developers of the HTA technique *(1,2,7)*, have previously shown that the migration of heteroduplexes relative to the homoduplex on gels are approximately proportional to the percent nucleotide divergence between two species, and therefore, the genetic distance between two species can be determined. Genetic rearrangements, deletions, and/or insertions can alter the migration of heteroduplexes in a manner that disturbs the direct relationship between relative migration and genetic distance. Typically, heteroduplexes of 0.176–1.8 kb containing >1.4–3% to ~30% nucleotide substitutions, which lack genetic alterations, can be identified as unique species on MDE gels *(1,4,6)*. The number and distribution of unique bands indicates the genetic complexity of viral species in each sample.

Two applications of HTA, which differ primarily by the choice of probe(s), are described in this chapter: genotype determination and quasispecies analysis. The partial core(C)/E1 region (444 nt) probes described in **Table 1** were specifically designed for HCV genotyping. RT-PCR products from patient or

Table 1
HTA RT-PCR Primers

	Primer	5'-3'[d]	PCR
Genotype (6)			
C170S[a]	CCTGGTTGCTCTTTCTCTATCT	508–529	I
E338A1	GATGGCTTGTGGGATCCGGAG	1032–1012	I
E338A2a	GATGACCTCGGGGACGCGCAT	1032–1012	I
E338A2b	GACCAGTTCTGGAACACGAGC	1032–1012	I
E338A3a	CAAGGTCTGGGGTAAACGCAG	1032–1012	I
E320A[b]	CCAGTTCATCATCATATCCCA	978–958	II
C179S1	TGGCCCTGCTCTCTTGCTTGAC	536–557	II
C179S2	TTGCTCTTCTGTCGTGCGTCAC	536–557	II
C179S3	TTGCTCTGTTCTCTTGCTTAAT	536–557	II
E2 HV[c]			
X(E2)14	GGTGCTCACTGGGGAGTCCT	1048–1067	I
(C) (G)			
X(E2)18J	CATTGCAGTTCAGGGCCGTGCTA	1291–1269	I
X(E2)4	TCCATGGTGGGGAACTGGGC	1087–1106	II
X(E2)19J	TGCCAACTGCCGTTGGTGTT	1262–1243	II

[a]C170S, universal sense primer for genotype determination.
[b]E320A, universal antisense primer for genotype determination.
[c]Suitable for type 1a and 1b HCV (9). The nucleotides given above X(E2)18J in parentheses are preferred in type 1b HCV.
[d]Nucleotide coordinates according to **ref. 15**.

blood donor sera are hybridized to five subtype specific probes (1a, 1b, 2a, 2b, 3a), which fail to crosshybridize to each other, in order to identify the genotype of the virus(es) in the sample. For example, a 3a probe formed a tight cluster of heteroduplexes with 7 of 15 patient samples in **Fig. 1A** (lanes 1–7), whereas a 1a probe failed to hybridize to any of the same 15 patient samples (**Fig. 1B**). Therefore, **Fig. 1** indicates seven type 3a and no type 1a HCV in the set of 15 samples analyzed. In addition, **Fig. 1A** shows that 2 samples, lanes 3 and 5, had two unique 3a species. The migration of a heteroduplex relative to a set of standard homoduplexes of known percent nucleotide divergence from the probe can be measured to determine the genetic distance between the sample and the probe without sequencing the PCR products more precisely.

For quasispecies analysis, two closely related techniques, HTA and heteroduplex mobility assay (HMA), have been described (1,2). In the HTA method, a probe derived from an RT-PCR product found in a particular individual can be used to track related sequences in the individual and/or popula-

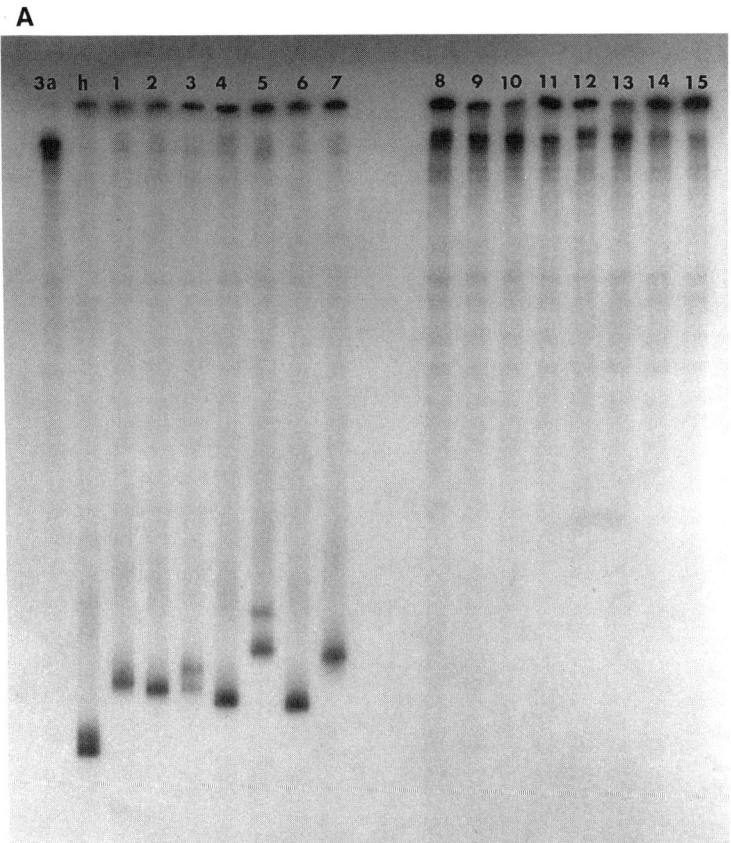

Fig. 1. Single-stranded probes (lanes 3a, 1a, and 2a in **A–C** respectively) were hybridized to PCR products from either the same control sample from which they were derived, forming homoduplexes (h), or from patient sera, which formed heteroduplexes (numbered lanes). Autoradiographs of the hybridization products electrophoresed on MDE gels are shown in (A–C).

tion over a period of time *(4,5)*. The predominant species, or "master" sequence, in the sample can be identified by cloning and sequencing the RT-PCR products *(4)* or by simply choosing a few clones as templates for making probes and observing which probe generates the most frequently represented pattern of heteroduplexes when hybridized to the population of RT-PCR products from which clone was derived. HMA involves hybridizing labeled or unlabeled, total PCR products from one sample to total PCR products from a particular individual or group of individuals over a period of time in order to evaluate shifting populations of viral genomes *(1)*. The choice of primers for HTA/HMA

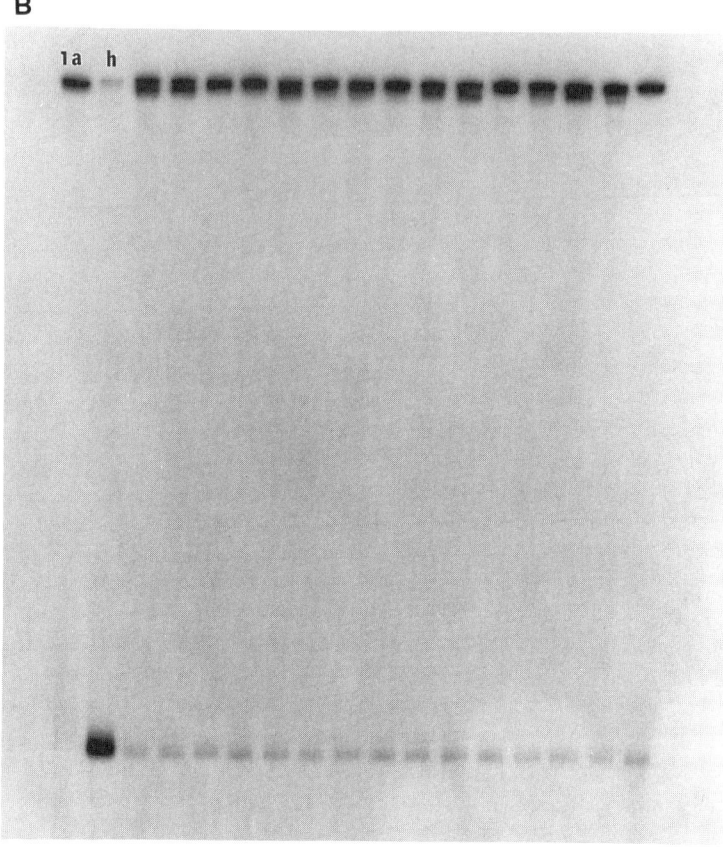

Fig. 1. **(B)**

depends on nature of the experimental questions being addressed. For example, Gretch et al. used RT-PCR primers from the E2HV (HVRI) region of the E2 *(8–10)* (*see* **Table 1**) to investigate quasispecies in liver transplant patients.

Alternatively, since substantial evidence suggests that the hypervariation in the E2HV domain most likely results from positive immune selection, other less mutable regions of the genome, such as the 5'-UTR, NS5, and E2(p7)/NS2, have been used to study quasispecies by DNA sequencing *(11,12)*. E1 primers, which were used for genotype determination, have also been used to demonstrate evolutionary diversity among type 2 HCV *(6)*. The degree of nucleotide heterogeneity and the genetic stability of the region are important factors in choosing appropriate RT-PCR fragments for HTA/HMA analysis.

C

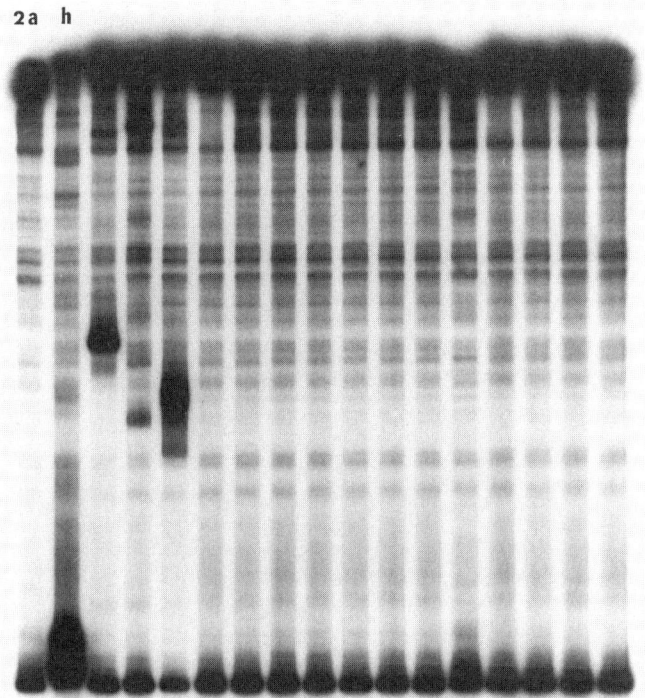

Fig. 1. (C)

In summary, HTA:

1. Offers a high degree of accuracy in determining genotype.
2. Is more easily performed than DNA sequencing.
3. Can detect related species that are up to 30–35% divergent.
4. Can detect coinfections where one genotype may not be detected by RFLP *(11)* or DNA sequencing *(6)*.

HTA results are more reliable than those obtained with SSCP, since the interpretation of SSCP gels may be complicated by the ability of the individual strands of dsPCR products to behave aberrantly in gels. Although HTA is not a large-scale genotyping assay, 60–100 samples can be analyzed weekly. In combination with RFLP prescreening (*see* **Note 1**), a larger number of samples could be processed. Discrepancies between HTA and RFLP are most likely to arise in cases where coinfections or new or diverging HCV subtypes, such as in type 2 HCV, occur.

HTA is particularly useful for tracking HCV variants without DNA sequencing. In contrast to SSCP, which is reported to detect a unique species at a frequency of 1/20 *(13)*, or DNA sequencing 10–30 clones, radioactively labeled HTA probes can identify a genetic variant that is represented at a frequency of approx 1/150 (D. Gretch, personal communication).

2. Materials (*see* Note 11)

All materials used in the following protocol, with the exception of single-strand probe preparation and hybridization buffers, are defined in the following commercially available kits (*see* **Note 2**):

1. RNA extraction: Strategene RNA Isolation Kit (#200345), QIAmp RNA Kit (Qiagen #29504).
2. cDNA synthesis: AMV-Reverse Transcriptase (RT) System (Gibco-BRL 8085SB).
3. PCR: Perkin Elmer #N801-0055.
4. 1X Blocking buffer: 0.1% BSA 1X PBS, pH 6.7.
5. Wash buffer: 5 mM Tris-HCl, pH 7.5, 0.5 mM EDTA, pH 8.0, 1.0 M NaCl.
6. STE: 0.1 M NaCl, 10 mM Tris-HCl, pH 8.0, 1 mM EDTA, pH 8.0.
7. 1X SSC: 0.15 M NaCl, 0.015 M Na citrate.
8. 10X TBE: 27.5 g boric acid (0.44 M), 162.0 g Trisma base (1.34 M), 9.5 g EDTA, tetrasodium salt (0.025 M) in 1 L distilled water (DIW) (1X = pH 8.8).
9. 10X Gel-loading buffer: 0.25 g bromophenol blue, 0.25 g xylene cyanol FF, 25.0 g Ficoll type 400, in 100 mL DIW.

3. Methods

3.1. RNA Extraction

1. Extract 100–200 µL plasma sample or sera using the Stratagene RNA Isolation Kit, QIAmp RNA kit, or alternative method, according to manufacturer's instructions. Resuspend RNA in 10 µL DEPC-treated, sterile DIW.

3.2. cDNA Synthesis

1. Using reagents provided in the AMV-RT cDNA synthesis kit, prepare the cocktail with the appropriate cDNA primer (**Table 1**). For each reaction (Rx), use 1–5 µL RNA. For 20 Rx:
       47–127 µL DIW (DEPC, autoclaved) (adjust DIW according to the amount of RNA/Rx)
       100 µL 5X RT buffer (500 mM Tris-HCl, pH 8.3, 50 mM MgCl$_2$, 50 mM DTT)
       100 µL 5X KCl (250 mM KCl)
       50 µL dNTP (10 mM each dNTP, pH 7.5)
       23 µL 10X KCl (500 mM)
       20 µL Antisense primer II (**Fig. 2**), 100 pmol/µL (*see* **Note 3**)

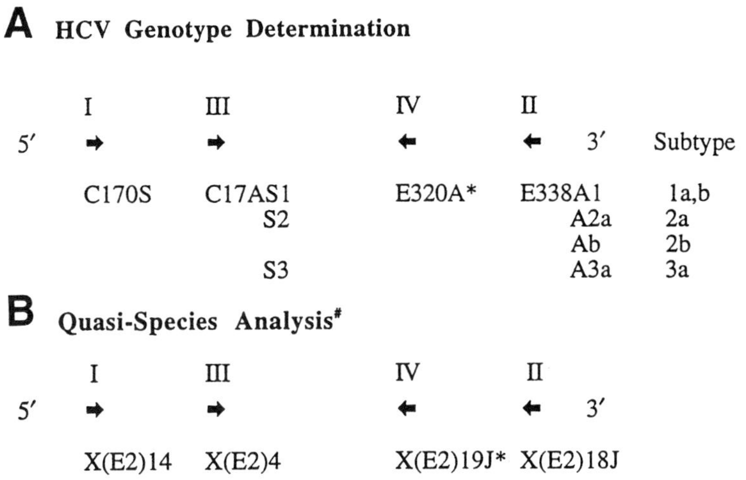

A HCV Genotype Determination

	I	III	IV	II	
5'	→	→	←	← 3'	Subtype
	C170S	C17AS1	E320A*	E338A1	1a,b
		S2		A2a	2a
				Ab	2b
		S3		A3a	3a

B Quasi-Species Analysis#

	I	III	IV	II
5'	→	→	←	← 3'
	X(E2)14	X(E2)4	X(E2)19J*	X(E2)18J

Fig. 2. Nested RT-PCR primers for genotype determination (**A**) (6) and/or quasispecies analysis (**B**) (9,4,5) are depicted graphically. Biotinylated (*) primers are used to generate ss probes.

20 µL RNasin (2500 U/40 µL)
40 µL AMV-RT (~2.5 U/µL)
Use 21 µL cocktail/reaction. Final reaction volume is 500 µL or 25 µL/Rx.
2. Incubate the samples for 1 h at 37°C or 30–45 min at 42°C.

3.3. Nested PCR (PCR I and II)

1. PCR I: Prepare the PCR I 3X cocktail. For 20 Rx:
   200 µL DIW
   150 µL 10X PCR buffer (500 mM KCl, 100 mM Tris HCl, pH 8.3, 15 mM MgCl$_2$, 0.1% gelatin)
   150 µL dNTP mix (200 µL DIW, 50 µL of each dNTP [1.25 mM]; final concentration is 200 µM of each dNTP)
   20 µL Sense primer I (**Fig. 2**), 100 pmol/µL (*see* **Note 3**)
   10 µL *Taq* polymerase (5 U/µL)
   Use 25 µL cocktail per reaction.
2. To each completed RT reaction, add 50 µL DIW. Heat at 94°C for 5 min, and then cool on ice for 2 min. Quick-spin samples. Add the resulting 75 µL of RT reaction mixture to a PCR reaction tube containing 25 µL of the PCR I 3X cocktail. Final reaction volume is 100 µL.
3. Perform PCR (*see* **Note 4**) in Perkin Elmer 9600 thermocycler. Forty cycles:
   94°C 10 s
   55°C 30 s (*see* **Note 5**)
   72°C 30 s
   72°C 7 min
   4°C

4. PCR II (*see* **Note 6**): Prepare reaction cocktail. For 1 Rx:
   63.5–72.5 µL DIW (adjust water according to the amount of DNA/Rx)
   1–10 µL DNA (PCRI)
   10 µL 10X PCR buffer
   16 µL dNTP mix
   0.5 µL *Taq* polymerase (5 U/µL)
   1 µL Sense primer (100 pmol/µL) (III, **Fig. 2**)
   1 µL Antisense primer (100 pmol/µL) (IV, **Fig. 2**)
   Final PCR reaction volume is 100 µL.
5. Repeat **step 3** except for the 1b reaction in which the annealing temperature is 45°C (*see* **Note 5**).
6. Check the yield of the method PCR product by loading 2–5 µL onto a 1.0-mm thick, 5% Tris-borate-EDTA polyacrylamide gel. A strong band of approx 50–100 ng should be visualized with ethidium bromide (*see* **Note 7**). The ratio of unlabeled PCR product (driver DNA) to the radiolabeled ss probe should be approx 100:1 in the hybridization reaction (**Subheading 5.3.**).

3.4. Single-Stranded Probes (from Eric Delwart, see Note 8)

PCR products from cloned DNA or RT-PCR I products from individual sera serve as the template for PCR II using a biotinylated primer (**Fig. 2**). The double-stranded (ds) biotinylated PCR product is then bound to washed, strepavidin-coated magnetic beads. The nonbiotinylated, single-stranded (ss) DNA is released into solution after denaturation in alkalai, neutralized with acid, subsequently labeled, and used as the HTA probe.

3.4.1. ssDNA

1. Remove primers from the PCR reaction using Wizard PCR prep or an alternative method, before adding PCR products to the streptavidin magnetic beads.
2. Wash beads by pipeting 50 µL of the streptavidin magnetic beads into an 1.5-mL Eppendorf tube, and place in a magnetic separator. After beads collect on the side of the tube, draw off the liquid with a pipet, and add 100 µL of blocking buffer. Mix well. Remove the blocking buffer after placing tubes in magnetic separator, and add 100 µL of 1X wash buffer. Mix well. Remove the 1X wash buffer after placing tube in magnetic separator, and add 50 µL of 2X wash buffer. Mix well.
3. Add ≤50 µL biotinylated PCR product (~1–2 µg) to 50 µL 2X wash buffer in tube. (Use 1X wash buffer to bring the total volume of the sample to 100 µL, if necessary). Mix well.
4. Incubate beads with PCR product at room temperature for 15 min. Remove buffer from the sample as in **step 2**.
5. Add 8 µL **freshly** prepared 0.1 *N* NaOH, mix, and incubate for 10 min at room temperature. Separate beads from liquid in magnetic separator, and transfer liquid into a fresh Eppendorf tube.

6. Add:
   40 µL DIW
   4 µL 0.2 N HCl
   1 µL 1 M Tris-HCl, pH 8.0

3.4.2. Radiolabeling ssDNA (Probe)

1. Reaction mixture:
   10 µL ss probe DNA (10–20 ng)
   2 µL 10X polynucleotide kinase buffer
   2 µL T4 polynucleotide kinase (PNK, 10 U/µL)
   5 µL ^{32}P-ATP, 10 mCi/mL
   Incubate for 1 h at 37°C. Add additional 3 µL PNK, and continue incubation for 1 h at 37°C.
2. Add 30 µL STE. Purify labeled ss probe with the G-50 spin column.
3. Count 2 µL PNK reaction in scintillation counter. A minimum of 10^6 cpm/µL are required for HTA hybridization (see **Note 9**).

3.5. Hybridization

1. Add the following reactants to a 1.5 mL Sarsteadt tube:
   1–3 µL PCR II product (≥50–200 ng, see **Note 10**)
   5 µL 2X SSC
   1–2 µL ^{32}P-ssProbe (0.5–2 ng)
   0–3 µL DIW
   Final volume is 10 µL.
   Overlay with mineral oil.
2. Place tubes in a 94°C heat block for 3 min. Transfer tubes to a 55°C heat block, and incubate for at least 2 h.

3.6. Gel Analysis of Hybridization Products

1. Siliconize glass plates using Baker Gel Slick.
2. Prepare a 33 cm × 42 cm, 1 mm thick sequencing gel using a 36-well standard comb (do not Shark's tooth, "v" shaped wells for DNA sequencing).
   66 mL DIW
   75 mL MDE Gel, 2X
   9 mL TBE, 10X
   50 µL TEMED
   0.5 mL ammonium persulfate, 10%
   Let the gel set for 1 h.
3. Set up sequencing gel apparatus. Use 0.6X TBE running buffer.
4. Pull two samples at a time from the heat block in order to avoid dropping the temperature of the reactions before they are loaded into the well. Quickly add 2 µL of 10X gel-loading buffer to each reaction and to do a quick spin in a microfuge. With clean P20 pipet tips, load sample onto the gel.

5. Run the gel at 400 mV for about 16 h. For consistent results, the dye front should stop at the same place on the gel if different gels will be compared. Adjust time if necessary.
6. Mount the gel onto a Whatman 3M chromotography paper. Drying in a heated gel (typically requires 45 min).
7. Remove dry gel and expose to film 5 min to 2 h, depending on the probe specific activity. Try a 2-h exposure initially and adjust as needed.

4. Notes

1. By performing RT-PCR using 5'-UTR primers and analyzing the products with RFLP *(11)*, a quick genotype estimate can be made and thereby reduce the number of subtype probes required for HTA. The drawback of this approach is that genotyping with the 5'-UTR may be inaccurate. The HTA result will, however, clearly (a) indicate whether the genotype is valid and (b) further indicate coinfections or highly divergent species.
2. Alternative kits or reagents for **Subheadings 3.1.–3.3.** may be equally suitable for the HTA assay, but were not tested in our laboratory. For example, one could substitute a "one-tube" RT-PCR method for cDNA synthesis. Note that systems such as Boehringer Mannheim Titan™ system (cat. #1-855-382, 25 reactions), utilize a 60% reverse transcription step, which may not work well for mismatched 1b primers.
3. We have used a variety of primer concentrations for cDNA (25–100 pmol) and PCR reactions (50–100 pmol), and have found equivalent results using the conditions described in **Subheadings 3.2. and 3.3.**
4. PCR conditions were designed for small, <0.5 kb, PCR products. For larger PCR products, we recommend using a proofreading *Taq* polymerase, such as Stratagene PFU or Perkin Elmer Ultima Taq polymerase. If multiple PCR products are observed on ethidum bromide gels, we recommend using Ampli Wax Gem 100 beads (Perkin Elmer N808-0100) or similar products to eliminate nonspecific priming events. The number of cycles can be reduced to 30 if the sample has a relatively high titer of HCV.
5. If a sample is known to be RT-PCR-positive using primers from the 5'-UTR, but PCR-negative using HTA primers, we suggest lowering the annealing temperature to identify potentially new or diverging HCV subtypes. If a primer is known to have a higher degree of mismatch in a related subtype than to other sequences of the same subtype, i.e., the 1a PCR II sense primer is mismatched with the corresponding concensus 1b sequence, reducing the annealing temperature can allow the use of that primer to amplify the mismatched sequence without having to synthesize a new primer specifically suited to the subtype in which mismatches were found.
6. The number of PCR II reactions required to obtain 1–2 µg of PCR II product depends on the yield of PCR I product. Since we typically do not know the titer of the sample being evaluated, we pool two to four PCR II reactions to ensure obtaining enough material to perform several HTA hybridizations. The amount of DNA added to the PCR II reaction should not exceed the amount that produces two bands (PCR I and II reaction products) on ethidium bromide-stained poly-

acrylamide gels after the PCR II reaction is completed. Typically, we introduce <10 ng DNA into the PCR II reaction.
7. To estimate roughly the amount of PCR product, electrophorese a known amount of a molecular standard that contains a fragment approximately the same size as the PCR product.
8. Production of ssDNA probes is a slightly modified, unpublished protocol generously given to us by Eric Delwart. Biotinylated primers, PCR products, and biotinylated probes should be stored in aliquots at –20°C (avoid freeze-thawing). We typically prepare fresh probe from either stored biotinylated DNA or from freshly synthesized biotinylated PCR products. Intact biotinylated DNA is important for generating good ss probes. DNA degradation during the production of ss probes can cause dsDNA contamination of the ss probe. Background resulting from degraded probe is illustrated in **Fig. 1A,C**.
9. For genotype determination, the probe should have a high enough specific activity (10^6 cpm/µL) to give rapid results (~5–15 min) and to avoid long exposures, which can result in high backgrounds (*see* **Fig. 1C**).
10. To generate heteroduplexes or homoduplexes, respectively, add PCR products from the experimental sample or the nonbiotinylated PCR products from which the probe was derived to the labeled, ss probe in individual reactions.
11. List of materials and suppliers:

AMV-Reverse Transcriptase (RT) system	Gibco-BRL 8085SB
Gel slick	J.T. Baker 4746-00
Gel 36-well Comb (1.0 mm)	J.T. Baker 4743-00
G-50 spin columns	Pharmacia, Cat. #275335-01
T4 Polynucleotide kinase	Promega #501-6412
Magnetic Bead Separator	Dynal (MPC-E1 [1 tube] or E [6 tubes])
MDE Gel, 2X	J.T. Baker, Cat. #4739-00
PCR kit	Perkin Elmer #N801-0055
^{32}P-ATP, 10 mC/mL	Amersham #PB, 10068
Polynucleotide kinase buffer	Fisher PRM 4101
QIAmp RNA Kit	Qiagen #29504
RNAsin	Promega, Fisher #PRN2111
RNA Isolation Kit	Stratagene #200345
Wizard PCR prep	Promega #A7170
Sarsteadt 1.5 ml tubes	Sarsteadt 726.92005
Sequencing Gel System	Gibco-BRL #21105-010
Streptavidin magnetic beads	Dynal #112.05

Acknowledgments

The authors are grateful to Eric Delwart for sharing his unpublished ssDNA probe production protocol. We also thank Jeff Wilson, Steve Polyak, and Kevin Crawford for technical assistance and helpful discussions. DNA sequencing was expertly performed by Chun Ting Lee. We also thank Peter Anderson for preparation of the manuscript. The work was supported by Chiron Vaccines.

References

1. Delwart, E. L., Shpaer, E. G., Louwagie, J., McCutchan, F. E., Grez, M., Rübsamen-Waigmann, H., et al. (1993) Genetic relationships determined by a DNA heteroduplex mobility assay. Analysis of HIV-1 *env* genes. *Science* **262,** 1257–1261.
2. Delwart, E. L., Busch, M. P., Kalish, M. L., Mosley, J. W., and Mullins, J. I. (1995) Rapid molecular epidemiology of HIV-1 transmission. *AIDS Res.* **11,** 1181–1193.
3. Kostrikis, L. G., Bagdades, E., Cao, Y., Zhang, L., Dimitriou, D., and Ho, D. D. (1995) Genetic analysis of human immunodeficiency virus type 1 strains from patients in Cyprus. Identification of a new subtype designated subtype I. *J. Virol.* **69,** 6122–6130.
4. Wilson, J. J., Polyak, S. J., Day, T. D., and Gretch, D. R. (1995) Characterization of simple and complex hepatitis C virus quasispecies by heteroduplex gel shift analysis. Correlation with nucleotide sequencing. *J. Gen. Virol.* **76,** 1763–1771.
5. Gretch, D. R., Polyak S. J., Wilson, J. J., Carithers, R. L., Perkins, J. D., and Corey, L. (1996) Tracking hepatitis C virus quasispecies major and minor variants in symptomatic and asymptomatic liver transplant recipients. *J. Virol.* **70,** 7622–7631.
6. Calvo, P. L., Kansopon, J., Sra, K., Quan, S., DiNello, R., Guaschino, R., et al. (1996) Diverging hepatitis C virus (HCV) genotype 2 isolates identified in Italian hemodialysis patients by heteroduplex tracking assay. *JCM*, submitted.
7. Delwart E. L., Sheppard, H. W., Walker, B. D., Goudsmit, J., and Mullins, J. I. (1994) Human immunodeficiency virus type 1 evolution in vivo tracked by DNA heteroduplex mobility assays. *J. Virol.* **68,** 6672–6683.
8. Weiner, A. J., Brauer, M. J., Rosenblatt, J., Richman, K. H., Tung, J., Crawford, K., et al. (1991) Variable and hypervariable domains are found in the regions of HCV corresponding to the flavivirus envelope and NS1 proteins and the pestivirus envelope glycoproteins. *Virology* **180,** 842–848.
9. Weiner, A. J., Geysen, H. M., Christopherson, C., Hall, J. E., Mason, T. J., Saracco, G., et al. (1992) Evidence for immune selection of hepatitis C virus (HCV) putative envelope glycoprotein variants: Potential role in chronic HCV infections. *Proc. Natl. Acad. Sci. USA* **89,** 3468–3472.
10. Hijikata, M., Kato, N., Ootsuyama, Y., Nakagawa, M., Ohkoshi, S., and Shimotohno, K. (1991) Hypervariable regions in the putative glycoprotein of hepatitis C virus. *Biochem. Biophys. Res. Commun.* **175,** 220–228.
11. Bukh, J., Miller, R. H., and Purcell, R. H. (1995) Genetic heterogeneity of hepatitis C virus: Quasispecies and genotypes. *Semin. Liver Dis.* **15,** 41–63.
12. Davidson, E., Simmonds, P., Ferguson, J. C., Jarvis, L. M., Dow, B. C., Follett, E. A. C., et al. (1995) Survey of major genotypes and subtypes of hepatitis C virus using RFLP of sequences amplified from the 5' non-coding region. *J. Gen. Virol.* **76,** 1197–1204.

13. Cabot, B., Esteban, J. I., Martell, M., Genescà, J., Vargas, V., Esteban, R., et al. (1997) Structure of replicating hepatitis C virus (HCV) quasispecies in the liver may not be reflected by analysis of circulating HCV virions. *J. Virol.* **71,** 1732–1734.
14. Enomoto, N., Kurosaki, M., Tanaka, Y., Marumo, F., and Sato, C. (1994) Fluctuation of hepatitis C virus quasispecies in persistent infection and interferon treatment revealed by single-strand conformation polymorphism analysis. *J. Gen. Virol.* **75,** 1361–1369.
15. Choo, Q.-L., Richman, K. H., Han, J. H., Berger, K., Lee, C., Dong, C., et al. (1991) Genetic organization and diversity of the hepatitis C virus. *Proc. Natl. Acad. Sci. USA* **88,** 2451–2455.

V

DETECTION OF HCV IN SITU

21

In Situ Detection of HCV

An Overview

Francesco Negro and Johnson Y. N. Lau

1. Introduction

Hepatitis C virus (HCV) is the agent responsible for the majority of cases of the parenterally transmitted non-A, non-B hepatitis. The major obstacles to its discovery were the low level of replication in the infected host, both natural and experimental, and the low immunogenicity of its proteins, making it difficult to characterize antigen–antibody systems associated with this virus *(1)*. The genome of HCV is a (+) single-stranded RNA of about 9400 nucleotides, genetically related to the flavi- and pestiviruses *(2)*. HCV RNA can be detected in infected individuals by reverse transcripterase (RT) and polymerase chain reaction (PCR)-based assays, which underscore the low replicative levels of HCV. The fine mechanisms of the pathogenesis of HCV-associated liver damage are unknown. This is owing both to the limited availability of experimental animal models (chimpanzees) and to the difficulties in reproducing in vitro infection models. The abovementioned low titer of the virus in clinical samples has hampered the studies on the viral life cycle in vivo. These problems are reflected by the conflicting results that have been reported by the investigators who attempted to localize HCV products in infected tissues by *in situ* hybridization (ISH), immunohistochemistry, and *in situ* PCR. The published data are sometimes discrepant and in some cases have been very difficult to reproduce. The scope of this chapter is to review the data reported in the literature, whereas the technical procedures are discussed in more detail elsewhere in this book. Critical reviews on the subject have appeared recently in the literature *(3,4)*.

2. In Situ Hybridization

ISH is aimed at identifying nucleic acid sequences in morphologically intact tissues. Therefore, ISH may assess the topographical correlations between the presence of a nucleic acid and both morphological and immunocytochemical features. In viral infections, ISH is used to define the tissue and cell tropism, the subcellular site of replication, and the relationship between viral replication and the host protein expression (e.g., adhesion molecules, proliferation markers) or with the cell damage (cytopathic effect, inflammatory infiltrate). ISH is therefore a very powerful tool, complementary to other molecular biology techniques, to study the pathobiology of an infectious agent.

The major problem in the study of the tissue expression of HCV RNA by ISH is the low level of HCV replication. The intrinsic sensitivity limit of ISH is probably not enough to detect HCV RNA in all infected cells. A second problem lies in the fact that the true cell tropism of HCV is hypothetical and can only be inferred by comparison with the somehow related flavi- and pestiviruses *(5,6)*. A priori, HCV should infect hepatocytes and the cells of the lymphoid system. However, given the spectrum of extrahepatic disorders associated with HCV infection (e.g., skin and thyroid diseases) *(7)*, one cannot exclude that the HCV cell tropism may be much more varied than expected. Despite these caveats, the availability of a sensitive, specific, and reproducible procedure to detect HCV RNA by ISH would be of unquestionable importance. Several issues of clinical relevance are still unanswered, such as the exact timing of the recurrent HCV infection in the transplanted liver, the site of ongoing HCV replication in the healthy HCV carriers, and the putative role of HCV in the extrahepatic manifestations in patients with acute and chronic hepatitis C.

An increasing number of investigators have reported on the detection of HCV RNA by ISH, both in the liver and in extrahepatic tissues, both in the peer-reviewed literature and as communications at scientific meetings *(8–31)*. Data are often conflicting with one another, and probably not a single protocol has been independently reproduced.

The evidence that HCV infects the hepatocytes is almost unanimous. However, in a single, unconfirmed report *(10)*, use of ^{125}I-labeled riboprobes representing about 35% of the HCV genome (thus a very sensitive approach) identified rare mononuclear cells as the only site of HCV replication. These cells were probably lymphocytes or macrophages close to portal tracts. The signal was shown to be specific by appropriate experiments. A few other investigators have reported the HCV infection of tissue mononuclear cells, other than from hepatocytes *(9,11,14,18)*, but the cell types involved were not further characterized. In one case *(14)* also the biliary epithelial cells were shown to be infected by HCV. This observation is intriguing, since HCV infection is often associated with biliary ducts damage. Again, these data have not been independently confirmed. There are also isolated reports decribing the HCV tropism for the skin *(17)* and the salivary gland epithelial cells *(27)*.

What is the proportion of infected cells, and what is the overall proportion of positive specimens? Once more, the answer in not univocal. Oddly enough, most authors, using differently labeled probes, usually covering a very small portion of the HCV genome (0.32–3.8%), report a diffuse signal, often involving the vast majority of hepatocytes *(8,16,21)*. This is in conflict with the known low level of viremia, whose detection invariably needs the RT-PCR amplification. A hypothetical restricted replication of HCV may not for this discrepancy, since HCV RNA needs to be amplified even when extracted from tissues. Interestingly, despite the alleged high sensitivity of some procedures, the proportion of totally negative specimens can be as high as 70% *(24)*. The likelihood of a sampling bias may therefore be a frequent event in assessing intrahepatic HCV replication. Other contradictory results have been reported on the peripheral blood mononuclear cells (PBMC). Using a radiolabeled probe, some authors have reported a very rare proportion of infected PBMC (1–3 out of 10,000) *(22)*. In contrast, using RNA probes labeled with digoxigenin and revealed by an immunohistochemical procedure (i.e., a less sensitive procedure), the proportion of infected PBMC was ranging from 30 to 50% *(18)*.

Another issue concerns the subcellular localization of HCV RNA, which may be of interest because of possible interactions with specific cell constituents. Despite the fact that the majority of investigators have described a cytoplasmic localization of HCV RNA, some authors have reported a nuclear staining, both with radioactive *(9,10)* and nonradioactive *(14)* probes. Although most immunohistochemistry data have localized HCV proteins in the cytoplasm of hepatocytes (*see* **Subheading 3.**), a nuclear phase of the viral replicative cycle cannot be ruled out, as shown also for some flaviviruses, which have been otherwise reported to replicate predominantly in the cytoplasm *(5)*.

What is the relationship with cell damage? This is a relevant issue, but the picture is again very hazy. In acutely infected chimpanzees, where the time-course of replication vs histopathology has been studied in detail *(8)*, infected hepatocytes appear to be healthy, and necrotic areas do not contain detectable amounts of HCV RNA. However, the extent of intrahepatic replication of HCV seems to vary in parallel with the serum alanine aminotransferases: a direct damage to the hepatocyte membrane has been hypothesized, although a sampling bias may be a likely explanation. Lack of cytopathic changes of the infected cells has been reported by almost all authors who have analyzed histopathology in detail. In a single report *(13)*, however, HCV RNA-positive hepatocytes often contained fat droplets, even though the significance of this association was not evaluated and a precise cause–effect relationship cannot be therefore established. HCV-induced liver damage is likely owing to the host immune reaction, as suggested by the finding that hepatocytes positive for HCV RNA are frequently associated with mononuclear cell infiltration *(16,21)*. The correlation between biliary epithelial cells infection and damage was anecdotally reported *(14)* but not confirmed.

The technical issues raised by ISH protocols are several. The most widely used fixation procedure involves a more or less prolonged passage in formalin. The formalin fixation creates tight crosslinks between macromolecules, and therefore a decreased diffusion of the probe. The Bouin fixation as well as other procedures using precipitating agents is very good for preserving morphology and may allow a better diffusion of large probes. However, this approach is not recommended to detect small RNA molecules by ISH, since their retention during the various steps of the ISH procedure is lower than with crosslinking fixatives. Another issue is represented by the activation of cellular RNases during the time interval between the collection of the specimen and its fixation. RNA degradation may also occur during the hot embedding procedure needed to melt the paraffin. For these reasons, embedding in water-soluble moieties followed by snap-freezing in liquid nitrogen is probably the best procedure. Formation of crystals can be avoided by tissue permeation by cryopreserving solutions (e.g., 30% sucrose) prior to freezing.

The choice of the reporter molecule for probe labeling is also a relevant issue. Since both biotin- and ^{35}S-labeled probes may give nonspecific staining, many authors have advocated the use of digoxigenin *(8,14,16–18,21,23–27,29–31)*. Digoxigenin is of plant origin, and antisera raised against this hapten are unlikely to bind nonspecifically to endogenous epitopes (*see* Chapter 23). An alternative approach exploits oligomers with polythymidine tails as probes. The UV-induced dimerization between two adjacent thymines creates an immunogenic structure that can be detected by specific antibodies *(11,12,15,19,28)*. Unfortunately, nonradioactive probes are also less sensitive than radioactive ones. To improve sensitivity, some authors have used oligonucleotide mixtures or a signal amplification system by the alkaline phosphatase/antialkaline phosphatase antibody (APAAP) complexes *(8,25)* (*see* Chapter 23). However, convincing results were reported *(16,21,26,29)* with a relatively insensitive approach, i.e., use of digoxigeninlabeled double-stranded DNA probes. A self-sustained signal amplification may be obtained with these probes if conditions are used that allow intermolecular network formation.

Our personal experience with ISH suggests that a major issue for a correct interpretation of the ISH results lies in the appropriate choice of control experiments. In fact, most currently used specificity experiments may not be sufficient. Normal liver tissue is not a good control, since it may not express specific RNAs abundant in diseased livers, independently of the etiology. Therefore, use of a large number of liver tissues covering a wide spectrum of pathologies should be consistently used. Predigestion of sections with nucleases is useful, but not critical. Unrelated probes are important and should be chosen of the same length and G + C content as the specific probe. When confronted with an unexpected positive signal in *bona fide* negative control tissues, an analysis of the hybrid T_m in both true and supposedly false-positive tissues should be performed. This is best accomplished by using a rather low temperature of hybridization followed by stringent washes performed at increasing temperatures *(32)*. Obviously, a perfectly matched hybrid is more stable than a mismatched one, and the optimization of the wash temperature may allow for a specific detection of the target molecule. If the signal disappears at the same washing temperature from the true-positive tissue section as well as from the falsely positive one, the signal is very probably owing to a nonspecific basepairing. Finally, within certain limits imposed by the intrinsic sensitivity of each procedure, the characteristics of a signal (localization, number of positive cells) should be consistent when varying the labeling technique while maintaining unaltered all other variables.

In conclusion, reported techniques are difficult to reproduce. Newly available procedures should probably be independently confirmed in order to assess their reliability. The possibility of sharing samples and reagents has been proposed, but it may be difficult to bring into effect *(32)*. The variability among different series of samples may be resolved by establishing a unique panel of tissue specimens well characterized from the clinical and virological points of view to be analyzed simultaneously by all investigators.

3. Immunohistochemistry

Several papers have described the successful immunocytochemical detection of HCV proteins in tissues *(21,23,33–45)*. As for the ISH, conflicting data and difficulties in reproducing consistent results are evident and somehow discouraging. However, with respect to ISH, there is a tendency toward more consistency at least as far as the cellular and subcellular localization of HCV proteins are concerned. Thus, immunohistochemistry (IHC) seems to be a more sensitive and reliable technique to identify HCV cell tropism, although the detection of viral proteins may not always identify the presence of a productive viral replication, as well as is described for other pathogens.

The reported procedures use chemically fixed, paraffin-embedded as well as frozen tissues. In the former case, use of crosslinking fixatives requires a limited proteolytic digestion or microwave treatment for retrieval of some antigens. Nonspecific enzyme activities that may interfere with the reporter system and nonspecific adsorption are then blocked with appropriate nonimmune serum. Primary antibodies are applied to interact with the viral antigens, and the detection can be accomplished by applying one or more layers of revealing antibodies. The successful and reliable detection of viral antigens by IHC depends on several factors. First, the binding affinity of an antibody to its antigen is usually lower than a molecular hybridization reaction. Therefore, a relatively large number of viral antigen molecules are required to be detectable. Second, detection of every single epitope is specifically fixation-dependent. Some antigens are destroyed or masked by strong crosslinking fixatives (e.g., formaldehyde). Thus, weaker crosslinkers (paraformaldehyde), a crosslinking agent together with linker molecules (paraformaldehyde/lysine/periodate), or a precipitating fixative (e.g., an organic solvent) can be tried. In general, fixation of frozen sections with precipitating agents is known to preserve several epitopes that are masked by crosslinking agents, but each single epitope requires a specific optimization of conditions. Third, highly specific, high-affinity antibodies are essential for a good sensitivity and an optimal signal-to-background ratio. Antibodies against conformational (natural) epitopes may perform better than those raised against linear (recombinant) epitopes. Fourth, the epitope recognized by the antibody should be unique in relation to the tissue under examination. Otherwise, crossreactivity with host epitopes may occur. Based on the above, detection of HCV antigens, as for any other pathogen, must be optimized for every single antigen–antibody system. Furthermore, an appropriate choice of specificity controls is critical, as for ISH.

Some studies reported data based only on a few patients. Thus, the detection rate of these techniques, as well as the clinical significance of the intrahepatic expression of these viral antigens cannot be assessed properly. Second, only a few papers described the optimization experiments involved (if any), and it was unclear whether the detection rate reported was optimal and whether the antibodies described could be used with different fixatives. Most studies reported the application of a protocol on frozen sections fixed with organic solvents. When different fixatives were systematically evaluated, an acetone–chloroform mixture was found to be the best to preserve HCV antigens *(41)*. An exception to this observation was the study by Blight et al. *(40)*, where an organic solvent fixation was worse than formaldehyde or no fixation at all. Interestingly, all studies that reported the successful detection of HCV antigens by IHC in paraffin-embedded liver tissue detected the nonstructural protein NS4 *(33,38,45)*. However, in a study *(23)*, the monoclonal antibody (MAb) Tordji-22, which is known to recognize an epitope of NS4, stained also host-derived epitopes. Conflicting results were reported with other antibodies. The anti-HCV peptide rabbit polyclonal antibodies, which were found to give a poor signal-to-background ratio in one study *(41)*, were reported to give a good and specific signal in another *(40)*. Discordant results such as these are difficult to understand, especially when the antibodies belong to the same batch.

The cellular and subcellular localization of all HCV antigens tested is rather consistent. All positive signals are in fact localized in the hepatocyte cytoplasms, with some exceptions, where the NS4 antigen was detected in the sinusoids *(45)* or in lymphocytes, essentially CD20+ B-cells and CD8+ T-cells *(40)*. Using various systems, a signal has been detected using antibodies against the core, E1, E2, NS3, NS4, and NS5 proteins. The detection rate, however, varies considerably, ranging from 23–100%. The majority of studies report a percentage of stained hepatocytes lower than 10% of the total. In two studies in which liver tissue from acute hepatitis cases was available (both from a chimpanzee and from patients), the proportion of stained hepatocytes was higher than that observed in chronic infection *(35,38)*. In the few studies were this parameter was analyzed, the proportion of stained hepatocytes was not unequivocally correlated with the viremia level *(36,42)*. The detection of HCV antigen may, however, be correlated with the disease stage and activity *(21,34,44)*. The HCV antigen expression was reduced by successful α-interferon therapy, but not by the ribavirin treatment *(36)*. This interesting observation provides insight into the different mechanism of action of these two drugs.

In conclusion, the detection of HCV antigens by IHC is still to be considered a research tool, and further technical improvements are required before it can be used as a diagnostic tool in the clinical setting. The low level of expression of HCV antigens will continue to represent the most significant obstacle in this effort.

4. *In Situ* PCR

Since the HCV replicative level is low, it was logical to pursue a more sensitive approach such as *in situ* PCR. The intracellular amplification of HCV RNA by RT-PCR has been described by several groups *(23,31,46–48)*. The so-called *in situ* PCR technique was introduced a few years ago to detect successfully *in situ* DNA present in low copy number, such as in some retroviral infections and in the human papillomavirus infection. Two major techniques have been described: the direct *in situ* PCR, where the labeled nucleotides are directly incorporated in the amplicon, and the indirect procedure, in which the in-cell PCR amplification is followed by a classical ISH using a labeled probe *(49)*. Although direct procedures are believed to pose the risk of a nonspecific, primer-independent incorporation of the label at sites of host DNA fragmentation, they have been successfully used by some investigators, at the price of extensive and cumbersome specificity experiments *(47)*. Predigestion of sections with DNase has been suggested *(46)*. Although indirect procedures may be theoretically more specific, their sensitivity seems lower.

The results published by the groups who attempted to detect HCV RNA by *in situ* PCR are very discordant. Some authors have reported data consistent with the observations performed by conventional ISH, i.e., a cytoplasmic localization of HCV RNA *(23,47,48)*. In contrast, in two additional reports, HCV RNA was detected as a perinuclear halo in some hepatocytes *(46)* or in the nuclei of the vast majority of cells, including mononuclear cells *(31)*. Infection of mononuclear cells was confirmed by others *(47)*. These discrepancies are very difficult to interpret. No correlation was found between the proportion of positive hepatocytes and the clinical and biochemical parameters of disease, or with the total and single activity scores of the histological activity index *(48)*. When patients were treated with interferon, the intrahepatic HCV RNA decreased in parallel with the response to therapy, but pretreatment levels were not predictive of success *(48)*.

Overall, the *in situ* PCR procedure is very cumbersome, requires technical skills, and its results must be constantly confronted with a large number of control experiments. These limitations have clearly deterred many investigators, thus hampering the diffusion of the procedure, whose costs (both in terms of reagents and labor) may be a significant issue.

5. Future Perspectives

Although ISH should be considered the gold standard technique, the analysis of the HCV replication at the tissue level can be alternatively and successfully performed by RT-PCR amplification of either HCV RNA strand (i.e., the genome and the putative replication intermediate) in total tissue RNA *(50,51)*. This technique does not allow, of course, the definition of the number and type of infected cells, but may provide critical information to understand the replicative status of HCV in a given tissue. As far as classical ISH protocols are concerned, signal-amplification procedures may still play an important role, especially those using APAAP complexes *(8)* or "branched" DNA systems, provided that technical improvements are developed to avoid background staining. An optimal fixation is crucial to combining good sensitivity, retention of the target RNA, and morphological preservation: a paraformaldehyde fixation combined with a cryopreserving procedure prior to snap-freezing seem to give the best results *(16)*.

In-cell amplification procedures are very interesting, but difficult to perform and require a great number of control experiments. Use of multiple primer pairs *(52)* or coamplification with housekeeping genes *(53)* may represent future, successful approaches, but the technical obstacles may be significant.

References

1. Kuo, G., Choo, Q. L., Alter, H. J., Gitnick, G. L., Redeker, A. G., Purcell, R. H., et al. (1989) An assay for circulating antibodies to a major etiologic virus of human non-A, non-B hepatitis. *Science* **244,** 362–365.

2. Miller, R. H. and Purcell, R. H. (1990) Hepatitis C virus shares amino acid sequence similarity with pestiviruses and flaviviruses as well as members of two plant virus subgroups. *Proc. Natl. Acad. Sci. USA* **87,** 2057–2061.
3. Blight, K. J. and Gowans, E. J. (1995) In situ hybridization and immunohistochemical staining of hepatitis C virus products. *Viral Hep. Rev.* **1,** 143–155.
4. Lau, J. Y. N., Krawczynski, K., Negro, F., and González-Peralta, R. P. (1996) *In situ* detection of hepatitis C virus—a critical appraisal. *J. Hepatol.* **24,** 43–51.
5. Westaway, E. G. (1987) Flaviviruses replication strategy. *Adv. Virus Res.* **33,** 45–90.
6. Nakao, S., Lai, C. J., and Young, N. S. (1989) Dengue virus, a flavivirus, propagates in human bone marrow progenitor and hematopoietic cell lines. *Blood* **74,** 1235–1241.
7. Gumber, S. C. and Chopra, S. (1995) Hepatitis C: a multifaceted disease. Review of extrahepatic manifestations. *Ann. Intern. Med.* **123,** 615–620.
8. Negro, F., Pacchioni, D., Shimizu, Y., Miller, R. H., Bussolati, G., Purcell, R. H., et al. (1992) Detection of intrahepatic replication of hepatitis C virus RNA by in situ hybridization and comparison with histopathology. *Proc. Natl. Acad. Sci. USA* **89,** 2247–2251.
9. Lamas, E., Baccarini, P., Housset, C., Kremsdorf, D., and Brechot, C. (1992) Detection of hepatitis C virus (HCV) RNA sequences in liver tissue by in situ hybridization. *J. Hepatol.* **16,** 219–223.
10. Blight, K., Trowbridge, R., Rowland, R., and Gowans, E. (1992) Detection of hepatitis C virus RNA by in situ hybridization. *Liver* **12,** 286–289.
11. Yamada, S., Koji, T., Nozawa, M., Kiyosawa, K., and Nakane, P. K. (1992) Detection of hepatitis C virus (HCV) RNA in paraffin embedded tissue sections of human liver of non-A, non-B hepatitis patients by in situ hybridization. *J. Clin. Lab. Anal* **6,** 40–46.
12. Endo, H., Yamada, G., Nakane, P. K., and Tsuji, T. (1992) Localization of hepatitis C virus RNA in human liver biopsies by in situ hybridization using thymine-thymine dimerized oligo DNA probes: improved method. *Acta Med. Okayama* **46,** 355–364.
13. Haruna, Y., Hayashi, N., Hiramatsu, N., Takehara, T., Hagiwara, H., Sasaki, Y., et al. (1993) Detection of hepatitis C virus RNA in liver tissues by an in situ hybridization technique. *J. Hepatol.* **18,** 96–100.
14. Nouri-Aria, K. T., Sallie, R., Sangar, D., Alexander, G. J. M., Smith, H., Byrne, J., et al. (1993) Detection of genomic and intermediate replicative strands of hepatitis C virus in liver tissue by in situ hybridization. *J. Clin. Invest.* **91,** 2226–2234.
15. Yamada, G., Nishimoto, H., Endou, H., Doi, T., Takahashi, M., Tsuji, T., et al. (1993) Localization of hepatitis C viral RNA and capsid protein in human liver. *Dig. Dis. Sci.* **38,** 882–887.
16. Tanaka, Y., Enomoto, N., Kojima, S., Tang, L., Goto, M., Marumo, F., et al. (1993) Detection of hepatitis C virus RNA in the liver by in situ hybridization. *Liver* **13,** 203–208.
17. Agnello, V., Abel, G., and Knight, G. (1993) The role of hepatitis C virus (HCV) in the pathogenesis of type II cryoglobulinemia (MC) [Abstract]. *Arthritis Rheum.* **36,** S241.

18. Töx, U., Kolbe, E., Tien, D., Krausslich, H. G., Hofmann, W. J., Muller, H. M., et al. (1993) Detection of hepatitis C virus RNA in liver paraffin sections by in situ hybridization: distribution and identification of infected cells (abstract). *Hepatology* **18,** 82A.
19. Kawai, H., Kaneko, S., Adachi, H., Unoura, M., Kobayashi, K., Nozawa, M., et al. (1993) Simultaneous detection of hepatitis C virus genome and HCV proteins in paraffin-embedded tissue sections. *Proceedings of the International Symposium on Viral Hepatitis and Liver Disease,* Tokyo, p. 176.
20. Marrone, A., Kleiner, D., Mahanev, K., Conjeeveran, H., Tedeschi, V., Hoofnagle, J. H., et al. (1994) The significance of hepatic HCV RNA: analysis by semiquantitative in situ hybridization [Abstract]. *Hepatology* **20,** 236A.
21. Tsutsumi, M., Urashima, S., Takada, A., Date, T., and Tanaka, Y. (1994) Detection of antigens related to hepatitis C virus RNA encoding the NS5 region in the livers of patients with chronic type C hepatitis. *Hepatology* **19,** 265–272.
22. Moldvay, J., Deny, P., Pol, S., Brechot, C., and Lamas, E. (1994) Detection of hepatitis C virus RNA in peripheral blood mononuclear cells of infected patients by in situ hybridization. *Blood* **83,** 269–273.
23. Komminoth, P., Adams, V., Roth, J., Saremaslani, P., Flury, R., Schmid, M., et al. (1994) Evaluation of methods for hepatitis C virus (HCV) detection in archival liver biopsies: comparison of immunohistochemistry, ISH, RT-PCR and in-situ RT-PCR. *Path. Res. Pract.* **190,** 1017–1025.
24. Lau, J. Y. N. and Davis, G. L. (1994) Detection of hepatitis C virus RNA genome in liver tissue by non-isotopic in-situ hybridization. *J. Med. Virol.* **42,** 268–271.
25. Gastaldi, M., Massacrier, A., Planells, R., Robaglia-Schlupp, A., Portal-Bartolomei, I., Bourlière, M., et al. (1995) Detection by in situ hybridization of hepatitis C virus positive and negative RNA strands using digoxigenin-labeled cRNA probes in human liver cells. *J. Hepatology* **23,** 509–518.
26. Tang, L., Tanaka, Y., Enomoto, N., Marumo, F., and Sato, C. (1995) Detection of hepatitis C virus RNA in hepatocellular carcinoma by in situ hybridization. *Cancer* **76,** 2211–2216.
27. De Vita, S., Sansonno, D., Dolcetti, R., Ferraccioli, G., Carbone, A., Cornacchiulo, V., et al. (1995) Hepatitis C virus within a malignant lymphoma lesion in the course of type II mixed cryoglobulinemia. *Blood* **86,** 1887–1892.
28. Ohishi, M., Sakisaka, S., Koga, H., Sasatomi, K., Koji, T., Nakane, P. K., et al. (1995) The localization of HCV and the expression of Fas antigen in the liver of HCV-related chronic liver disease [Abstract]. *Hepatology* **22,** 274A.
29. Kojima, S., Tanaka, Y., Enomoto, N., Marumo, F., and Sato, C. (1996) Distribution of hepatitis C virus RNA in the liver and its relation to histopathological changes. *Liver* **16,** 55–60.
30. Cho, S. W., Hwang, S. G., Han, D. C., Jin, S. Y., Lee, M. S., Shim, C. S., et al. (1996) In situ detection of hepatitis C virus RNA in liver tissue using a digoxigenin-labeled probe created during a polymerase chain reaction. *J. Med. Virol.* **48,** 227–233.
31. Walker, F., Lehy, T., Hervatin, F., Dazza, M. C., Sobhani, I., Boucher, O., et al. (1996) In situ gene amplification greatly improves the in situ hybridization detection of HCV in liver and HPVs in anal lesions [Abstract]. *Gastroenterology* **110,** A1041.

32. Negro, F. and Hadengue, A. (1997) Detection of hepatitis C virus RNA by in situ hybridization: a critical appraisal. *Gastroenterol. Clin. Biol.* **21**, 93–97.
33. Infantolino, D., Chiaramonte, M., Zanetti, A., Lesniewski, R. R., and Bonino, F. (1990) Localization of hepatitis C antigen(s) by immunohistochemistry on fixed-embedded liver tissue. *Ital. J. Gastroenterol.* **22**, 198,199.
34. Hiramatsu, N., Hayashi, N., Haruna, Y., Kasahara, A., Fusamoto, H., Mori, C., et al. (1992) Immunohistochemical detection of hepatitis C virus-infected hepatocytes in chronic liver disease with monoclonal antibodies to core, envelope and NS3 regions of the hepatitis C virus genome. *Hepatology* **16**, 306–311.
35. Krawczynski, K., Beach, M. J., Bradley, D. W., Kuo, G., Di Bisceglie, A. M., Houghton, M., et al. (1992) Hepatitis C virus antigen in hepatocytes: immuno-morphologic detection and identification. *Gastroenterology* **103**, 622–629.
36. Di Bisceglie, A. M., Krawczynski, K., Brazzeal, D., and Hoofnagle, J. H. (1993) hepatitis C viral antigen (HCV Ag) in the liver: effect of antiviral therapy. *Gastroenterology* **105**, 858–862.
37. Yap, S. H., Willems, M., Van den Oord, J., Habets, W., Middeldorp, J. M., Hellings, J. A., et al. (1994) Detection of hepatitis C virus antigen by immunohistochemical staining: a histological marker of hepatitis C virus infection. *J. Hepatology* **20**, 275–281.
38. Sansonno, D. and Dammacco, F. (1993) Hepatitis C virus c100 antigen in liver tissue from patients with acute and chronic infection. *Hepatology* **18**, 240–245.
39. Blight, K., Rowland, R., de la Hall, P. M., Lesniewski, R. R., Trowbridge, R., LaBrooy, J. T., et al. (1993) Immunohistochemical detection of the NS4 antigen of hepatitis C virus and its relation to histopathology. *Am. J. Pathol.* **143**, 1568–1573.
40. Blight, K., Lesniewski, R. R., LaBrooy, J. T., and Gowans, E. J. (1994) Detection and distribution of hepatitis C-specific antigens in naturally infected liver. *Hepatology* **20**, 553–557.
41. González-Peralta, R. P., Fang, J. W. S., Davis, G. L., Gish, R. G., Tsukiyama-Kohara, K., Kohara, M., et al. (1994) Optimization for the detection of hepatitis C virus antigens in the liver. *J. Hepatol.* **20**, 143–147.
42. González-Peralta, R. P., Fang, J. W. S., Davis, G. L., Gish, R. G., Kohara, M., Mondelli, M. U., et al. (1995) Significance of hepatic expression of hepatitis C viral antigens in chronic hepatitis C. *Dig. Dis. Sci.* **40**, 1595–1601.
43. Sansonno, D., Cornacchiulo, V., Iacobelli, A. R., Di Stefano, R., Lospalluti, M., and Dammacco, F. (1995) Localization of hepatitis C virus antigens in liver and skin tissues of chronic hepatitis C virus-infected patients with mixed cryoglobulinemia. *Hepatology* **21**, 305–312.
44. Gane, E. J., Naoumov, N. V., Qian, K.-P., Mondelli, M. U., Maertens, G., Portmann, B. C., et al. (1996) A longitudianl analysis of hepatitis C virus replication following liver transplantation. *Gastroenterology* **110**, 167–177.
45. Gretch, D. R., Bacchi, C. E., Corey, L., dela Rosa, C., Lesniewski, R. R., Kowdley, K., et al. (1995) Persistent hepatitis C virus infection after liver transplantation: clinical and virological features. *Hepatology* **22**, 1–9.

46. Nuovo, G. J., Lidonnici, K., MacConnell, P., and Lane, B. (1993) Intracellular localization of polymerase chain reaction (PCR)-amplified hepatitis C cDNA. *Am. J. Surg. Pathol.* **17,** 683–690.
47. Lau, G. K. K., Fang, J. W. S., Wu, P. C., Davis, G. L., and Lau, J. Y. N. (1994) Detection of hepatitis C virus genome in formalin-fixed paraffin-embedded liver tissue by in situ reverse transcriptase-polymerase chain reaction. *J. Med. Virol.* **44,** 406–409.
48. Lau, G. K. K., Davis, G. L., Wu, S. P. C., Gish, R. G., Balart, L. A., and Lau, J. Y. N. (1996) Hepatic expression of hepatitis C virus RNA in chronic hepatitis C: a study by in situ reverse-transcription polymerase chain reaction. *Hepatology* **23,** 1318–1323.
49. Komminoth, P. and Long, A. A. (1993) In-situ polymerase chain reaction. An overview of methods, applications and limitations of a new molecular technique. *Virchows Arch. B Cell. Pathol.* **64,** 67–73.
50. Lanford, R. E., Sureau, C., Jacob, J. R., White, R., and Fuerst, T. R. (1994) Demonstration of in vitro infection of chimpanzee hepatocytes with hepatitis C virus using strand-specific RT/PCR. *Virology* **202,** 606–614.
51. Lerat, H., Berby, F., Trabaud, M.-A., Vidalin, O., Major, M., Trepo, C., et al. (1996) Specific detection of hepatitis C virus minus-strand RNA in hematopoietic cells. *J. Clin. Invest.* **97,** 845–851.
52. Haase, A. T., Retzel, E. F., and Staskus, K. A. (1990) Amplification and detection of lentiviral DNA inside cells. *Proc. Natl. Acad. Sci. USA* **87,** 4971–4975.
53. Embleton, M. J., Gorochov, G., Jones, P. T., and Winter, G. (1992) In-cell PCR from mRNA: amplifying and linking the rearranged immunoglobulin heavy and light chain V-genes within single cells. *Nucleic Acid Res.* **20,** 3831–3837.

22

In Situ Detection of Hepatitis C Viral Antigens

Regino P. González-Peralta and Krzysztof Krawczynski

1. Introduction

A reliable detection system for HCV antigens in liver tissue may be used to identify the HCV cellular tropism and subcellular sites of viral replication. Also, it can be used to study the relationship between viral expression and disease activity. Finally, it can facilitate the study of host–viral interactions at the cellular level (1).

The *in situ* detection of viral proteins by immunohistochemistry requires, among other parameters, the presence of many antigen molecules (*see* Chapter 21). HCV replicates at a low rate, and therefore, the amount of HCV antigens in the liver is small, rendering its detection difficult. Immunohistochemical studies conducted before the discovery of HCV claimed detection of non-A, non-B-associated antigens in the liver. However, Krawczynski et al. were the first to demonstrate specific immunofluorescent staining of HCV antigens, which was confirmed with blocking and absorption experiments (2).

In this chapter, immunohistochemical methods will be described that have been used to detect specifically HCV antigens in the liver. The techniques that will be outlined are the result of optimization experiments done in our laboratories, in which different tissue processing, fixatives, antibodies, and detection schemes have been tested (3) (**Table 1**). Using these techniques, HCV core, nonstructural (NS) 3, and NS4 antigens have been detected in 60–90% of patients with chronic HCV infection (2–5). However, most liver sections with detectable HCV antigens contain <5% of immunoreactive hepatocytes. Positive staining has been confined to the cytoplasm of hepatocytes, and has not been observed in either sinusoidal cells or bile duct epithelia (**Figs. 1** and **2**).

Table 1
Immunohistochemical Conditions Studied and Those Found to Be Optimal

Condition studied	Optimal condition
Cryostat	Cryostate sections
Paraffin sections	
Proteolytic digestion	
Antigen retrieval system	
Fixatives (cryostat samples)	
Acetone	Chloroform
Acetone/chloroform	Acetone/chloroform
Acetone/chloroform/methanol	
Ethanol	
Paraformaldehyde	
Zamboni's solution	
Antibodies	
Mouse anticore monoclonal	Mouse anticore monoclonal
Group A (aa 26–45)	Group A
Group B (aa 39–74)	
Human anti-NS4 monoclonal	Human anti-NS4 monoclonal (digoxigenin/labeled)
Rabbit polyclonals:	
Anti-core	
Anti-E2/NS1	
Anti-NS3/anti-NS4	
Anti-NS5	
Detection system	
Three- and five-step PAP	Five-step PAP
Immunofluorescence	Immunofluorescence
Avidin–biotin	

2. Materials

2.1. HCV Antigen Detection Using Polyclonal Human Immunoglobulin (Anti-HCVAg)

1. Reagent-grade chloroform (Fisher Scientific, Pittsburgh, PA).
2. Phosphate-buffered saline (PBS, pH 7.4): Prepare stock solution (20X)—dissolve 23 g Na_2HPO_4, 4.0 g KH_2PO_4, and 160 g NaCl in deionized water/L of solution. Adjust to appropriate pH with NaOH or HCl. Prepare fresh PBS (1X) on the day of use.
3. Primary antibody: purified polyclonal human IgG, fluorescein isothiocyanate (FITC) labeled at 10–12 mg/mL of protein concentration (*see* **Notes 1–3**).

In Situ Detection of HCV Antigens

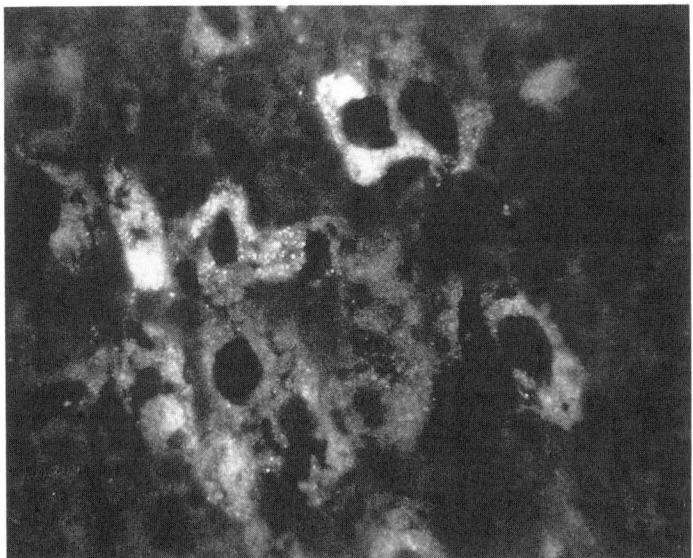

Fig. 1. HCV Ag in the cytoplasm on hepatocytes in a frozen section, identified by a one-step staining procedure using FITC-labeled polyclonal human IgG anti-HCVAg (2). A group of HCVAg-positive hepatocytes with granular and more homogeneous deposits of the antigen. Liver biopsy from HCV-positive patient with chronic hepatitis (original magnification 8 × 63).

4. Mounting medium: 50% glycerol in PBS.
5. Coplin jars and humid slide chamber.

2.2. HCV Antigen Detection Using Monoclonal Antibodies (MAbs)

1. Reagent-grade acetone and chloroform (Fisher): Prepare acetone/chloroform fixative by adding equal volumes of these reagents. The reaction is mildly exothermic; allow mixture to cool to room temperature before use (see **Note 4**).
2. Tris-HCl buffer saline (TBS, pH 7.6): Prepare stock solution (10X)—dissolve 60.6 g Tris-HCl, and 85.3 g NaCl in deionized water/L of solution. Adjust to appropriate pH with NaOH or HCl. Prepare fresh TBS (1X) on the day of use.
3. Crystalline bovine serum albumin (BSA) (Sigma Chemicals, St. Louis, MO): Prepare solution at 1% (used for primary MAbs) and 3% (used for diluting blocking solutions) in TBS.
4. Quenching solution: Prepare 1% hydrogen peroxide (Fisher) in methanol.
5. Blocking solution: Prepare 10% rabbit serum in 3% BSA (by volume).
6. Primary antibodies: Mouse monoclonals anti-HCV core (200 µg/mL), human monoclonal anti-NS4 (80 µg/mL), digoxigenin labeled (see **Note 5**).
7. Secondary antibodies: Peroxidase-labeled rabbit antimouse and rabbit antisheep IgG (1:50 and 1:100, Dako Corporation, Carpinteria, CA), sheep antidigoxigenin IgG

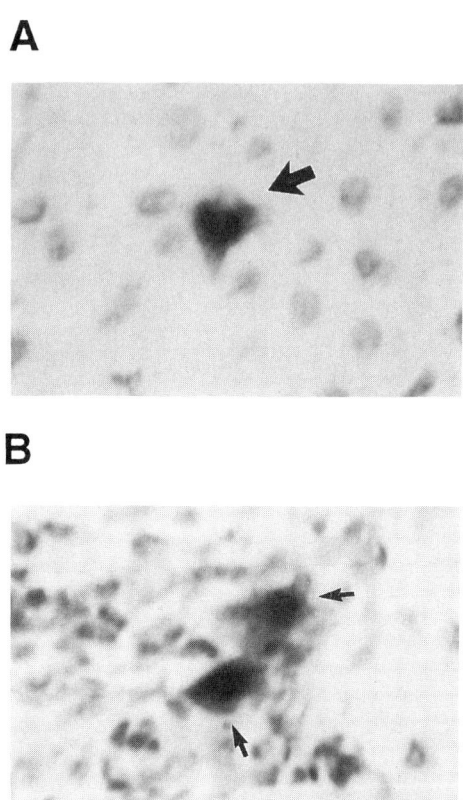

Fig. 2. *In situ* detection of **(A)** HCV core and **(B)** HCV NS4 (using mouse and human MAbs, respectively); note the low level of background and exclusive cytoplasmic staining (original magnification 10 × 40).

    (1:500, Boehringer-Mannheim, Indianapolis, IN), mouse and sheep peroxide–antiperoxidase complex (PAP, 1:50 and 1:100, Dako).
8. Washing solution: Prepare Triton X-100 (0.5% in TBS, Fisher).
9. Developing solution: Prepare 3′, 3′ diaminobenzidine (DAB) solution (mix 6 mg DAB [Fisher], 2 µL of 30% hydrogen peroxidase [Fisher] in 10 mL deionized water).
10. Counterstain solution: Prepare Carazzi's hematoxylin by dissolving 0.5 g hematoxylin in 100 mL glycerol and 25 g potassium alum in 300 mL of deionized water. Allow these solutions to dissolve overnight with continuous mixing. Slowly add alum solution to the hematoxylin solution with careful mixing. Dissolve 0.1 g potassium iodate in 100 mL of deionized water, and mix with the hematoxylin–alum solution. This solution is stable for up to 6 mo.
11. Mounting medium: Permount (Fisher).

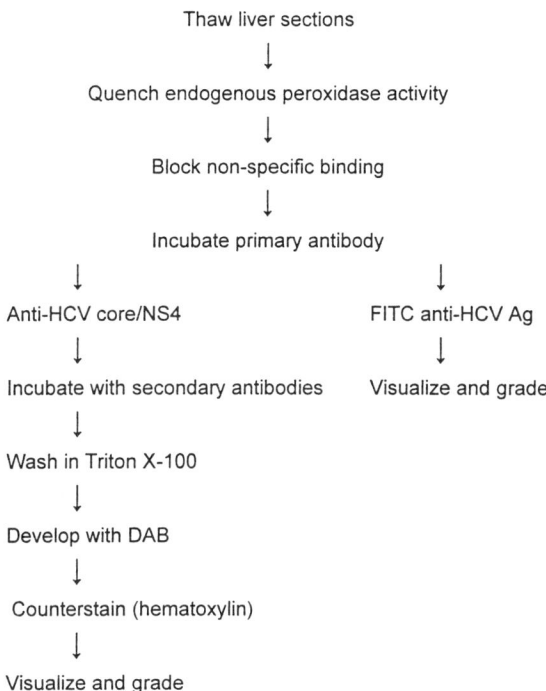

Fig. 3. Flow diagram for *in situ* detection of HCV antigens. Abbreviations as in text.

3. Method

3.1. HCV Antigen Detection Using Anti-HCVAg (See *Protocol Flowchart in Fig. 3*)

1. Obtain liver specimens by standard percutaneous technique using a Jamshidi needle (16-gage), or other biopsy needle. Our liver biopsy samples from patients measure on average 3–5 cm; at least 2 cm of the samples are fixed in 10% formaldehyde saline and processed for routine histopathology. The spare biopsy specimens, usually >1.5 cm, are embedded in OCT compound (Tissue-Tek, Miles Inc, Elkhart, IN), immediately snap-frozen in liquid nitrogen-cooled isopentane, and stored at −70°C.
2. Cut 2–4 μm tissue sections using a cryotome. Fix sections in chloroform for 5 min at room temperature, and allow to air-dry.
3. In a humid slide chamber, overlay liver sections with 60 μL of appropriately diluted FITC-labeled antibody for 40 min at room temperature.
4. Place slides in a Coplin jar, and wash three times with PBS (7 min each).
5. Mount slides using 50% glycerol in PBS.
6. Visualize under conventional microscopy. The grading scale used to semi-quantitate *in situ* HCV antigen expression is 0 = none, 1 + = <5%, 2 + = 5–20%, 3 + = >20% of positive hepatocytes.

3.2. HCV Antigen Detection Using MAbs (See Flowchart in Fig. 3)

1. Obtain liver biopsy specimens as mentioned above.
2. Cut 4–6 µm tissue sections using a cryotome, and place them on either positively stained (Fisher Scientific) or 0.1% poly-L-lysine-treated slides. Fix sections in acetone/chloroform for 10 min at room temperature. Wash extensively in PBS to remove fixative. If sections are not to be immediately stained, wrap slides "back-to-back" (2/packet) in aluminum foil, and store at –70°C.
3. Thaw cryostat liver sections for 10 min at room temperature. Draw a circle around the tissue sections on the slide with a wax pen to create a physical barrier and prevent antibody runoff.
4. Place slides in Coplin jars and quench endogenous peroxidase activity by incubating in 1% methanol peroxide for 10 min. Rinse three times in TBS.
5. Place slides on a slide chamber, and overlay sections with blocking solution for 30 min. Flickoff solution (see **Note 6**). Do not rinse in TBS.
6. Overlay sections with 50–100 µL of appropriately diluted primary antibody (mouse anti-HCV core monoclonal, or digoxigenin-labeled human anti-HCV NS4). Incubate for 1 h at room temperature and then at 4°C overnight. Avoid drying of antibody solutions on sections (see **Note 7**). Rinse three times in TBS.
7. Sequentially incubate sections with 50–100 µL of secondary antibodies at room temperature with rinsing three times in TBS, between applications. For HCV core antigen: rabbit antimouse peroxidase (1:50, 45 min), mouse PAP (1:100, 45 min), rabbit antimouse peroxidase (1:100, 30 min), and mouse PAP (1:200, 15 min). For HCV NS4 antigen: sheep antidigoxigenin (1:500, 45 min), rabbit antisheep peroxidase (1:80, 45 min), sheep PAP (1:160, 30 min), rabbit antisheep peroxidase (1:160, 15 min).
8. Place slides in Coplin jar, rinse three times in TBS and incubate in 0.5% Triton X-100 for 15 min to reduce nonspecific antibody binding.
9. Add DAB to each section and carefully monitor developing reaction (see **Note 8**). Rinse with tap water.
10. Counterstain with Carrazzi's hematoxylin for 5 min, and rinse with tap water (see **Note 9**).
11. Dehydrate sections through graded ethanol, clear through xylene, and mount slides.
12. Visualize under conventional microscopy. The grading scale that is used to semiquantitate *in situ* HCV antigen expression is 0 = none, 1 + = <1%, 2 + = 2–5%, 3 + = 6–20%, 4 + = >20% of positive hepatocytes (see **Notes 10** and **11**).

4. Notes

1. The anti-HCV Ag was derived from serum from patients or chimpanzees with HCV infection. Before use, it was purified by immunoprecipitation and ion-exchange chromatography, and FITC-labeled by the dialysis method *(6)*. Finally, the anti-HCV Ag was adsorbed with mouse acetone liver powder and diluted in normal human serum.

2. The specificity of the anti-HCV Ag antibody was confirmed by blocking experiments using liver sections known to be strongly positive for hepatic HCV Ag. For these experiments, equal amounts of FITC-labeled anti-HCVAg and blocking serum were mixed and used as primary antibodies. Samples used for blocking included paired sera obtained before and during the acute or chronic phase of HCV infection in chimpanzees and paired samples of human serum obtained before and after HCV seroconversion.
3. The specificity of the anti-HCV Ag was also confirmed with absorption studies. For these experiments, anti-HCV Ag was mixed with HCV structural (c22, E1 and E2) and nonstructural (c200 [NS3/NS4], a fusion of c33c and c100) proteins expressed in yeast *(2)*. Immunofluorescent staining was performed on selected liver samples before and after absorption with the HCV proteins. Based on results of these studies, the reactivity of the human anti-HCV Ag has been shown to be specific for proteins encoded within the HCV NS3/NS4 regions *(2)*.
4. Tissue processing is an important factor for immunohistochemical detection of viral antigens. Many tissue fixatives and fixation schemes have been used to localize HCV antigens (*5,6*, and references contained within). However, we have observed that acetone/chloroform fixation (at room temperature for 10 min) yields the best results using the MAbs described above. Using MAbs, we have not been able to detect specifically HCV antigens in paraffin-embedded tissue, despite using mild proteolytic digestion and microwave antigen-retrieval protocols *(4)*.
5. The primary MAbs used were derived from different sources. First, the combination of anti-HCV core monoclonals used were produced by conventional myeloma fusion technique. They have been shown to recognize amino acid sequence (aa) 26–45 (GGGQIVGGVYLLPRRGPRLG) of the HCV core region *(7)*. Second, the human anti-HCV NS4 monoclonal was produced by Epstein-Barr virus-transformed cell lines, and it has been demonstrated to recognize aa 1700–1705 (VLYREF) of the HCV NS4 region *(8)*. To enhance specificity, the anti-HCV NS4 antibody was labeled with digoxigenin (a steroid present in plants only) using the digoxigenin-NHS-ester method as recommended by the manufacturer and purified in a Sephadex G50 column (Sigma Chemicals).
6. The amount of HCV antigens in the liver is small, so that high concentrations of primary anti-HCV antibodies are need for detection of viral antigens. This leads to nonspecific antibody binding and results in high background staining. To reduce this, blocking with appropriate animal serum becomes very important. Further, we have observed improved signal-to-background levels with a final detergent wash. Although we have routinely used Triton X-100 for this purpose, other non-ionic detergents can probably be used.
7. It is important to avoid drying of antibody solutions on the tissue sections, since this leads to increased background. Thus, during overnight incubation with primary antibody, a wet paper towel is placed in the slide chamber used.
8. Carefully monitoring the development reaction is important to avoid under- or overstaining, which may result in false-negative detection and high background, respectively. Thus, we routinely do not develop more than 10 sections at a time. For added convenience, we use an inverted microscope to monitor DAB reaction.

9. Counterstaining highlights antigen expression. We prefer Carazzi's hematoxylin because of its precise nuclear specificity without staining cytoplasmic structures (where HCV is believed to replicate). Its short staining time is also advantageous.
10. To ensure immunohistochemical specificity of HCV antigen detection using the MAbs, positive and negative controls (omitting the primary antibodies and testing liver sections from patients with non-HCV liver diseases) are included with all experiments.
11. Using the immunohistochemical methods described, HCV core and NS4 have been detected in 60 and 80% of patients with chronic HCV infection, respectively. However, most liver sections with detectable HCV antigens contain <5% of immunoreactive hepatocytes.

Acknowledgments

R. P. G. P. is supported, in part, by grants from the National Institutes of Health (KO8AI01486), the Blowitz-Ridgeway Foundation Health Scholar Award, the Children's Miracle Network Research Fund, and the Division of Sponsored Research of the University of Florida (DSR-D8-95-96).

References

1. González-Peralta, R. P. and Lau, J. Y. N. (1995) Pathogenesis of hepatocellular damage in chronic hepatitis C virus infection. *Semin Gastrointest. Dis.* **6**, 28–34.
2. Krawczynski, K., Beach, M., Bradley, D. W., Kuo G., DiBisceglie, A. M., Houghton, M., et al. (1992) Hepatitis C virus antigen in hepatocytes: immuno–morphologic detection and identification. *Gastroenterology* **103**, 622–629.
3. González-Peralta, R. P., Fang, J. W. S., Davis, G. L., Gish, R. G., Tsukiyama-Kohara, K., Kohara, M., et al. (1994) Optimization for the detection of hepatitis C viral antigens in the liver. *J. Hepatol.* **20**, 143–147.
4. DiBisceglie, A. M., Krawczynski, K., Brazzeal, D., and Hoofnagle, J. H. (1993) Hepatitis C viral antigen (HCVAg) in the liver: effect of antiviral therapy. *Gastroenterology* **105**, 858–862.
5. González-Peralta, R. P., Fang, J. W. S., Davis, G. L., Gish, R. G., Kohara, M., Mondelli, M. U., et al. (1995) Significance of hepatitis C virus antigens in the liver. *Dig. Dis. Sci.* **40**, 2595–2601.
6. Clark, H. F. and Shepard, C. C. (1963) A dialysis technique for preparing fluorescent antibody. *Virology* **20**, 642–644.
7. Mizokami, M., Orito, E., Hasegawa, A., Ohba, Y., Kohara, M., and Lau, J. Y. N. (1995) Two overlapping immunodominant B-cell epitopes in HCV core antigen identified by monoclonal antibody mapping [Abstract]. *Gastroenterology* **108**, A1124.
8. Cerino, A. and Mondelli, M. U. (1991) Identification of an immunodominant B cell epitope on the hepatitis C virus nonstructural region defined by human monoclonal antibodies. *J. Immunol.* **147**, 2692–2696.

23

In Situ Hybridization and the Detection and Localization of HCV RNA

Francesco Negro, Donatella Pacchioni, and Gianni Bussolati

1. Introduction

The procedure described below was originally reported to detect the hepatitis C virus RNA (genomic strand) by nonradioisotopic *in situ* hybridization in formalin-fixed, paraffin-embedded liver tissue of two acutely infected chimpanzees, in a collaborative study conducted with R. H. Purcell, at the National Institute of Allergy and Infectious Diseases, Bethesda, MD *(1)*. Briefly, a synthetic DNA 50-mer was end-labeled with a digoxygenin-conjugated dUTP *(2)* and hybridized to liver sections. After washing, hybrides were detected by a specific antidigoxigenin antibody and the antigen–antibody reaction revealed by alkaline phosphatase-based enzymatic reaction, through a signal amplification procedure *(3)*. Although the probe represented only 0.5% of the target sequences, the procedure was sensitive enough to detect the low amounts of genomic HCV RNA present in the acutely infected livers, probably owing to both the multistep amplification of the enzymatic reaction and to the prehybridization treatment of the tissue sections, intended to facilitate the diffusion of both the probe and the revealing system molecules.

2. Materials

1. The oligodeoxyribonucleotide has the sequence 5'-CGGGGCACTCGCAAGC-ACCCTATCAGGCAGTACCACAAGGCCTTTCGCGA-3' and is complementary to bases 252–301 of the 5' noncoding region of the HCV genome *(4)*.
2. Digoxigenin-11-dUTP (Boehringer Mannheim, Mannheim, Germany): this labeled nucleotide is provided by the manufacturer as 10X solution containing 1 mM dATP, dCTP, dGTP (each), 0.65 mM dTTP, and 0.35 mM digoxigenin-11-dUTP *(2)*.

3. Terminal deoxynucleotydil transferase, 20 U/μL (Promega Biotech, Madison, WI).
4. Poly-L-lysine-coated microscope slides: a 0.1% solution of poly-L-lysine (Sigma Chemicals Co., St. Louis, MO) is layered onto glass microscope slides and allowed to dry.
5. Xylene and absolute ethanol and ethanol dilutions in water (Fluka Chemie AG, Buchs, Switzerland).
6. Phosphate-buffered saline (PBS): 10X stock is 137 mM NaCl, 2.7 mM KCl, 4.3 mM Na$_2$HPO$_4$, 1.4 mM KH$_2$PO$_4$, pH 7.3.
7. Proteinase K, DNase- and RNase-free (Merck, Darmstadt, Germany).
8. PBS containing 0.1 M glycine (Sigma).
9. Deionized formamide: take 500 mL of formamide (Fluka), add 50 g of resin (AG 501-X8, 20–50 mesh, Bio-Rad, Glattsbrugg, Switzerland), stir for 30 min at room temperature, filter through Whatman 2, and store in 50-mL aliquots at –20°C, protecting from light.
10. Standard saline citrate (SSC): 20X stock is 3 M NaCl, 0.3 M Na$_3$citrate, pH 7.0.
11. 50X Denhardt's solution: 5 g Ficoll 400, 5 g polyvinyl pyrrolidone, 5 g bovine serum albumin (Pentax Fraction V, Miles Laboratories, Kankakee, IL) in 500 mL H$_2$O; filter sterilize and store in aliquots at –20°C.
12. 10 mg/mL herring sperm DNA (Promega).
13. 10 mg/mL yeast tRNA (Sigma).
14. TN buffer: 100 mM Tris-HCl, pH 7.5, 150 mM NaCl.
15. Normal sheep serum (Dakopatts, Copenhagen, Denmark).
16. Triton X-100 (Sigma).
17. Primary antibody: sheep antidigoxigenin antibody, conjugated to calf intestinal alkaline phosphatase (Boehringer Mannheim).
18. Secondary antibody: monoclonal mouse antialkaline phosphatase antibody (Zymed Laboratories, San Francisco, CA).
19. 10% Bovine serum albumin stock solution.
20. Tertiary antibody: goat antimouse antibody (Techno-Genetics-Recordati, Trezzano sul Naviglio, Italy).
21. Amplification complexes: calf intestinal alkaline phosphatase complexed to saturation with mouse monoclonal antialkaline phosphatase antibody (APAAP complexes) (Dakopatts).
22. PBS containing 10 mM MgCl$_2$.
23. TNM buffer: 100 mM Tris-HCl, pH 9.5, 100 mM NaCl, 50 mM MgCl$_2$.
24. Development solution: add 45 μL of nitroblue tetrazolium salt, 100 mg/mL in dimethylformamide (Boehringer Mannheim), 35 μL of 5-bromo-4-chloro-3-indolyl-phosphate, 50 mg/mL solution in dimethylformamide (Boehringer Mannheim), 0.024% tetramisole (Sigma) to 10 mL of TNM buffer; prepare immediately before use.
25. Stopping buffer: 10 mM Tris-HCl, pH 8.0, 1 mM EDTA.
26. Methyl green (Sigma).
27. Mounting medium (Entellan™, Merck).

3. Method

1. Label 25 pmol of the oligomer with digoxigenin-11-dUTP using 30 U of TdT for 1 h at 37°C. Store at −20°C until use (up to 3 mo).
2. Deparaffinize tissue sections in xylene twice for 10 min.
3. Rehydrate to PBS through a standard series of ethanols (absolute, twice for 5 min, then 95% for 5 min and 70% for 5 min).
4. Digest in proteinase K, 0.15–0.5 mg/mL in PBS for 15 min at 37°C (*see* **Note 1**).
5. Block digestion in ice-cold PBS, 0.1 M glycine, twice for 5 min.
6. Rinse in 2X SSC for 3 min.
7. Denature for 5 min at 65°C in 70% formamide, 0.1X SSC.
8. Stop in 2X SSC for 5 min.
9. Prehybridize for 1 h at room temperature in a mixture containing 50% formamide, 5X SSC, 1X Denhardt's solution, 0.5 mg/mL herring sperm DNA, 0.25 mg/mL yeast tRNA.
10. Tap excess prehybridization mixture and hybridize overnight at 37°C in a wet chamber with the same mixture as above containing the digoxigenin-labeled probe at a final concentration of 100 nM.
11. Wash for 1 h at room temperature in 2X SSC, then 1 h in 1X SSC, then 30 min at 42°C in 0.5X SSC, and finally 1 h at room temperature in 0.1X SSC (unless specified, all subsequent steps are to be performed at room temperature).
12. Rinse briefly in TN buffer.
13. Incubate the sections with TN buffer containing 2% normal sheep serum and 0.3% Triton X-100 for 30 min. **Do not allow the sections to dry at any time.**
14. Tap excess buffer and incubate the sections with TN buffer containing 1% normal sheep serum, 0.3% Triton X-100, and 0.2% sheep antidigoxigenin antibody for 2 h.
15. Wash the sections for 5 min in PBS.
16. Incubate for 30 min with the monoclonal mouse antialkaline phosphatase antibody diluted 1:100 in PBS containing 0.1% bovine serum albumin.
17. Wash for 5 min in PBS.
18. Incubate for 30 min with the goat antimouse antibody diluted 1:50 in PBS.
19. Wash in PBS twice for 3 min.
20. Incubate for 30 min with the APAAP complex diluted 1:50 in PBS and 10 mM MgCl$_2$.
21. Wash in PBS twice for 3 min.
22. Repeat once **steps 18–21**.
23. Wash in TN buffer twice for 15 min.
24. Incubate for 2 min in TNM buffer.
25. Develop for 20–40 min in the developing mixture, checking from time to time the intensity of the cytoplasmic staining with the microscope. **Do not allow the sections to dry at any time.**
26. Block the development for 5 min with 10 mM Tris-HCl, pH 8.0, and 1 mM EDTA.
27. Countercolor with 1% methyl green.
28. Rinse in water, dehydrate (passage in 95% ethanol should be quick because it may destain the section), and mount.

4. Notes

1. The proteinase K concentration used to pretreat the sections cannot be predetermined, since it depends on the amount of crosslinks formed during the formalin fixation. In general, the longer the tissue has been kept in the fixative, the tighter the crosslinks are, and therefore, the higher the protease concentration *(5)*. This step is critical in allowing an optimal accessibility of the target to the probe as well as to the revealing system macromolecules. The optimal protease concentration can only be established empirically, trying different conditions in a preliminary experiment. Excessive digestion will result in loss of morphological details as well as poor retention of small tissue molecules (including the target RNA) during the hybridization and the other steps.
2. The above detailed method was shown to detect specifically the genomic strand of HCV in the hepatocyte cytoplasms by use of appropriate controls *(1)*. HCV RNA was found in the liver early after inoculation, the staining intensity (ranging from 0–100% of hepatocytes) being correlated with the alanine aminotransferase fluctuations. With progression to the persistent phase of infection, intrahepatic HCV RNA could not be detected any longer, at least by the above procedure. Disappointingly enough, this method has consistently failed to detect HCV RNA in the liver of chronically infected humans (Negro et al., unpublished observations), and this in contrast with the data reported (using different protocols) by other investigators (*see* Chapter 21 for an overview). The diffuse, but short-lived intrahepatic expression of genomic HCV RNA, as detected by the above *in situ* hybridization procedure, was, however, confirmed in a further experimentally infected chimpanzee (Negro and Prince, unpublished observations).
3. Considering the low levels of HCV viremia in the infected host, the detection of HCV RNA in the vast majority of hepatocytes reported in the acutely infected chimpanzee is clearly surprising *(1)*. However, in a study conducted on the duck hepatitis B virus (DHBV), high levels of intrahepatic DHBV DNA were detected by *in situ* as well as by Southern blot hybridization in the absence of detectable viremia, suggesting a block in the secretion of viral particles *(6)*. The same could be true for HCV, at least in the particular setting of the acute experimental infection. It has to be noted that in both animals analyzed, on some occasions, as serum alanine aminotransferase levels decreased, the pattern of HCV RNA staining shifted from a diffusely cytoplasmic to a more submembranous appearance. This intracellular distribution was interpreted as consistent with a maturation stage of virus particles preceding their release into circulation. However, an alternative interpretation could be represented by an impaired secretion of virion particles, with their accumulation induced, for instance, by the local production of interferon(s). This phenomenon has been reported for some murine tumor viruses *(7,8)* and might well apply to HCV. The livers of both animals considered in the above study were shown to express the 48-1 antigen in typical microtubular structures *(9,10)*, known for being specifically induced by interferon-α *(11)*. These structures are rarely found in human livers infected with HCV. Unfortunately, the abundant intrahepatic expression of HCV RNA in this

peculiar setting was not studied by Northern blot hybridization. In other settings, notably the human chronic infection, this approach has consistently failed to detect high levels of intrahepatic HCV replication. Again, the two models may be considerably different in terms of viral–host interactions. Therefore, the chimpanzee data may not be directly applicable to the human infection.

4. A modification of the above reported *in situ* hybridization procedure was recently and successfully applied to detect HCV RNA in livers from chronically infected humans *(12)*. Basically, the method differs from the original in that it uses digoxigenin-labeled riboprobes covering a more important portion of the target RNA. These data, however, although interesting, have not been independently confirmed.

References

1. Negro, F., Pacchioni, D., Shimizu, Y., Miller, R. H., Bussolati, G., Purcell, R. H., et al. (1992) Detection of intrahepatic replication of hepatitis C virus RNA by in situ hybridization and comparison with histopathology. *Proc. Natl. Acad. Sci. USA* **89,** 2247–2251.
2. Schmitz, G. G., Walter, T., Seibl, R., and Kessler, C. (1991) Nonradioactive labeling of oligonucleotides in vitro with the hapten digoxigenin by tailing with terminal transferase. *Anal. Biochem.* **192,** 222–231.
3. Cordell, J. L., Falini, B., Erber, W. N., Ghosh, A. K., Abdulaziz, Z., Macdonald, S., et al. (1984) Immunoenzymatic labeling of monoclonal antibodies using immune complexes of alkaline phosphatase and monoclonal anti-alkaline phosphatase (APAAP complexes). *J. Histochem. Cytochem.* **32,** 219–229.
4. Han, J. H., Shyamala, V., Richman, K. H., Brauer, M. J., Irvine, B., Urdea, M. S., et al. (1991) Characterization of the terminal regions of hepatitis C viral RNA: identification of conserved sequences in the 5' untranslated region and poly(A) tails at the 3' end. *Proc. Natl. Acad. Sci. USA* **88,** 1711–1715.
5. Polak, J. M. and McGee, J. O. D. (eds.) (1990) *In Situ Hybridisation.* Oxford University Press, Oxford, UK.
6. Jilbert, A. R., Wu, T. T., England, J. M., Hall, P. M., Carp, N. Z., O'Connell, A. P., et al. (1992) Rapid resolution of duck hepatitis B virus infections occurs after massive hepatocellular involvement. *J. Virol.* **66,** 1377–1388.
7. Salzberg, S., Bakhanashvili, M., and Aboud, M. (1978) Effect of interferon on mouse cells chronically infected with murine leukaemia virus: kinetic studies on virus production and virus RNA synthesis. *J. Gen. Virol.* **40,** 121–130.
8. Sen, G. C. and Sarkar, N. H. (1980) Effects of interferon on the production of murine mammary tumor virus by mammary tumor cells in culture. *Virology* **102,** 431–443.
9. Shimizu, Y. K., Oomura, M., Abe, K., Uno, M., Yamada, E., Ono, Y., et al. (1985) Production of antibody associated with non-A, non-B hepatitis in a chimpanzee lymphoblastoid cell line established by in vitro transformation with Epstein-Barr virus. *Proc. Natl. Acad. Sci. USA* **82,** 2138–2142.

10. Shimizu, Y. K., Weiner, A. J., Rosenblatt, J., Wong, D. C., Shapiro, M., Popkin, T., et al. (1990) Early events in hepatitis C virus infection of chimpanzees. *Proc. Natl. Acad. Sci. USA* **87,** 6441–6444.
11. Shimizu, Y. K. and Purcell, R. H. (1989) Cytoplasmic antigen in hepatocytes of chimpanzees infected with non-A, non-B hepatitis virus or hepatitis delta virus: relationship to interferon. *Hepatology* **10,** 764–768.
12. Gastaldi, M., Massacrier, A., Planells, R., Robaglia-Schlupp, A., Portal-Bartolomei, I., Bourlière, M., et al. (1995) Detection by in situ hybridization of hepatitis C virus positive and negative RNA strands using digoxigenin-labeled cRNA probes in human liver cells. *J. Hepatology* **23,** 509–518.

24

The *In Situ* Detection of PCR-Amplified Hepatitis C RNA

Gerard J. Nuovo and Maria Lynn Alfieri

1. Introduction
1.1. Introductory Statement

The discovery of PCR in 1985 has had an enormous impact on the field of molecular diagnostics. However, an important drawback of solution-phase PCR is that one cannot localize the target of interest to a specific cell type owing to the obligatory tissue destruction required for DNA extraction. This problem has been circumvented by the field of *in situ* PCR. This chapter will describe the theoretical basis of *in situ* PCR using hepatitis C as a model system. The goals of this manuscript are:

1. To describe the various DNA synthesis pathways that may be operative during *in situ* PCR.
2. To describe the key preparatory steps of reverse transcriptase (RT) *in situ* PCR.
3. To describe the actual protocol of RT *in situ* PCR.
4. To discuss potential problems when doing RT *in situ* PCR and how to resolve these problems, using hepatitis C infection of liver tissues as the model system.

1.2. DNA Synthesis

In order to comprehend fully the technique of RT *in situ* PCR, a basic knowledge of the biological synthesis of DNA is needed. Each nucleotide of DNA has two ends, the triphosphate group end (5'), and the hydroxyl (OH) group end (3'). When the nucleotides combine, the 5' triphosphate group of one nucleotide joins the 3' OH group of the other. This results in the release of pyrophosphate, and the end result is a dinucleotide that contains an unoccupied 3' OH group on one side opposing an unoccupied 5'-triphosphate on the other *(1)*.

The phosphodiester bond is catalyzed by DNA polymerase, which can only combine the unoccupied 5' triphosphate group of the single nucleotide to the 3' OH group of the growing, longer chain. DNA synthesis therefore can only occur 5' to 3'. The complete product is the replication of two complementary strands of DNA which are synthesized in opposing directions.

During PCR, several different DNA synthesis pathways may be operative. One category, the primer dependent pathways, requires the presence of a primer that, after annealing to a strand of DNA, can dictate DNA synthesis by the DNA polymerase. The primer-dependent pathways include primer oligomerization, mispriming, and target-specific amplification *(1–3)*. The other category, often called DNA repair, is primer-independent. This latter pathway serves as an essential control for RT *in situ* PCR, and its persistence after DNase digestion with suboptimal protease digestion can lead to a false-positive signal *(1,2)*. Because of its importance in RT *in situ* PCR, we will discuss the primer independent DNA synthesis pathway first.

1.3. Primer-Independent DNA Synthesis

The occurrence of DNA repair during *in situ* PCR is dependent on specific conditions. For example, it will not be operative in cytospin preparations or frozen, fixed tissues unless these are exposed to dry heat of 55°C or greater prior to amplification *(1,2)*. Primer independent DNA synthesis can be readily induced during *in situ* PCR by heating the tissue sample to 55°–65°C prior to doing the procedure. Paraffin-embedded tissue has invariably been heated to 65°C for 4 h during tissue processing, and, thus, will always demonstrate the primer independent pathway during *in situ* PCR (**Fig. 1**). This can be demonstrated by using any paraffin-embedded tissue and performing *in situ* PCR without primers and using a labeled reporter nucleotide, such as digoxigenin dUTP. Under these conditions, all cell types will show an intense nuclear-based signal *(1,2)*. This most likely represents the filling in of DNA gaps that were induced by the prior heating, which in turn become "surrogate endogenous primers" during cycling. As noted above, the primer-independent signal is not apparent in frozen, fixed tissues, if they have not been exposed to dry heat prior to cycling (**Fig. 1**). The DNA repair signal can also be averted if one uses unheated cytospins preparations. This allows one to do target-specific direct incorporation for DNA target in cytospin preparations or frozen, fixed tissues *(1,2)*. However, clearly one cannot do target-specific direct incorporation of the reporter nucleotide for DNA targets when using paraffin-embedded tissues.

Further evidence for the mechanism of the primer-independent signal with paraffin-embedded tissues comes from experiments where such tissue is pretreated with *taq* polymerase and a dideoxy nucleotide after optimal protease digestion and prior to *in situ* PCR. This, too, can suppress the nonspecific signal

In Situ Detection

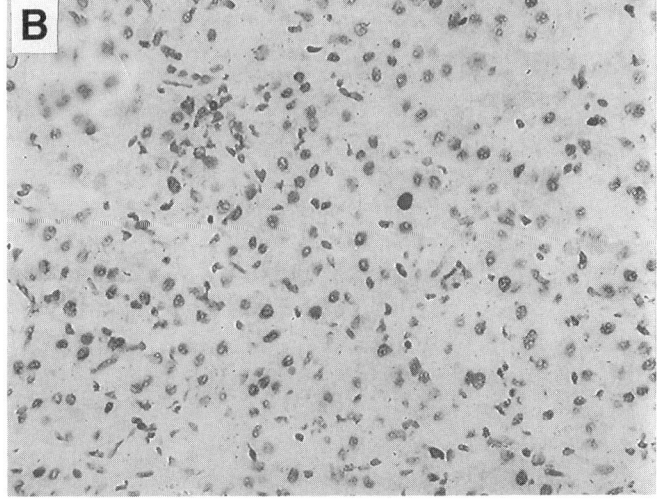

Fig. 1. The primer-independent signal with *in situ* PCR is dependent on prior heating of the tissue. No signal was evident in this frozen, fixed tissue from the CNS if *in situ* PCR was done without primers (**A**). A strong signal is evident from the reporter nucleotide digoxigenin dUTP if paraffin-embedded liver was used; tissue is heated to 65°C during the paraffin embedding process (**B**).

caused by DNA repair in a process analogous to sequencing DNA; incorporation of the dideoxynucleotide in the pretreatment step prevents further nucleotide incorporation during amplification *(1,2)*. However, this requires meticulous attention to optimizing protease digestion time to avoid a false-positive signal, which will be discussed shortly under the category of DNase digestion.

1.4. Primer-Dependent DNA Synthesis

1.4.1. Mispriming

The nonspecific primer-dependent pathway of mispriming is the result of the primer binding to nontarget DNA. In order to study the effects of mispriming, the primer-independent DNA repair pathway must be inactivated. This can be done by using frozen, fixed tissue and primers that do not have any corresponding target in the sample. Under these conditions, the nonspecific signal is only present during *in situ* PCR if the *taq* polymerase is added before the temperature increase of the cycling block. The signal is eliminated if the *taq* polymerase is added after the thermal cycler reaches 55°C; i.e., if the hot-start maneuver is used *(1,2)* (**Fig. 2**). Similar inhibition of nonspecific DNA synthesis (with a concomitant augmented target-specific DNA synthesis) with the hot-start maneuver is seen in solution-phase PCR *(1–3)*. The poor homology between hybridized primer and nontarget DNA can lead to the denaturing of these complexes by simply raising the reaction temperature to at least 55°C prior to DNA synthesis, while preserving target–primer hybrids.

1.4.2. Primer Oligomerization

The discussion on mispriming presupposed that primer oligomerization is not operative in the cell during *in situ* PCR. This would seem an unlikely statement given the observation by anyone who has done solution-phase PCR that primer oligomerization can be a dominant pathway during the amplification step. Primer oligomerization during *in situ* PCR can be studied after eliminating DNA repair and mispriming. This can be accomplished by using paraffin-embedded tissue that has been adequately digested with protease and pretreated with DNase. One could also perform these experiments using frozen, fixed tissue and the hot-start maneuver. In either case, one must employ primers that do not have a corresponding target in the sample to be tested. We performed such experiments with paraffin-embedded liver tissue and frozen, fixed gerbil brain tissue; in each case, human papillomavirus (HPV) specific primers were used—neither tissue can be infected by HPV. By doing "cold start" *in situ* PCR, we were able to induce primer oligomerization in the amplifying solution. However, no intracellular signal was apparent under these conditions if one did a high-stringency post-PCR wash (**Fig. 2**) *(1,2)*.

It is not clear why primer oligomerization does not appear to be operative inside a cell, even when it is occurring robustly in the overlying amplifying solution. An obvious difference between the two milieus is that the nucleus contains a high concentration of nucleic acids and proteins. It has been demon-

In Situ Detection

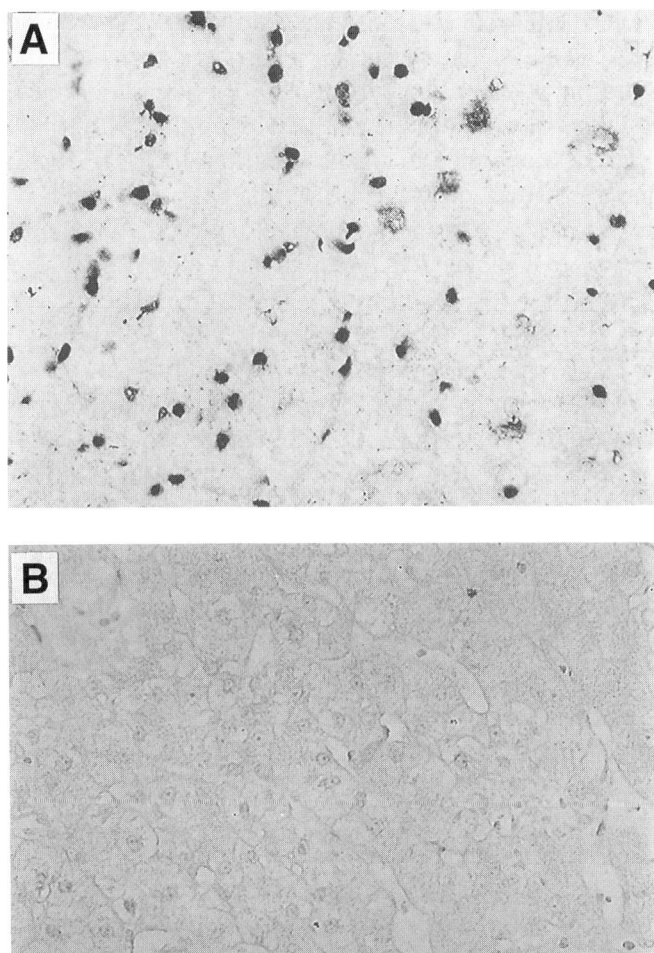

Fig. 2. Mispriming and primer oligomerization during *in situ* PCR. A signal is evident in the frozen, fixed CNS tissue if irrelevant (HPV) primers and the other reagents are added at room temperature (**A**). The signal was lost if the *taq* polymerase was withheld until the block temperature reached 55°C (not shown). If DNA repair and mispriming are eliminated by DNase digestion after optimal protease digestion, no signal is evident using irrelevant primers (**B**) despite documentation of robust primer oligomerization in the amplifying solution.

strated in solution-phase PCR that certain proteins can strongly inhibit primer oligomerization *(1,2)*. The apparent lack of primer oligomerization in the cell has an important practical consideration for those doing *in situ* PCR. In solution-phase PCR, if one wishes to detect the amplicon with a hybridization step, one must use a probe that is internal to the primers or risk obtaining a false-positive signal from primer oligomerization. Such oligoprobes, which are usually from 20–40 bp in size, are difficult to work with for *in situ* hybridization because of their narrow range of signal to background *(1)*. However, with *in situ* PCR, one can use a full-length probe that spans the entire region of the amplicon. Such full length probes, optimal at between 90 and 150 bp, have a much broader range of signal to background. On a practical level, one can do a posthybridization wash of 60°C in 15 m*M* NaCl with 0.2% bovine serum albumin (BSA) for 15 min, and be assured that background will be minimal and the signal preserved. These conditions would certainly eliminate the signal as well as the background with an oligoprobe. For an oligoprobe, a typical post hybridization wash would be 50°C in 150 m*M* NaCl with 0.2% BSA for 10 min. Depending on conditions, such as probe size, purity, the hybridization time, and probe concentration, this could result in background or even loss of signal *(1)*. Trial and error are needed to determine what the proper temperature and salt concentration should be of the posthybridization wash when using an oligoprobe.

1.4.3. Target-Specific Amplification

The final pathway of primer-dependent DNA synthesis is target-specific amplification. This pathway results in the binding of the primer to a specific target, achieving 100% homology among its basepairs. The differentiation between target-specific amplification and primer-independent signal is easily appreciated by either pretreating the tissues in the dideoxy-containing solution after optimal protease digestion, or using frozen, fixed tissues fixed in 10% buffered formalin after cryostat sectioning with the hot-start manuever, as mentioned previously. Under these conditions, one can easily demonstrate target-specific incorporation of the reporter nucleotide in viral-infected tissue by knowing the specific tropism of the virus. For example, HPV infects only the squamous epithelium in vulvar and penile tissues. If one is using frozen, fixed tissue and the hot start maneuver, then the viral DNA localizes only the superficial squamous epithelium; if one omits the hot-start manuever, all cell types demonstrate a signal *(1,2)*. Alternatively, one can detect target-specific amplification of a DNA target with a labeled probe, in a process called PCR *in situ* hybridization. For RNA targets, such as hepatitis C, the DNase digestion step allows one to do target-specific incorporation of the labeled nucleotide into the PCR-amplified cDNA (after the RT step) in a process called RT *in situ* PCR, which will be discussed in detail shortly.

With regard to RT *in situ* PCR, it is very important to realize that there are two histologic markers of specificity:

Table 1
The Effect of Protease Digestion Time on the Primer-Independent Signal During *In Situ* PCR as a Function of the Time of Fixation in 10% Buffered Formalin (Modified from Ref. 4)[a]

Fixation time	Pepsin (2 mg/mL) digestion time						
	0 min	15 min	30 min	45 min	60 min	75 min	90 min
4 h	0	2+	Overdigested				
6 h	0	3+	2+	Overdigested			
8 h	0	0	1+	3+	—	—	—
15 h	0	0	0	1+	1+	2+	3+
48 h	0	0	0	0	1+	2+	3+
1 wk	0	0	0	0	1+	1+	2–3+

[a]The signal was scored as follows: 0, 1+ (<25% of cells positive), 2+ (25–50% cells positive), and 3+ (>50% of cells positive = optimal).

1. The RNA-based target specific signal should not be pan-nuclear, whereas the DNA-based signal for the positive control (no DNase digestion, from DNA repair) should be pan-nuclear.
2. The RNA-based target signal should involve specific cell types, whereas the DNA-based signal for the positive control should involve all cell types.
   These two important points will be stressed in the discussion of hepatitis C RNA detection by RT *in situ* PCR.

1.4.4. Determination of the Optimal Protease Digestion Time

Optimal protease digestion is the key for successful RT *in situ* PCR. It is a function of the type of tissue and, more importantly, the length of time that the tissue was fixed in formalin *(1,4)*. It needs to be determined by trial and error. A general and important principle is that the longer the fixation time, the broader the window of optimal protease digestion time. If one knows the length of time that a tissue was fixed in 10% buffered formalin, the optimal protease digestion time can be estimated from **Table 1**. However, in most cases, one does not know the length of time that the tissue was fixed in 10% buffered formalin. Furthermore, at times formalin is not the fixative that is used; for example, a weaker crosslinking fixative, such as 2% paraformaldehyde, may be used. In these instances, one must first determine the optimal protease digestion time. The protocol that the authors recommend to use is presented in **Fig. 3**. Assume that one sees the most intense signal in the greatest percentage of cells after 60 min of digestion in 2 mg/mL of pepsin. The next step is to confirm that this is the optimal protease digestion by demonstrating the loss of the signal with overnight digestion in DNase. From a practical viewpoint, the

1. Place 3 Tissue Sections on a Silane Coated Glass Slide

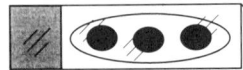

2. Remove Paraffin with 5 Min. Wash In Xylene, 5 Min. Wash In 100% ETOH, Then Air-Dry

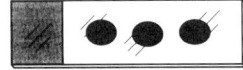

3. Protease Digest for 30 Min., 60 Min., and 90 Min. with Pepsin (2 mg/ml)

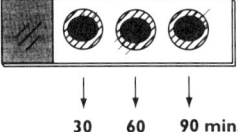

4. Remove Protease, do in situ PCR for 20 Cycles, a 3+Signal Denotes Optimal Digestion Time

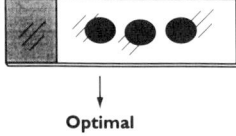

Fig. 3. A recommended start-up protocol for *in situ* PCR. The start-up protocol relies on the primer-independent signal to generate an intense signal dependent on the optimal protease time for the particular sample.

protease digestion time that gives an intense signal in the majority of cells usually will allow for the complete loss of the signal with overnight digestion in DNase. To summarize:

Optimal protease digestion time: The definition of optimal protease digestion time is the amount of time in protease that produces an intense signal in most cells with *in situ* PCR (i.e., using direct incorporation of the reporter nucleotide). This protease digestion time should lead to a complete loss of signal with overnight digestion in DNase prior to *in situ* PCR.

Suboptimal protease digestion time: Suboptimal protease digestion time is recognized as a weak-to-moderate signal in some cells with *in situ* PCR. The signal persists after DNase digestion, and is usually stronger than the corresponding tissue that is not pretreated in DNase.

Protease overdigestion time: Over protease digestion time is recognized as a weak-to-absent signal with loss of the cytoplasmic and nuclear detail. The loss of cellular detail is evident as poor staining with the counterstain (nuclear fast red for 5-bromo-4-chloro-3-indolyl-phosphate [NBT/BCIP]) and prominent basement membranes.

1.5. Outline of Procedures Involved When Doing In Situ PCR

1. Place tissue sections on silane-coated slides.
2. Remove paraffin.
3. Determine optimal protease digestion time.
4. Do optimal protease digestion, and then DNase-digest two of three tissue samples/slide.
5. Using the rTth system, do RT and *in situ* PCR with direct incorporation of the reporter nucleotide. The no DNase section is the positive control, the DNase, no RT (or RT with HPV primers) is the negative control, and the DNase, RT with hepatitis C primers is the test.
6. High-stringency wash.
7. Detect digoxigenin using alkaline phosphatase conjugate and nitroblue tetrazolium and 5-bromo-4-chloro-3-indolyl-phosphate (NBT/BCIP) as chromogen.
8. Counterstain in nuclear fast red; coverslip.

2. Materials

1. Silane-coated glass slides: These are available from ONCOR, Gaithersburg, MD. Whenever possible, place three 4-µ sections/glass slide. This allows one to do the positive and negative controls on the same glass slide as the test. Slides can be stored after sectioning at room temperature for at least 10 yr. If one uses the Perkin Elmer 1000 thermal cycler, one must use the slides made by Perkin Elmer (Norwalk, CT). Regular thickness slides are too thin for the 1000 thermal cycler, and will either break or lose reagent with the Perkin Elmer thermal cycler.
2. Xylene and ethanol: These are available from many sources, including Fisher Scientific (Pittsburgh, PA). They can be stored at room temperature in a flame-retardant storage area.
3. Protease: One can use many different protease solutions and obtain good results with RT *in situ* PCR. We prefer either a trypsin or a pepsin solution: 20 mg pepsin (Digene Diagnostics, Silver Spring, MD), plus 9.5 mL DEPC water (Research Genetics, Birmingham, AL) and 0.5 mL of 2 NHCl. Freeze 1-mL aliquots for 1 wk; thaw and use immediately. We perform protease digestion at room temperature. For PCR *in situ* hybridization, 30 min are adequate for most samples. For RT *in situ* PCR, the optimal protease digestion time must be determined empirically, as described in detail above.
4. DNase digestion: To prepare the DNase solution, per tissue sample use 1 µL of PCR buffer II (Perkin Elmer, GeneAmp kit) and add 1 µL of RNase-free DNase (Boehringer Mannheim, Indianapolis, IN) and 8 µL of DEPC water. Prepare fresh. Cover with autoclaved polypropylene coverslip (Fisher Scientific) and place in humidity chamber at 37°C overnight.

5. EZ PCR kit (Perkin Elmer): Store all reagents at 4°C, except for the rTth enzyme, which should be stored at –20°C.
6. Thermal cycler: Perkin Elmer 1000 *in situ* PCR machine, which comes with ampliclips and amplicovers. Alternatives include using the "aluminum boat method" with any aluminum block thermal cycler *(1,5)* or the Self-seal method with the MJ Research Laboratory (Watertown, MA). For those who already have an aluminum block thermal cycler, it is recommended that they either use the aluminum boat method or use the self-seal (or frame-seal) containment system from MJ Research, and place the glass slide directly on the block. For the latter, one should not exceed 88°C for denaturation.
7. Buffers for *in situ* PCR: The buffers are from the *in situ* hybridization kit from Digene Diagnostics. Similar materials are available from the *in situ* hybridization made by Enzo Diagnostics (Farmingdale, NY). Buffer #1: 0.1 M Tris, pH 7.5, 0.1 M NaCl (for antidigoxigenen solution); buffer #2: 0.1X SSC and 2% BSA (post-RT PCR wash); buffer #3: 0.1 M Tris-HCl, pH 9.5, 0.1 M NaCl, 0.05 M $MgCl_2$ (for NBT/BCIP solution); store all buffers at 4°C.
8. Antidigoxigenin–alkaline phosphatase conjugate: The stock solution from Boehringer Mannheim (Indianapolis, IN) should be stored at 4°C and made fresh before use by diluting 1:150 in buffer 1.
9. Nuclear fast red: Store at room temperature indefinitely. It can be reused for up to 1 yr. It is recommended that one purchase nuclear fast red (Enzo Diagnostics or Digene Diagnostics).

3. Methods
3.1. Tissue Preparation

1. Cut three 4-µm sections, and place on a silane-coated glass slides. Heat slide for 15–30 min at 65°C, and then store at room temperature.
2. To deparaffinize the tissue sections, wash slides in xylene for 5 min, 5 min in 100% ethanol, and then air-dry.
3. Protease digestion: Digest each tissue section in pepsin 2 mg/mL for the optimal time determined as described above.
4. Remove protease by washing slide in sterile DEPC water for 1 min, 100% ethanol for 1 min, then air dry.
5. DNase digest 2 of the 3 tissue sections overnight at 37°C (10 µL/section, with 10 U of DNase/section). Overlay with sterile coverslip.
6. Remove coverslip, wash in sterile DEPC water, 100% ethanol for 1 min, and air-dry.

3.2. RT-PCR

1. Add 15 µL (for the aluminum boat method or self-seal method) or 50 µL (for the Amplicover or frame-seal method) of the following RT-PCR solution to each sample: 10 µL EZ buffer, 1.6 µL each dATP, dCTP, dGTP, dTTP (10 mM), 1.6 µL 2% BSA, 1.6 µL RNasin (10 U/µL), 0.6 µL digoxigenin dUTP (1 mM), 12.4 µL Mn acetate (10 mM), 14.0 µL DEPC water, 3.0 µL hepatitis C primers (20 µM stock solution), and 2.0 µL rTth enzyme (5 U/µL).

Table 2
Hepatitis-Specific Primers

Primer	Orientation	Sequence
JH51	Antisense	CCCAACACTACTCGGCTA
JH52	Antisense	AGTCTTGCGGCCGCAGCGCCAAATC
JH93	Sense	TCCGCGGCCGCACTCCACCATGAATCACTCCCC

Table 3
HPV 16-Specific Sequence

Primer	Position of first nt[a]	Sequence
HPV16-1 (5')	110	CAGGACCCACAGGAGCGACC
HPV16-2 (3')	559	TTACAGCTGGGTTTCTCTAC

[a]nt nucleotide.

The hepatitis C-specific primers we use are as in **Table 2** *(6,7)*. For the negative control, either omit the primers or use irrelevant primers. A recommended pair of negative primers for hepatitis C work is the following HPV 16-specific sequence shown in **Table 3** *(1,8)*.

2. Do RT step at 65°C for 30 min. This should be followed by denaturation at 94°C for 3 min, and then cycle at 60°C for 1 min, and 94°C for 45 s for 20 cycles.

3.3. Detection

1. If using the aluminum boat method, remove mineral oil with 5 min in fresh xylene, and 5 min in 100% ethanol. Then air-dry. If using the self-seal method, place slides in water for 5 min to remove coverslip, followed by dip in 100% ethanol, and then air-dry. If using the Perkin Elmer amplicover system, dip slide in 100% ethanol, and then air-dry.
2. Post hybridization wash—Place slides at 60°C for 15 min in buffer 2. Using a Kleenex, remove buffer 2 from the back of the slide and from around the edge of the front of the slide. Using a hydrophobic pen (PapPen, Jersey Glove and Lab Supplies, Mount Laurel, NJ), circle the perimeter of the front of the slide. Place the slide in a humidity chamber; do not let the slide dry out.
3. Make antidigoxigenin–streptavidin alkaline phosphatase conjugate, 100 μL/slide. Take 150 μL of buffer 1 and add 1 μL of the stock solution of the alkaline phosphatase conjugate. Incubate at 37°C for 30 min in the humidity chamber, making certain it is level so the conjugate does not migrate off of the slide.
4. Take 15 mL of buffer 3, and add to it 50 μL substrate 1 and 50 μL substrate 2. Buffer 3 should be warmed to 37°C prior to adding the chromogen, or the latter

may precipitate. Incubate in the chromogen solution for 5–15 min. Periodically check the slide under the microscope, and stop the reaction when the positive control (no DNase) shows an intense signal.
5. Rinse in water, nuclear fast red for 3 min, water, 100% ethanol, xylene, permount, and coverslip.

4. Notes

1. Sections fall off: Possible causes of this unusual problem include water under the tissue, tissue being poorly cut (e.g., dry), tissue not being baked after sectioning, or not using silane-coated slides.
2. Slides not clear after PCR step: This is caused by xylene and ethanol contaminated by water. The slide appears milky or has a thin film on it. Use fresh xylene and ethanol.
3. Signal with negative control: A nuclear signal with negative control (DNase, no RT, or RT with HPV primers) is indicative of the most common problem with RT *in situ* PCR: underprotease digestion. Redo the experiment, increasing time of protease digestion (**Fig. 4**).
4. No signal or weak signal with poor tissue morphology: This reflects overprotease digestion. Redo the experiment, decreasing the time of protease digestion (**Fig. 4**).
5. High background: Background refers to cytoplasmic membrane staining with the negative control; it often will be evident in the positive control and test section as well. This is owing to the primer oligomers that form in the amplifying solution sticking nonspecifically to cellular proteins. This is caused by a post-PCR wash that is at too low a temperature or not of sufficient time. This can be rectified by washing at 60°C for 15 min in 15 mM salt.

    Another cause of background is the source of the NBT/BCIP. In the authors' experience, NBT/BCIP from certain companies (e.g., Boehringer Mannheim) can produce high background. This has not been the case with the chromogen from other vendors (e.g., Digene) *(1)*.
6. No signal with the positive control: This has many potential causes. The two most likely in our experience are: inadequate/inactive protease and inactive antidigoxigenin–alkaline phosphatase conjugate. The latter can be caused by placing the conjugate in the freezer.
7. Hepatitis C as a model system for RT *in situ* PCR: This final section will demonstrate the principles of the methodology of RT *in situ* PCR using hepatitis C detection as the model system. This will be followed by a brief discussion of data about the pathogenesis of hepatitis C infection as determined by RT *in situ* PCR. RT *in situ* PCR: detection of hepatitis C. Three possible outcomes account for most of the results when testing for hepatitis C:
    a. Desired result: Negative control—no signal; positive control—intense nuclear signal in most cells and in all cell types; test—no signal or perinuclear/cytoplasmic signal in hepatocytes and Kuppfer cells. This result demonstrates that protease digestion time was optimal (**Fig. 4**).

In Situ Detection

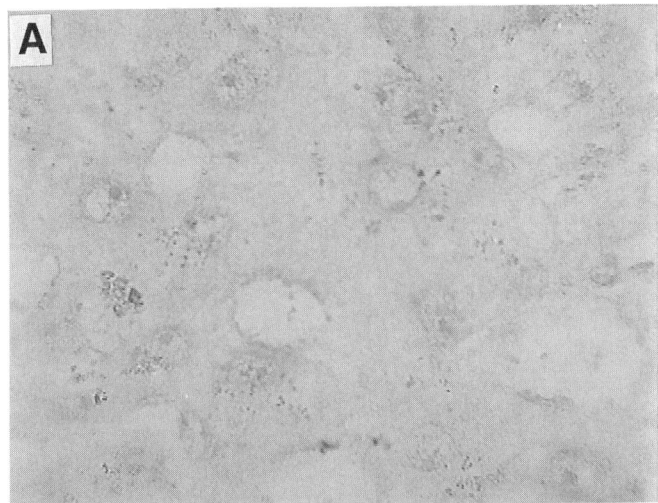

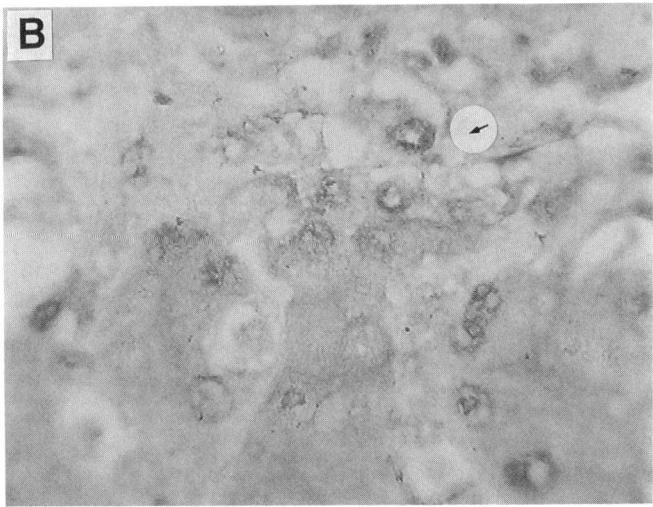

Fig. 4. Suboptimal, optimal, and over protease digestion in the analysis for hepatitis C by RT *in situ* PCR. With optimal protease digestion, no signal is noted in the negative control (DNase, RT with HPV primers) **(A)**. A strong nuclear signal was evident in the positive control (*see* **Fig. 1B**). A nuclear membrane and cytoplasmic signal were evident in some hepatocytes after RT *in situ* PCR analysis for hepatitis C after optimal protease digestion **(B)** *(continued)*.

  b. Undesired result #1 (suboptimal protease digestion): Negative control—nuclear based signal in all cell types; positive control—nuclear signal in all cell types that is usually weaker than the signal evident with the negative

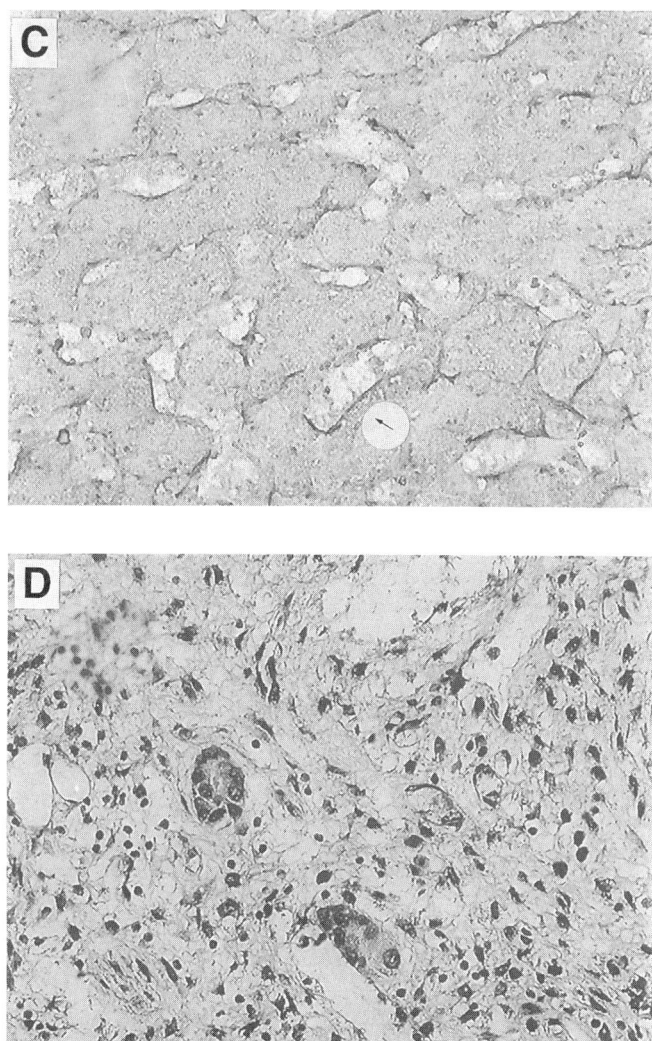

Fig. 4. *(continued)* If the protease time was too long, the signal was lost; note the prominent sinusoidal basement membranes, loss of cellular detail, and high background (**C**). If the protease digestion time was too short, a nuclear-based signal is seen in all cell types in the negative control (**D**).

control; test—nuclear signal in all cell types. This result indicates suboptimal protease digestion. The nuclear-based signal in the negative control and the test will demonstrate that the signal is nonspecific (owing primarily to primer-independent DNA synthesis). The problem can be corrected by increasing the time of protease digestion (**Fig. 4**).

c. Undesired result #2 (over protease digestion): Negative control—no or weak signal; positive control—no or weak signal, or cytoplasmic signal, poor nuclear and cytoplasmic detail, prominent basement membranes in the sinusoids and the central vein region; test—no signal. This result indicates over protease digestion. The nuclear fast red counterstain binds to cellular nucleic acids and proteins, and thus, will stain weakly if the proteins have been degraded. The problem can be corrected by decreasing the time of protease digestion (**Fig. 4**).

8. Clinicopathologic data on Hepatitis C infection as determined by RT *in situ* PCR: We performed two studies *(6,8)* comparing the serological analysis for hepatitis C infection using the recombinant immunoblot assay (RIBA™-Chiron) to the direct *in situ* localization of the hepatitis C viral genome using the RT *in situ* PCR technique. Concurrent sera and liver biopsies from 42 patients with clinical and histologic evidence of chronic liver disease were studied. Antibodies against hepatitis C-specific antigens were demonstrated by RIBA in the sera of 39/42 (92%), and PCR-amplified viral cDNA was detected in the biopsies of 21 (54%) of the 39 seropositive patients. The detection rate using standard *in situ* hybridization for the tissues known to be viral-positive with RT *in situ* PCR was 9/21 (42%). This study demonstrated that:
   a. RT *in situ* PCR was more sensitive than standard *in situ* hybridization for the detection of hepatitis C RNA.
   b. About one-half of patients with chronic hepatitis and serologic evidence of hepatitis C infection will not have virus detectable in their liver biopsy even with a highly sensitive PCR-based technique. Whether inteferon therapy is contraindicated in the viral-negative people will require further study.
   c. The viral RNA localized to the hepatocyte and Kuppfer cell (liver macrophage). In rare instances, a signal was evident in biliary epithelium.

References

1. Nuovo, G. J. (1996) *PCR In Situ Hybridization: Protocols and Applications,* 3rd ed. Lippincott-Raven, New York.
2. Nuovo, G. J., Gallery, F., Hom, R., MacConnell, P., and Bloch, W. (1993) Importance of different variables for optimizing in situ detection of PCR-amplified DNA. *PCR Method. Applic.* **2,** 305–312.
3. Nuovo, G. J., Gallery, F., MacConnell, P., Becker, J., and Bloch, W. (1991) An improved technique for the detection of DNA by *in situ* hybridization after PCR-amplification. *Am. J. Pathol.* **139,** 1239–1244.
4. Nuovo, G. J., Gallery, F., and MacConnell, P. (1994) Analysis of non-specific DNA synthesis during in situ PCR. *PCR Method Applic.* **4,** 342–349.
5. Nuovo, G. J. (1996) *Keys to Successful In Situ PCR: Video.* Lippincott-Raven, New York.
6. Nuovo, G. J., Lidonocci, K., MacConnell, P., and Lane, B. (1993) Intracellular localization of PCR-amplified hepatitis C cDNA. *Am. J. Pathol.* **17,** 683–690.

7. Han, J. H., Shyamala, V., Richman, K. H., Brauer, M. J., Irvine, B., Urdea, M. S., et al. (1991) Characterization of the terminal regions of hepatitis C viral RNA: Identification of conserved sequences in the 5' untranslated region and poly(A) tails at the 3' end. *Proc. Natl. Acad. Sci. USA* **88,** 1711–1715.
8. Lidonnici, K., Lane, B., and Nuovo, G. J. (1995) A comparison of serologic analysis and *in situ* localization of PCR-amplified cDNA for the diagnosis of hepatitis C infection. *Diagn. Mol. Pathol.* **4,** 98–107.

25

Immunoelectron Microscopic Characterization of HCV

Shozo Watanabe, Masahiko Kaito, and Michinori Kohara

1. Introduction

The improvement of instruments and technology enabled the first visualization of viral particles by means of electron microscopy in 1939 *(1)*. In particular, the negative staining technique provided high-resolution electron microscopic images of viral particles. This technique utilizes the principle of surrounding viral particles with electron-dense heavy metal atoms, whereby viral particles are recognized as negative contrast against a dark background of heavy metal atoms. The disadvantage of the so-called negative staining technique is that only small amounts of the sample are examined. Therefore, a highly concentrated virus suspension is usually required in order to visualize the viral particles. Since electron microscopic detection of virus in general requires particle concentrations in the range of 10^9–10^{12} particles/mL *(2)*, and most clinical specimens contain a concentration of viral particles much less than this range, additional procedures are required to increase the concentration of viral particles before visualization. The addition of specific antibody to the specimen may produce antigen–antibody aggregates and enhance viral concentrations within the immune complex, thereby facilitating electron microscopic detection. This immunoelectron microscopic procedure improves the sensitivity of electron microscopy by approx 1000-fold, and offers the advantage of identifying the immunologic specificity of the viruses *(3)*.

Blood-borne non-A, non-B hepatitis was first recognized in 1974 *(4)*. Since then, many investigators have tried to identify the causative agent of this type of hepatitis in sera and liver samples from humans and experimental animals using conventional electron microscopy and/or immunoelectron microscopy. A variety of virus-like particles, morphologically resembling parvovirus, togavirus, picornavirus, hepadonavirus, paramyxovirus, papovavirus and retrovirus, have been reported as candidate etiologic agents *(5,6)*, but none have been universally accepted as the etiologic agent. In 1989, a breakthrough was achieved by the successful cloning of the genome of hepatitis C virus (HCV), a major etiologic agent of non-A, non-B hepatitis, from highly infectious chimpanzee plasma *(7)*. Analysis of the structure of this HCV genome suggested that it is closely related to pesti- and flaviviruses. However, the morphology of HCV remained unknown.

We attempted to identify viral particles in plasma from HCV-infected patients using conventional electron microscopy, and were able to observe small clusters of various forms of virus-like particles in specimens prepared by sucrose density gradient centrifugation from concentrated HCV-positive plasma samples. Successive immunoaggregation testing of these specimens using convalescent serum of a patient who recovered from posttransfusion acute hepatitis C or with antibodies specific to the putative HCV envelope 1 protein revealed large aggregates of these particles, but the specificity of the immune reaction was not clear, because the aggregates were composed of various forms of virus-like particles in the specimen before the addition of the antibodies. In order to visualize clearly the antigen–antibody reaction on the surface of individual virus-like particles, we have employed indirect immunogold electron microscopy using the method described by Murti and Webster *(8)* with minor modifications. Using polyclonal antibodies and monoclonal antibodies (MAbs) specific to the HCV envelope 1 protein, this technique enabled the discrimination of HCVs from other particles by the immunogold labeling, which allowed the clarification of the morphology of HCV, which was shown to be 55–65 nm spherical particles with delicate surface projections of approx 6 nm in length *(9)*. Here, we describe our indirect immunogold electron microscopic procedure for immunological identification and characterization of HCV in human plasma.

2. Materials

1. Virus-containing specimens: Large volume of plasma from patients with high HCV RNA titers.
2. TEN buffer: 100 mM Tris-HCl, pH 8.0, 1 mM EDTA Na$_2$, 100 mM NaCl.
3. TE buffer: 100 mM Tris-HCl, pH 8.0, 1 mM EDTA Na$_2$.
4. Phosphate-buffered saline (PBS), pH 7.4.
5. Polyclonal antibodies and MAbs to putative HCV envelope 1 protein: Antibodies used for our experiments were generated through immunization with antigens expressed by recombinant vaccinia virus carrying HCV cDNAs of the putative envelope 1 gene of HCV, encoding the whole gp35 of HCV envelope 1 glycoprotein *(10)*.
6. Secondary antibodies for indirect immunogold electron microscopy: Goat antirabbit IgG-conjugated colloidal gold particles and protein A-conjugated

colloidal gold particles (Super EM Grade, 5 nm diameter, BioCell Research Laboratories, Cardiff, UK).
7. Tris-buffered saline (TBS): 100 mM Tris-HCl, pH 7.6, 150 mM NaCl is prepared and sterilized by autoclaving, and stored at 4°C.
8. TBS containing 2% bovine serum albumin (TBS-BSA) is prepared immediately before use by adding 2 g of BSA (Fraction V, Sigma Chemical Co., St. Louis, MO) to 100 mL of TBS, and filtering through a 0.22-µm nitrocellulose filter.
9. TBS containing 3% gelatin (Sigma) is also prepared immediately before use and filtered through a 0.22-µm nitrocellulose filter.
10. Adjust 2% solution of phosphotungstic acid (TAAB Laboratories Equipment Ltd., Berkshire, UK) in distilled water to pH 6.5.

3. Methods
3.1. Preparation of Virus-Containing Specimen (See Note 1)

1. Centrifuge 100 mL of plasma from patients with high HCV RNA titers at 75,000g for 6 h in a Hitachi RPS 27-2 rotor at 4°C.
2. Resuspend the pellet in TEN and centrifuge again at 150,000g for 2.5 h in a Hitachi RPS 40T rotor at 4°C.
3. Prepare an approx 1000-fold concentrated suspension of the sample in TEN, and then layer on a 20–60% linear sucrose density gradient in TE buffer.
4. Centrifuge the sample at 100,000g for 16 h in a Hitachi RPS 40T rotor at 4°C.
5. Collect 500-mL fractions from the bottom of the tube and assay HCV RNA titers in each fraction by competitive PCR *(11,12)*.
6. Dilute fractions positive for high titers of HCV RNA (>5 × 10^7 copies/mL) in PBS and centrifuge at 150,000g for 2.5 h in a Hitachi RPS 40T rotor at 4°C to prepare 1000-fold concentrated specimens for immunoelectron microscopic examination.
7. Suspend the pellet in 100 µL of PBS and store at –80°C until use.

3.2. Immunoelectron Microscopic Study

The procedure for visualizing HCV particles using indirect immunogold electron microscopy is shown in **Fig. 1**.

1. Apply 2–3 µL of concentrated virus-containing specimen to a Formvar-coated and carbon-vaporized 300-mesh copper grid using an Eppendorf pipet.
2. Allow the specimen to sit for 10–15 min at room temperature until it becomes semidry to allow virus absorption onto the grid.
3. Using a pair of fine forceps, invert the grid and bring it into contact with the surface of a drop of TBS-BSA placed on parafilm in a moist chamber (*see* **Note 2**).
4. Allow the grid to float on the drop of TBS-BSA for 5 min at room temperature.
5. Then put the grid on top of a drop of TBS containing 3% gelatin for 30 min.
6. Place the grid on top of a drop of TBS-BSA to wash away the excessive gelatin.
7. Float the grid on a drop of primary antibody solution (diluted 1:10 to 1:100 in TBS-BSA) and incubate for 60 min at room temperature (*see* **Note 3**).

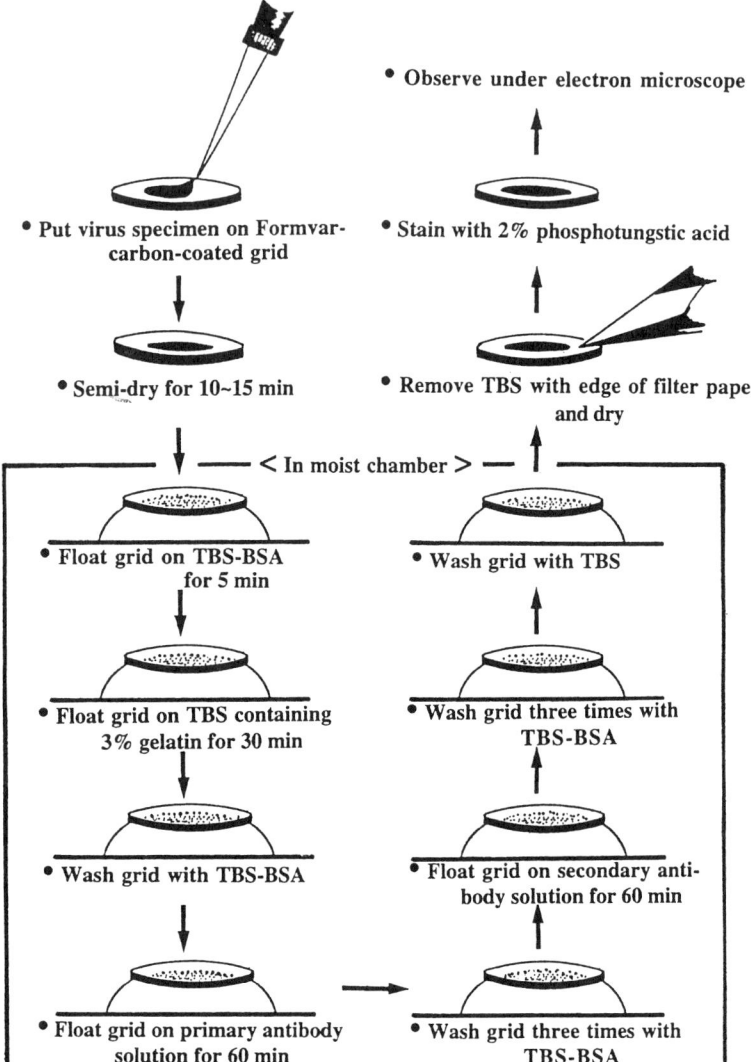

Fig. 1. Flowchart of the indirect immunogold electron microscopic procedure. Abbreviations are given in text.

8. Wash the grid three times on three separate drops of TBS-BSA.
9. Float the grid on a drop of secondary antibody solution (diluted 1:20 in TBS-BSA) and incubate for 60 min at room temperature (*see* **Note 4**).
10. Wash the grid three times on three separate drops of TBS-BSA.
11. Wash the grid on a drop of TBS.

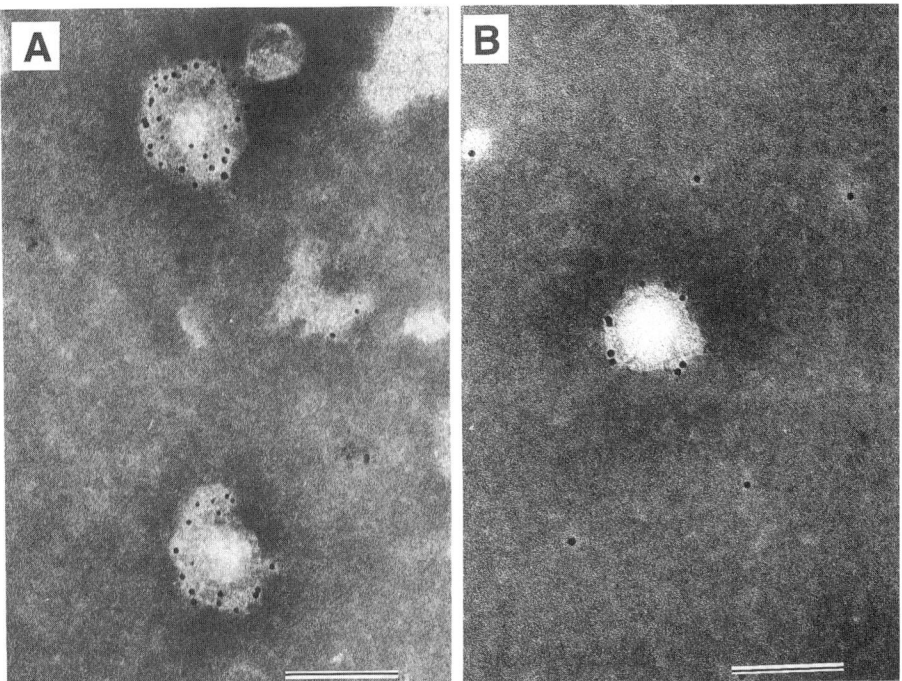

Fig. 2. Immunoelectron micrographs of HCV particles from human plasma, as detected using (A) polyclonal, and (B) MAbs to HCV envelope 1 protein. Specific gold (5 nm) labeling to antibody haloes is noted. Scale bar represents 100 nm.

12. Remove the grid from the moist chamber and remove the excessive TBS by touching the edge of the grid with a filter paper.
13. After drying the grid for 10 min, add a drop of 2% phosphotungstic acid on the specimen surface, and allow the grid to sit for 40 s at room temperature.
14. Remove the excess stain with the edge of a filter paper and dry the stained specimen thoroughly.
15. Evaluate the stained grid using a Hitachi H-800 electron microscope operated at 100 kV.
16. **Figure 2** shows images of HCV particles detected with (A) polyclonal antibodies and (B) MAbs to the putative HCV envelope 1 protein (*see* **Notes 5** and **6**).

4. Notes

1. Efficient immunolabeling of virus particles largely depends on specimen preparation. Although plasma HCV RNA titers are generally $<10^8$ copies/mL in most patients with chronic HCV infection, selecting HCV RNA-rich ($>10^7$ copies/mL) plasma samples and raising virus concentration by 3 logs are advisable for

immunogold electron microscopic detection. The distribution of peak titers of HCV RNA in fractions obtained from sucrose density gradient centrifugation varies among plasma samples. Therefore, measurement of HCV RNA titer in every sucrose fraction is required to assist the selection of fractions with the highest titers. It is also recommended that specimens prepared for indirect immunogold electron microscopy should be dispensed into small aliquots and stored at –80°C until use.

2. Both BSA and gelatin are used as blocking agents to prevent nonspecific binding of the antibodies to the Formvar-carbon-coated grid surface and the contaminating proteins. Two percent BSA and 3% gelatin are usually good enough for minimizing nonspecific background staining. We did preliminary tests to ascertain optimal gold labeling and minimal background by using a series of 10 times serially diluted primary and secondary antibodies. The procedure for immunolabeling should be carried out in a moist chamber to avoid drying of the specimen, which will drastically increase nonspecific labeling.

3. Genetic analysis has identified different HCV genotypes. Amino acid diversities among HCV genotypes can be observed in the region that encodes viral envelope proteins. This diversity is probably responsible for differences in the antigenicity of HCV envelope proteins from genotype to genotype. Therefore, the HCV genotype of the plasma sample to be tested should be the same as the immunogen used to raise the antibodies.

4. Immunogold labeling of HCV particles is performed using a combination of the primary antibody and its corresponding secondary antibody. The principle is as follows: specific antibody haloes on the surface of HCV particles, resulting from primary immune reaction of rabbit polyclonal antibody to the HCV envelope 1 protein at a dilution of 1:100, are traced by secondary immunolabeling with goat antirabbit IgG-conjugated colloidal gold particles (5 nm) at a dilution of 1:20, as shown in **Fig. 2A**. In the case of mouse MAbs, a dilution of 1:10 is used, followed by secondary immune reaction with protein A-conjugated colloidal gold particles (5 nm) at a dilution 1:20, and specific gold labeling of the HCV particle is detected as shown in **Fig. 2B**. In the latter case, immunolabeling with mouse MAbs, the binding affinity of protein A varies depending on the immunoglobulin subclasses, and mouse IgG_1 has low affinity to protein A. Fortunately, protein G–gold conjugate is available for specific gold labeling to every subclass of mouse MAbs and it can also be used as a tracer.

5. Specificity of immunogold labeling should be confirmed by performing a number of negative control tests, for example, by replacing the primary antibody with preimmune normal rabbit serum, serum from a rabbit infected with wild type vaccinia virus, and mouse MAb to human blood type A antigen, or by omitting the use of the primary antibody. The secondary antibody tracer should also be controlled with antibodies reactive against immunoglobulin from a different species.

6. The Formvar-carbon-coated surface membrane on a copper grid should be tough enough to endure all the steps involved in the indirect immunogold electron microscopic procedure as well as the impact of the electron beam.

References

1. Kausche, G. A., Pfankuch, E., and Ruska, H. (1939) Die sichtbarmachung von pflanzlichen virus im übermikroskop. *Naturwissenchaften* **18,** 292–299.
2. Horne, R. W. (1965) Negative staining methods, in *Techniques for Electron Microscopy* (Kay, D. H., ed.) Blackwell Scientific Publications, Oxford, pp. 328–355.
3. Feinstone, S. M., Kapikian, A. Z., and Purcell, R. H. (1973) Hepatitis A: detection by immune electron microscopy of a virus-like antigen associated with acute illness. *Science* **182,** 1026–1028.
4. Prince, A. M., Brotman, B., Grady, G. F., Kuhns, W. J., Hazzi, C., Levine, R. W., and Millian, S. J. (1974) Long-incubation post-transfusion hepatitis without serological evidence of exposure to hepatitis B virus. *Lancet* **ii,** 241–246.
5. Dienstag, J. L. (1983) Non-A, non-B hepatitis. II. Experimental transmission, putative virus agents and markers, and prevention. *Gastroenterology* **85,** 743–768.
6. Bradley, D. W. and Maynard, J. E. (1986) Etiology and natural history of post-transfusion and enterically-transmitted non-A, non-B hepatitis. *Semin. Liver Dis.* **6,** 56–66.
7. Choo, Q.-L., Kuo, G., Weiner, A. J., Overby, L. R., Bradley, D. W., and Houghton, M. (1989) Isolation of a cDNA clone derived from a blood-borne non-A, non-B viral hepatitis genome. *Science* **244,** 359–362.
8. Murti, K. G. and Webster, R. G. (1986) Distribution of hemagglutinin and neuraminidase on influenza virions as revealed by immunoelectron microscopy. *Virology* **149,** 36–43.
9. Kaito, M., Watanabe, S., Tsukiyama-Kohara, K., Yamaguchi, K., Kobayashi, Y., Konishi, M., et al. (1994) Hepatitis C virus particle detected by immunoelectron microscopic study. *J. Gen. Virol.* **75,** 1755–1760.
10. Kohara, M., Tsukiyama-Kohara, K., Maki, N., Asano, K., Yamaguchi, K., Miki, K., et al. (1992) Expression and characterization of glycoprotein gp35 of hepatitis C virus using recombinant vaccinia virus. *J. Gen. Virol.* **73,** 2313–2318.
11. Kaneko, S., Murakami, S., Unoura, M., and Kobayashi, K. (1992) Quantitation of hepatitis C virus RNA by competitive polymerase chain reaction. *J. Med. Virol.* **37,** 278–282.
12. Yoshioka, K., Kakumu, S., Wakita, T., Ishikawa, T., Itou, Y., Takayanagi, M., et al. (1992) Detection of hepatitis C virus by polymerase chain reaction and response to interferon-α therapy: relationship to genotypes of hepatitis C virus. *Hepatology* **16,** 293–299.

VI

MOLECULAR BIOLOGIC CHARACTERIZATION

26

Cloning and Assembly of Complex Libraries of Full-Length HCV cDNA Clones

Alexander A. Kolykhalov, Karen E. Reed, and Charles M. Rice

1. Introduction

Many studies of the molecular biology of hepatitis C virus (HCV) begin by obtaining representative cDNA clones of the viral genome. Most cloning strategies have been devised to deal with the low levels of HCV RNA present in starting material used for RNA isolation and cDNA synthesis. Typical sources include patient sera, liver samples, sera and tissues from infected chimpanzees, or in some cases, viral RNA obtained after replication in cell culture. Thus far, patient samples are the most common source of HCV RNA for cDNA cloning. Titers of HCV RNA in patient sera are low, typically ranging from 10^3 to 10^8 mol/mL. Except for a few instances, where cDNA libraries were obtained directly by isolating RNA from large volumes of high-titer sera *(1,2)*, PCR is used for amplifying HCV cDNA prior to cloning. Since this procedure requires smaller amounts of HCV RNA, it is more generally useful for construction of complex cDNA libraries from a wide variety of HCV-containing samples.

HCV studies may involve cloning of short (100–1000 nt) regions or the entire genome. Amplification of and cloning of a short region are usually easier, require less viral RNA, and in some cases may be done on as little as a single HCV RNA molecule, isolated from serum, cell culture, or liver tissue. Amplification of longer regions is often more problematic, and requires optimization and higher levels of input RNA. We routinely amplify short regions of HCV genomic RNA from patient sera or liver tissue with titers of 10^3–10^8 RNA equivalents (per mL of serum or mg total liver RNA), and have also cloned nearly the entire genome of the genotype 1a HCV-H strain by amplifying overlapping regions 1200–3800 nt in length. Cloning the extreme 5' and 3' ends of the HCV genome requires special techniques (*see* **refs.** *3–5* for examples).

Highlighted below are the specific methods used for isolation of RNA, cDNA synthesis, polymerase chain reaction (PCR) amplification, and PCR assembly of a full-length library for the genotype 1a HCV-H strain.

1.1. Isolation of HCV RNA

Two methods of RNA purification are widely used: SDS solubilization and proteinase K digestion followed by phenol-chloroform extraction, or lysis and extraction using a guanidine thiocyanate (GuSCN)/phenol mixture *(6,7)*. Both methods have proven successful, but the latter method is preferable because of its simplicity. Commercial GuSCN/phenol mixtures are manufactured by several biotechnological and chemical companies that provide reagents for molecular biology (e.g., RNAzol B [Tel Test, Friendswood, TX] and TRIzol [Gibco-BRL, Gaithersburg, MD]).

Proper handling of virus-containing serum is important for preserving the integrity of genomic RNA prior to extraction, especially since HCV virion RNA is usually present at very low quantities (10^7 virions contain ~50 pg RNA). Serum kept frozen in aliquots at $-80°C$ can maintain biological activity and is the storage method of choice for recovering intact RNA. Viral RNA appears to be reasonably stable in the virion, but can be rapidly degraded by serum RNases after breakdown of virus particles. To prevent exposure of the viral RNA to serum RNases, the GuSCN/phenol mixture, which efficiently inactivates RNases, is added directly to the frozen serum sample. Following extraction, RNA is collected by alcohol precipitation. Most sera contain sufficient polysaccharides or other alcohol-insoluble materials to allow efficient precipitation of the HCV RNA. However, for small amounts of RNA, it may be necessary to add carrier glycogen as a coprecipitant. We prefer to use glycogen as a carrier, rather than tRNA, since excessive carrier RNA tends to inhibit the amplification of longer products (perhaps owing to false priming by the carrier).

Since even trace quantities of RNases will destroy viral RNA, all reagents used in subsequent work should be RNase-free. The preparation of RNase-free reagents as well as general precautions for working with RNA are described in **refs.** *6,7*.

1.2. Reverse Transcription (RT)

Various enzymes have been used for the RT step, including the reverse transcriptase purified from avian myeloblastosis virus (AMV), from bacteria overexpressing murine leukemia virus reverse transcriptase, or various RNase H deletion variants of the latter enzyme, such as Superscript II (Gibco-BRL). Although one enzyme may be superior to others for specific applications, we have had the most success with AMV RT, and this enzyme is specified in the protocols below.

A key issue for the RT step is the selection of primers. We have found that many primers used successfully for PCR or sequencing are not useful for RT (especially for the subsequent generation of large PCR products). Experiments with different concentrations of random hexamer primers revealed that complete omission of the primer in the RT reaction resulted in the best yield of long PCR products (Kolykhalov, unpublished data). Two phenomena may explain this efficient "self-priming" of HCV genomic RNA during RT. We found that the stable hairpin structure at the 3' terminus of HCV genome RNA *(3)* efficiently self-primes cDNA synthesis (Kolykhalov, unpublished data). In addition, short oligonucleotides, which appear to be present in most HCV RNA preparations from human serum, may serve as primers in RT (Kolykhalov, unpublished data).

1.3. PCR

Perhaps the most important parameter in the establishment of an efficient PCR amplification protocol is the selection of primers. For example, primer pairs capable of amplifying fragments up to 9.3 kb in length from purified plasmid DNA may not work when small amounts of unpurified cDNA are used as template. Primer pairs are selected empirically by testing different combinations. The best model template for identifying useful primer pairs is an in vitro synthesized full-length RNA transcript of the same or a closely related HCV genotype (*see* **Note 1**). It is advisable to start with a level of transcript RNA that is 10-fold lower than the expected amount of input HCV genomic RNA. For the genotype 1a HCV-H isolate, optimized primer pairs and amplifed regions are shown in **Table 1** and **Fig. 1**, respectively. If synthetic test RNA is not available, then the HCV RNA sample to be cloned can be used for primer pair selection and optimization.

Another variable in the PCR reaction is the thermostable DNA polymerase. Many companies now sell different formulations of enzyme(s) designed to amplify long fragments. The major breakthrough allowing PCR amplification of long fragments was the use of thermostable enzymes containing a proof-reading activity or mixtures of highly processive enzymes with an enzyme possessing proof-reading activity *(8)*. Commercial claims demonstrating PCR amplification of long segments are typically based on experiments using purified DNA templates and high levels of starting material. Even so, only low levels of amplification are obtained (10^3- to 10^5-fold after 30–40 cycles). For HCV cDNA, where starting material is limited and greater overall amplification is required, it is necessary to perform pilot experiments comparing enzymes from different sources. In our experiments, we used a 4:1 mixture of the highly processive KlenTaq *(8)* and Pfu polymerase (which contains proof-reading activity).

Table 1
Oligonucleotides Used for Amplification of HCV-H cDNA

Name	Sequence, 5' to 3'	Position in HCV-H and orientation
SF49	GGCGACACTCCACCATAGATC	(+) 18–38
SF128	TGGCACTACCCTCCAAGACC	(+) 1800–1819
SF162	ATGACACAAGGGGGCGCTCCGCACACT	(−) 2027–2053
SF131	TCCTGCTTGTGGATGATG	(+) 2538–2555
SF152	TAGTTTGGTGATGTCA	(−) 2999–3014
PCL10067	ACATAGGTGCCAGTAAG	(−) 3171–3187
PCL10066	CTGGCAACGTGCATCA	(+) 3549–3564
CMR115	GGGTGAGAACAATTACCA	(+) 4183–4200
CMR117	ATTGATGCCCAATGCG	(−) 4565–4580
SF140	ACTGCCTGGGATTCCCT	(+) 6347–6363
SF137	CATTCAGAGTAGGACTCC	(+) 6778–6795
SF156	CATGGACGTCAACACG	(−) 6848–6863
CMR120	AGGTAGGGTTGATTCGGT	(−) 7347–7364
PCL23660	GGCATGGCAACGGACGTCTTTTGC	(−) 7914–7937
SF1045	AATCTTCACCGGTTGGGGAGGAGGTAGATG	(−) 9353–9391

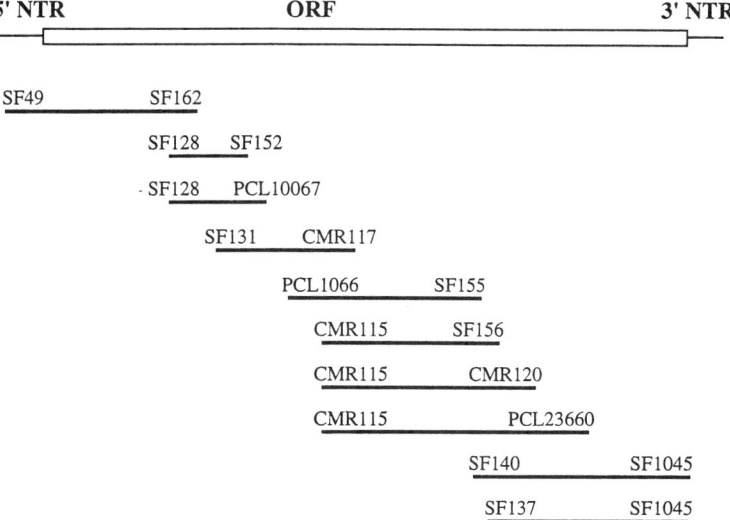

Fig. 1. Amplified regions of the HCV genome and primers used for the amplification of cDNA. A diagram of the HCV genomic RNA is shown at the top. Single lines correspond to nontranslated regions (5' NTR and 3' NTR); the open reading frame is shown by an open box. Primers used for amplification of each subregion (thick lines) are indicated above.

In the construction of cDNA libraries, it is always important to maintain desired levels of complexity at all steps. Theoretical limits of library complexity will initially be set by the number of independent cDNA molecules amplified by PCR. This can be measured directly by quantitative methods, such as competitive PCR, or a rough measure can be made by determining the dilution of cDNA that can still be amplified under optimized conditions. For our HCV-H library, at least a 10-fold dilution of each cDNA used for library construction could still be amplified, indicating representation of at least 10 independent cDNA molecules. To obtain representative libraries of highly variable regions of the HCV genome (such as E2 HVR1), even greater complexity (amplification of more independent cDNAs) is required (*see* **Note 2**). Alternatively, to maintain complexity, multiple independent PCR reactions could be performed, and the products pooled or analyzed separately, but this approach is much more labor-intensive.

1.4. Assembling by PCR

PCR fragments can be cloned directly, each fragment analyzed separately, and then assembled into longer cDNA clones by the use of convenient restriction enzymes. However, for assembling of complex libraries of full-length HCV cDNA clones, it is preferable to leave cloning until the last step. By using PCR assembly, complex mixtures of long cDNA segments can be easily handled prior to isolation and analysis of individual clones. These combinatorial libraries have the advantage that new combinations, not present in the original virus population, can be assembled and screened. However, this combinatoral approach can also be seen as a disadvantage if coselected mutations in a single genome are required for assembly of a functional clone. One can argue, however, that a library of sufficient complexity should contain the appropriate combinations.

Figure 2 shows an outline of the assembly PCR method. Two overlapping gel-purified PCR fragments are mixed in equimolar amounts together with primers. Following denaturation, the plus strand of one fragment anneals to the minus strand of the other within the overlapping region. After the first cycle of PCR, the resulting longer fragment is then a template for amplification by the primers. To prevent the accumulation of errors, the fragment concentration should be kept high, minimizing the number of cycles. The difficulties that can be encountered in the original PCR amplification of small amounts of HCV cDNA are not applicable in this assembly procedure, since it is possible to start the assembly reaction with large quantities of purified DNA. In our experience, most combinations of fragments result in efficient amplification of the desired longer products. False priming does occur, but shorter products do not usually dominate, and the desired product can be easily separated by gel puri-

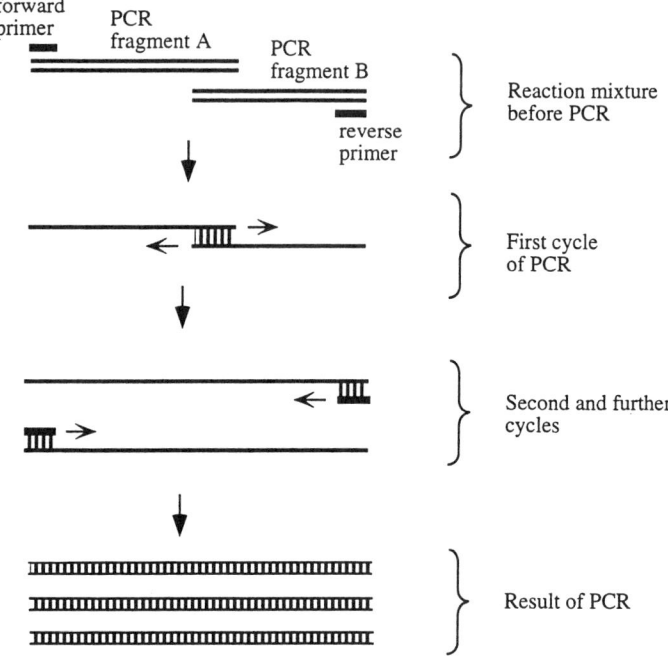

Fig. 2. Scheme of assembly by PCR.

fication and used in the next step of assembly or, finally, for cloning. For assembly of 9.4 kb of HCV-H cDNA, which encompasses nearly the whole genome, we used PCR fragments with overlapping regions as short as 80 nt or as long as 2780 nt.

1.5. Cloning of cDNA

Any general method for cloning PCR fragments can be used for cloning HCV *(6,7)*. In the case of our HCV-H full-length library, an internal restriction fragment encompassing 8.6 kb was cloned into a recipient vector containing the 5'- and 3'-terminal HCV sequences flanked by the T7 RNA polymerase promoter and a restriction site that could be used for production of synthetic HCV genome RNA. Problems with toxicity and stability of cDNA cloned in bacteria have been encountered in earlier efforts to obtain full-length functional clones for other members of the *Flaviviridae*. Although difficult to predict or control, such problems can sometimes be identified and avoided by transforming the same ligation mixture into different bacterial strains and utilizing the host that gives the highest proportion of clones with the correct structure, as determined by restriction digestion.

2. Materials

1. RNazol B, Tel Test.
2. TRIzol, total RNA isolation reagent (Gibco-BRL).
3. Chloroform, analytical grade (Mallinckrodt, Paris, KY).
4. Glycogen, molecular-biology-grade (Boehringer Mannheim, Indianapolis, IN).
5. Isopropanol, analytical-grade (Mallinckrodt).
6. Ethanol, 200 proof (Quantum, Tuscola, IL).
7. RNasin, 40 U/µL (Promega, Madison, WI). Store at –20°C.
8. AMV reverse transcriptase, 5 U/µL (Promega).
9. dNTP mix, 25 mM each of dATP, dGTP, dCTP, and dTTP (Gibco-BRL). Store aliquoted at –20°C.
10. PCR buffer, 10X: 200 mM Tris-HCl (pH 9.1 at 25°C), 1.5 mg/mL bovine serum albumin, 160 mM $(NH_4)_2SO_4$, 35 mM $MgCl_2$. Keep aliquoted at –20°C.
11. KlenTaqLA *(8)*, obtained from W. Barnes, Washington University, St. Louis, MO. May be kept aliquoted at –80°C for at least 2 yr.
12. Pfu DNA polymerase, 2.5 U/µL (Stratagene, La Jolla, CA).
13. Gel-loading buffer, 10X: 10 M urea (ICN, Aurora, OH) in water, 0.01% bromophenol blue (Sigma, St. Louis, MO). Store at room temperature.
14. DNA size marker(s): 100-bp ladder (Gibco-BRL) and λ-*Hin*dIII (NEB, Beverly, MA) or a mixture of λ-*Hin*dIII with ØX174-*Hae*III. Dilute with 1X gel-loading buffer to 10 ng/µL, and keep at 4°C for up to a month, or at –20°C for longer periods of time.
15. Agarose, ultrapure (Gibco-BRL).
16. Ethidium bromide (Sigma). Prepare a 10 mg/mL stock in water, and keep it in the dark at room temperature.
17. LMT agarose: low-melting-point agarose, ultrapure (Gibco-BRL).
18. DNA extraction buffer: 100 mM Tris-HCl, pH 8.0, 500 mM NaCl, 100 mM $MgCl_2$. Keep at 4°C for up to a month or at –20°C for a longer time.
19. Phenol, buffer-saturated (pH 8.0) (Amresco, Solon, OH). Keep at 4°C.
20. DNA mass ladder (Gibco-BRL). Dilute with 1X gel-loading buffer in proper concentrations (usually 1–10 ng/µL/2000 nucleotide band). Store at –20°C.

3. Methods

3.1. RNA Purification

Warning! HCV-containing material is potentially infectious and should be handled with proper precautions. A biological safety cabinet must be used, and a lab coat and gloves worn all times. All contaminated materials and equipment must be treated with bleach or autoclaved to inactivate any virus. All waste must be collected separately and autoclaved before disposal.

1. To 50 µL of frozen serum in a 0.6–2.0 mL microcentrifuge tube, add 500 µL RNazol B or TRIzol, and vortex for 30–60 s until the mixture becomes homogenous. Incubate at room temperature for 2 min.

2. Add 50 µL of chloroform, mix by vortexing for 10 s, and keep on ice for 5 min.
3. Centrifuge for 5 min at 16,000g. Two phases will form: a colorless aqueous phase, containing the RNA, and a heavier organic phase with a blue (RNazol B) or red (TRIzol) color. The volume of the aqueous phase is expected to be 50 µL (serum volume) plus 250 µL (half the volume of the added RNazol B or TRIzol) for a total of 300 µL.
4. Carefully transfer the upper phase into a new tube. Add 10 µg of glycogen, if necessary, and 300 µL of isopropanol. Mix by vortexing.
5. Incubate for 2–24 h at 4°C.
6. Pellet by centrifugation for 3 min at 16,000g.
7. Carefully remove the supernatant using a pipetman without disturbing the pellet (*see* **Note 3**).
8. Add 200 µL of 100% ethanol, and wash the pellet by gently flicking the tube (*see* **Note 4**).
9. Centrifuge for 1 min to bring the pellet to the bottom. Remove the supernatant with a pipetman.
10. Air-dry the pellet.
11. Resuspend the RNA pellet in 10 µL RNase-free water, and store frozen at –80°C or use immediately for cDNA synthesis (*see* **Note 5**).

3.2. cDNA Synthesis

1. To 10 µL RNA add 9.3 µL of the following mixture:
   2 µL RT buffer, 10X, supplied with the enzyme.
   2 µL DTT, 10X, supplied with the enzyme.
   0.2 µL RNasin, 40 U/µL.
   0.4 µL dNTP mix.
   4.7 µL water.
2. Heat 2 min at 75°C (*see* **Note 6**).
3. Cool the reaction by putting the tube on ice. Add another 0.2 µL of RNasin and 0.5 µL AMV reverse transcriptase (5 U/µL). Mix and incubate as follows:
   20 min at 37°C.
   20 min at 42°C.
   20 min at 48°C.
4. Inactivate the RT by heating the reaction for 3–5 min at 96°C. Spin the tube briefly to collect condensed liquid, mix, and store the resulting cDNA at –20°C (stable for at least 6 mo).

3.3. Polymerase Chain Reaction and Purification of Amplified DNA

3.3.1. Polymerase Chain Reaction

1. Aliquot 0.2 and 2 µL of cDNA into two thin-walled PCR tubes. Add 1.8 µL water into the tube with the 0.2-µL sample. Store on ice.

2. On ice prepare the following mixture:
   80.2 μL water.
   10 μL PCR buffer, 10X.
   0.8 μL dNTP mix.
   2 μL forward primer, 25 pmol/μL.
   2 μL reverse primer, 25 pmol/μL.
   0.8 μL KlenTaqLA.
   0.2 μL Pfu.
   Mix by vortexing and spin briefly. Aliquot 48 μL into each of the tubes containing cDNA. Store on ice (*see* **Note 7**).
3. Start the PCR machine with the following program:
   a. Incubation at 95°C for 2 min followed by 35 cycles:
      1 min at 95°C.
      1 min at 55°C.
      5 min at 72°C.
   b. Complete the PCR with a 10-min incubation at 72°C to complete all unfinished ends.
4. When the temperature of the heating block reaches 85°C, insert the tubes containing the reaction mixtures and tighten the heated lid (*see* **Note 8**). The PCR is now in progress.

3.3.2. Analysis of PCR Products by Agarose Gel-Electrophoresis

1. Aliquot 5 μL of the PCR reaction into a microcentrifuge tube, add 3 μL of 10X gel-loading buffer, mix and load on a 1% agarose gel *(6,7)*. In a neighboring well(s), load 10 μL of DNA size marker(s).
2. Electrophorese at 5–10 V/cm until the bromophenol blue tracer dye reaches the bottom of the gel.
3. Stain the gel in 1 μg/μL ethidium bromide solution for 10 min. **Warning!** Ethidium bromide is a mutagen. Use gloves and dispose of ethidium bromide waste properly *(6,7)*.
4. Visualize the DNA band(s) using a long-wave UV light source, taking pictures if desired *(6,7)*. **Warning!** Exposure to UV light is dangerous for the skin and, especially, for the eyes. Use the precautions specified for the UV box or UV lamp.

3.3.3. Purification of the PCR Products

1. To 15 μL of the PCR reaction add 10 μL of 10X gel-loading buffer, mix, and load on a 0.8% low-melting-point (LMP) agarose gel.
2. Electrophorese until the bromophenol blue dye reaches the bottom of the gel, or farther, if necessary.
3. Stain the gel and visualize the DNA bands as described in **Subheading 3.3.2.**, **steps 3** and **4**.
4. With a new single-edged razor blade, excise the DNA band with minimal extra agarose, and transfer it into a 1.5-mL microcentrifuge tube. Add enough water to bring the volume up to 180 and 20 μL of DNA extraction buffer (*see* **Note 9**).

5. Incubate the tube for 5 min at 70°C, mix the contents by vortexing, and incubate an additional 5 min.
6. The DNA can now be purified using a commercial DNA purification kit. Alternatively, follow **steps 7–11**.
7. To the hot melted agarose–DNA mixture add 200 μL phenol (not phenol-chloroform!), and mix by vortexing for 1 min. The agarose becomes insoluble.
8. Centrifuge for 5 min at 16,000g. Agarose forms a white fluffy interface, but DNA stays in the upper aqueous phase. Carefully transfer the aqueous phase into a new tube. Add an equal volume of phenol, vortex, centrifuge, and transfer the aqueous phase into a new tube. If desired, the aqueous phase can be extracted once with an equal volume of chloroform to remove residual phenol.
9. To the aqueous phase, add 0.25 μL (5 μg) of glycogen as carrier, sodium acetate to a final concentration of 0.2 M, and 3 vol 100% ethanol. Mix and cool to –20°C for 20 min.
10. Centrifuge at 16,000g for 3 min. A small pellet will be visible at the bottom of the microfuge tube. Remove the supernatant carefully by aspiration, wash the pellet with 100% ethanol, remove the ethanol, and air-dry the pellet for 5–10 min.
11. Resuspend the pellet in 10 μL water. To check recovery and concentration, add 1 μL of purified DNA to 8 μL water and 1 μL 10X gel-loading buffer. Load on a 1% agarose gel. To allow estimation of the amount of DNA recovered, load different dilutions of a DNA mass ladder in neighboring lanes.
12. Run the electrophoresis, and visualize the DNA as described in **Subheading 3.3.2.**, **steps 2–4**.

3.4. Assembling of PCR Fragments

1. In a thin-walled PCR tube mix the following components on ice:
    10 ng of the longer of two overlapping fragments that need to be assembled.
    x ng of the shorter fragment, where x = 10 (size of shorter fragment/size of longer fragment).
    5 μL PCR buffer, 10X.
    0.4 μL dNTP mix.
    1 μL Forward PCR primer, 25 pmol/μL.
    1 μL Reverse PCR primer, 25 pmol/μL. Water to 50 μL.
    0.4 μL KlenTaq.
    0.1 μL Pfu.
2. Perform the PCR as described in **Subheading 3.3.1.**, **steps 3** and **4**. Analyze the PCR products as described in **Subheading 3.3.2.**
3. Repeat the steps in **Subheadings 3.3.3.** and **steps 1** and **2** in this subheading until the desired region is assembled.

3.5. Cloning

Cloning of HCV cDNA could be performed by digestion with convenient restriction nucleases and cloning in an appropriate vector(s) as described in **refs.** *6,7*, by polishing the fragments' ends and blunt-end cloning *(6,7)*, or by addition of desired linker-adapters. Note that A-T cohesive end cloning using commercial kits designed specifically for cloning PCR products may not work efficiently for PCR products made in the presence of polymerases with proofreading activity.

4. Notes

1. If an appropriate plasmid exists for making synthetic HCV test RNAs for RT and PCR primer selection and long PCR optimization, it will be necessary to remove plasmid template DNA. The following method has worked well in our hands. After in vitro transcription in the presence of ^{3}H-UTP (see **refs. 6,7,9** for methods), digest the DNA for 30 min with 1 U of RQ DNase (RNase-free, Promega) per microgram of DNA using the conditions recommended by the manufacturer, extract with an equal volume of phenol-chloroform, add sodium acetate to 0.3 M, and precipitate the RNA by adding 0.6 vol of isopropanol. After 10 min at room temperature, centrifuge for 5 min at 16,000g, remove the supernatant, and resuspend the RNA pellet in water. Add 10 M urea/0.01% bromophenol blue to a final urea concentration of 4 M, and load on a 1% nondenaturing LMP agarose gel. Electrophorese until the dye reaches the bottom of the gel. Stain the gel for 1 min with ethidium bromide (1 µg/mL in water), and visualize the RNA band with long-wavelength UV light. Excise the RNA band from the gel, transfer the gel slice into a microcentrifuge tube, and heat the tube in a 70°C water bath for 5 min. Add an equal volume of phenol (not phenol-chloroform!) to the melted agarose, vortex 1 min, and centrifuge at 16,000g for 5 min. Transfer the aqueous phase into a new tube, and precipitate the RNA as described above. Wash with 100% ethanol. Air-dry the pellet. Resuspend the RNA in a small volume of water, digest a second time with DNase (1/10 the amount of DNase used in the first digestion), extract with phenol-chloroform, and precipitate as above. Wash the pellet with 100% ethanol and air-dry. Resuspend the purified RNA in an appropriate volume. Check the integrity of the RNA by denaturing agarose-gel electrophoresis and subsequent autoradiography *(6,7)*, and calculate the amount of RNA by measuring the level of incorporated radioactivity. Check for the absence of DNA by amplifying different amounts of RNA without the RT step. Usually, amplification of a sample containing 10^7–10^8 mol of RNA results in no PCR products after such purification. If necessary, purify the RNA again by agarose-gel electrophoresis. When the RNA is prepared, store aliquots at –80°C.
2. For some regions, like the hypervariable region of the E2 protein, it is necessary to generate even more complex libraries to be representative. In this case, even greater dilutions of cDNA (e.g., 1/100) should be tested for successful amplification to ensure preservation of a desired level of complexity for subsequent analyses (*see* **Subheading 1.3.**).
3. The RNA pellet is visible on the bottom side of the tube, but it is small and quite unstable after precipitation with isopropanol. Vacuum aspiration of the supernatant is not recomended.

4. Residual GuSCN as well as phenol can inhibit the reverse transcription reaction. Therefore, it is necessary to wash the RNA pellet with 70–100% ethanol. We prefer 100% ethanol vs 70%, because both GuSCN and phenol are fairly soluble in 100% ethanol, but the pellet is more visible and stable after washing with 100% ethanol.
5. Resuspension of the pellet in water may sometimes be difficult, especially when the resuspension volume is small. Make sure that the RNA is completely solubilized by gentle pipeting up and down until nothing remains on the bottom of tube and the viscosity of all liquid is the same.
6. RNA is unstable in the presence of Mg^{2+} ions at high temperatures, so where possible, avoid high temperatures and long denaturing steps.
7. If a PCR machine without a heated lid is used, overlay reaction mixtures with 30 µL of mineral oil (light, Sigma) or paraffin (Baxter, or Perkin Elmer).
8. Within 3–5 s, the block temperature will reach more than 100°C, and then drop to 95°C. Tubes should be transferred to the block when it reaches 85°C, so that the temperature inside the tube will rise quickly, decreasing exposure of the reaction mixture to low temperatures, and consequently, low-temperature false priming. Alternatively, "hot-start" reagents can be used.
9. In low salt, double-stranded DNA melts during prolonged incubation at temperatures higher than 70°C. Decreasing the melting temperature to 65°C or below often results in less efficient recovery of DNA. Therefore, Mg^{2+} is added to stabilize double-stranded DNA during recovery from LMT.

References

1. Kato, N., Hijikata, M., Ootsuyama, Y., Nakagawa, M., Ohkoshi, S., Sugimura, T., et al. (1990) Molecular cloning of the human hepatitis C virus genome from Japanese patients with non-A, non-B hepatitis. *Proc. Natl. Acad. Sci. USA* **87**, 9524–9528.
2. Takamizawa, A., Mori, C., Fuke, I., Manabe, S., Murakami, S., Fujita, J., et al. (1991) Structure and organization of the hepatitis C virus genome isolated from human carriers. *J. Virol.* **65**, 1105–1113.
3. Kolykhalov, A. A., Feinstone, S. M., and Rice, C. M. (1996) Identification of a highly conserved sequence element at the 3' terminus of hepatitis C virus genome RNA. *J. Virol.* **70**, 3363–3371.
4. Tanaka, T., Kato, N., Cho, M.-J., Sugiyama, K., and Shimotohno, K. (1996) Structure of the 3' terminus of the hepatitis C virus genome. *J. Virol.* **70**, 3307–3312.
5. Yamada, N., Tanihara, K., Takada, A., Yorihuzi, T., Tsutsumi, M., Shimomura, H., et al. (1996) Genetic organization and diversity of the 3' noncoding region of the hepatitis C virus genome. *Virology* **223**, 255–261.
6. Ausubel, F. M., Brent, R., Kingston, R. E., Moore, D. D., Seidman, J. G., Smith, J. A., et al. (eds.) (1993) *Current Protocols in Molecular Biology.* Greene Publishing Associates, New York.

7. Sambrook, J., Fritsch, E., and Maniatis, T. (1989) *Molecular Cloning: A Laboratory Manual.* Cold Spring Harbor Laboratory, Cold Spring Harbor, NY.
8. Barnes, W. M. (1994) PCR amplification of up to 35-kb DNA with high fidelity and high yield from l bacteriophage templates. *Proc. Natl. Acad. Sci. USA* **91,** 2216–2220.
9. Rice, C. M., Grakoui, A., Galler, R., and Chambers, T. J. (1989) Transcription of infectious yellow fever virus RNA from full-length cDNA templates produced by in vitro ligation. *New Biol.* **1,** 285–296.

27

Use of the Vaccinia Virus/T7 Expression System for Studying HCV Protein Processing

Eugene V. Agapov, Karen E. Reed, and Charles M. Rice

1. Introduction

HCV and related viruses are now classified as a separate genus in the family *Flaviviridae (1)*, which includes two other genera, Flavivirus *(2)*, and Pestivirus *(3)*. The positive-strand HCV genome RNA is approx 9.4 kb in length and contains a highly conserved 5' noncoding region followed by a long open reading frame encoding a polyprotein of 3010–3033 amino acids *(4,5)*. Recently, it was determined that the 3' end contains another highly conserved noncoding region approx 100 bp in length *(6–8)*. Because a cell-culture system supporting efficient HCV replication is lacking, efforts to define potential HCV-encoded polypeptides have utilized expression of HCV cDNA in cell-free translation systems and in cell cultures. The HCV polyprotein appears to be cleaved at multiple sites to produce at least 10 structural and nonstructural (NS) proteins *(9)*. The order and nomenclature of these cleavage products for the HCV-H strain are NH_2-C-E1-E2-p7-NS2-NS3-NS4A-NS4B-NS5A-NS5B-COOH, where C, E1, and E2 are putative structural proteins and the remaining NS proteins are believed to be replicase components *(9–12)*. Host signal peptidase in the endoplasmatic reticulum lumen appears to catalyze cleavages in the structural-NS2 region (C/E1, E1/E2, E2/p7, and p7/NS2 sites) *(9,13)*, whereas an HCV-encoded serine proteinase located in the N-terminal one-third of the NS3 protein is responsible for four cleavages in the NS region (3/4A, 4A/4B, 4B/5A, and 5A/5B sites) *(11,14–16)*. Autocatalytic cleavage at the 2/3 site is mediated by a second HCV-encoded proteinase that encompasses the NS2 region and the NS3 serine proteinase domain *(12,16)*.

Heterologous expression systems have been widely used to study HCV proteins and protein processing in lieu of an efficient method for establishing HCV

From: *Methods in Molecular Medicine, Vol. 19: Hepatitis C Protocols*
Edited by: J. Y. N. Lau © Humana Press Inc., Totowa, NJ

infections in cell culture. One of the most commonly used systems is the vaccinia virus/T7 hybrid transient expression system *(17)*. In this system, foreign genes are inserted into a plasmid vector under the control of a strong bacteriophage T7 RNA polymerase promoter and are followed by a signal for transcriptional termination. The foreign gene often is also positioned just downstream of the internal ribosome entry site (IRES) of encephalomyocarditis virus (EMC), which forms a complex secondary structure in the 5'-untranslated region of the RNA transcript that acts as a landing pad for ribosomes and thereby enhances translation *(18,19)*. Plasmid DNA containing the foreign gene and the regulatory elements described above is transfected into cells that have been infected with a vaccinia virus recombinant (vTF7-3) that encodes the bacteriophage T7 RNA polymerase continuously expressed from the early/late vaccinia virus P7.5 promoter. Once the plasmid enters the cell, T7 RNA polymerase expressed by vTF7-3 specifically recognizes the T7 promoter of the plasmid and transcribes large quantities of RNA containing the foreign gene. The IRES sequence ensures that the resulting transcripts are efficiently translated by cellular ribosomes. Alternatively, the same plasmids used for transient expression can be used to generate recombinant vaccinia viruses that carry genes of interest downstream of the T7 promoter. When cells are coinfected with one of these recombinants and vTF7-3, the gene of interest is transcribed by T7 RNA polymerase and translated as described above. The plasmids pTM1 and pTM3 each contain segments of the vaccinia virus thymidine kinase (TK) gene, which flank the expression cassette; thus, the TK$^-$ phenotype can be used as the basis for selection of recombinant viruses. Although the level of gene expression from such recombinants may be higher than that obtained from the corresponding plasmids because of viral DNA replication, more time is required for selection, plaque purification, and production of large-scale virus stocks. Using cationic liposomes, the transfection efficiency of plasmid DNA can be very high, and most cells express the desired gene at levels sufficient for detection and analysis of the expression products. Although the generation of recombinant vaccinia viruses is usually not necessary, they may be useful for some purposes, and have been used by some researchers to study the processing of HCV proteins *(10)*.

The highly active and specific nature of T7 RNA polymerase coupled with the translational efficiency provided by the EMC IRES usually results in abundant expression of the foreign gene product. Another advantage of this system is the cytoplasmic location of vaccinia virus replication and transcription, which may be especially important for the expression of proteins from viruses thought to replicate in the cytoplasm, such as HCV. The nuclear location of RNA synthesis in other transient expression systems could pose problems for HCV-derived RNA processing or transport, e.g., the potential recognition of RNA sequences and cleavage by the nuclear splicing machinery.

In order to express HCV polyproteins using the vaccinia virus/T7 system, the region of interest is inserted into a suitable expression vector, such as pTM1, pTM3 *(19)*, or pCITE (Novagen, Madison, WI). The chosen region is usually inserted so that the unique *Nco*I site provides the initiating methionine codon for translation. A multiple cloning site downstream of the *Nco*I site provides a number of restriction sites for cloning the 3'-end of the insert. Once the region of interest has been inserted into the expression vector, a high-quality DNA stock of the resulting expression construct is usually prepared. Although DNA purified on some commercially available columns may give adequate expression, we usually purify DNA by banding on CsCl gradients. The DNA purity may be increased by repeated bandings, although this is usually not necessary for high-copy-number plasmids like pTM1, pTM3, and pCITE.

Virus stocks of vTF7-3 should also be prepared in advance of actual expression. For this purpose, BSC40 or other suitable cells are infected with a starting inoculum of vTF7-3 at a low multiplicity of infection (MOI), incubated until complete cytopathic effect is observed, and harvested by scraping the cells into a small volume of medium, centrifuging them, and lysing the cell pellet by Dounce homogenization, since vaccinia virus remains cell-associated rather than being released into the medium like certain other viruses. The virus is then partially purified by low-speed ultracentrifugation through a sucrose cushion. The viral titer is determined by infecting separate wells of cells with serial dilutions of the stock, incubating them to allow plaque formation, and staining the cells to facilitate plaque counting.

Once a DNA stock of the expression construct and a virus stock of vTF7-3 have been prepared, the system is ready for use. BHK-21 or other suitable cells are infected with vTF7-3 at a high MOI to ensure nearly 100% infection. The cells are then transfected with the expression construct DNA using a mixture of cationic and neutral liposomes. The mechanism of uptake is not well understood, but negatively charged phosphate groups on DNA are thought to bind to positively charged liposomes, which may bind to negatively charged sialic acid residues on the cell surface and fuse with the plasma membrane. Following the transfection period, the cells are washed to remove the DNA/liposome mixture, which is toxic to the cells after prolonged exposure, and the proteins are labeled with a semicrude preparation of ^{35}S-labeled methionine. At the end of the expression period, the cells are washed to remove excess label and lysed in buffer containing sodium dodecyl sulfate (SDS). The lysates are passaged several times though a small-bore needle to shear cellular genomic DNA and heated to denature the proteins. Portions of lysate are diluted in a buffered salt solution containing nonionic detergent, which forms mixed micelles with the diluted SDS and prevents antibody denaturation, and then mixed with antiserum that recognizes one or more of the HCV polyprotein cleavage products.

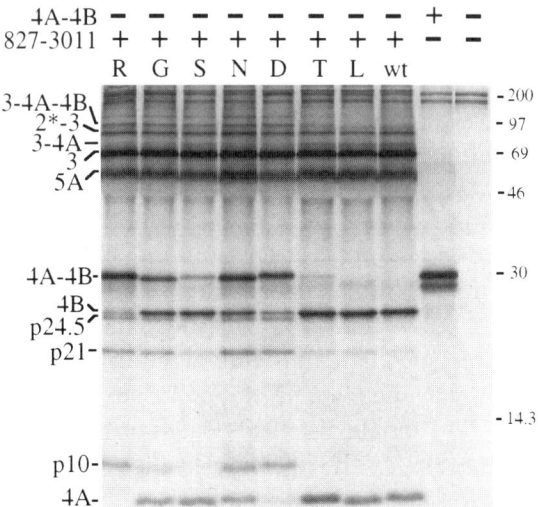

Fig. 1. Processing of 827-3011 polyproteins containing substitutions at the P1 position of the 4A/4B site. vTF7-3-infected BHK-21 cell monolayers were transfected with plasmids expressing the indicated parental (wt) or mutant (in the single-letter code) 827-3011 polyproteins, or pGEM 3Zf(+) as a negative control, and labeled for 4 h with ^{35}S-protein-labeling mixture as described in **Subheading 3.** Cell lysates were prepared, immunoprecipitated with patient JHF serum, and products separated by SDS-12% PAGE. Figure taken from **ref. 24**. Truncated NS2* and NS5B were not seen, since the patient serum used for this immunoprecipitation does not recognize these proteins.

Immune complexes are precipitated by the addition of the *Staphylococcus aureus* Cowan I strain, which on its surface bears protein A, which binds with high affinity to the F_c region of IgG antibody molecules. The immunoprecipitates are washed a few times in buffer containing detergent to remove nonspecifically adsorbed protein, and once in buffer without detergent to prevent interference by the nonionic detergent in the next step, which is solubilization in protein sample buffer. The samples are then analyzed by SDS-PAGE followed by autoradiography (for illustration of this approach, see **Fig. 1** *[10]*).

2. Materials
2.1. Preparation of DNA Stock
1. Luria-Bertani medium (LB): To 950 mL of distilled water (dH$_2$O), add 10 g tryptone, 5 g yeast extract, and 10 g NaCl. Stir until ingredients are dissolved; adjust the pH to 7.4 with NaOH, and adjust the final volume to 1 L with dH$_2$O. Sterilize by autoclaving for 20 min at 15 psi on liquid cycle.

2. Ampicillin, sodium salt (Sigma, St. Louis, MO, cat. # A-9518): 50 mg/mL in H_2O. Filter-sterilize and store in small aliquots at $-20°C$.
3. STE: 25 mM Tris-HCl, pH 7.5, 10 mM EDTA, 15% sucrose. Use sterile technique in preparation; store at room temperature.
4. Bacterial lysis solution: 0.2 N NaOH, 1% SDS. Make up fresh each time at room temperature.
5. 3 M Na$^+$/5 M OAc$^-$: Add 23 mL glacial acetic acid/200 mL final volume 3 M NaOAc. Store at room temperature.
6. Isopropanol. Store at room temperature.
7. TE: 10 mM Tris-HCl, pH 7.5; 1 mM EDTA. Store at room temperature.
8. CsCl. Store at room temperature.
9. Ethidium bromide, 10 mg/mL in H_2O. Store at 4°C in a dark bottle.
10. Isopropanol saturated with NaCl: Mix equal volumes of isopropanol and 5 M NaCl. Prepare in advance, and allow phases to separate completely before use. Store at room temperature.
11. Absolute ethanol.
12. 70% Ethanol.
13. Double-distilled or distilled-deionized H_2O (ddH_2O).

2.2. Preparation of vTF7-3 Stock

1. Solution A: 137 mM NaCl, 2.7 mM KCl, 4.3 mM Na_2HPO_4, 1.4 mM KH_2PO_4. Store at room temperature.
2. Fetal bovine serum (FBS). Heat at 56°C for 30 min; store at $-20°C$.
3. Minimal Essential Medium (MEM) (Gibco-BRL, Gaithersburg, MD cat. # 11095-072). Store at 4°C.
4. 100X Nonessential amino acids (NEAA) (Gibco-BRL, cat. # 11140-019).
5. 1000X Penicillin-streptomycin solution (Gibco-BRL, cat. # 15140-015).
6. 10 mM Tris-HCl, pH 9.0.
7. 36% (w/v) Sucrose in 10 mM Tris-HCl, pH 9.0.
8. 7% (v/v) Formaldehyde.
9. Crystal violet stain: 1% (w/v) crystal violet in 5% (v/v) ethanol.

2.3. Expression of the HCV Proteins

1. Solution A (*see* **Subheading 2.2.**).
2. FBS (*see* **Subheading 2.2.**).
3. MEM (*see* **Subheading 2.2.**).
4. Lipofectamine (Gibco-BRL, cat. # 18324-012). Store at 4°C. Alternatively, Transfectam (Promega, Madison, WI) or the transfection reagent DOTAP (Boehringer Mannheim, Indianapolis, IN) may be used.
5. MEM lacking methionine (Sigma, cat. # M-3911). Store at 4°C.
6. ^{35}S protein labeling mix (Du Pont/NEN Research Products, Boston, MA, cat. # NEG-072; ICN, Costa Mesa, CA, cat. # 51006, or Amersham, Arlington Heights, IL, cat. # SJQ 0079). Store in small aliquots at $-80°C$.

2.4. Cell Lysis, Immunoprecipitation, and Analysis of HCV Proteins

1. Solution A (*see* **Subheading 2.2.**)
2. Cell lysis solution: 50 mM Tris-HCl, pH 7.5, 1 mM EDTA, 0.5% SDS. Store at room temperature, but chill prior to use.
3. TNA: 50 mM Tris-HCl, pH 7.5, 150 mM NaCl; 1 mM EDTA, 0.5% (v/v) Triton X-100; 0.66 mg/mL bovine serum albumin. Store at 4°C.
4. Antiserum raised against HCV proteins. Store in small aliquots at –20°C.
5. TNAS: Prepare using the recipe for TNA, but include 0.1% (w/v) SDS. Store at 4°C.
6. PANSORBIN cells (Calbiochem, La Jolla, CA). Store at 4°C.
7. TNE: 50 mM Tris-HCl, pH 7.5, 150 mM NaCl, 1 mM EDTA. Store at 4°C or room temperature, but chill prior to use.
8. Protein sample buffer: 62.5 mM Tris-HCl, pH 6.8, 2% (w/v) SDS, 10% (v/v) glycerol, 5% (v/v) β-mercaptoethanol, 0.01% (w/v) bromphenol blue.

3. Methods
3.1. Preparation of DNA Stock

1. Using sterile technique, inoculate 200 mL LB containing 50 µg/mL ampicillin with a single colony of bacteria containing pTM1, pTM3, or pCITE with the HCV region of interest.
2. Grow the culture overnight at 37°C on an orbital shaker at 275–300 rpm.
3. Transfer the culture to a 250-mL centrifuge bottle, and centrifuge 10 min at 8000 rpm in a Sorvall GSA rotor at 4°C to pellet the bacteria.
4. Remove the medium, and resuspend the pellet in 10 mL STE.
5. Add 20 mL bacterial lysis solution; mix gently by inverting the bottle several times to avoid shearing the genomic DNA, and incubate at room temperature for 10 min.
6. Add 15 mL 3 M Na$^+$/5 M OAc$^-$, and mix gently by inversion; incubate for 10 min on ice.
7. Centrifuge for 10 min at 10,000 rpm in a Sorvall GSA rotor at 4°C.
8. Pour the supernatant into a clean 250-mL centrifuge bottle through cheesecloth or a cotton ball placed in a funnel to remove any flocculent material remaining in the supernatant.
9. Add 22.5 mL isopropanol; mix vigorously, and spin for 10 min at 10,000 rpm in a Sorvall GSA rotor.
10. Remove the supernatant, and dissolve the pellet in 4.5 mL TE; add 5 g CsCl, and mix until the CsCl is dissolved as well. Add 0.1 mL 10 mg/mL ethidium bromide; mix, and centrifuge at 1000–2000g for 5 min at room temperature to remove some cellular debris. Transfer the supernatant to a Quick-Seal polyallomer centrifuge tube (Beckman, Palo Alto, CA, cat. # 342412) (*see* **Note 2**).
11. Heat-seal the tube, and spin at 78,000 rpm for 4 h or at 60,000 rpm overnight in a Beckman NVT90 rotor at 20°C.

12. After removing the tubes from the rotor, insert an 18-gage needle into the top of the tube, making a single puncture. Leave this needle in the tube, and insert a 1-mL syringe attached to a 20-gage needle into the tube a few millimeters below the band with the beveled tip facing upward and positioned at the bottom edge of the band. A long-wave, handheld UV illuminator may facilitate this process. Slowly withdraw the DNA band by gently pulling back on the syringe plunger. Withdraw the syringe, hold it in an inverted position, remove the needle, and inject the contents into a 1.5-mL microcentrifuge tube.
13. Remove the ethidium bromide by extracting five times with isopropanol saturated with NaCl. For each extraction, add an equal volume of isopropanol saturated with NaCl, vortex, spin at top speed for 2 min in a microcentrifuge, and remove the top layer.
14. Transfer the DNA solution to a larger centrifuge tube with a 10–30-mL capacity; add 2 vol of dd H_2O, mix, add 6 vol of absolute ethanol, and vortex.
15. Centrifuge 10 min at 10,000 rpm in a Sorvall SS-34 or SA-600 rotor at 4°C.
16. Remove the supernatant, add 2 mL of 70% ethanol, and vortex.
17. Centrifuge at 10,000 rpm for 10 min in a Sorvall SS-34 or SA-600 rotor at 4°C.
18. Remove the supernatant, and allow the pellet to air-dry completely.
19. Dissolve the pellet in an appropriate volume of TE, e.g., 0.5 mL, and determine the DNA concentration by measuring the optical density at a wavelength of 260 nm (OD_{260}) (*see* **Note 2**).

3.2. Preparation of vTF7-3 (see Note 1)

1. Plate BSC40, CV-1, VERO, L, or HeLa cells in five 150-mm dishes, and grow them until confluent monolayers are established.
2. Wash each plate once with 10 mL of solution A.
3. Infect the cells at an MOI of 0.01 PFU/cell in 5 mL of solution A containing 1% FBS and 1 m*M* $MgCl_2$ (*see* **Note 1**). Incubate them for 1 h at room temperature in a cell-culture hood, rocking every 15 min to prevent drying of the cells.
4. Remove the inoculum, add 25 mL of MEM containing 10% FBS, 1X NEAA, and 1X penicillin/streptomycin to each plate, and place them in a 37°C cell incubator with 5% CO_2 until complete cytopathic effect is observed, usually at 48–72 h postinfection.
5. Aspirate all except 5 mL of medium from each plate, scrape the cells off of the bottom of each plate, and pool them in a sterile, 50-mL conical tube.
6. Centrifuge at 500*g* for 5 min at 4°C to pellet the cells.
7. Aspirate the supernatant carefully and discard it. Resuspend the pellet in 2.5 mL (0.5 mL/plate) of 10 m*M* Tris-HCl, pH 9.0.
8. Lyse the cells with 25 strokes of a tight-fitting Dounce homogenizer.
9. Centrifuge at 500*g* for 10 min at 4°C to pellet the nuclei.
10. Carefully remove the milky supernatant, and save it on ice. Resuspend the nuclear pellet in 2.5 mL 10 m*M* Tris-HCl, pH 9.0, and homogenize it as described above.
11. Centrifuge the second homogenate at 500*g* for 10 min at 4°C, and pool the resulting supernatant with the first supernatant.

12. Add 10 mM Tris-HCl, pH 9.0, to a final volume of 12 mL, and layer 6 mL of the homogenate onto 6-mL cushions of 36% sucrose in 10 mM Tris-HCl, pH 9.0, in each of two Beckman polyallomer ultracentrifuge tubes (cat. # 331372). The tubes have a 12-mL capacity, so they should be almost completely full after this step.
13. Centrifuge at 18,000 rpm for 80 min in an SW41 rotor at 4°C.
14. Remove the supernatant, and resuspend the pellet in 0.2 mL/plate of 10 mM Tris-HCl, pH 9.0 with a pipet, transfer the solution to a sterile tight-fitting Dounce homogenizer, and finish resuspending the pellet with 30 strokes.
15. The resulting partially purified stock is stored in small aliquots at –80°C.
16. To titer the vTF7-3 stock, prepare 10^{-4}, 10^{-5}, 10^{-6}, 10^{-7}, and 10^{-8} dilutions of the vTF7-3 stock in solution A containing 1% FBS and 1 mM MgCl$_2$, and infect individual wells of a six-well dish of BHK-21 cells (or another cell line to be used for expression) with 200 µL of solution A containing 1% FBS and 1 mM MgCl$_2$, or a mixture containing 10 µL of the above dilutions plus 190 µL of solution A containing 1% FBS and 1 mM MgCl$_2$. Incubate the cells at room temperature for 1 h in a cell-culture hood, rocking them every 15 min.
17. Remove the inoculum, add 2 mL of MEM containing 2% FBS, 1X NEAA, and 1X penicillin/streptomycin, and place them in a 37°C cell incubator for 24–48 h.
18. Pipet 2 mL of 7% formaldehyde into each well, and incubate at room temperature for 10 min.
19. Remove the medium plus formaldehyde, add 2 mL of crystal violet stain to each well, and incubate at room temperature for 10 min.
20. Remove the stain for reuse, and rinse the cells gently with water to remove the excess stain, drain them, and count the plaques to determine the titer of virus stock.

3.3. Expression of the HCV Proteins

1. Plate BHK-21 cells or another suitable cell line into the desired number of six-well dishes, and grow them to approx 50% confluency (*see* **Note 3**).
2. Wash the cells once with 2 mL/well of solution A.
3. Infect each well with 0.2 mL of solution A containing 1% FBS, 1 mM MgCl$_2$, and vTF7-3 at an MOI of 5–10 PFU/cell for 1 h at room temperature in a cell-culture hood with the blower turned off, rocking every 15 min.
4. During the infection period, mix 0.2 mL of MEM and 1 µg of DNA in a 1.5-mL microcentrifuge tube while mixing 0.3 mL of MEM and 8 µL of Lipofectamine in a separate tube (*see* **Note 4**). Next, combine the contents of the two tubes, and incubate the MEM/DNA/liposome mixture for 20–30 min at room temperature before transfection.
5. Wash the cells once with 2 mL/well of MEM.
6. Gently add the MEM/DNA/liposome mixture to the cells, and place them in a 37°C cell incubator for 2.5 h.
7. Wash the cells once with 2 mL/well of MEM lacking methionine.
8. Add 0.5 mL of MEM lacking methionine that contains 2% FBS, 40–100 µCi/mL of ^{35}S protein-labeling mix, and 1/40 vol of regular MEM to the cells, and place them in a 37°C cell incubator for 4 h (*see* **Note 5**).

3.4. Cell Lysis, Immunoprecipitation, and Analysis of HCV Proteins (see Notes 6 and 8)

1. Wash the cells twice with cold solution A to remove unincorporated label.
2. Lyse the cells in 0.3 mL of cell lysis buffer, and transfer the lysate to a 1.5-mL microcentrifuge tube.
3. Passage the lysate at least twice through a 27.5-gage needle to shear the DNA and reduce its viscosity. The lysates may be frozen at this point, or heated at 70°C for 10 min and used immediately for immunoprecipitation.
4. Mix 150 µL of lysate with 600 µL of TNA, and then add an appropriate amount of an antiserum that recognizes HCV proteins. The optimal amount should be determined empirically. We typically use a maximum of 5 µL of rabbit polyclonal antiserum or 1 µL of a monoclonal antibody (MAb) for 50 µL of starting lysate.
5. Incubate the lysate and antiserum at 4°C with rocking for a period ranging from 2 h to overnight, depending on the antiserum.
6. Wash PANSORBIN cells by pelleting them for 20 s at top speed in a microcentrifuge and resuspending them in the same volume of cold TNAS; repeat this cycle four more times for a total of five washes. After the last wash, resuspend the PANSORBIN cells in the original volume, add an appropriate amount of the prewashed PANSORBIN cells to the lysates that were incubated overnight with the antiserum, and incubate 2 h more at 4°C. As a general rule, the volume of the 10% (w/v) PANSORBIN used (*see* **Note 7**) should be 20 times the volume of antiserum suspension.
7. Wash the immunoprecipitates three times with cold TNAS as described above for the PANSORBIN cells, once with cold TNE, and resuspend them in 20–50 µL of protein sample buffer.
8. Heat the samples at 90°C for 5 min, pellet the PANSORBIN cells as described above, and transfer the supernatant to a new microcentrifuge tube. The samples may be frozen or analyzed immediately by SDS-PAGE followed by autoradiography.

4. Notes

1. Work carefully and follow biosafety level 2 (BL-2) practices when working with vaccinia virus. According to recommendations from the Centers for Disease Control (CDC) and National Institutes of Health (NIH), all personnel who come in contact with vaccinia virus should be vaccinated every 10 yr *(20,21)*. Also, several approaches have been taken to enhance the safety of work with poxvirus vectors. One of these is based on using the highly attenuated vaccinia virus Ankara strain (MVA) and another is based on using an avianpox (fowlpox) virus. Utilization of an attenuated virus, such as MVA, enables work to be performed under biosafety level 1 (BL-1) conditions without vaccination. Although both viruses are unable to multiply in human and most mammalian cells, viral proteins are synthesized normally. Virus stocks can be prepared in avian cells *(22,23)*.
2. Since both DNA and RNA absorb light with a wavelength of 260 nm, a portion of the DNA should be checked on an agarose gel for RNA contamination, which

can interfere with the calculation of DNA concentration from the OD_{260} and reduce transfection efficiency. DNA purified on some commercially available columns (e.g., Promega or Qiagen, Chatsworth, CA) gives the same result as CsCl-purified DNA.
3. Density of the monolayer is a critical parameter. Maximal efficiency of transfection can be achieved when cells are nonadjacent (around 50–80% confluency).
4. To maximize the efficiency of transfection for cells other than BHK-21, the optimal ratio of DNA and liposomes (lipofectamine) has to be determined experimentally.
5. If there is a need to express a full-length DNA copy of HCV with 5'- and 3'-flanking regions, the labeling time should be extended to 6 h.
6. The methods presented in this chapter utilize denaturing conditions for cell lysis and immunoprecipitation, because rabbit antisera are usually raised against denatured antigens. However, the substitution of nonionic detergents, such as Triton X-100 or Nonidet-P40, for SDS may facilitate antigen recognition by some antisera, such as those collected from human HCV patients.
7. Utilization of protein A coupled to Sepharose often helps to reduce nonspecific binding of cell proteins.
8. Starting with plasmid containing the gene of interest cloned in the pTM3 vector, the entire procedure from infection to harvesting and analysis of the expressed product requires 2 d and an overnight exposure of film.

References

1. Rice, C. M. (1996) Flaviviridae: the viruses and their replication, in *Fields Virology*, vol. 1 (Fields, B. N., Knipe, D. M., and Howley, P. M., eds.), Lippincott-Raven, Philadelphia, pp. 931–959.
2. Monath, T. P. and Heinz, F. X. (1996) Flaviviruses, in *Fields Virology*, vol. 1 (Fields, B. N., Knipe, D. M., and Howley, P. M., eds.), Lippincott-Raven, Philadelphia, pp. 961–1034.
3. Thiel, H. J., Plagemann, P. G. W., and Moennig, V. (1996) Pestiviruses, in *Fields Virology*, vol. 1 (Fields, B. N., Knipe, D. M., and Howley, P. M., eds.), Lippincott-Raven, Philadelphia, pp. 1059–1073.
4. Houghton, M., Weiner, A., Han, J., Kuo, G., and Choo, Q.-L. (1991) The hepatitis C virus encodes a serine protease involved in processing of the putative nonstructural proteins from the viral polyprotein precursor. *Hepatology* **14,** 381–388.
5. Matsuura, Y. and Miyamura, T. (1993) The molecular biology of hepatitis C virus. *Semin. Virol.* **4,** 297–304.
6. Kolykhalov, A. A., Feinstone, S. M., and Rice, C. M. (1996) Identification of a highly conserved sequence element at the 3' terminus of hepatitis C virus genome RNA. *J. Virol.* **70,** 3363–3371.
7. Tanaka, T., Kato, N., Cho, M.-J., and Shimotohno, K. (1995) A novel sequence found at the 3' terminus of hepatitis C virus genome. *Biochem. Biophys. Res. Commun.* **215,** 744–749.

8. Tanaka, T., Kato, N., Cho, M.-J., Sugiyama, K., and Shimotohno, K. (1996) Structure of the 3' terminus of the hepatitis C virus genome. *J. Virol.* **70**, 3307–3312.
9. Lin, C., Lindenbach, B. D., Prágai, B., McCourt, D. W., and Rice, C. M. (1994) Processing of the hepatitis C virus E2-NS2 region: identification of p7 and two distinct E2-specific products with different C termini. *J. Virol.* **68**, 5063–5073.
10. Grakoui, A., Wychowski, C., Lin, C., Feinstone, S. M., and Rice, C. M. (1993) Expression and identification of hepatitis C virus polyprotein cleavage products. *J. Virol.* **67**, 1385–1395.
11. Grakoui, A., McCourt, D. W., Wychowski, C., Feinstone, S. M., and Rice, C. M. (1993) Characterization of the hepatitis C virus-encoded serine proteinase: determination of proteinase-dependent polyprotein cleavage sites. *J. Virol.* **67**, 2832–2843.
12. Grakoui, A., McCourt, D. W., Wychowski, C., Feinstone, S. M., and Rice, C. M. (1993) A second hepatitis C virus-encoded proteinase. *Proc. Natl. Acad. Sci. USA* **90**, 10,583–10,587.
13. Hijikata, M., Kato, N., Ootsuyama, Y., Nakagawa, M., and Shimotohno, K. (1991) Gene mapping of the putative structural region of the hepatitis C virus genome by in vitro processing analysis. *Proc. Natl. Acad. Sci. USA* **88**, 5547–5551.
14. Bartenschlager, R., Ahlborn-Laake, L., Mous, J., and Jacobsen, H. (1993) Nonstructural protein 3 of the hepatitis C virus encodes a serine-type proteinase required for cleavage at the NS3/4 and NS4/5 junctions. *J. Virol.* **67**, 3835–3844.
15. Eckart, M. R., Selby, M., Masiarz, F., Lee, C., Berger, K., Crawford, K., et al. (1993) The hepatitis C virus encodes a serine protease involved in processing of the putative nonstructural proteins from the viral polyprotein precursor. *Biochem. Biophys. Res. Commun.* **192**, 399–406.
16. Hijikata, M., Mizushima, H., Akagi, T., Mori, S., Kakiuchi, N., Kato, N., et al. (1993) Two distinct proteinase activities required for the processing of a putative nonstructural precursor protein of hepatitis C virus. *J. Virol.* **67**, 4665–4675.
17. Fuerst, T. R., Niles, E. G., Studier, F. W., and Moss, B. (1986) Eukaryotic transient-expression system based on recombinant vaccinia virus that synthesizes bacteriophage T7 RNA polymerase. *Proc. Natl. Acad. Sci. USA* **83**, 8122–8126.
18. Elroy-Stein, O., Fuerst, T. R., and Moss, B. (1989) Cap-independent translation of mRNA conferred by encephalomyocarditis virus 5' sequence improves the performance of the vaccinia virus/bacteriophage T7 hybrid expression system. *Proc. Natl. Acad. Sci. USA* **86**, 6126–6130.
19. Moss, B., Elroy-Stein, O., Mizukami, T., Alexander, W. A., and Fuerst, T. R. (1990) New mammalian expression vectors. *Nature (Lond.)* **348**, 91,92.
20. Richmond, J. Y. and McKinney, R. W. (1993) Biosafety, in *Microbiological and Biomedical Laboratories*, US Department of Health and Human Services, Washington, DC, p. 177.
21. Moss, B. (1996) Genetically engineered pox viruses for recombinant gene expression, vaccination, and safety. *Proc. Natl. Acad. Sci. USA* **93**, 11,341–11,348.

22. Britton, P., Green, P., Kottier, S., Mawditt, K. L., Penzes, Z., Cavanagh, D., et al. (1996) Expression of bacteriophage T7 RNA polymerase in avian and mammalian cells by a recombinant fowlpox virus. *J. Gen. Virol.* **77,** 963–967.
23. Sutter, G. and Moss, B. (1992) Nonreplicating vaccinia vector efficiently expresses recombinant genes. *Proc. Natl. Acad. Sci. USA* **89,** 10,847–10,851.
24. Kolykhalov, A. A., Agapov, E. V., and Rice, C. M. (1994) Specificity of the hepatitis C virus serine proteinase: Effects of substitutions at the 3/4A, 4A/4B, 4B/5A, and 5A/5B cleavage sites on polyprotein processing. *J. Virol.* **68,** 7525–7533.

28

Use of a Discistronic Vector for the Quantitation of HCV IRES Activity

Joyce A. Feller and Johnson Y. N. Lau

1. Introduction

The 5'-untranslated region of hepatitis C virus (HCV) has been shown to function as an internal ribosomal entry site, or IRES. The biological function of the HCV IRES has been shown to be essential for initiation of translation of the viral proteins by host ribosomes. With this critical role in HCV replication, the IRES makes an attractive target for the development of antiviral compounds. Furthermore, since eukaryotic translation is not initiated via an IRES, agents that specifically interfere with function of the HCV IRES may be relatively nontoxic to the host. Fundamental to the testing of any of these antivirals is a system to evaluate their efficacy. This chapter describes the use of a dicistronic vector in an in vitro system to assess the translational initiation efficiency of isolated HCV IRES elements.

The most convenient way to assay the activity of a regulatory element, such as an IRES, is to place it in control of a reporter gene. A reporter gene is simply one that encodes a protein that can be easily detected. Many common reporter genes, such as β-galactosidase, luciferase and chloramphenicol acetyl transferase (CAT), produce enzymes whose activity can be measured by simple quantitative assays. Alternatively, these proteins can be analyzed by electrophoresis in SDS-polyacrylamide gels, which have the added benefit of showing the sizes of the proteins and their relative abundance in a sample. Using this second method, even protein that is not enzymatically active (i.e., owing to problems with processing, compartmentalization, and so forth) can be detected and measured.

Since assays may be done for both enzymatically active and total protein, this sort of reporter construct is quite flexible. In addition, it can be used both in in vitro transcription/translation systems and in transfected tissue-culture cells. However, in the cell-based system, it is only practical to measure enzymatically active protein, since polyacrylamide gels of those samples will also contain proteins derived from the many endogenous cellular messages, potentially making it very difficult to identify the reporter protein. This will force the investigator to perform immunoprecipitations or Western blots, both of which are time-consuming and impractical for use in processing a large number of samples. For at least the initial round of screening of antiviral compounds, Promega's cell-free coupled transcription/translation system is faster, simpler, and more easily controlled. Therefore, this chapter details only the protocol for use of reporter plasmids in a cell-free system.

The general structure of a reporter plasmid is shown in **Fig. 1**. It consists of a promoter to initiate transcription of the messenger RNA (*see* **Note 1**), followed by the IRES/reporter gene cassette. A plasmid that contains only the promoter and an IRES region immediately 5' to a reporter gene constitutes a monocistronic vector, since the plasmid contains a single open reading frame (cistron) (**Fig. 1A**). This sort of vector can give valuable information about IRES function, but may be difficult to use to generate accurate, reproducible results. For example, in one experiment, a monocistronic IRES vector may produce less reporter protein in the presence of an inhibitor than in its absence. This could mean that the inhibitor is specifically interfering with translational initiation from the IRES. However, unless a second, independent factor is used to normalize between samples from the two conditions, there is no way to exclude the possibility that this result is simply an artifact, reflecting some unaccounted for difference between the samples or an unrelated secondary effect of the antiviral agent (e.g., perhaps either an effect of the inhibitor on transcription or total inhibition of translation, regardless of whether it is initiated by an IRES or a 5' cap structure).

An alternative is to use a dicistronic reporter vector, as diagrammed in **Fig. 1B**. In this system, the plasmid contains the genes for two different reporter proteins, encoded within one transcriptional unit (*see* **Note 2**). This will generate a single messenger RNA containing two separate coding regions. In a eukaryotic milieu, translation of the 5'-open reading frame will be initiated by the standard cap-dependent method. This begins by recognition of the 5'-cap structure and assembly of the ribosome, followed by ribosomal scanning to the first AUG codon in context of a Kozak consensus sequence, a sequence that greatly enhances initiation of translation *(1–3)*. On reaching the gene's termination codon, the ribosome dissociates from the RNA, releasing the protein.

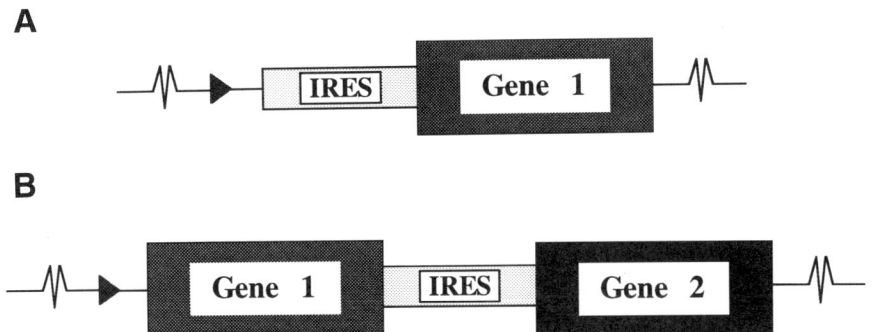

Fig. 1. Generalized structure of mono- and dicistronic IRES reporter plasmids. (**A**) Basic monocistronic reporter plasmid. The triangle represents a promoter to provide transcription of the cassette, the IRES box is the internal ribosomal entry site from HCV, and Gene 1 denotes any reporter gene. The IRES element controls initiation of translation of the single reporter gene. (**B**) Basic dicistronic reporter plasmid. Here, the promoter directs transcription of both reporter genes as a single message. Translation of the first reporter gene would be initiated by a cap structure, but translation of the second reporter would require IRES function. The first gene thereby serves as an IRES–independent internal control.

Unlike prokaryotic systems, eukaryotic ribosomes will not normally reinitiate translation at an internal start codon on a messenger RNA (3), so that the 3'-reporter gene cannot be translated. However, the presence of the IRES 5' to the second reporter gene directs the ribosomes to reinitiate translation of the dicistronic RNA and synthesize the second reporter protein. In this system it is possible to use the 5' reporter protein as an IRES-independent internal control to normalize between samples, which allows the distinction between a global or IRES-specific effect on translation.

2. Materials
2.1. In Vitro Transcription/Translation

1. A relatively clean stock of DNA of known concentration from a dicistronic reporter plasmid (**Fig. 1B**), assembled by standard cloning techniques (*see* **Note 3**).
2. TNT T7 coupled transcription/translation system (Promega, Madison, WI) (*see* **Note 4**). These kits are stable for at least 6 mo at –70°C.
3. RNasin ribonuclease inhibitor (Promega).
4. Translational grade [α^{35}S]-methionine, such as #NEG 009A from NEN Life Science Products (Boston, MA). Aliquots of the radiolabeled amino acid are fairly stable at –70°C as long as freeze–thaw cycles are kept to a minimum, but it must be remembered that the half-life of ^{35}S is only 87 d. This component is a radiation hazard and should be treated as such.

2.2. SDS-PAGE

Unless otherwise noted, reagents were purchased from Fisher Scientific (Pittsburgh, PA):

1. 30% acrylamide/1% *bis*-stock: Dissolve 30 g acrylamide (99% pure; Bio-Rad, Hercules, CA) and 1 g *N,N'*-methylene-*bis*-acrylamide (e.g., Sigma, St. Louis, MO) in ~60 mL deionized water, and bring volume to 100 mL. Filter solution through a 0.2 μm filter, store at 4°C. Note that acrylamide is a toxic chemical and should be handled accordingly.
2. 10% (w/v) SDS: Dissolve 10 g SDS in ~75 mL deionized water with gentle stirring, bring volume to 100 mL. Solution may be autoclaved or 0.2-μm filtered. Store at room temperature; if stored cold, the SDS will precipitate. Note that aerosolized SDS powder is extremely irritating on inhalation.
3. 1 M Tris-HCl, pH 6.8: Dissolve 121.1 g Tris (hydroxymethyl) aminomethane in ~70 mL deionized water, and pH to 6.8 with concentrated HCl. Bring volume to 100 mL, and autoclave. Store at room temperature.
4. 1 M Tris-HCl, pH 8.7: Dissolve 121.1 g Tris (hydroxymethyl) aminomethane in ~80 mL deionized water, adjust pH to 8.7 with concentrated HCl. Bring volume to 100 mL, and autoclave. Store at room temperature.
5. 10% (w/v) Ammonium persulfate: Dissolve 0.1 g ammonium persulfate in 1 mL deionized water. For best results, make fresh each day.
6. *N,N,N',N'*-Tetramethylethylenediamine (TEMED).
7. 2X sample buffer: 125 mM Tris-HCl, pH 8.7, 20% glycerol, 4% SDS, 5% 2-mercaptoethanol, and 0.02% bromophenol blue.

1 M Tris-HCl, pH 8.7	12.5 mL
Glycerol	20 mL
SDS	4 g
2-mercaptoethanol	5 mL
Bromophenol blue	0.02 g
Deionized water	to 100 mL

8. 10X running buffer: 25 mM Tris, 192 mM glycine, 0.1% SDS.

Tris	30.3 g
Glycine	144.1 g
SDS	10.0 g
Deionized water	~700 mL

    Bring volume to 1 L. **Do not** adjust the pH. Dilute to 1X for electrophoresis; the volume needed will depend on the electrophoresis apparatus used.
9. Vertical polyacrylamide gel electrophoresis apparatus, such as the Protean II xi system from Bio-Rad (Hercules, CA).
10. A protein molecular mass marker for sizing of the products on the gel. For the effort and time they save, The authors prefer prestained markers, particularly Bio-Rad's kaleidoscope marker.

2.3. Solutions for Fluorography

1. Dimethylsulfoxide (DMSO).
2. 22.2% PPO in DMSO: Dissolve 111 g of PPO (2,5-Diphenyloxazole; Amersham Life Science Products, Arlington Heights, IL) in 400 mL of DMSO, and adjust volume to 500 mL with DMSO. Because PPO is insoluble in water, the glassware used for this solution must be dry. Store at room temperature (*see* **Note 5**). This solution may be reused many times with no detectable effect on the gels. Note that DMSO is readily absorbed through the skin and may also facilitate the absorption of other chemicals, so proper precautions should be taken.
3. Vacuum gel drying system, autoradiography film, and cassettes.

3. Methods

3.1. TNT T7 Coupled Transcription/Translation Reactions

1. First, determine how many reactions will be required, including both a positive control (the luciferase plasmid provided with the kit) and a negative control (water alone, no plasmid). Label a 0.5-mL microcentrifuge tube for each reaction and an appropriately sized tube for the premix *(see below)*.
2. Thaw the components of the kit following the company's directions, and set up the premix as follows, mixing gently with the pipet after each addition: (*see* **Notes 6** and **7**):

    For 1 reaction*:
TNT reaction buffer	2 µL
Amino acid mix minus methionine	0.5 µL
TNT T7 RNA polymerase	0.5 µL
RNasin ribonuclease inhibitor	0.5 µL
[α^{35}S]-methionine	0.8 µL (10 µCi)
TNT reticulocyte lysate	12.5 µL
	16.8 µL

    *Make enough premix for two reactions more than the number of samples to account for any volume lost to bubbles and minor pipet inaccuracies. Dispense 16.8 µL of the completed premix into each of the labeled tubes.
3. For each plasmid, determine the volume of stock needed to contain 0.5 µg DNA. Add 0.5 µg each DNA to its premix tube, along with sterile deionized water to bring each reaction to 25 µL. The combined volume of DNA plus water added to each tube will be 8.2 µL. (Very dilute plasmids can be concentrated by ethanol precipitation and resuspended in a smaller volume of TE [10 mM Tris-HCl, 1 mM Na$_2$EDTA, pH 8.0]). Gently mix the reactions, and briefly spin the tubes in a microcentrifuge to remove any bubbles generated (*see* **Note 8**). Incubate the reactions for 1–2 h at 30°C.

3.2. SDS-PAGE

1. Based on the predicted sizes of your reporter proteins, determine which gel percentage will give the best separation. Recipes are given for 7.5 and 10% separat-

ing gels, which resolve 40–200 and 21–100 kDa, respectively. If necessary, recipes for other percent separating or gradient gels are readily available from manufacturers of electrophoresis reagents and in laboratory manuals. (Alternatively, although they are relatively expensive, precast gels are commercially available in a variety of percents and formulations.)
2. Prepare the glass plate sandwich, per the manufacturer's instructions. Begin making the separating gel by combining the first four components in a 50-mL screw-cap tube, and mixing by gently inverting the tube. After this, add the APS and TEMED, and gently mix the solution; it will be necessary to work moderately quickly once the APS and TEMED have been added.

	7.5% gels	10% gels
30:1 Acrylamide/*bis* stock	12.5 mL	16.6 mL
1 *M* Tris-HCl, pH 8.7	18.75 mL	18.75 mL
10% SDS	500 μL	500 μL
Deionized water	18.0 mL	13.8 mL
10% APS	500 μL	500 μL
TEMED	20 μL	20 μL

Using this relatively large volume of APS, there is no need to degas the gel prior to pouring.
3. Pour or pipet the gel into the glass sandwich to a level of ~1.5 cm below where the bottom of the wells will be. Then use a small syringe and needle to overlay the gel gently with water or water-saturated butanol, to give a sharp upper boundary.
4. After the separating gel has set (30 min–1 h) (*see* **Note 9**), pour off the overlay and insert the comb into the sandwich. Prepare a 10-mL 4% stacking gel in the same manner as the separating gel, using the following recipe:

30:1 Acrylamide/*bis* stock	1.33 mL
1 *M* Tris-HCl, pH 6.8	3.75 mL
10% SDS	100 μL
Deionized water	4.76 mL
10% APS	100 μL
TEMED	10 μL

5. Use a 5-mL pipet to run the stacking gel down one of the side spacers to minimize bubbles. Continue until the gel solution brims over the top of the shorter glass plate. Let the stacker set for 30–60 min.
6. While the stacking gel is setting, the samples may be prepared for electrophoresis. To do this, pipet an aliquot of the TNT reaction into a 0.5-mL microcentrifuge tube along with an equal volume of 2X sample buffer. Using the TNT kit with a T7 promoter, 2.5 μL (10%) of the reaction regularly gives dark bands from an overnight exposure. However, the first time a reporter plasmid is used, it may be wise to run several volumes of the reaction on a gel to determine the optimum. When using only small amounts of the TNT reaction, the total sample volume to be loaded onto the gel may be increased by adding equal proportions of sterile deionized water and 2X sample buffer to the aliquot.

7. Once the samples have been diluted to the desired volume in sample buffer, close the tubes tightly, and boil the samples for 2–3 min in a water bath. Remember also to boil an aliquot of the protein molecular mass marker, which will be run on the gel. There is no need to quench the heated samples.
8. Finally, remove the comb from the polymerized gel and assemble the completed electrophoresis apparatus. Add 1X running buffer to the level recommended by the manufacturer. Using a Pasteur pipet or a syringe and needle, rinse the wells thoroughly with the running buffer. Also remove any bubbles trapped under the glass plate sandwich.
9. The samples may now be loaded and electrophoresed (*see* **Note 10**). It is often most convenient to run the gel overnight; a 20 cm gel can be run at 60 V for at least 15 h. In the morning, run the gel at a higher voltage (see the manufacturer's limits for that apparatus) until the purple dye front just migrates off the bottom of the gel.

3.3. Fluorography

1. In order to shorten exposure times for the relatively weak $[^{35}S]$-methionine, the gels are impregnated with the fluor PPO, which amplifies the signal from the labeled amino acid (*see* **Note 11**). Once the gel has been run to completion, disassemble the apparatus and open the glass sandwich. Using a sharp scalpel, cut off the stacking gel and put it in the radioactive waste. Place the gel in a shallow container (glass baking dishes work well).
2. Put the gel into enough fixer to cover its surface thoroughly (at least 200 mL). Gently rock for 15 min at room temperature. Discard the used fixer and repeat once. After the second incubation, take care to pour off as much of the fixer as possible.
3. Pour about 200 mL DMSO into the baking dish, and rock for 30 min at room temperature. Do not be alarmed if the gel curls slightly as the DMSO dehydrates it. Pour the DMSO into a bottle for chemical waste, and repeat once (*see* **Note 12**).
4. Pour 200–250 mL of the PPO-DMSO solution onto the dehydrated gel and rock for 30 min at room temperature. It may be wise to cover the glass dish with foil at this point, since the PPO is light-sensitive. After the incubation, the PPO-DMSO can be returned to its bottle for reuse. Pour off as much as possible.
5. Run a gentle stream of tap water over the gel. At this point, the PPO impregnated into the gel will precipitate, causing the gel to become opaque white. It may appear blotchy at first, but with continued rinsing the gel should turn evenly white. Continue to rinse the gel under gently running tap water for 1 h. (Alternatively, the gel may placed in water and rocked for 1 h, with one or two changes of the water.)
6. Dry the rinsed gel onto a thick paper stock in a vacuum gel drier for 2 h at 55–60°C.

3.4. Autoradiography and Quantitation

After it has cooled, the dried gel may then be exposed to either X-ray film or the plate of a phosphorimager to visualize the labeled proteins. For quantitation, a phosphorimager is ideal. However, these systems can be expensive, so if one is unavailable, a densitometer may be used to scan films that are not overexposed. Exposing films beyond their linear range can give artificially low readings.

4. Notes

1. Many promoter elements have now been identified, characterized, and isolated from bacteriophages, other viruses, bacteria, yeast and eukaryotes. Many companies sell plasmids that contain a promoter followed by a multicloning region, which can be used as the beginning of a reporter vector. Indeed, for most applications, there is likely to be a promoter construct available that will generate the desired level of transcription in the appropriate environment. In choosing a promoter, it can be decided whether transcription is to be constitutive or inducible, high or low level. However, it is crucial to keep in mind that when a promoter is placed in a nonnative environment, such as the bacteriophage T7 promoter in a eukaryotic system, the RNA polymerase that recognizes the promoter may not be present and would have to be added to the system separately.
2. As with promoters, there is a wide spectrum of reporter gene combinations that can be used in a dicistronic construct. However, care must be exercised in their selection. Points to consider include the ease of obtaining and subcloning the DNA for each coding region, the broadness of applicability and complexity of the enzymatic assays to quantitate the reporter proteins (not described in this chapter, but practical to keep in mind for other potential uses of your construct), and the expected sizes of the mature proteins. If gel analysis is to be used to study the protein products, they must be of sufficiently different sizes that they can be clearly resolved on a polyacrylamide gel. If it is necessary to generate the DNA regions by polymerase chain reaction (e.g., to add restriction sites), the resulting fragments must be sequenced or tested for activity prior to using the construct to rule out *Taq*-induced errors that may affect protein structure and function. Finally, if the 3'-reporter protein is to be expressed as a fusion protein with the 5'-end of the HCV core (i.e., if the HCV IRES cassette to be used in the construct extends downstream past the virus' natural ATG start codon), the second coding region must be in frame with the HCV start codon. Unfortunately, it is possible that N-terminal fusion with the HCV core peptide may significantly alter the normal folding or processing of some reporter proteins; in this case, a literature search on the chosen reporter gene will be useful before beginning the cloning.
3. In general, the cleaner the plasmid DNA, the more reproducible the results will be. Many commercial alkaline lysis-based plasmid purification kits, such as those from Qiagen (Chatsworth, CA), are simple to use and give DNA that is reportedly as pure as cesium chloride banding. However, the kits are much faster and easier than centrifugation through cesium chloride gradients.

4. The Promega TNT coupled transcription/translation kit is much easier and less time-consuming than doing separate transcription and translation reactions. Advantages of this protocol over the traditional two-step method include:
   a. There is no need to purify large amounts of linearized DNA for transcription.
   b. There is no need to analyze and purify the resultant RNA.
   c. There will be no possibility of the RNA intermediate degrading upon storage.
   The only potential disadvantage of the TNT kit involves the inability to isolate large quantities of the transcribed RNA, so that if a problem arises, it may be more difficult to isolate the step that is not working.
5. On occasion, during storage the PPO will precipitate out of solution. The solution can be revived by adding small amounts of DMSO (5–10 mL at a time) with stirring until the PPO goes back into solution. The small change in volume does not appreciably affect the function of the solution.
6. Using the T7 promoter, half-scale (25-µL) reactions should give ample product to run at least eight gels. This means that one kit can be used for 80 reactions, decreasing the cost per reaction. Further scaling down of the reactions may also be possible with cassettes that express well.
7. It may be easiest to add the components in the order shown, for the following reasons: The proteinaceous lysate is prone to generation of bubbles in the solution on even the most gentle pipetting, so it is best added last. The radioactive methionine is added just prior to the lysate to reduce the number of radioactive tips generated and the likelihood of radioactive contamination of the work area.
8. Some bubbles can be very difficult to remove, especially those that will not rise to the surface of the reaction. This can be alleviated by firmly rapping the bottom of the closed tube on a sturdy plastic surface prior to centrifugation. Ensure that the tubes are tightly closed, keeping in mind that the contents of the tubes are radioactive.
9. When the gel is set, the boundary line between it and the overlay will be much more obvious. However, the easiest way to see whether the gel has set is to save any excess gel solution in the screw-cap tube, and simply tip the tube slowly on its side. As it sets, the gel excludes water from its matrix, so do not be surprised that a small amount of the solution will still appear to flow after the majority of the gel has formed a firm plug.
10. When loading the samples, it is best to follow a predetermined order. Points to consider include: It is impossible to tell the front of a gel from its back, so be sure that the samples are not symmetric in the gel. Otherwise, it will be necessary to cut a corner off of the gel for orientation prior to taking apart the sandwich. The luciferase control from the kit is very efficient, so it is best run in one of the end wells next to the marker or negative control rather than next to a valuable sample.
11. Although the PPO-DMSO method described here requires little hands-on time and is easy to master, there are faster reagents on the market, such as Amplify from Amersham Life Science Products, Inc. (Arlington Heights, IL). However, the cost of these alternatives is many times that of PPO.

12. There is one minor change that will save some money and slow the production of chemical waste. Label a bottle "once-used DMSO" for DMSO that has been used in one dehydration step. This may be stored indefinitely at room temperature. The once-used DMSO can be used for the first wash of the next gel, after which it should be put into chemical waste. The second wash of the gel should always use fresh DMSO, so that there is no water in it. DMSO from the second wash can go into the once-used bottle to be the first rinse of the next gel.

References

1. Kozak, M. (1986) Point mutations define a sequence flanking the AUG initiator codon that modulates transcription by eukaryotic ribosomes. *Cell* **44,** 283–292.
2. Kozak, M. (1989) The scanning model for translation: an update. *J. Cell. Biol.* **108,** 229–241.
3. Lodish, H., Baltimore, B., Berk, A., Zipursky, S. L., Matsudaira, P., and Darnell, J. (1995) *Molecular Biology of the Gene*, 3rd ed. Scientific American Press, New York.

29

Expression and Dimerization of Hepatitis C Virus Core Protein in *E. coli*

Shih-Yen Lo and Jing-Hsiung Ou

1. Introduction

Hepatitis C virus (HCV) is a positive-stranded RNA virus with a genome size of about 9–10 kb. The genome of this virus encodes a polyprotein with a length of over 3000 amino acids. This polyprotein is cleaved by cellular and viral proteases to generate at least 10 viral gene products. Recent reports have indicated that there are extensive interactions between various HCV proteins: the core (capsid) protein can interact with itself *(1)* and with the E1 envelope protein *(2)*; E1 protein can interact with the E2 envelope protein *(3,4)* which in turn can be covalently linked to its following p7 protein and interact with another integral membrane protein named NS2 *(5)*; NS2 can also interact with NS5A and NS5B nonstructural proteins *(6)*; and NS3 proteinase/helicase has also been shown to complex with the NS4A protein *(6,7)*. Thus, most of the known HCV proteins interact with at least another HCV protein. These interactions are presumably very important for morphogenesis and replication of HCV.

As mentioned above, it has recently been demonstrated that the HCV core protein can interact with itself. This interaction which occurs in yeast and in mammalian cells, allows the core protein to form homodimers and oligomers *(1)*. We have been able to verify this observation by performing the crosslinking experiments using the HCV core protein expressed in *Escherichia coli*. Based on these crosslinking experiments, we found that the HCV core protein expressed in *E. coli* could indeed form a homodimer. In addition, we found that removal of the core protein sequence downstream of amino acid (aa) 127 did not affect the dimerization of the core protein. This finding, which indicates that the dimerization domain of the core protein resides in the sequence upstream of aa 127, is consistent with the previous report *(1)*. In this chapter, we will describe the procedures of these crosslinking experiments. In the first half of this chapter, we will describe the procedures for expressing HCV core proteins in *E. coli* and in the second half, we will describe the crosslinking procedures that we used to study the dimerization of the HCV core protein.

2. Materials

1. LB broth: Dehydrated LB broth is from Difco Laboratories (Detroit, MI; #0446-17-3). This broth should be reconstituted with water to a concentration of 25 gm/L and autoclaved. For LB-amp plate or LB-amp culture, ampicillin is added to a final concentration of 100 µg/mL.
2. Phosphate-buffered saline (PBS, catalog #20012-019, Life Technologies [Gibco-BRL, Gaithersburg, MD]).
3. Tris (Hydroxymethyl) aminoethane (catalog #BP152), isopropyl thio-β-D-galactoside (IPTG) (catalog #BP1620-10) and glycerol (catalog #G33-1) are from Fisher Scientific (Pittsburgh, PA).
4. 2X Laemmli sample buffer: 0.135 M Tris-HCl, pH 6.8, 6% SDS, 20% glycerol, and 10% 2-mercaptoethanol.
5. NitroPlus nitrocellulose (NC) membrane (#W02HY450F5) from Micron Separation Inc. (Westboro, MA).
6. The primary antibody used is an anti-HCV serum isolated from an HCV patient.
7. Alkaline phosphatase-conjugated goat antihuman IgG (#605 415) from Boehringer Mannheim Corporation (Indianapolis, IN).
8. Alkaline phosphatase-conjugate substrate kit (#170-6432) from Bio-Rad Laboratories (Hercules, CA).
9. Carnation nonfat dry milk purchased from the supermarkets. Other brands of the nonfat powdered milk can also be used.
10. The construction of the DNA plasmid pET-RC has been described previously *(8)*. This plasmid contains the entire core protein coding sequence (191 aa) of the HCV-RH isolate *(8)*. The expression of the HCV-RH core protein in this plasmid is under the control of the T7 phage promoter. The plasmid pET-RC127 is identical to pET-RC, except that the core protein sequence downstream of aa 127 is deleted.
11. The BL21(DE3) strain of *E. coli* contains the T7 RNA polymerase gene of which the expression is under the control of the Lac UV5 promoter *(9)*. The preparation of the BL21(DE3) transformation competent cells is as follows: inoculate a fresh colony of BL21(DE3) into a tube containing 2 mL of the LB broth, and incubate the culture overnight in a 37°C air shaker; inoculate this overnight culture into a flask containing 100 mL LB broth; allow cells to grow until A_{600} = 0.6; split the culture into two 50-mL conical tubes and centrifuge cells in a Sorvall HS4 rotor at 4000g for 5 min; resuspend the cell pellet in 50-mL of ice-cold 0.1 M Ca$_2$Cl, and centrifuge cells again in an HS4 rotor at 4000g for 5 min; resuspend the cell pellet again in 7 mL of ice-cold 0.1 M Ca$_2$Cl and incubate cells on ice for 4–6 h; add 1.4 mL of ice-cold 90% glycerol in cells and mix gently; freeze cells in

100 µL aliquots in the microfuge tubes that have been prechilled in liquid nitrogen; store cells frozen at –80°C until use.

3. Methods
3.1. Expression of HCV Core Proteins in E. coli

1. Thaw a tube of competent BL21(DE3) cells on ice, and add 10 ng of pET-3a, pET-RC, or pET-RC127 (*see* **Note 1**). Incubate cells on ice for 30 min and subsequently heat-shock cells at 42°C for 2 min. Add 1.4 mL of the LB broth to the tube, and further incubate cells at 37°C for 30 min. Plate 100 µL of transformed cells on an LB-amp plate. This transformation procedure should generate enough colonies on the plate after an overnight incubation at 37°C.
2. Inoculate a fresh colony of transformed cells into a 20-mL LB-amp culture. Incubate the culture overnight at 37°C in an air shaker.
3. Transfer the overnight culture to a 500-mL LB-amp culture. Incubate the culture at 37°C in an air shaker until A_{600} = 0.6 (*see* **Notes 2–4**).
4. Induce the expression of core protein with 1 mM IPTG (final concentration) for 3 h at 37°C.
5. Pellet bacterial cells in a GSA rotor at 8000g for 10 min.
6. Resuspend the bacterial pellet in 10 mL PBS containing 1% Triton X-100. Transfer cells to a 50-mL conical centrifuge tube.
7. Sonicate cells for 10 s on ice. Repeat sonication for a total of 18 times. Pause for 10 s between each sonication step to prevent cell lysates from heating up.
8. Centrifuge at 8000g for 10 min to pellet cell debris and insoluble proteins (*see* **Notes 5** and **6**). Save the supernatant for the crosslinking study.

3.2. Crosslinking of HCV Core Protein

1. Dilute glutaraldehyde to 0.05% or higher concentrations with water.
2. Add 1 µL of 0.05% glutaraldehyde to 9 µL of *E. coli* lysate (the supernatant prepared in **step 8** of **Subheading 3.1.**). Incubate at room temperature for 30 min.
3. Add 10 µL of 2X Laemmli sample buffer to the reaction. Incubate the sample at 95°C for 5 min.
4. Load the sample on a 12.5% SDS-PAGE.
5. The procedures for protein gel electrophoresis and for Western blot transfer of proteins to NC membrane have been described in detail elsewhere *(10)* and, thus, will not be repeated here.
6. The NC membranes containing the protein samples were preblocked with Tris-buffered saline (TBS): 10 mM Tris-HCl, pH 7.0, 150 mM NaCl, containing 1% nonfat powdered milk at room temperature for 3 h.
7. Remove the preblocking milk solution. Dilute primary antibody 1:1000 in TBS containing 1% milk and 0.1% NP40. Add this diluted antibody solution to the preblocked NC membrane. Rock on a platform shaker at room temperature for 3 h.
8. Wash the membrane in TBS by rocking at room temperature for 10 min.
9. Wash the membrane in TBS containing 0.1% NP40 by rocking at room temperature for 10 min.

10. Wash the membrane in TBS by rocking at room temperature for 10 min.
11. Dilute alkaline phosphatase-conjugated secondary antibody 1:500 in TBS containing 1% milk and 0.1% NP40. Add this secondary antibody solution to the membrane. Rock at room temperature for 1 h.
12. Repeat washing **steps 8–10**.
13. Develop the signal using the Bio-Rad alkaline phosphatase conjugate substrate kit. Mix 20 mL AP color buffer with 0.2 mL reagent A and 0.2 mL reagent B. AP color buffer and reagents A and B are supplied in the kit. Rock until color is apparent.
14. A typical crosslinking result is shown in **Fig. 1**. This result revealed that the HCV core proteins expressed in *E. coli* could be crosslinked by glutaraldehyde to form dimers (**Fig. 1A**). In addition, since removal of the core protein sequence downstream of aa 127 did not affect dimerization of the truncated core protein (**Fig. 1B**), the dimerization domain of the HCV core protein must be located in the amino terminus. This result is consistent with what has been previously reported *(1)* (*see* **Notes 7** and **8**).

4. Notes

1. For the preparation of the TC cells, we have found that the transformation efficiency can be substantially increased if the TC cells are aliquoted into microfuge tubes that have been immersed in liquid nitrogen.
2. The protocol for the expression of HCV core proteins described above is for the large-scale preparation. For minipreps, simply inoculate a colony into a 3-mL culture, and grow the miniculture to A_{600} = 0.6. The miniculture can then be induced with 1 m*M* IPTG for 3 h. After IPTG induction, 1.5 mL of the culture is then transferred to a microfuge tube and centrifuged in a microfuge at full speed. The cell pellet is then resuspended in 50 µL 2X Laemmli buffer or 25 µL PBS containing 1% Triton X-100. Cells are then sonicated as described above.
3. Depending on the size of the colony used for inoculation, it may take up to 6 h for the miniculture of *E. coli* containing the HCV core protein to grow to an A_{600} of 0.6. This slow growth rate may be owing to leaky expression of the core protein and the toxicity of this protein to cells. In comparison, BL21(DE3) transformed by the control vector plasmid pET-3a has a much higher growth rate. It usually takes about 3 h for this control *E. coli* culture to reach an A_{600} of 0.6.
4. For the expression of HCV core proteins, it is advisable to pick several colonies for minipreps prior to conducting the large scale preparation, because based on our past experience, not all the colonies will express the HCV core protein. Save an aliquot of the miniculture prior to IPTG induction to make a glycerol stock. The glycerol stock is prepared by adding glycerol to the culture to a final concentration of 15% (e.g., add 100 µL 90% glycerol to 500 µL of the *E. coli* culture). Vortex well to mix the glycerol with the *E. coli* culture. This glycerol stock, which can be used to streak out colonies on an LB-amp plate for the large prep, is stored at –80°C in a freezer until use.

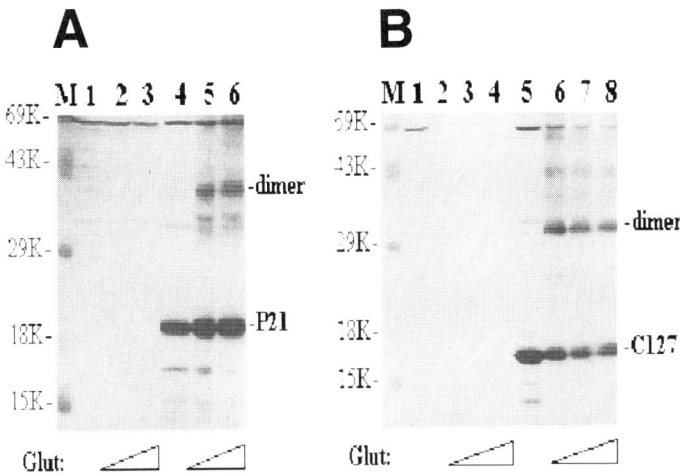

Fig. 1. Crosslinking of the HCV core protein expressed in *E. coli*. **(A)** Analysis of the full-length HCV core protein. *E. coli* carrying pET-3a (lanes 1–3) or pET-RC (lanes 4–6) was lysed by sonication and crosslinked with 0% (lanes 1 and 4), 0.005% (lanes 2 and 5), or 0.02% glutaraldehyde and subjected to Western blot analysis. The locations of the full-length core protein (P21) and its dimer are indicated. **(B)** Analysis of the 127 aa truncated HCV core protein. Lanes 1–4, *E. coli* cells carrying pET-3a; lanes 5–8, *E. coli* cells carrying pET- RC127. Lanes 1 and 5, 0% glutaraldehyde added; lanes 2 and 6, 0.005% glutaraldehyde added; lanes 3 and 7, 0.02% glutaraldehyde added; lanes 4 and 8, 0.05% glutaraldehyde added. C127 indicates the location of the core protein truncated at aa 127. Glut: glutaraldehyde.

5. After sonication, a substantial fraction of the HCV core protein will be insoluble and pelleted by centrifugation. However, a significant fraction of the HCV core protein will remain in the supernatant after centrifugation. In our experience, truncated HCV core proteins lacking all or part of the carboxy-terminal hydrophobic sequence are more soluble than the full-length core proteins.
6. No significant difference in protein solubility was observed when *E. coli* cells were sonicated in TBS containing 1% NP40 or directly in water. However, the core protein solubility is substantially increased, if 1% SDS is used to replace NP40 or Triton X-100.
7. As shown in **Fig. 1**, 0.005% of glutaraldehyde was sufficient to generate a clear dimerized core protein signal. Further increase of the glutaraldehyde concentration did not increase the signal of the dimerized core protein. In fact, the core protein signal appeared to be slightly reduced when the glutaraldehyde concentration was further increased. The reduction of the core protein signal by the high concentration of glutaraldehyde may be owing to the formation of core protein oligomers *(1)* and/or the crosslinking of the core protein to other nonspecific *E. coli* proteins.

8. Similar expression experiments have also been conducted to express core proteins truncated at various locations between aa 191 and 127. Protein species equivalent in size to the homodimer of their respective truncated core proteins were also observed.

References

1. Matsumoto, M., Hwang, S. B., Jeng, K.-S., Zhu, N., and Lai, M. M. C. (1996) Homotypic interaction and multimerization of hepatitis C virus core protein. *Virology* **218**, 43–51.
2. Lo, S.-Y., Selby, M. J., and Ou, J.-H. (1996) Interaction between hepatitis C virus core protein and E1 envelope protein. *J. Virol.* **70**, 5177–5182.
3. Dubuisson, J., Hsu, H. H., Cheung, R. C., Greenberg, H. B., Russel, D. G., and Rice, C. M. (1994) Formation and intracellular localization of hepatitis C virus envelope glycoprotein complexes expressed by recombinant Vaccinia and Sindbis viruses. *J. Virol.* **68**, 6147–6160.
4. Matsuura, Y., Suzuki, T., Suzuki, R., Sato, M., Aizaki, H., Saito, I., et al. (1994) Processing of E1 and E2 glycoproteins of hepatitis C virus expressed in mammalian and insect cells. *Virology* **205**, 141–150.
5. Selby, M. J., Glazer, E., Masiarz, F., and Houghton, M. (1994) Complex processing and protein:protein interactions in the E2:NS2 region of HCV. *Virology* **204**, 114–122.
6. Hijikata, M., Mizushima, H., Tanji, Y., Komoda, Y., Hirowatari, Y., Akagi, T., et al. (1993) Proteolytic processing and membrane association of putative nonstructural proteins of hepatitis C virus. *Proc. Natl. Acad. Sci. USA* **90**, 10,773–10,777.
7. Failla, C., Tomei, L., and Francesco, R. D. (1995) An amino-terminal domain of hepatitis C virus NS3 protease is essential for the interaction with NS4A. *J. Virol.* **69**, 1769–1777.
8. Lo, S.-Y., Masiarz, F., Hwang, S. B., Lai, M. M. C., and Ou, J.-H. (1995) Differential subcellular localization of hepatitis C virus core gene products. *Virology* **213**, 455–461.
9. Rosenberg, A. H., Lade, B. N., Chui, D.-S., Lin, S.-W., Dunn, J. J., and Studier, F. W. (1987) Vectors for selective expression of cloned DNAs by T7 RNA polymerase. *Gene* **56**, 125–135.
10. Sambrook, J., Fritsch, E., and Maniatis, T. (1989) *Molecular Cloning: A Laboratory Manual.* Cold Spring Harbor Laboratory, Cold Spring Harbor, NY.

30

Expression and Characterization of the HCV NS2 Protease

Karen E. Reed and Charles M. Rice

1. Introduction

Heterologous expression systems have been widely used to study hepatitis C virus (HCV) proteins in lieu of an efficient method for establishing HCV infections in cell culture. Studies of HCV polyprotein processing in both mammalian-cell-based and cell-free expression systems have shown that host signalase is responsible for cleavages between the structural proteins and at the N-terminus of NS2 *(1–4)*, whereas a chymotrypsin-like serine protease located in the N-terminal region of NS3 is responsible for most cleavages between the nonstructural proteins, including the 3/4A, 4A/4B, 4B/5A, and 5A/5B sites *(5–10)*. However, two observations indicated that the 2/3 site is cleaved by a distinct virus-encoded protease, known as the NS2, NS2-3, or Cpro-2 protease: (1) mutation of the catalytic serine at amino acid (aa) 1165 of NS3 abolished cleavage at all sites in the nonstructural polyprotein except the 2/3 site, and (2) two mutations in NS2 located more than 30 residues from the NS2-NS3 junction abolished cleavage at the 2/3 site, but had little or no effect on downstream cleavages catalyzed by the serine protease *(8,11)*. The minimal region required for cleavage at the 2/3 site has been mapped to aa 898 on the N-terminal side *(8)* and aa 1207 on the C-terminal side *(11)* (numbers refer to HCV 1a and 1b isolates). Although a single construct extending from aa 898 to 1207 has never been tested for proteolytic viability, cleavage with an efficiency similar to that of polypeptides containing full-length NS2 and NS3 has been demonstrated for truncated constructs extending from aa 898 to 1233 or 827 to 1207 *(8, 11)*. This region overlaps with the serine protease domain even though cleavage at the 2/3 site does not require catalytic activity of the serine protease. Site-directed mutagenesis of residues surrounding the 2/3 cleavage site (L_{1026}/A_{1027}) has

From: *Methods in Molecular Medicine, Vol. 19: Hepatitis C Protocols*
Edited by: J. Y. N. Lau © Humana Press Inc., Totowa, NJ

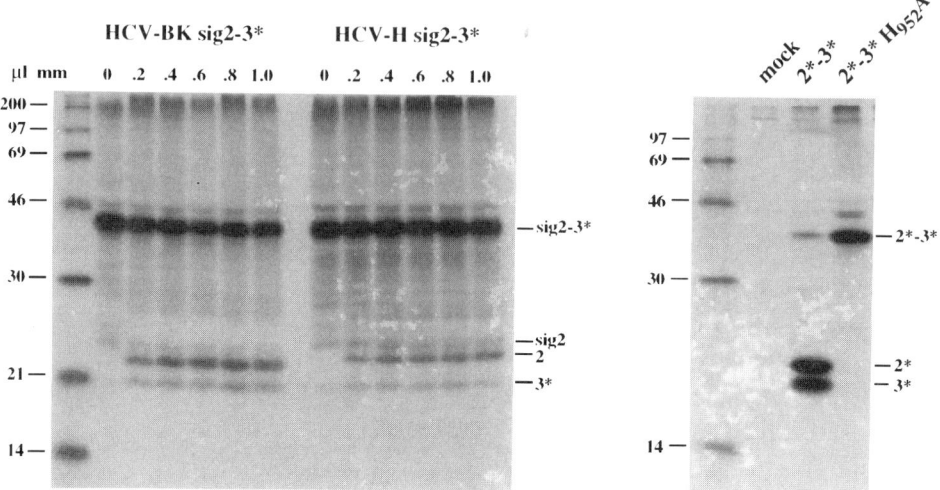

Fig. 1. Comparison of cleavage at the HCV 2/3 site in vitro and in cultured cells. **(A)** Uncapped RNA transcripts (100 ng) derived from pTM3/HCV-BK 785-1207 or pTM3/HCV-H 785-1207 (numbers refer to amino acid positions in the HCV polyprotein) were translated in rabbit reticulocytes in the absence or presence of increasing amounts of microsomal membranes. Reactions were incubated at 30°C for 1 h, denatured by heating at 70°C for 10 min in buffer containing 0.5% SDS, and immunoprecipitated with the antiserum WU43 *(19)*, which is specific for both NS2 and NS3. **(B)** BHK-21 cells infected for 30 min with the vaccinia virus/T7 RNA polymerase recombinant vTF7-3 were transfected for 2 h with 1 µg of pTM3 (mock), pTM3/HCV 827-1207 (2*-3*), or pTM3/HCV 827–1207 $H_{952}A$ (2*-3* $H_{952}A$), labeled 3 h with EXPRE^{35}S^{35}S protein-labeling mix (NEN, Boston, MA), lysed in 50 mM Tris-HCl, pH 7.5, 1 mM EDTA, 0.5% SDS, and 20 µg/mL phenylmethylsulfonyl fluoride, sheared by passage through a 27.5-gage needle, denatured by heating at 70°C for 10 min, and immunoprecipitated with antiserum WU43. The asterisk denotes truncated proteins.

shown that the NS2 protease tolerates most single amino-acid substitutions *(12,13)*, with the exception of proline at certain positions, suggesting that regional conformation may be an important cleavage determinant.

Cleavage at the 2/3 site is stimulated in cell-free translation systems by the addition of microsomal membranes or detergents *(8,11,14,15)*. The degree of stimulation may vary among HCV isolates *(14)*, but the efficiency of cleavage in vitro is usually much lower than in mammalian cells, even when microsomal membranes are present (**Fig. 1**). The necessity of microsomal membranes for signalase cleavage at the N-terminus of NS2 or evidence suggesting that NS2 is an integral membrane protein *(14)* may explain the increased cleavage efficiency observed in the presence of membranes. $ZnCl_2$ has also been shown to stimulate cleavage at the 2/3 site in vitro *(8)*, which is a characteristic of metalloproteases. However, no homology has been found between the HCV NS-2 region and known metalloproteases. In particular, the NS2-3 region lacks an HEXXH or HXXEH motif that is present in all known metalloproteases and forms part of the active center of these enzymes *(15,16)*. Recent comparison of NS2 with the catalytic domains of viral or cellular cysteine proteases has led to the suggestion that NS2 is a cysteine protease. If so, zinc may have a structural rather than catalytic function. In any case, definitive classification of the HCV NS2-3 protease and clarification of the role of zinc await further biochemical and structural studies.

For the analysis of mammalian proteins, expression systems based in mammalian cells are often superior to *Escherichia coli* or cell-free systems in terms of stability, protein folding, authenticity of posttranslational modifications, and biological activity; therefore, they may be preferable for studies of HCV NS2 protease activity. Although stably transfected cell lines may be useful for some purposes, transient transfections typically require less labor and produce more protein. The HCV NS2 protease has previously been analyzed in mammalian cells by transient transfection of the plasmids containing the region of interest under the control of promoters recognized by the cellular RNA polymerase II complex or the exogenous bacteriophage T7 RNA polymerase. T7 polymerase is introduced into permissive transfected cells by infection with a recombinant vaccinia virus that encodes the polymerase in its genome *(17)*. The vaccinia virus/T7 hybrid system has all of the aforementioned advantages of mammalian cell-based transient expression systems plus some additional benefits. The use of the highly specific and active T7 RNA polymerase for transcription, coupled with the enhanced translational efficiency provided by an internal ribosome entry site (IRES) located in the 5'-untranslated region of transcripts encoding the region of interest, usually results in levels of expression that are higher than those obtained from systems that rely on the host machinery for transcription, capping, and eventual translation. Another advantage of this system is the cytoplasmic location of vaccinia virus replication, which may be especially important for the expression of proteins from viruses thought to replicate in the cytoplasm, such as HCV. The nuclear location of RNA synthesis in other transient expression systems could pose problems for HCV-derived RNA processing or transport, e.g., the potential recognition and cleavage of RNA sequences by the nuclear splicing machinery. For all of the reasons discussed above, we prefer to use the vaccinia virus/T7 hybrid system for expression of the HCV NS2 protease. Please refer to Chapter 27 for more information regarding the specific methods involved in the use of this system.

Cell-free expression systems may be more amenable to certain applications, however, such as the analysis of divalent cation requirements or the effects of protease inhibitors on HCV NS2 protease activity. In one of the most commonly used cell–free expression systems, mRNA encoding a region of interest is synthesized in vitro and translated in a lysate prepared from rabbit reticulocyte lysates in the presence of radiolabeled methionine. Almost any plasmid vector that contains a promoter for the DNA-dependent bacteriophage T7 or SP6 RNA polymerases followed by one or more cloning sites for the insertion of a region of interest can be used. The highly active and specific nature of these transcriptases combined with their commercial availability makes them the enzymes of choice for in vitro transcription. Although many vectors can be used for cell-free expression, pTM1, pTM3 *(18)*, and pCITE (Novagen, Madison, WI) are particularly advantageous, because they contain a T7 promoter for in vitro synthesis of mRNA containing the region of interest, an IRES to enhance translation of the ensuing transcript, and they can be used for expression in both the cell-free and vaccinia virus/T7 hybrid systems. The vectors pTM1 and pTM3 are identical, except that pTM3 also contains a guanine phosphoribosyltransferase (gpt) expression cassette, which can be used for the selection of vaccinia virus recombinants.

In order to express the HCV NS2 protease using the rabbit reticulocyte system, the region of interest, e.g., aa 785–1207, which includes the signal sequence at the N-terminus of NS2, is inserted into a suitable expression vector. The resulting construct is linearized prior to transcription in vitro to ensure that mRNAs of a finite length are produced. Linearization is advisable even for such vectors as pTM1, pTM3, and pCITE that contain a transcriptional termination signal because recognition of this signal seems to be reduced in vitro. Once the DNA is linearized, it is extracted with phenol/$CHCl_3$ to inactivate and remove the restriction enzyme and any ribonucleases (RNases) that may be present; then it is concentrated by ethanol precipitation.

For in vitro transcription, the linearized DNA is dissolved in a small volume of water and incubated in a reaction mixture containing a suitable buffer, free ribonucleotides, ribonuclease (RNase) inhibitor to prevent degradation of newly synthesized RNA by contaminating ribonucleases, the appropriate bacteriophage RNA polymerase, dithiothreitol (DTT) to reduce disulfide linkages and stimulate activity of the polymerase and RNase inhibitor, and ^{3}H uridine triphosphate (UTP) to label the RNA for later quantitation. The quality of the synthesized RNA may be checked by agarose-gel electrophoresis and the yield determined by measuring the percentage of ^{3}H UTP incorporation. This measurement is made by spotting small, equal portions of the reaction mixture on duplicate pieces of diethylaminoethyl (DEAE) cellulose ion-exchange chromatography paper, which provides a positively charged matrix for binding the negatively charged RNA, and washing one of the spotted samples in a sodium phosphate solution of medium ionic strength to elute the unincorporated nucleotides, including ^{3}H UTP, by competing electrostatic interactions. The other sample is dried without washing, the amount of ^{3}H in each sample is determined by scintillation counting, and the percentage of ^{3}H UTP incorporation is calculated by dividing the number of counts in the RNA polymer (washed sample) by the total counts in the reaction mixture (unwashed sample).

Once mRNA of sufficient quantity and integrity has been synthesized, it is translated by incubation at 30°C in a rabbit reticulocyte lysate supplemented with a mixture of exogenous amino acids lacking methionine, ^{35}S-labeled methionine to allow visualization of the resulting translation products by autoradiography, RNase inhibitor to slow degradation of the input RNA, and DTT to maintain the stability and activity of the RNase inhibitor. Although rabbit reticulocyte lysates may be obtained from a number of commercial sources, they are usually prepared by some variation of the method developed by Pelham and Jackson *(19)*. First, rabbits are injected with the hemolytic agent phenylhydrazine hydrochloride, which causes anemia and increases the proportion of reticulocytes in the blood. The translational capability of these cells is very high, because as precursors to mature erythrocytes, they are adapted for the large-scale synthesis of hemoglobin. The reticulocytes are usually harvested about 8 d after the initial dose of phenylhydrazine hydrochloride, pelleted by centrifugation, washed in saline solution, and incubated in cold water for hypotonic lysis. The plasma membranes and mitochondria are removed by centrifugation, and the supernatant is treated with a calcium-dependent nuclease, such as micrococcal nuclease, to remove endogenous mRNA. The nuclease is then inactivated by the addition of ethylene glycol-*bis*(2-aminoethyl ether)-N,N'-tetra-acetic acid (EGTA), a fairly specific calcium chelator. Two components of an ATP-producing reaction, phosphocreatine and phosphocreatine kinase, are added to the lysate to regenerate ATP depleted during translation, and calf liver tRNA is added to compensate for the uneven composition of the endogenous tRNA pool, which is biased toward the amino-acid content of hemoglobin. Hemin is also added to the reticulocyte lysate to prevent the inhibition of translational initiation by the heme-regulated inhibitor (HRI), a protein kinase that phosphorylates the α subunit of the translation initiation factor eIF2. Phosphorylation of eIF2 increases its affinity for the guanine nucleotide exchange factor eIF2B, which is then trapped in an inactive eIF2 complex that can no longer facilitate binding between the methionyl initiator tRNA and the small ribosomal subunit. Since there is less eIF2B than eIF2 in the reticulocyte, phosphorylation of eIF2 can result in the inactivation of all of the available eIF2B and the arrest of translation.

Once the mRNA has been translated in vitro in the rabbit reticulocyte system, the resulting translation products are analyzed by sodium dodecyl sulfate-polyacrylamide gel electrophoresis (SDS-PAGE) followed by autoradiography.

The background of polypeptides translated from endogenous mRNAs tends to be fairly low owing to nuclease treatment of the reticulocyte lysate, so polypeptides translated from the input RNA can usually be analyzed by mixing a portion of the translation reaction with an equal volume of 2X protein sample buffer and subjecting it directly to SDS-PAGE. However, the background may be further reduced by immunoprecipitating a portion of the translation mixture with antisera specific for NS2 and/or NS3 prior to analysis by SDS-PAGE.

2. Materials
2.1. Linearization of the DNA Template

1. Appropriate restriction enzyme: Store at –20°C.
2. Appropriate 10X restriction enzyme buffer: Store at –20°C.
3. Phenol/CHCl$_3$: Mix equal volumes of phenol that has been equilibrated with Tris-HCl, pH 7.9 (AMRESCO, Solon, OH, cat. #0945-400) and CHCl$_3$, and allow the phases to separate. Store at 4°C in a dark bottle.
4. 3 M sodium acetate, adjusted to pH 5.2 with glacial acetic acid: Store at room temperature.
5. Absolute ethanol: Store at room temperature.
6. 70% ethanol: Store at room temperature.
7. Sterile distilled-deionized H$_2$O (ddH$_2$O).
8. Materials for agarose-gel electrophoresis:
   a. Agarose. Store at room temperature.
   b. 50X TAE: Dissolve 242 g of Tris base in a final volume of 1 L of distilled H$_2$O containing 57.1 mL glacial acetic acid and 100 mL 0.5 M EDTA, pH 8.0. Store at room temperature.
   c. Ethidium bromide, 10 mg/mL. Store in a dark bottle at 4°C.

2.2. Transcription of RNA In Vitro

1. ^{3}H UTP (Du Pont/NEN Research Products, Boston, MA, cat. #NET-380): Store at –20°C.
2. 10X T7 transcription buffer: 400 mM Tris-HCl, pH 7.5, 60 mM MgCl$_2$, 100 mM NaCl, 20 mM spermidine. Store in small aliquots at –20°C.
3. 4 mM rNTPs. Store in small aliquots at –20°C.
4. 400 mM dithiothreitol (DTT). Store in small aliquots at –20°C.
5. RNasin (Promega, Madison, WI, cat. #N2511). Store at –20°C.
6. T7 RNA polymerase (Epicentre, Madison, WI, cat. #T7910k). Store at –20°C.
7. TE: 10 mM Tris-HCl, pH 7.5, 1 mM EDTA: Store at room temperature.
8. ddH$_2$O.
9. DEAE ion-exchange chromatography paper, DE81 grade (Whatman, Fairfield, NJ, cat. #3658-323).
10. 0.5 M Na$_2$HPO$_4$: Store at room temperature.

2.3. Cell-Free Translation of In Vitro Transcripts

1. Rabbit reticulocyte lysate system, nuclease-treated (Promega, cat. # L4970). Store in aliquots under liquid nitrogen (*see* **Note 1**).
2. RNasin: Store at –20°C.
3. ^{35}S methionine (Amersham, Arlington Heights, IL, cat. #SJ1515). Store in small aliquots at –80°C (*see* **Note 2**).
4. Sterile ddH$_2$O.
5. Canine pancreatic microsomal membranes (Promega, cat. #Y4041): Store in small aliquots under liquid nitrogen.
6. RNase A, 10 mg/mL: Store at –20°C.
7. Cycloheximide, 6 mg/mL: Store in small aliquots at –20°C.
8. Non-radiolabeled methionine, 6 mM: Store in small aliquots at –20°C.

2.4. Immunoprecipitation of Proteins Translated In Vitro

1. Denaturation buffer: 50 mM Tris-HCl, pH 7.5, 1 mM EDTA, 0.5% SDS: Store at 4°C or room temperature, but chill prior to use.
2. TNA: 50 mM Tris-HCl, pH 7.5, 150 mM NaCl, 1 mM EDTA, 0.33% (v/v) Triton X-100, 0.66 mg/mL bovine serum albumin, Fraction V: Store at 4°C.
3. Antiserum specific for HCV NS2 and/or NS3: Store in small aliquots at –20°C.
4. PANSORBIN cells (Calbiochem, La Jolla, CA, cat. #507861): Store at 4°C.
5. TNAS: Prepare using the recipe for TNA, but include 0.1% (w/v) SDS: Store at 4°C.
6. TNE: 50 mM Tris-HCl, pH 7.5, 150 mM NaCl, 1 mM EDTA: Store at 4°C or room temperature, but chill prior to use.
7. Protein sample buffer: 62.5 mM Tris-HCl, pH 6.8, 2% (w/v) SDS, 10% (v/v) glycerol, 5% (v/v) β-mercaptoethanol, 0.01% bromphenol blue. Store at –20°C.
8. Materials for SDS-PAGE and autoradiography:
   a. 40% acrylamide, 37.5:1 ratio of acrylamide to *bis*-acrylamide (Fisher Scientific, Pittsburgh, PA, cat. #BP1410-1): Store at 4°C.
   b. 1.5 M Tris-HCl, pH 8.8: Store at room temperature.
   c. ddH$_2$O.
   d. Ammonium persulfate, 10%: Make up fresh each time, or store at 4°C for up to 1 mo.
   e. TEMED (Sigma Chemical Co., St. Louis, MO, cat. # T-8133): Store at room temperature or 4°C.
   f. 40% Acrylamide, 19:1 ratio of acrylamide to *bis*-acrylamide (Fisher Scientific, cat. # BP1406-1): Store at 4°C.
   g. 0.5 M Tris-HCl, pH 6.8: Store at room temperature.
   h. Electrophoresis buffer: 50 mM Tris base, 384 mM glycine, 0.1% SDS. Store at room temperature.
   i. Fixative: 30% methanol, 10% glacial acetic acid.
   j. X-OMAT™ AR5 scientific imaging film (Eastman Kodak Company, Rochester, NY).

3. Methods

3.1. Linearization of the DNA Template

1. Digest 5 μg of the expression plasmid construct in a total reaction volume of 50 μL for 1–2 h with a restriction enzyme that cleaves at a unique site located just downstream of the translational stop codon (or poly A tail for pCITE derivatives). Use the buffer and incubation temperature recommended by the enzyme supplier.
2. Extract the digest twice with an equal volume of a 1:1 mixture of chloroform and phenol that has been equilibrated with Tris-HCl, pH 7.9.
3. Precipitate the DNA by mixing it with a 1/10 vol of 3 M sodium acetate, pH 5.2, followed by 2.5 vol of absolute ethanol and incubating it for 20 min at –20°C (*see* **Note 3**).
4. Pellet the DNA by microcentrifugation for 10 min at top speed.
5. Remove the supernatant, and wash the pellet by vortexing it in 300 μL of 70% ethanol.
6. Pellet the DNA again by microcentrifugation for 8 min at top speed.
7. Remove the supernatant, and dry the pellet by lyophilizing it briefly or by allowing it to air-dry.
8. Dissolve the dried pellet in 25 μL of sterile ddH_2O.
9. To check the extent of linearization and recovery of the template, mix 8 μL of dd H_2O and 1 μL of 10X DNA sample buffer with 1 μL of linearized DNA, and analyze it by agarose-gel electrophoresis.

3.2. Transcription of RNA In Vitro

1. Mix 1 μL of 10X T7 RNA polymerase buffer, 2.5 μL of 4 mM rNTPs, 0.5 μL of 400 mM DTT, 0.5 μL of RNasin, 0.2 μL of ^{3}H UTP, and 0.5 μL of T7 RNA polymerase; then add 4.8 μL of the linearized template, mix, and incubate the reaction at 37°C for 1 h (*see* **Notes 4–7**).
2. Dilute the reaction mixture by adding 40 μL of TE containing 0.5 μL of 400 mM DTT and 0.25 μL of RNasin. The transcribed RNA may be analyzed immediately or stored at –80°C.
3. Mix 6.5 μL of sterile ddH_2O and 1 μL of 10X DNA sample buffer with 2.5 μL of the diluted reaction mixture, and analyze it by normal agarose-gel electrophoresis. A band corresponding to the DNA template should still be visible, but a bright band corresponding to the RNA transcript should now be present below it.
4. To begin quantitation of the RNA yield, spot 0.5 μL of the diluted reaction mixture on duplicate pieces of DE81 paper. Allow the spotted sample to dry on the first piece as a representative of the total amount of ^{3}H UTP, but place the second piece immediately after the sample has been spotted into approx 50 mL of 0.5 M Na_2HPO_4, and incubate it for 5 min with agitation.
5. Wash the second piece of DE81 paper three times by changing the sodium phosphate solution and agitating each time for 5 min to remove unincorporated nucleotides.

6. Rinse the washed DE81 paper once briefly in dd H_2O to remove salt and once briefly in 95% ethanol to accelerate subsequent evaporation.
7. Submerge the dried pieces of DE81 paper in separate vials containing scintillation fluid, and determine the amount of ^3H present in each by scintillation counting. Also count a blank vial containing scintillation fluid only for background determination.
8. The concentration of RNA transcribed during the reaction equals the moles of ribonucleotides present in the reaction multiplied by the average molecular weight of an incorporated ribonucleotide (320 g/mol) and the percent incorporation, divided by the volume of the diluted reaction mixture. For example, the concentration of RNA in ng/µL produced in the reaction described above is:

$$(4 \text{ mmol rNTP/1 L}) \times (1 \text{ L}/1 \times 10^6 \text{ µL}) \times 2.5 \text{ µL} \times$$
$$(1 \times 10^6 \text{ nmol}/1 \text{ nmol}) \times (320 \text{ ng/mol}) \times \% \text{ incorporation} \times (1/50 \text{ µL})$$

3.3. Cell-Free Translation of In Vitro Transcripts

1. For in vitro translation of the synthesized mRNA, mix 7 µL of rabbit reticulocyte lysate, 0.2 mL of RNasin, 0.2 µL of an amino acid mixture lacking methionine (this mixture is included in the rabbit reticulocyte system purchased from Promega), 12 µCi of ^{35}S methionine, 50–100 ng of the RNA transcript, and enough sterile ddH_2O to bring the final reaction volume to 10 µL. Incubate the translation reaction at 30°C for 1 h (*see* **Notes 8–11**).
2. Terminate translation by adding RNase A, cycloheximide, and cold methionine to final concentrations of 10, 300, and 44.8 mg/mL (0.3 m*M*), respectively.
3. The translation products may be analyzed immediately by direct SDS-PAGE and autoradiography of a mixture containing 2 µL of the translation reaction and 2 µL of 2X protein sample buffer, by immunoprecipitation prior to SDS-PAGE and autoradiography, or they may be stored at –80°C for later analysis (*see* **Note 12**).

3.4. Immunoprecipitation of Proteins Translated In Vitro

1. Mix 23 µL of denaturation buffer with 2 µL of the translation reaction (*see* **Note 13**), heat the sample for 10 min at 70°C, add 100 µL of TNA, and mix the sample before adding an appropriate amount of an antiserum that recognizes HCV NS2 and/or NS3. The optimal amount of antiserum should be determined empirically, but we typically use 2.5 µL of a polyclonal rabbit antiserum.
2. Incubate the diluted translation products and antiserum 4–20 h at 4°C with rocking to allow the formation of immune complexes.
3. Wash an appropriate amount (*see* **Subheading 3.4.4.**) of PANSORBIN cells by pelleting them for 20 s at top speed in a microcentrifuge and resuspending them in 0.5 mL of cold TNAS; repeat this cycle four more times for a total of five washes.
4. After the PANSORBIN cells have been washed for the last time, resuspend them in enough TNAS to restore their original volume, add 50 µL of the pre-washed PANSORBIN cells to the samples containing the immune complexes, and incubate for 1–2 h more at 4°C.

5. Wash the immunoprecipitates three times with cold TNAS as described above for the PANSORBIN cells, once with cold TNE, and resuspend them in 30 μL of protein sample buffer.
6. Heat the sample for 5 min at 90°C, pellet the PANSORBIN cells as described above, and transfer the supernatant to a new microcentrifuge tube. The samples may be frozen or analyzed immediately by SDS-PAGE followed by autoradiography. If the samples are frozen, they should be reheated immediately before SDS-PAGE.

4. Notes

1. Rabbit reticulocytes have been reported to lose activity rapidly at –20°C and more slowly, but progressively, when stored at –80°C. However, activity is said to be retained for years when the lysates are stored in small aliquots under liquid nitrogen without multiple cycles of freezing and thawing *(19)*.
2. ^{35}S methionine is sensitive to decomposition by sulfoxide formation, with a rate proportionate to the temperature. Storage in small aliquots at –80°C with a minimum number of freeze/thaw cycles helps to preserve the ^{35}S methionine by delaying the process of oxidation.
3. Beginning with this step and for every step afterward until termination of the translation reaction, great care must be taken to avoid contamination by RNases, which are extremely stable and highly active enzymes that do not require cofactors. Once the DNA template has been extracted with phenol/chloroform, which removes and inactivates RNases in addition to other proteins, all materials used for preparation of the DNA template and the transcription and translation reactions must be RNase-free. Only sterile, disposable plasticware or baked glassware should come in contact with the samples and solutions. The water used for preparation of solutions should be distilled, deionized, and free from microbial contamination. Chemicals should be measured in sterile, disposable weigh boats and should not be touched by a spatula unless it has been baked. If the pH of a solution needs to be adjusted, remove small aliquots for pH measurements, and dispose of them after contact with the probe. Treatment with diethyl pyrocarbonate (DEPC), which inactivates many proteins, including RNases, by chemical modification, is sometimes recommended for the preparation of RNase-free solutions. However, DEPC is difficult to remove, and any that remains can also modify RNA by carboxymethylation on purine residues, which can significantly reduce the efficiency of that RNA as a template for translation in cell-free systems.
4. The ^{3}H UTP is supplied in 50% ethanol, which can inhibit the transcription reaction unless added to a final ethanol concentration of <1%.
5. The presence of DTT is essential for the stability and activity of RNasin, so it should always be mixed into a solution before RNasin is added.
6. The template should be added to the reaction mixture last to prevent precipitation of DNA by the spermidine present in the 10X T7 transcription buffer.

7. Translation from in vitro transcripts lacking an IRES sequence may be improved by the addition of cap analog (m^{7}G[5']ppp[5']G) to the transcription reaction. The optimal amount should be determined empirically, using a concentration of 0.5 mM as a reference point.
8. The use of pure ^{35}S methionine in the translation reaction rather than a crude metabolic label is important for the efficient incorporation of radioactivity into nascent polypeptides.
9. Remember that any experiments that require the addition of Ca^{2+} to the reticulocyte lysate may result in reactivation of micrococcal nuclease and degradation of the input RNA.
10. At temperatures >30°C, the lysate usually fails to maintain a linear incorporation rate, perhaps owing to the gradual activation of HRI.
11. Since some level of endogenous mRNA translation persists after nuclease treatment, a mock translation reaction should always be performed without input RNA so that polypeptides of interest can be distinguished from the endogenous background.
12. Rabbit reticulocyte lysates contain a large amount of globin, which usually migrates at a position close to that of the 14-kDa lysozyme standard present in many protein mol-wt markers and distorts the migration of similarly sized proteins. If proteins that migrate in the vicinity of globin are to be analyzed, the translation reaction should be immunoprecipitated to remove globin prior to electrophoresis. Alternatively, load a smaller amount of the translation reaction on the gel and expose the autoradiograph longer to obtain an equivalent signal with less distortion.
13. The methods presented in this chapter utilize denaturing conditions for immunoprecipitation, because rabbit antisera are usually raised against denatured antigens. However, the substitution of nonionic detergents, such as Triton X-100 or Nonidet P-40, for SDS may facilitate antigen recognition by some antisera, such as those collected from human HCV patients.

References

1. Hijikata, M., Kato, N., Ootsuyama, Y., Nakagawa, M., and Shimotohno, K. (1991) Gene mapping of the putative structural region of the hepatitis C virus genome by in vitro processing analysis. *Proc. Natl. Acad. Sci. USA* **88,** 5547–5551.
2. Lin, C., Lindenbach, B. D., Prágai, B., McCourt, D. W., and Rice, C. M. (1994) Processing of the hepatitis C virus E2-NS2 region: identification of p7 and two distinct E2-specific products with different C termini. *J. Virol.* **68,** 5063–5073.
3. Mizushima, H., Hijikata, H., Asabe, S.-I., Hirota, M., Kimura, K., and Shimotohno, K. (1994) Two hepatitis C virus glycoprotein E2 products with different C termini. *J. Virol.* **68,** 6215–6222.
4. Selby, M. J., Glazer, E., Masiarz, F., and Houghton, M. (1994) Complex processing and protein:protein interactions in the E2:NS2 region of HCV. *Virology* **204,** 114–122.

5. Bartenschlager, R., Ahlborn-Laake, L., Mous, J., and Jacobsen, H. (1993) Nonstructural protein 3 of the hepatitis C virus encodes a serine-type proteinase required for cleavage at the NS3/4 and NS4/5 junctions. *J. Virol.* **67**, 3835–3844.
6. Eckart, M. R., Selby, M., Masiarz, F., Lee, C., Berger, K., Crawford, K., Kuo, C., Kuo, G., Houghton, M., and Choo, Q.-L. (1993) The hepatitis C virus encodes a serine protease involved in processing of the putative nonstructural proteins from the viral polyprotein precursor. *Biochem. Biophys. Res. Comm.* **192**, 399–406.
7. Grakoui, A., McCourt, D. W., Wychowski, C., Feinstone, S. M., and Rice, C. M. (1993) Characterization of the hepatitis C virus-encoded serine proteinase: determination of proteinase-dependent polyprotein cleavage sites. *J. Virol.* **67**, 2832–2843.
8. Hijikata, M., Mizushima, H., Akagi, T., Mori, S., Kakiuchi, N., Kato, N., et al. (1993) Two distinct proteinase activities required for the processing of a putative nonstructural precursor protein of hepatitis C virus. *J. Virol.* **67**, 4665–4675.
9. Manabe, S., Fuke, I., Tanishita, O., Kaji, C., Gomi, Y., Yoshida, S., Mori, S., et al. (1994) Production of nonstructural proteins of hepatitis C virus requires a putative viral protease encoded by NS3. *Virology* **198**, 636–644.
10. Tomei, L., Failla, C., Santolini, E., De Francesco, R., and La Monica, N. (1993) NS3 is a serine protease required for processing of hepatitis C virus polyprotein. *J. Virol.* **67**, 4017–4026.
11. Grakoui, A., McCourt, D. W., Wychowski, C., Feinstone, S. M., and Rice, C. M. (1993) A second hepatitis C virus-encoded proteinase. *Proc. Natl. Acad. Sci. USA* **90**, 10,583–10,587.
12. Hirowatari, Y., Hijikata, M., Tanji, Y., Nyunoya, H., Mizushima, H., Kimura, K., et al. (1993) Two proteinase activities in HCV polypeptide expressed in insect cells using baculovirus vector. *Arch. Virol.* **133**, 349–356.
13. Reed, K. E., Grakoui, A., and Rice, C. M. (1995) Hepatitis C virus-encoded NS2-3 protease: cleavage-site mutagenesis and requirements for bimolecular cleavage. *J. Virol.* **69**, 4127–4136.
14. Santolini, E., Pacini, L., Fipaldini, C., Migliaccio, G., and La Monica, N. (1995) The NS2 protein of hepatitis C virus is a transmembrane polypeptide. *J. Virol.* **69**, 7461–7471.
15. Pieroni, L., Santolini, E., Fipaldini, C., Pacini, L., Migliaccio, G., and LaMonica, N. (1997) In vitro study of the NS2-3 protease of hepatitis C virus. *J. Virol.* **71**, 6373–6380.
16. Jiang, W. and Bond, J. S. (1992) Families of metalloendopeptidases and their relationships. *FEBS Lett.* **312**, 110–114.
17. Fuerst, T. R., Niles, E. G., Studier, F. W., and Moss, B. (1986) Eukaryotic transient-expression system based on recombinant vaccinia virus that synthesizes bacteriophage T7 RNA polymerase. *Proc. Natl. Acad. Sci. USA* **83**, 8122–8126.
18. Moss, B., Elroy-Stein, O., Mizukami, T., Alexander, W. A., and Fuerst, T. R. (1990) New mammalian expression vectors. *Nature (London)* **348**, 91,92.
19. Pelham, H. R. B. and Jackson, R. J. (1976) An efficient mRNA-dependent translation system from reticulocyte lysates. *Eur. J. Biochem.* **67**, 247–256.
20. Grakoui, A., Wychowski, C., Lin, C., Feinstone, S. M., and Rice, C. M. (1993) Expression and identification of hepatitis C virus polyprotein cleavage products. *J. Virol.* **67**, 1385–1395.

31

Expression and Characterization of HCV NS3 Protease

Eric D'Souza, Norman Gray, Malcolm Ellis, and Berwyn E. Clarke

1. Introduction

The overexpression of a gene in a heterologous system is often the prelude to or the prerequisite of the elucidation and characterization of a given protein, in particular where the protein is difficult to obtain in sufficient quantity from natural sources. Prokaryotic expression systems, in particular *Escherichia coli* have been exploited successfully for a number of viral proteins. A large number of *E. coli* expression systems are currently commercially available that offer the investigator a large number of choices with regard to promoter choice, site of expression, fusions, and so forth. Since the variety and number of expression systems available are extensive, it is not within the scope of this chapter to discuss them fully, and the final choice of expression system used, is often arrived at empirically and often reflects the investigator's "favored system."

Hepatitis C virus (HCV) NS3 protease is processed from the viral polyprotein by the action of two viral coded proteases. The cleavage to release the N-terminal of NS3 is carried out by a metallo-protease coded for by sequences contained in NS2 and NS3 *(1,2)*. The release of the C-terminal of NS3 is a *cis*-cleavage event, and is mediated by the serine protease contained within the N-terminal third of the NS3 gene product *(3–5)*. All subsequent processing of the non-structural portion of the polyprotein are *trans*-cleavage events, and are also carried out by the serine protease contained in the NS3 gene product. The C-terminal two-thirds of the NS3 gene contains a NTP-ase dependent RNA-helicase activity *(6,7)*. Studies have demonstrated that the two enzymatic functions of NS3 function independently and that deletion of the helicase domain does not affect the protease activity *(8)*. The protease domain can be defined as amino acid 1-181, of the NS3 gene. The first 22 amino acids are not essential for cleavage activity. These N-terminal residues are, however, involved in interactions with NS4A, a cofactor for NS3 mediated cleavages in particular the NS4A/NS4B, and NS4B/NS5A cleavage sites *(9–11)*.

A fragment of the NS3 gene coding for amino acids 1–183 was cloned into the vector pET19B downstream of a T7 promoter and used to transform BL21 (DE3) strain of *E. coli*. Fermentations were carried out at 37°C and inductions achieved using 1 mM IPTG (final concentration). The protease when expressed under these conditions is produced as insoluble aggregates within inclusion bodies. Measuring the activity of NS3 protease prepared in this way is made possible by refolding or renaturing the protein. The refolding conditions have been optimized and are described in **Note 4**.

The enzyme assay routinely used depends on the proteolytic cleavage by NS3 protease of a peptide that mimics the NS3-dependent NS5A/NS5B cleavage site in the HCV polyprotein. Enzyme activity is assessed by reversed-phase high performance liquid chromatography (HPLC) analysis of the cleavage products. The rate of cleavage is enhanced by adding NS4A peptide cofactor in a 1:1 molar ratio with the enzyme. This biochemical assay allows for the measurement of the kinetic parameters of the proteolytic cleavage and the evaluation of compounds that inhibit the enzyme reaction. The HPLC peptide assay can also be used to study the NS3-dependent cleavage of the NS4A/NS4B and NS4B/NS5A junctions in the HCV genome, using synthetic peptides based on the natural sequences. The efficient cleavage of these substrates is more dependent on the presence of the NS4A cofactor in the reaction than is the cleavage of the NS5A/NS5B substrate.

In this chapter we describe the extraction, purification, refolding, and assay conditions for obtaining catalytically active HCV protease from inclusion bodies produced in *E. coli*.

2. Materials

2.1. Cell Breakage

1. Cell paste (*see* **Subheading 3.1.**).
2. E-64 (Sigma Chemical Co. Ltd., Poole, Dorset, UK).
3. 3,4-DCI (Sigma).
4. *N*-Acetyl pepstatin (Sigma).
5. Leupeptin (Sigma).
6. Cell breakage buffer: 25 mM Tris-HCl, pH 8.0, 150 mM NaCl, 2 mM β-mercaptoethanol, 0.01% (v/v) Triton X-100, 10 μM E-64, 1 μM 3,4-DCI, 5 μM *N*-acetyl pepstatin, and 20 μM leupeptin.
7. Brandon 'Sonfier 450' cell sonicator with a 1 cm probe.

2.2. Inclusion Body Extraction

1. Urea, sequential-grade (Pierce & Warriner, Chester, Cheshire, UK); store at 4°C (*see* **Note 4**).
2. Washing buffer: 25 mM HEPES, pH 7.5, and 2 mM β-mercaptoethanol.
3. Solubilizing buffer: 25 mM HEPES, pH 7.5, 8 M urea, and 20 mM β-mercaptoethanol.

2.3. Protein Purification

1. FPLC (Pharmacia, St Albans, Hertfordshire, UK).
2. Resource Q (6 mL) column (Pharmacia).
3. Resource S (6 mL) column (Pharmacia).
4. HEPES, MES, β-mercaptoethanol, and NaCl (Sigma).
5. Urea, sequenal grade (Pierce & Warriner), store at 4°C (*see* **Note 4**).
6. Superdex 200 Hi-load 26/60 column (Pharmacia).
7. MES-urea-mecaptoethanol buffer: 25 mM MES, pH 5.5, 8 M urea and 2 mM β-mercaptoethanol.

2.4. Refolding

1. 3-(3-Cholamidopropyl-dimethylamio)-1-propane-sulfonate (CHAPS) (Sigma).
2. Refolding buffer: 50 mM Tris-HCl, pH 7.4, 2 mM dithiothreitol, 50% (v/v) glycerol, 10 mM CHAPS, and 10 mM MgSO$_4$.

2.5. Proteolytic Cleavage Assay

1. NS3 stock solution (3 mg/mL), stored at –70°C. (type 1a).
2. NS4A peptide cofactor: H-KKGSVVIVGRVVLSGKK-OH, 200 μM stock prepared in 0.5 M Tris-HCl, pH 7.4, stored at –20°C.
3. 5A/5B peptide substrate, Ac-EDVVPCSMSY-NH2, purchased from Peptide & Protein Research (PPR) Consultants, Washington, Singer Laboratories, University of Exeter, 2 mM stock prepared in 0.5 M Tris-HCl pH 7.4, stored at –20°C.
4. HPLC reagents:
   a. Trifluoroacetic acid (Fisher HPLC-Grade, Loughborough, UK).
   b. Acetonitrile (Rathburn HPLC-grade S, Walkerburn, UK).
5. HPLC column: Brownlee reverse phase HPLC column, 100 × 4.6 mm Spheri-5 ODS 5 μi.

3. Methods

3.1. Cell Breakage

1. The cell paste (10 g wet weight) was thawed by mixing with 40 mL of ice-cold cell breakage buffer prior to sonication (*see* **Note 1**).
2. The sonication probe should be placed just below the surface of the cell suspension and sonicated at 40 cycles/s using five 30 s bursts with 60 s cooling between each burst (*see* **Note 2**).
3. The broken cell suspension should be checked under a microscope to confirm that the cells are broken.

3.2. Inclusion Body Extraction

The broken cell suspension is brought up to 20% (v/v) with glycerol and the spun at 10,000g for 20 min at 4°C (*see* **Note 3**).

1. Carefully decant the supernatant (*see* **Note 3**) and resuspend the pellet in 25 mM Tris-HCl, pH 8.0, 20% glycerol (v/v), 2 mM β-mercaptoethanol and 0.01% (v/v) Triton X-100.
2. Spin at 10,000g for 20 min at 4°C and carefully decant the supernatant.
3. Resuspend the pellet in washing buffer, and spin at 10,000g for 20 min at 4°C.
4. Decant the supernatant and remove the pellet for weighing. Solubilize the pellet in solubilizing buffer to a final concentration of 2–3 mg/mL using a magnetic stirrer with gentle agitation (*see* **Note 4**).
5. If, after 60 min the solution is still cloudy, it should be spun at 30,000g for 20 min and the supernatant carefully decanted.

3.3. Protein Purification

The resolubilised NS3 was loaded onto a Resource Q column that had been equilibrated with solubilizing buffer. The unbound protein was pooled and the column cleaned with 5 column volumes of the same buffer with the addition 2 M NaCl (*see* **Note 5**). The pH of unbound protein pool is lowered to 5.5 by adding MES solid and diluted four-fold using 8 M urea and 2 mM β-mercaptoethanol (*see* **Note 6**). The protein was loaded onto a Resource S column that had been equilibrated in MES-urea-mercaptoethanol buffer. The column was washed with 5 column volumes of the above buffer and eluted from the column with a 0–0.4 M linear gradient of NaCl in 20 column volumes, collecting 5 mL fractions (*see* **Note 6**). The NS3 elutes at approx 0.2 M NaCl. The fractions were analyzed by SDS-PAGE and those containing the NS3 pooled. If purity of >95% is desired, the NS3 can be further purified by gel permeation chromatography. This involves the use of a Superdex 200 column equilibrated in MES-urea-mercaptoethanol buffer with 150 mM NaCl (*see* **Note 7**).

The purified NS3 should be diluted to 3 mg/mL in MES-urea-mercaptoethanol buffer with 150 mM NaCl, aliquoted, and then stored at –70°C until required (*see* **Note 8**).

3.4. Refolding

Refolding of NS3 is carried out in refolding buffer. The stock solution of NS3 (3 mg/mL) is slowly added to the refolding buffer at 4°C (*see* **Note 9**) and gently mixed. The mixture is kept on ice for >1 h before use (*see* **Note 10**).

Substrate

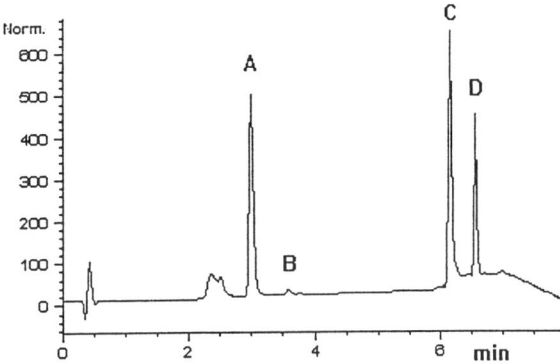

Substrate + NS3

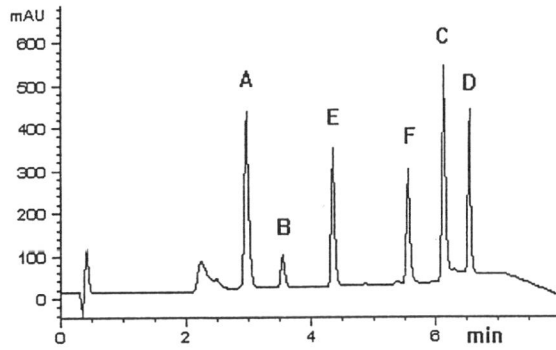

Fig. 1. HPCL profiles before (**top**) and after (**bottom**) NS3 cleavage of 5A/5B substrate, with 3 h incubation. The peaks are (**A,B**) DTT; (**C**) Ac-EDVVPCSMSY-NH2; (**D**) CHAPS; (**E**) C-terminal cleavage product SMSY-NH2 (4.4 min); and (**F**) N-terminal cleavage product Ac-EDVVPC (5.6 min).

3.5. Proteolytic Cleavage Assay

1. After the refolding period the concentration of DTT is increased to 10 mM and 1 Eq of NS4A peptide (*see* **Note 11**) added. The mixture is aliquoted into the required volumes for assay (typically 75 µL) and the enzyme is preincubated with NS4A for 15 min at 30°C. The enzyme reaction is initiated by the addition of NS5A/NS5B peptide substrate, normally at 200 µM (**Note 12**). The reaction mixture is incubated for 1–2 h at 30°C (**Note 13**).
2. The reaction is stopped by the addition of 0.2% TFA. The samples are kept on ice or frozen until analysis by reversed-phase HPLC, using a gradient of 0.5–55% acetonitrile over 8 min, at a flow rate of 3 mL/min. UV detection is at 214 nm (**Fig. 1**).

4. Notes
4.1. Cell Breakage

1. The cell breakage buffer is a fairly standard mixture with the inclusion of proteinase inhibitors (E-64, 3,4-DCI, *N*-acetyl pepstatin and leupeptin) being a precautionary measure to avoid unwanted proteolysis (the proteinase inhibitor cocktail is available from Boehringer-Mannheim in tablet form; this saves time in preparing stock solutions). Maintaining the temperature at 4°C should normally be adequate, since inclusions are resistant to proteolysis.
2. The crucial factors to obtain efficient cell breakage during sonication are not to exceed 20% (v/v) wet wt cells to cell breakage buffer, avoid frothing, and maintaining 4°C. To aid cooling during sonication, it is useful to add salt to the ice surrounding the sonication vessel. The speed of cooling can also be enhanced by placing the sonication vessel on dry ice for 30–60 s (if the contents freeze, thaw before the next round of sonication). Lysozyme, when added at 0.5 mg/mL for a minimum of 30 min prior to sonication, can enhance cell breakage. If, after sonication, the broken cell suspension appears extremely viscous, the suspension can be sonicated again to shear the released DNA or treated with DNase (add $MgCl_2$ to 10 mM followed by 5 μg/mL of DNase I) for 30–60 min. For preparative work (above 50 mL) it may be necessary to use a different technique of cell breakage, e.g., homogenization (Mantin-Gaulin) or bead milling.
3. The 20% glycerol has the effect of maintaining a large proportion of the cell debris in suspension while allowing the denser inclusion bodies to pellet. The supernatant from the first spin should be stored at 4°C in order to determine if significant inclusion bodies remain. If significant inclusion bodies remain in the supernatant, it should be recentrifuged 20,000g for 20 min. It is a sensible precaution to retain all supernatants until they can be checked by SDS-PAGE. Careful washing of inclusion bodies can result in a final pellet in which the expressed protein is of >75% purity. This can ease the downstream purification procedure.

4.2. Inclusion Body Extraction

4. The use of ultrapure urea is essential, since the formation of cyanate ions, which react with amino groups on the NS3, will result in the formation of carbamylated derivatives. If sequenal-grade urea is not available, use ultrapure urea and pass the solution through a mixed-bed ion-exchanger, e.g., AG 501-X8 (D) resin (Bio-Rad Laboratories Ltd, Hemel Hempstead, Herts, UK). Dissolution of urea is fairly endothermic but the use of heating to speed up solvation should be avoided, since this enhances the formation of cyanate ions. The inclusion body pellet was solubilized in urea, since the uncharged nature of urea allows the use of ion-exchange as a purification procedure. The high level of β-mercaptoethanol is to ensure that all the NS3 is in a reduced state.

4.3. Protein Purification

5. The use of an anion-exchange column (Resource Q) binds many of the contaminating *E.coli* proteins while allowing the NS3, which possess a relatively high theoretical pI of 9.8, to pass through the column. At this stage, the NS3 will be approx 80–90% pure as assessed by SDS-PAGE.
6. In order to bind the NS3 to the cation-exchange column (Resource S), the pH has to be lowered to 5.5. It is important to dilute the sample in order to lower the conductivity; otherwise, the NS3 will not bind to the cation-exchange column. This step increases purity to 90–95% and concentrates the NS3 to approx 15–20 mg/mL.
7. The gel-permeation chromatography step may not be necessary, since purity of >95% is frequently achieved with the two ion-exchange steps. The loading range of the Superdex 200 Hi-load 26/60 is 3–15 mL (the use of a 16/60 or HR10/30 columns are suitable for lower loadings).
8. The stock concentration of NS3 at 3 mg/mL is convenient for refolding. It is stable for at least 12 mo at $-70°C$.

4.4. Refolding

9. The factors that exert most influence over refolding of NS3 are protein concentration, temperature, pH, detergent (CHAPS), and reducing agent (dithiothreitol). They all reduce the degree of aggregation and maintain NS3 in an active state. It is vital to ensure that the refolding temperature is 4°C since even a temperature three or four degrees higher will result in increased aggregation. Refolding on a small scale (up to 20 mL) can be achieved by gently adding the NS3 and then refluxing carefully in a pipet. For larger volumes care needs to be given to ensure adequate mixing during the period of addition, since the NS3 will collect at surface of the refolding buffer (owing to the presence of 50% glycerol) and aggregation will occur.
    a. The detergent CHAPS, at 10mM, is above its critical micelle concentration. It increases enzyme activity, possibly by incorporating the NS3 into the micelles during refolding and stabilizing the protein. A high concentration of glycerol provides an hydrophobic environment for the enzyme and is the most important factor for observing good activity. It was found that the enzyme concentration could not greatly be increased beyond 40 µg/mL before seeing protein precipitation. The limits of solubility should always be checked with each new enzyme preparation.
    b. An excessive amount of 8 M urea added with the enzyme will interfere with activity. Usually no more than 1 µL 8 M urea/100 µL reaction mixture is added.
10. Refolded enzyme can be stored. It was found to be stable for 6–8 h at room temperature, up to 5 d at 4°C and >1 mo at $-20°C$.

4.5. Proteolytic Cleavage Assay

11. The NS4A peptide includes residues 21–34 of the complete 1a Glasgow NS4A protein. This region has been shown to be sufficient for cofactor activity. To increase solubility, lysine residues have been added at each end, and amino acid 22 has been changed from cysteine to serine. NS4A is added in stoichiometric amounts to the enzyme. It does not greatly stimulate the NS5A/NS5B cleavage, but its presence in the reaction becomes more important when examining the cleavage of peptides based on the NS4A/NS4B and NS4B/NS5A NS3-dependent sites of proteolysis.
12. The natural NS5A/NS5B substrate has a cysteine residue in the P2 position. The NS5A/NS5B peptide used in the assay contains proline in the P2 position to increase solubility and make synthesis of the peptide easier.
13. Because of the small volumes of extra DTT, NS4A peptide, and peptide substrate added, the levels of the other reagents in the final reaction mixture are essentially the same as in the refolding mixture.

References

1. Hijikata, M., Mizushima, H., Akagi, T., Mori, S., Kakiuchi, N., Kato, N., et al. (1993) Two distinct protease activities required for the processing of a putative non-structural precursor protein of Hepatitis C Virus. *J.Virol.* **67**, 4665–4675.
2. Grakoui, A., McCourt, D. W., Wychowski, C., Feinstone, S. M., and Rice, C. M. (1993) A second Hepatitis C virus-encoded proteinase. *Proc. Natl. Acad. Sci. USA* **90**, 10,583–10,587.
3. D'Souza, E. A., O'Sullivan, E., Amphlett, E. M., Rowlands, D. J., Sangar, D. V., and Clarke, B. E. (1994) Analysis of NS3-mediated processing of Hepatitis C virus non-structural region in vitro. *J. Gen. Virol.* **75**, 3469–3476.
4. Grakoui, A., McCourt, D. W., Wychowski, C., Feinstone, S. M., and Rice, C. M. (1993) Characterisation of Hepatitis C virus-encoded serine proteinase: Determination of proteinase-dependent polyprotein cleavage sites. *J. Virol.* **67**, 2832–2843.
5. Bartenschlager, R., Ahlborn-Laake, L., Mous, J., and Jacobsen, H. (1993) Nonstructural protein 3 of the Hepatitis C virus encodes a serine-type proteinase required for cleavage at the NS3/4 and NS4/5 Junction. *J. Virol.* **67**, 3835–3844.
6. Bartenschlager, R., Ahlborn-Laake, L., Yasargil, K., Mous, J., and Jacobsen, H. (1995) Substrate determinants for cleavage in *cis* and *trans* by the Hepatitis C virus NS3 proteinase. *J.Virol.* **69**, 198–205.
7. Lin, C., Pragai, B. M., Grakoui, A., Xu, J., and Rice, C. M. (1994) Hepatitis C virus NS3 serine proteinase: trans-cleavage requirements and processing kinetics. *J. Virol.* **68**, 8147–8157.
8. Han, D. S., Hahm, B., Rho, H., and Jang, S. K. (1995) Identification of the protease domain in NS3 of Hepatitis C virus. *J. Gen. Virol.* **76**, 985–993.
9. Bartenschlager, R., Lohmann, V., Wilkinson, T., and Koch, J. O. (1995) Complex formation between the NS3 serine-type proteinase of the Hepatitis C

virus and NS4A and its importance for polyprotein maturation. *J. Virol.* **69,** 7519–7528.
10. Lin, C. and Rice, C. M. (1995) The Hepatitis C virus NS3 serine proteinase and NS4A cofactor: Establishment of a cell-free trans-processing assay. *Proc. Natl. Acad. Sci. USA.* **92,** 7622–7626.
11. Failla, C., Tomei, L., and De Francesco, R. (1994) Both NS3 and NS4A are required for proteolytic processing of Hepatitis C virus nonstructural proteins. *J. Virol.* **68,** 3753–3760.

32

Expression and Characterization of the HCV NS3 Helicase Domain

Frank Preugschat, Mary H. Hanlon, Martin J. Rink, Berwyn E. Clarke, and David J. T. Porter

1. Introduction

The hepatitis C virus (HCV) NS3 protein has two distinct biochemical domains. The N-terminal 20 kDa has serine protease activity (*see* Chapter 31) and the C-terminal 50 kDa has both nucleoside triphosphatase (NTPase) and helicase activities *(1–4)*.

Helicases are essential for DNA and RNA metabolism *(5)*. They disrupt basepairing of duplex nucleic acid, translocating along the nucleic acid in either a 3' or 5' direction, with concomitant hydrolysis of NTPs *(6)*. Because helicases are conserved components of viral replication complexes, they are attractive targets for antiviral therapy. In order to study the biochemistry and the mechanism of these essential viral and cellular enzymes, a large supply of pure, active protein is required. This chapter concentrates on the optimization of expression through fermentation (**Subheadings 2.1.** and **3.1.**) and on the characterization of active enzyme (**Subheadings 3.3.–3.5.**).

The choice of expression system for the protein is dictated by the needs of the investigator. For example, Chapters 6 and 10 of this volume describe the use of viral and cellular systems for producing HCV proteins. We have chosen an *Escherichia coli* expression system for HCV helicase to produce a large amount of protein. The reader is referred to **ref.** 7 for the factors that go into selection of a suitable expression vector for *E. coli*.

Production of high levels of recombinant protein in *E. coli* can be limited by the availability of oxygen. In most fermenters, the metabolic rate of *E. coli* exceeds the rate of transport of oxygen across the air–water interface *(8)*. If oxygen becomes limiting, the culture switches from aerobic to anaerobic metabolism. Under anaerobic growth conditions, glucose is metabolized to organic acids that can inhibit cell growth and recombinant protein production *(9–11)*. Consequently, careful control of dissolved oxygen tension, cell-culture density, growth rates, pH, temperature, and media composition are important for high yields of recombinant protein. A standard method to obtain high yields of recombinant protein is to grow a culture quickly to high density, and then induce protein expression at low temperatures *(12)*. **Subheadings 3.1. and 4.1.** describe procedures used for optimization of expression of HCV helicase. The quality and quantity of recombinant protein can be rapidly assayed by Western blotting *(13)*. By iteratively changing growth conditions and monitoring the effects on overall protein production, expression conditions for the protein of interest can be rapidly optimized.

The object of an enzyme purification protocol is to isolate the activity of interest with maximal yield and purity. A successful purification protocol exploits the differences in charge, solubility, size, and specific binding sites between the enzyme and impurities. A simple purification scheme was developed for the HCV helicase domain expressed in *E. coli (1)*. The catalytic activity of the protein is determined by monitoring the rate of conversion of substrate to product under defined conditions, and the purification is carried out until the specific activity of a preparation reaches a constant value.

Proteins that are judged to be homogeneous by standard analytical methods (SDS-PAGE, quantitative amino acid analysis, N-terminal sequencing) may not retain catalytic activity. Consequently, it is important to characterize the purified enzyme not only by monitoring catalytic activity, but also by active site titration. A rapid and sensitive method for measuring the catalytic activity of a preparation of HCV helicase is to determine the number of ATP molecules hydrolyzed per unit of time. ATPase activity can be monitored by the oxidation of NADH coupled to the formation of ADP, as described by **Eqs. 1** and **2**.

Pyruvate kinase

$$ADP + phosphoenolpyruvate \rightarrow ATP + pyruvate \qquad (1)$$

Lactate dehydrogenase

$$Pyruvate + NADH \rightarrow Lactate + NAD^+ \qquad (2)$$

The oxidation of NADH is monitored by the associated absorbance change at 340 nm (using a $\Delta A_{340} = 6.22$ mM^{-1}/cm) *(14)*. **Subheading 3.3.** describes methods used to determine ATP hydrolysis by purified HCV helicase.

During the catalytic cycle, helicases bind nucleic acid. HCV helicase binds nucleic acid with high affinity (<10 nM in the absence of ATP) and with an approximate binding site size of 12 nucleotides. The enzyme undergoes a conformational change on binding nucleic acid that is associated with quenching of intrinsic tryptophan fluorescence *(1)*. By titrating protein fluorescence with a defined nucleic acid, the K_d and the concentration of binding sites present in a protein preparation can be estimated. Site concentration and the protein concentration (obtained by quantitative amino acid sequence analysis or UV absorbance) define the fraction of competent protein in a preparation. **Subheading 3.4.** describes methods used for estimating the fraction of correctly folded HCV helicase.

HCV helicase unwinds duplex RNA, duplex DNA, and RNA:DNA hybrids that have a 3' single-stranded tail of more than three nucleotides *(1,10)*. Typical helicase assays use a partially duplex substrate that has one radiolabeled-strand. The product (displaced radiolabeled strand) is separated from the substrate by electrophoresis through nondenaturing polyacrylamide gels and is detected by autoradiography. The displaced strand can also be detected in a scintillation proximity assay (SPA) format that does not require separation of the single-stranded product (ssDNA) from the duplex substrate. In a commercially available SPA helicase assay kit (Amersham Life Science), HCV helicase unwinds a short tritiated oligonucleotide, [^{3}H]ssDNA, annealed to M13 DNA. The assay conditions suggested by the manufacturer have been refined for the HCV helicase as described in **Subheading 3.5.** Because the DNA substrate is stable and the reagents are commercially available, this assay is convenient for routine monitoring of helicase activity.

Methods presented herein describe optimization of expression and characterization of HCV helicase. Using these methods, the investigator can quantitatively compare independent protein preparations to determine if differences in genotype or expression constructs physically alter the biochemical properties of the enzyme. This basic knowledge will facilitate the identification of potent and selective inhibitors of HCV helicase.

2. Materials

2.1. Fermentation

1. Bacto-tryptone, Bacto-yeast extract, Bacto-agar (Difco, Detroit, MI).
2. $(NH_4)_2SO_4$ (Gibco-BRL, Gaithersburg, MD).
3. KH_2PO_4, NaOH, NaCl, and 40% (w/v) glucose, steam-sterilized for 15 min at 121°C. (store at 4°C) (Baker, Phillipsburg, NJ).
4. Polypropylene glycol (M_r = 4000) (Aldrich, Milwaukee, WI).
5. IPTG (store at –20°C) (Boehringer Mannheim, Indianapolis, IN).
6. 5 g/L tetracycline in 50% ethanol (light-sensitive, filter-sterilized; store at 4°C) and 50 g/L ampicillin (filter-sterilized, store at –20°C) (Sigma Chemical Co., St. Louis, MO).

7. 10 L working volume, sterilize-in-place fermenter, equipped with pH, dissolved oxygen sensors, variable-speed agitator, and compressed air sparger (i.e., B. Braun, BIOSTAT ED-10, H/D ratio 3:1).

2.2. Western Blotting

1. 14% Tris-glycine gels (store at 4°C), Tris-Glycine SDS sample buffer (Novex part # LC2676), Tris-glycine SDS running buffer (Novex part # LC2675), carbonate transfer buffer (Novex part # LC2675), nitrocellulose membrane, and XCell II Mini-Cell and Blot module (Novex, San Diego, CA).
2. Prestained SDS-PAGE standards, low-mol-wt range (store at –20°C) (Bio-Rad, Hercules, CA).
3. β-Mercaptoethanol, Tris, NaCl, and Tween 20 (Sigma).
4. Anti-HCV mixed-titer performance panel (store at –20°C, **biohazard!**) (Boston Biomedica, Boston, MA).
5. Carnation Nonfat Dry Milk (Nestlé Food Co., Glendale, CA).
6. ECL Western blotting detection reagents, horseradish peroxidase linked (HRP)-protein A (store at 4°C), and Hyperfilm ECL (Amersham Corporation, Arlington Heights, IL).
7. Bleach (The Clorox Co., Oakland, CA).

2.3. ATPase Assay

1. Rabbit muscle pyruvate kinase and rabbit muscle lactate dehydrogenase (store at 4°C), and NADH (store desiccated at 4°C, and protect from light), phosphoenolpyruvate, MOPS, and $MgCl_2$ (Sigma).
2. ATP (store desiccated at –20°C), and poly(rU) (60 mM base solution in RNase-free water, store at –20°C) (Pharmacia Biotech, Piscataway, NJ).
3. Purified HCV helicase (store at –20°C).
4. SigmaPlot® (Jandel Scientific, San Rafael, CA).
5. UV/VIS adjustable-wavelength spectrometer, with kinetics software.

2.4. Binding Site Titration

1. Adjustable-wavelength fluorescence spectrometer.
2. $(rU)_{15}$ (in RNase-free water, store at –20°C), (Oligo Therapeutics, Inc., Wilsonville, OR).
3. Helicase and SigmaPlot® (*see above*).

2.5. Helicase Reagents

1. SPA plates: 96-well microtiter plates, such as Wallac (part #1450-410/512) or Costar (part # 3632). The plates must have a clear bottom and opaque sides.
2. Assay kit: Helicase [^{3}H]-SPA enzyme assay system (part #TRKQ7030, Amersham Life Science).
3. Radioactivity plate reader: 1450 Microbeta™ (Wallac) or equivalent liquid scintillation counter.

4. Helicase solution: 3 μM enzyme (A_{280} = 0.27) in 0.5 M NaCl, 50 mM MOPS, pH 7.0, and 3.5 mM MgCl$_2$. Store the solution in 100-μL aliquots at –20°C. Aliquots may be thawed and refrozen up to 20 times without loss of activity.
5. 5X assay buffer: 1 M ATP, 17.5 mM MgCl$_2$, 12.5 mM DTT, 0.125% Triton-X-100, and 250 mM MOPS, adjusted to pH 7.0 with 1 N NaOH. After filter sterilization (Corning part #25942-500), aliquot buffer into volumes sufficient for daily work, and store frozen (–70°C). Thaw buffer as needed, and keep on ice during the day. Buffer can be frozen and thawed multiple times.
6. Helicase working solution: Mix 1 mL deionized water, 1 mL 5X assay buffer, and 1 mL helicase solution. This solution may be kept on ice during the day without loss of activity.
7. Working substrate solution: Mix 1 mL 5X assay buffer, 4 mL deionized water, and 80 mL substrate solution (from assay kit). Make fresh daily.
8. EDTA/NaCl: Add 34.8 g NaCl to 100 mL 0.5 M EDTA, pH 8.0 (Gibco-BRL part #15575-088). Store at room temperature.
9. Stop solution: Mix 1.5 mL EDTA/NaCl and 1.5 mL stop/capture solution from assay kit (which contains 90 nM biotinylated DNA).
10. 5 M NaCl: Filter-sterilize (Corning 25942-500 filter system), and store at room temperature.
11. SPA beads: Add 10 mL 5 M NaCl to 100 mL SPA beads from the assay kit.

3. Methods
3.1. Fermentation

1. Transform expression plasmid into XL1-Blue cells (Stratagene, San Diego, CA), and plate onto Luria broth (10 g Bacto-tryptone, 10 g NaCl, 10 g Bacto-agar, 5 g Bacto-yeast extract/L, adjust to pH 7.5 with NaOH) and ampicillin (50 μg/mL)/tetracycline plates (15 μg/mL). Incubate at 37°C overnight.
2. Load the fermenter with rich nitrogen medium (300 g Bacto-tryptone, 150 g Bacto-yeast extract, 30 g [NH$_4$]$_2$SO$_4$, and 10 g KH$_2$PO$_4$, to 10 L with deionized water). Adjust to pH 7.0 with NaOH. Remove 100 mL into a baffled 500-mL erlenmeyer inoculum flask, and autoclave for 15 min at 121°C. Sterilize the fermenter for 20 min at 121°C.
3. Inoculate 100 mL of rich nitrogen medium, containing 0.3 mL of tetracycline and 0.1 mL of ampicillin, with a colony isolate from the transformation plate prepared above. Incubate in a shaker-incubator at 30°C, 300 rpm, for 14–18 h (final A_{600} should be ~1.5, using a water blank).
4. Set fermenter to initial fermentation conditions: temperature = 37°C, air flow = 4.00 STD L/minute, agitation = 100 rpm. Set dissolved oxygen tension at 100% of initial growth conditions. Since the oxygen demand increases during cell growth, maintain a dissolved oxygen level of 65% (relative to initial conditions) by varying agitator speed (*see* **Note 2**).
5. Transfer the inoculum flask to the fermenter. Add 30 mL of tetracycline, 10 mL of ampicillin, and 50 mL of glucose to the fermenter (final concentrations are: 15 μg/mL, 50 μg/mL, and 0.2% [w/v], respectively).

6. When the culture in the fermenter reaches an $A_{600} = 1.5$ (~4–5 h), reduce the temperature set point to 15°C.
7. When the culture reaches the induction density of $A_{600} = 1.8$–2.0 (~2 h later), mix 0.6 g IPTG into 50 mL of glucose, and add the solution to the fermenter (final concentration, 250 µM IPTG).
8. Allow the cells to incubate for 20 h. Remove 1-mL samples for Western blot analysis at 0, 3, and 20 h postinduction.
9. Harvest the cells by centrifugation, and freeze the cell pellet at –80°C.

3.2. Western Blotting

1. Resuspend 0-, 3-, and 20-h postinduction cell pellets in 250 µL of 1X SDS sample buffer containing 250 mM β-mercaptoethanol. Heat to 95°C for 5 min.
2. Assemble a 14% Tris-glycine gel in an XCell II apparatus, as described by the manufacturer. Fill the anode and cathode buffer chambers with 1X Tris-glycine running buffer, and rinse the wells.
3. Load 15 µL of denatured, reduced sample/lane. Load a marker lane containing 10 µL of prestained mol-wt standards, and run at 35 mA constant current until the bromophenol blue dye reaches the bottom of the gel.
4. Disassemble the apparatus. Trim the bottom of the gel with a razor blade (to remove excess acrylamide), and carefully transfer the gel to a large glass baking dish containing 1 L of 1X carbonate transfer buffer.
5. Equilibrate gel, nitrocellulose membranes, Whatman 3M paper and Scotchbrite® pads in 1X carbonate buffer. Assemble a gel sandwich using two Scotchbrite® pads, one sheet of 3M paper, and one sheet of nitrocellulose for each side of the gel. Be careful to avoid bubbles between the gel and the nitrocellulose membranes. Assemble the blotting apparatus. Transfer protein using a constant current of 200 mA for 2 h.
6. Disassemble the apparatus, and remove the sheet of nitrocellulose with the prestained markers (cathode). Block nonspecific protein binding sites by incubating the filter in 50 mM Tris, pH 7.5, 150 mM NaCl, 0.2% Tween 20, 5% (w/v) nonfat milk (TBST/milk) overnight at 4°C (*see* **Notes**).
7. Incubate the blocked filter in 30 mL of TBST/milk containing a 1:500 dilution of primary human anti-HCV serum, for 30 min at room temperature, using a rotary shaker (*see* **Notes 4** and **5**).
8. Remove the primary serum solution, placing it in a beaker containing 100 mL of 100% bleach (*see* **Subheading 4.**). Wash liberally with TBST/milk, and dispose of wash into the bleach beaker. Wash three times for 15 min each, and inactivate washes in bleach beaker.
9. Add 30 mL of TBST/milk containing a 1:3000 dilution of HRP-protein A, and incubate for 30 min with shaking at room temperature.
10. Remove 2° detection reagent, and wash three times with TBST/milk and one final wash using TBST. Inactivate washes in bleach beaker.
11. Develop image using the Amersham ECL kit reagents, per manufacturer's instruction (*see* **Notes 6** and **7**).

3.3. ATPase Assay

1. Make fresh 50X NADH (10 mM), 50X phosphoenol pyruvate (100 mM), 50X MgCl$_2$ (175 mM), 100 mM ATP, and 10X MOPS, pH 7.0, in RNase-free water. Thaw enzyme and poly(U). Keep on ice.
2. Make an appropriate volume of 1X reaction buffer containing 50 mM MOPS, pH 7.0, 3.5 mM MgCl$_2$, 200 µM NADH, 2 mM phosphoenol pyruvate, 600 µM base poly(U) (*see* **Note 8**), 40 U/mL of pyruvate kinase and lactate dehydrogenase, and 10 nM HCV helicase. Equilibrate 1X reaction buffer at room temperature (*see* **Note 8**).
3. Turn on the spectrophotometer and temperature control units. Set temperature to 25°C and wavelength/kinetic programs to read at 340 nm. Set baseline against 50 mM MOPS buffer, and then read the absorbance of 1X reaction buffer (A_{340} should be ~1.2).
4. Using the kinetics program of the spectrophotometer, take a reading of the initial rate of oxidation of NADH. This is the basal background rate in the absence of ATP.
5. Read initial rates of oxidation for at least 10 concentrations, spanning a concentration range of 25 µM to 1.5 mM.
6. Using SigmaPlot®, open a new spreadsheet and enter the x-values (0–1500 µM ATP). Enter the corresponding absolute y values (ΔA_{340}min^{-1}). Mathematically transform the y values into turnover numbers by dividing y values by the product of (0.0062) (concentration of helicase in µM). These transformed y values (V/E$_t$) are the turnover numbers in min^{-1} for each x value. Divide these numbers by 60, if s^{-1} units are desired (*see* **Note 10**).
7. Plot the transformed V/E$_t$ values against the x values. The curve should resemble a rectangular hyperbola in shape (*see* **Note 10**). Fit Eq. 3 to the data with:

$$y = c + [ax/(K + x)] \qquad (3)$$

where $a = (V_{max} - V_0)$, $c = V_0$, $K = K_m$, with x = substrate.

3.4. Binding Site Titration

1. Take absorbance scans of helicase and (rU)$_{15}$ in 50 mM MOPS, pH 7.0, 3.5 mM MgCl$_2$, from 230 to 500 nm. Use the extinction coefficient provided by the supplier to calculate the ([rU]$_{15}$). Check for impurities in the (rU)$_{15}$ that absorb or increase scatter at 290 nm. Using 290 nm as the excitation wavelength, take an emission scan of a 50-nM solution of helicase in 50 mM MOPS, pH 7.0, 3.5 mM MgCl$_2$, from 300 to 500 nm. The emission maximum should be at 340 nm.
2. Set 290 and 340 nm as excitation/emission wavelengths. Set up a cuvet containing a magnetic flea and 2.0 mL of 50 mM MOPS, pH 7.0, and 3.5 mM MgCl$_2$. Activate the stirrer function of the fluorescence spectrometer, and set temperature at 25°C. Read the observed fluorescence at 340 nm. This is the buffer control blank. Add 50 nM helicase, and read at 340 nm. This is your initial y value. Add increasing amounts of (rU)$_{15}$ to the cuvet, spanning a concentration range of 0–150 nM. Record the fluorescence values for each concentration. Repeat

the titration using 100 and 200 nM helicase. The fluorescence should be quenched approx 45% at 150 nM (rU)$_{15}$.
3. Using SigmaPlot®, open a new spreadsheet and enter the x values (0–150 nM [rU]$_{15}$). Correct these values for dilution. Enter the corresponding y values. Mathematically transform the y values into fractional fluorescence by
   a. Ssubtracting the buffer control blank from the observed y values (y_a).
   b. Correct the y_a values for dilution (y_b).
   c. Transform the y_b values to fractional fluorescence (f) by dividing by the blank-corrected initial y_a value. The f value is the fractional fluorescence of the enzyme–nucleic acid complex {F([NA]$_t$)} and is related to the total concentation of added nucleic acid ([NA]$_t$) by **Eq. 6** (*see* **Note 11**).
4. Plot the f values against the x values. Fit **Eq. 4** to the data (*see* **Note 11**),

$$f = 1 - [[F_\infty/2(E_t)] \cdot ([x + (E_t) + K_d] + [x + (E_t) + K_d]^2 - 4(E_t)x\}/2] \quad (4)$$

where f = fractional observed fluorescence (corrected for background and dilution), F_∞ is the maximal fractional change in fluorescence, x is the concentration of (rU)$_{15}$ (nM), K_d (nM) is the observed dissociation constant, and [E_t] (nM) is the concentration of helicase. Curve fitting is an iterative procedure that requires the user to specify initial estimates for K_d, and F_∞. Estimates of these parameters can be obtained by visually inspecting an initial plot of the observed f vs x values. Fix [E_t] to derive fitted values for K_d, and F_∞ (*see* **Note 12**).

3.5. Helicase Assay

1. Incubate assay mixture (15 μL water, 10 μL helicase working solution, and 25 μL working substrate solution) at room temperature in a 96-well SPA microtiter plate (*see* **Notes 13 and 14**). Final reagent concentrations are: 0.5 nM DNA substrate, 0.3 nM HCV helicase, 200 μM ATP, 3.5 mM MgCl$_2$, 2.5 mM DTT, 0.025% Triton X-100, 50 mM MOPS, pH 7.0 (*see* **Note 5**).
2. Terminate the assay after 30 min by adding 10 μL of stop solution. The 60 μL of stopped-assay mixture contain 75 mM EDTA and 500 mM NaCl, both of which serve to inhibit (reversibly) HCV helicase, and 7.5 nM of a biotinylated ssDNA, which is complementary to the [^{3}H] ssDNA assay product. The biotinylated ssDNA traps the [^{3}H] ssDNA assay product and (by competition) minimizes its reannealing to M13 DNA.
3. After 15 min, add 100 μL of a suspension of streptavadin–SPA beads to each assay well. The streptavadin–SPA beads bind the biotinylated DNA:[^{3}H] DNA duplex.
4. After 2 h at room temperature, place the microtiter plate in a radioactivity plate reader to determine dpm/well (*see* **Note 6**). A signal is generated in wells that contain [^{3}H] ssDNA product bound to the streptavadin–SPA beads. Wells with enzyme will have about 6000 dpm. Background in wells with no enzyme or inactivated enzyme will be about 1000 dpm (*see* **Note 17**).
5. Subtract background dpm from assay dpm to determine signal from enzyme-catalyzed unwinding of the partially duplex DNA substrate.

4. Notes
4.1. Fermentation

1. It is always possible through further medium development and optimization of conditions to increase levels of microbial expression. Vary the parameters discussed in **Subheading 1.** and the references to determine empirically the optimal conditions for the protein of interest.
2. One way to maintain the dissolved oxygen tension at the set point is to "cascade" the dissolved oxygen tension value into the agitation control, so that the agitation speed set point increases as the dissolved oxygen tension drops to the set point. Conversely, the agitation speed set point will decrease as the dissolved oxygen tension rises above the set point.

4.2. Western Blotting

3. Nonfat milk is an excellent source of protein for blocking nonspecific protein binding sites on nitrocellulose. Overnight blocking at 4°C works best, but shorter blocking times (1–2 h) can be used.
4. HCV-positive serum should be treated as a biosafety level 2 pathogen *(15)*. As a precaution, we routinely heat serum that has been supplemented with 0.2% (v/v) NP40 for 60 min at 50°C. Work is conducted inside a laminar flow hood, and universal precautions are observed. Gloves, labcoat, and safety glasses are worn at all times. All liquid and solid waste is bleach-treated prior to removal from the hood, and solid waste is autoclaved prior to disposal.
5. It is important to test lots of human sera for reactivity against *E. coli* proteins. Evaluate sera at several different dilutions to test for signal response in a Western blot. Selected HCV-positive sera contain high titers of anti-NS3 antibodies, and with the appropriate serum and conditions, it is possible to detect quantitatively HCV helicase.
6. In order to minimize background resulting from excess development reagent, it is important to remove as much of the reagent from the surface of the nitrocellulose membrane as possible prior to film or phosphorimager exposure. Marking the side of nitrocellulose that contains the prestained mol-wt markers with permanent ink is useful for aligning film.
7. As an alternative to using Amersham ECL film, a Storm phosphorimager (Molecular Dynamics, Sunnyvale, CA) can be used to visualize and quantitate chemiluminescence.

4.3. ATPase Assay

8. Poly(U) is the most labile component of the 1X reaction buffer, but it will remain at maximal stimulatory levels for at least 2 h at room temperature (the K_m for poly[U] is 8 µM base in the presence of saturating concentrations of ATP). Add poly(U) just before starting the ATPase assays. The K_m for ATP (K_{ATP}) at saturating poly(U) concentration is 95 µM. Bracket this concentration with at least 5 data points to generate a representative data set. Use an extinction coefficient of 64 mM^{-1}/cm to calculate the concentration of helicase *(1)*.

9. The addition of 50 µM ADP to the 1X reaction buffer will cause the oxidation of 50 µM NADH within 20 s. Check to confirm that doubling or halving the concentration of each reagent has no effect on the ATPase activity. Check to confirm that poly(U) does not inhibit the coupling enzymes.
10. SigmaPlot® uses nonlinear regression to fit the equation to the data. Fitting y values to x values is an iterative procedure, and it requires that the user specify initial estimates for K_{ATP}, V_{max}, and V_0. Estimates of these parameters can be obtained from an initial plot of the observed y vs x values. Reasonable K_{ATP}, V_{max}, and V_0 values for a helicase preparation should be 95 µM, 60 s^{-1}, and 4 s^{-1}, respectively. A V_{max} <10X V_0 is an indication that the helicase preparation is not pure or is not completely active.

4.4. Binding Site Titration

11. The fluorescence of HCV helicase is quenched on formation of the helicase–(rU)$_{15}$ complex (E · NA). The fractional fluorescence ($F[\{NA\}_t]$) remaining is related to the total concentration of added nucleic acid ([NA]$_t$) by **Eq. 5**:

$$F[(NA)_t] = 1 - \Delta F_\infty [(E \cdot NA)/(E_t)] \qquad (5)$$

in which ΔF_∞ is the fractional fluorescence decrease resulting from complete conversion of E to E · NA. Because the concentration of enzyme was comparable to the dissociation constant, the concentration of E · NA was related to [NA]$_t$ by **Eq. 6**. **Equations 5** and **6** are combined in **Eq. 4**, which is used to fit the titration data with a given

$$(E \cdot NA) = [(NA)_t + (E_t) + (K_d)]/2 - (\{[(NA)_t + (E_t) + K_d]^2 - 4(E_t)(NA)_t\}/2) \qquad (6)$$

enzyme concentration to yield the K_d of helicase for NA and the F_∞ value. Using the values obtained from fitting **Eq. 4** to the data, fix the K_d and F_∞ values, and allow [E$_t$] to vary. The fitted [E$_t$] value should be identical to the initial fixed [E$_t$] value (within the experimental error). If the fitted value it is not within the experimental error, then it suggests that only a fraction of the helicase preparation is competent to bind nucleic acid.
12. Global fitting of data sets with multiple concentrations of E$_t$ reduces the covariance between E$_t$ and K_d.

4.5. Helicase Assay

13. As a background control, the assay should include four wells with either no enzyme or enzyme that has been inactivated by the inclusion of 0.5 M NaCl in the 50 µL reaction buffer. The average background dpm is subtracted from assay wells.
14. The assay is not linear with time and enzyme when more than 60% of the substrate is unwound. Therefore, assay conditions should be kept such that at least 40% of the substrate remains at the end of the assay. The percent of substrate unwound can be determined as follows. Prepare 200 µL of assay buffer in a 1.5-mL microcentrifuge tube. Add 40 µL stop solution, and heat for 10 min in a boiling water

bath or a 100°C sand bath to dissociate the substrate. After cooling to room temperature, centrifuge briefly, and distribute 60-µL aliquots into wells of an SPA microtiter plate. Add 100 µL SPA beads and count radioactivity. This is the total dpm for completely unwound substrate, dpm in helicase assay wells should be <60% of this value.
15. The assay can be started with enzyme or substrate. DTT may be omitted from the assay.
16. Scintillation proximity assays can be read in a conventional liquid scintillation counter. Assays are done in 1.5-mL microcentrifuge tubes. The tubes are held upright in conventional 10-mL glass vials for counting.
17. The signal in the assay wells increases with time. After 24 h, background and sample wells will have increased to about 2000 and 7000 dpm, respectively. Because of this, all assay plates should include appropriate controls.

References

1. Preugschat, F., Averett, D. R., Clarke, B. E., and Porter, D. J. T. (1996) A steady-state and pre-steady-state kinetic analysis of the NTPase activity associated with the hepatitis C virus NS3 helicase domain. *J. Biol. Chem.* **271,** 24,449–24,457.
2. Porter, D. J. T., Short, S. A., Hanlon, M., Preugschat, F., Wilson, J. E., Willard, D. H., et al. (1997) A Steady-state and pre-steady-state kinetic analysis of the DNA unwinding activity associated with the hepatitis C virus NS3 helicase domain. Submitted for publication.
3. Suzich, J. A., Tamura, J. K., Palmer-Hill, F., Warrener, P., Grakoui, A., Rice, C. M., et al. (1993) Hepatitis C virus NS3 protein polynucleotide-stimulated nucleoside triphosphatase and comparison with the related pestivirus and flavivirus enzymes. *J. Virol.* **67,** 6152–6158.
4. Tai, C-L., Chi, W-K., Chen, D-S., and Hwang, L-H. (1996) The helicase activity associated with hepatitis C virus nonstructural protein 3 (NS3). *J. Virol.* **70,** 8477–8484.
5. Matson, S. W. and Kaiser-Rogers, K. A. (1990) DNA helicases. *Ann. Rev. Biochem.* **59,** 289–329.
6. Lohman, T. M. (1993) Helicase-catalyzed DNA unwinding. *J. Biol. Chem.* **268,** 2269–2272.
7. Gold, L. (1991) Expression of heterologous proteins in *Escherichia coli*, in *Methods in Enzymology*, vol. 185. Academic, San Diego, CA, pp. 11–14.
8. Preugschat, F. (1995) *Principles of Fermentation Technology*, 2nd ed., *Aeration and Agitation*. Elsevier Science, Tarryton, NY, pp. 243–272.
9. Anonymous (1987) Escherichia coli *and* Salmonella typhimurium, *Anaerobic Dissimilation of Pyruvate*. American Society for Microbiology. Washington, DC, pp. 151–155.
10. Lischke, H. H., Brandes, L., Wu, X., and Schuegerl, K. (1993) Influence of acetate on the growth of recombinant *Escherichia coli* JM103 and product formation. *Bioprocess Eng.* **9,** 155–157.
11. Han, K., Lim, H. C., and Hong, J. (1992) Acetic acid formation in Escherichia coli fermentation. *Biotechnol. Bioeng.* **39,** 663–671.

12. Hockney, R. C. (1994) Recent developments in heterologous protein production in *Eschericia coli. Tibtech* **12,** 456–463.
13. Towbin, H., Staehelin, T., and Gordon, J. (1979) Electrophoretic transfer of proteins from polyacrylamide gels to nitrocellulose sheets: procedure and some applications. *Proc. Natl. Acad. Sci. USA* **76,** 4350–4354.
14. Kayne, F. (1973) Pyruvate kinase. *Enzymes* **8,** 353–382.
15. Anonymous (1989) *Biosafety in the Laboratory. Prudent Practices for the Handling and Disposal of Infectious Materials.* National Academy Press, Washington, DC, pp. 34–42.

33

Hepatitis C Virus RNA-Dependent RNA Polymerase (NS5B Polymerase)

Curt H. Hagedorn

1. Introduction

The hepatitis C virus (HCV) chronically infects approx 4 million patients in the United States alone, and constitutes a major cause of chronic liver disease and hepatocellular carcinoma *(1–3)*. Current antiviral therapies for chronic hepatitis C remain relatively ineffective and have significant side-effects in many patients. Moreover, the lack of an easily reproducible tissue-culture system to propagate HCV has hampered the development of new antiviral therapies. Although detailed studies of several recombinant HCV nonstructural proteins have been initiated, our knowledge of the HCV NS5B polymerase that encodes an RNA-dependent RNA polymerase (RDRP) is rudimentary *(4–8)*. RNA-dependent RNA polymerases represent a class of viral enzymes that replicate the genomic RNA of plus strand RNA viruses *(9–11)*. A model enzyme of this group, the poliovirus RDRP encoded by the 3D^{pol} gene, has been extensively studied *(12–17)*. However, studies of recombinant hepatitis C virus RDRP (or NS5B polymerase) have only recently begun, and there is much to learn. A method is presented here for assaying HCV RDRP activity based on this laboratory's experience with recombinant NS5B expressed in *Escherichia coli* and the experience of others studying NS5B expressed in insect cells *(5–8)*.

RNA-dependent RNA polymerases interact with the plus-strand genomic RNA of the virus and synthesize negative strands (or replicative intermediates). The replicative intermediates generally serve as templates for the synthesis of a quantitatively larger number of plus strands of genomic RNA, which provide templates for viral protein synthesis and genomic RNA for the production of progeny virus. Plus-strand RNA viruses that have been propagated in tissue culture have provided evidence that relatively few copies of the replicative intermediates are synthesized compared to the number of plus strands of genomic RNA *(10,11)*. Even with poliovirus, a model system of studying RDRPs, the details of the switch in using plus as opposed to minus strands as templates remains to be determined *(16)*. In general, the catalytic subunit of RNA-dependent RNA polymerases (3D^{pol} for poliovirus and NS5B for HCV) can make copies of nonviral RNA templates *(10,18)*. This raises questions regarding factors that might provide specificity for viral RNA templates in vivo. In several studies, small proteins derived from the poliovirus polyprotein have been described that play a role in the interaction of the polio 3D^{pol} with viral RNA templates *(12,15–17)*. The observation that HCV NS5B polymerase can replicate globin mRNA when it is provided as a template suggests that either host or viral derived proteins may provide template specificity in vivo *(6,8)*. Furthermore, the observation that recombinant NS5B does not specifically bind to a representative 3'-end of genomic RNA suggests a role for additional factors regarding template specificity *(7)*. To study the replication of the HCV genome in detail, such specificity factors will eventually need to be identified and included in assay systems. The method described to quantitate the RNA-dependent RNA polymerase activity of recombinant HCV NS5B is modeled after those used to study recombinant poliovirus RDRP (3D^{pol}) *(19)*.

2. Materials
2.1. Polymerase Assay

1. [^{3}H]UTP: SA of 37 Ci/mmol (cat. no. 24061, ICN Pharmaceuticals, Costa Mesa, CA).
2. 1 M HEPES buffer, pH 8.0.
3. ATP, CTP, GTP: 10 mM each (Calbiochem-Novabiochem, San Diego, CA).
4. 0.5 mM ZnCl$_2$.
5. 0.1 M DTT.
6. 0.5 M Magnesium acetate.
7. Poly(A)$_{460–600}$: 1 mg/mL deionized H$_2$O (Pharmacia Biotech Inc., Piscataway, NJ).
8. Oligo(U)$_{12}$ or oligo(dT)$_{12}$: 1 mg/mL deionized H$_2$O (Pharmacia).
9. Actinomycin D: 80 µg/mL in ethanol.
10. Calf thymus DNA.
11. Sodium pyrophosphate/HCl wash: 0.1 M Na$_4$P$_2$O$_7$; 1 N HCl. 180 g sodium pyrophosphate (Na$_4$P$_2$O$_7$ · 10 H$_2$O; F.W. 446.06); 345 mL of concentrated HCl added dropwise; in a final volume of 4 L with deionized H$_2$O.
12. 20% TCA (prepare fresh): 1 vol 100% solution of TCA (stored at 4°C); 4 vol H$_2$O.
13. 0.45-µm Whatman (Clifton, NJ) GF/C filters.
14. Millipore (Bedford, MA) vacuum manifold.
15. Centricon concentrators (Amicon, Inc., Beverly, MA).
16. β-counter (LKB/EG+G Wallace Model 1218, Gaithersburg, MD).
17. ScintiSafe™ 30% (Fisher [Springfield, NJ], or another suitable biodegradable scintillation solution).

2.2. Analysis of [^{32}P]RNA Products by Formaldehyde/Agarose Gel Electrophoresis

1. Equilibrated phenol.
2. Phenol/chloroform (chloroform/isoamyl alcohol = 24/1).
3. High-quality agarose.
4. Deionized 37% formaldehyde (pH >4.0).
5. Formamide.
6. Sterile glycerol.
7. Sterile 500 mM EDTA (pH 8.0).
8. DEPC-treated deionized H$_2$O: Add 1% DEPC to Mill-iQ™ deionized H$_2$O; incubate overnight at 37°C (vented); autoclave.
9. 5X formaldehyde (MOPS) gel-running buffer: 100 mM MOPS (pH 7.0), 40 mM sodium acetate; and 5 mM EDTA.
10. Formaldehyde gel-loading buffer: 50% glycerol, 1 mM EDTA, 0.25% bromophenol blue, and 0.45% xylene cyanol FF (optional).
11. RNA standards (Life Technologies, Gaithersburg, MD).
12. 10 × 14 cm horizontal submarine gel electrophoresis system with power supply (Life Technologies).
13. Speed-Vac (Savant Instruments, Inc., Farmingdale, NY).
14. Gel dryer (e.g., Bio-Rad Laboratories, Hercules, CA).
15. Intensifying screen and autoradiography supplies.

3. Methods

3.1. Incubations

1. Use the following quantities of stock solutions for each incubation (50 μL final volume):

1 M HEPES, pH 8.0	2.5 μL/incubation
10 mM (each) ATP, CTP, GTP	2.5 μL/reaction
0.5 M Magnesium acetate	1 μL/reaction
0.5 mM ZnCl$_2$	6 μL/reaction
0.1 M DTT	2 μL/reaction
poly(A) 1 mg/mL	1 μL/reaction
oligo(U) 1 mg/mL	1 μL/reaction

2. Add the appropriate quantity of each stock solution to a tube ("stock mixture"), mix, and keep on ice. For example, for a total of 10 incubations add 25 μL of HEPES stock solution, and so forth. *See* **Notes 1** and **5** regarding templates/primers.
3. To a separate tube add 2.5 μL of the actinomycin D stock solution/incubation plus 20 μCi of ^{3}H-UTP per incubation.
4. Partially dry this mixture in a Speed-Vac to evaporate most of the ethanol (reduce to approximately one-third of the original volume).
5. Add the "stock mixture" to the ^{3}H-UTP/actinomycin D solution, and adjust the volume to 48 μL/incubation (this final preparation is subsequently referred to as reaction mixture).

6. Assays are 50 μL in final volume and contain 20 μg/mL poly(A); 10 μg/mL oligo(U); 50 mM HEPES (pH 8.0); 500 μM each ATP, CTP, and GTP; 4 mM DTT, 10 mM magnesium acetate; 5 mM KCl (from enzyme preparation); 60 μM $ZnCl_2$; and 4 μg/mL of actinomycin D. [^{3}H]UTP is at a final concentration of 11 μM (see **Notes 1** and **2**).

3.2. Starting Incubations

1. Incubations are started by adding 48 μL of the reaction mixture to a 1.5-mL microfuge tube followed by 2 μL of enzyme preparation. To add the enzyme, it is helpful to use a fixed volume 2 μL pipet, prewet the pipet tip, and "rinse" the pipet tip after ejecting the enzyme sample into the reaction mix (see **Note 3**).
2. Mix and incubate at 30°C.

3.3. Sample Collection and Analysis for Poly(U) Polymerase Activity

1. At the desired time (e.g., 30 and 60 min), remove 20 μL of the incubation mixture and pipet it into a 1.5-mL microfuge tube containing 0.8 mL of calf thymus DNA (100 μg/mL deionized H_2O). Rinse the pipet tip in the carrier DNA solution and mix.
2. To the same tube add 0.45 mL of 20% TCA, and keep the tubes on ice for at least 30 min.
3. Place GF/C glass filters in a Millipore vacuum manifold, and prewet each filter with 1 mL of sodium pyrophosphate/HCl wash.
4. Transfer samples containing carrier DNA and TCA to filters with the vacuum on, rinse the tube with 1 mL of the sodium pyrophosphate/HCl wash solution, transfer this rinse to the same filter. Rinse each filter five times with 3–5 mL of the sodium pyrophosphate/HCl wash. Washes can be done faster using a squeeze/wash bottle.
5. Rinse filters twice with 10 mL of 95% ethanol. Let the filters dry for approx 5 min under full vacuum and then in scintillation vials under a fume hood prior to the addition of scintillation cocktail (e.g., ScintiSafe™ 30%). ^{3}H-UTP incorporation into poly(U) is quantitated by scintillation spectrometry and fmoles of UTP incorporation calculated using the specific activity of the ^{3}H-UTP present in incubations, background values obtained using incubations without enzyme or a "zero time point" from a complete incubation (subtracted from data), and the results of a ^{3}H scintillation spectrometry standard.

3.4. Sample Collection and Analysis for Size of [^{32}P]RNA Products

The following modification can be made when using [α-^{32}P]UTP and a model heteropolymeric RNA (e.g., globin mRNA) or full-length HCV RNA as template (see **Note 5** regarding percentage of agarose gels).

3.4.1. Phenol Extraction and Concentration (for 50 μL Incubations in 1.5 mL Siliconized Microfuge Tubes)

1. Add 50 μL of carrier-tRNA (20 μg) stock solution (400 μg/mL in sterile 10 mM Tris-HCl, pH 7.6, 1 mM EDTA, and 100 mM NaCl).

2. Add an equal volume (100 μL) of equilibrated phenol, mix, centrifuge (16,000g) for several minutes, and transfer the aqueous phase (top) to a new tube.
3. Add an equal volume (100 μL) of phenol/chloroform (chloroform/isoamyl alcohol = 24/1), mix, centrifuge for several minutes, and transfer the aqueous phase to a new tube.
4. Add an equal volume (100 μL) of chloroform (chloroform/isoamyl alcohol = 24/1), mix, centrifuge for several minutes, and transfer the aqueous phase to a new siliconized tube.
5. The [^{32}P]RNA products are precipitated by adding 1/5 vol (20 μL for a 100 μL sample) of 3 M ammonium acetate (pH 5.2) and 2.5 vol (250 μL for a 100 μL initial sample) of ice-cold 95–100% ethanol.
6. The sample is mixed thoroughly by inversion and stored at –20°C for at least 15 min (or overnight). The precipitated RNA needs to be desalted by washing with 75% ETOH to avoid artifacts during formaldehyde/agarose gel electrophoresis.
7. Samples are centrifuged at 16,000g for 15 min at 4°C. Discard the ethanol with radioactive liquid waste.
8. Wash the pellets with 75% ethanol two to three times (centrifuge as above).
9. Briefly dry samples in a Speed-Vac, resuspend the RNA in nuclease-free water, and analyze them by formaldehyde/agarose gel electrophoresis as outlined below. Avoid drying the samples completely because this can make the pellets difficult to resuspend.

3.4.2. Formaldehyde/Agarose Gel Electrophoresis and Autoradiography

1. [^{32}P]RNA products produced when globin mRNA was used as a model heteropolymeric RNA template were analyzed by 1.5% formaldehyde/agarose gel electrophoresis (*see* **Note 5**) *(6,8)*.
2. This gel system, 11 × 14 cm, uses a final formaldehyde concentration of 0.66 M which appears to be as effective as the 2.2 M concentration that is frequently cited.
3. Agarose (1.5 g) in 75 mL of DEPC-treated deionized water is completely melted in a microwave oven and then kept at 55–66°C in a water bath.
4. Following temperature equilibration, add 20 mL of prewarmed 5X MOPS buffer and 5.5 mL of prewarmed 37% formaldehyde (all work with formaldehyde is done using gloves in a chemical hood). The agarose solution can be kept at 55–66°C (sealed) until casting the gel.
5. A horizontal submarine gel apparatus (11 × 14 cm gels) and comb that have been soaked with 3% H_2O_2 and then rinsed extensively with DEPC-treated deionized water is used to cast the gel (done in a chemical hood).
6. Immerse the gel in 1X MOPS gel-running buffer once it has solidified.
7. Gels are prerun for 5 min at 5 V/cm submerged in 1X MOPS gel-running buffer immediately before loading samples.
8. [^{32}P]RNA samples are prepared by mixing (micropipeting) in a sterile microfuge tube the RNA (4.5 μL), 2 μL of 5X MOPS gel-running buffer, 3.5 μL of formaldehyde, 10 μL of formamide.
9. Samples are incubated at 65°C for 15 min and then chilled on ice.

10. A 5–10-s centrifugation is done to collect all the liquid sample at the bottom of the tube after heating/cooling, and 2 µL of sterile formaldehyde gel-loading buffer are added.
11. After the samples and RNA standards are loaded, gels are run at 70 V for 2 h in a chemical hood.
12. At the end of the run, the lanes containing RNA markers may be cut from the gel and visualized by staining with ethidium bromide (0.5 µg/mL in 100 mM ammonium acetate) for 30 min.
13. Prior to drying gels for autoradiography, they need to be soaked in DEPC-treated deionized water or 1X MOPS gel-running buffer to remove formaldehyde (two to three changes over 15–20 min). Gels may be dried on DEAE paper to increase the recovery of [^{32}P]RNA and decrease contamination of the gel-drying apparatus.

4. Notes

1. An alternative template/primer to pol(A)/oligo(U)$_{12}$ is poly(C)/oligo(G)$_{12}$ or poly(C)/oligo(dG)$_{12}$ *(7)*. Appropriate changes in the NTPs need to be made, and [^{3}H], [^{35}S], or [α-^{32}P]-GTP needs to be included. Control incubations with the template RNA alone and primers alone should be done. Recent studies indicate that HCV NS5B polymerase does not encode a terminal nucleotidyl transferase activity; however, cellular extracts do contain TNTases that may contaminate enzyme preparations *(5–8)*. The incubation conditions described may be modified based on additional studies of recombinant NS5B polymerases that are being conducted at this time.
2. Assays are done under conditions where product formation is linear with time and enzyme protein concentration *(8)*.
3. When comparing different samples, it is necessary to control for salt concentrations, buffers, or other reagents in enzyme preparations. We have generally done this by concentrating, diluting, and reconcentrating chromatography fractions in the desired buffer using Centricon concentrators *(8,20)*. For example, if there is concern about altering the pH of the final incubation, then it should be measured in a mock incubation (minus radiolabeled nucleotide) that contains the quantity of enzyme buffer that will be added.
4. Precautions should be taken to prepare and maintain all reagents and tubes free of RNase. For example, store stock solutions frozen in small aliquots if possible. Microfuge tubes are autoclaved, but it is not generally necessary for them to be DEPC-treated. An alternative to DEPC is treatment with 0.5 N NaOH for 5 min, followed by thorough rinsing with sterile deionized water.
5. If full-length HCV RNA is being used as template and the product size is being analyzed, then a 0.8–0.6% formaldehyde/agarose gel should be used instead of the 1.5% gels described for analyzing products when globin mRNA is used as a template *(8)*. If the full-length HCV RNA includes a representative 3'-end of genomic HCV RNA, then the presence of primers is not necessarily based on the studies of Lohmann et al. *(7,21,22)*.

References

1. Bradley, D. W., Maynard, J. E., Popper, H., Cook, E. H., Ebert, J. W., McCaustland, K. A., Schable, C. A., and Fields, H. A. (1983) Postransfusion non-A, non-B hepatitis: Physicochemical properties of two distinct agents. *J. Infect. Dis.* **148**, 254–265.
2. Choo, Q.-L., Kuo, G., Weiner, A. J., Overby, L. R., Bradley, D. W., and Houghton, M. (1989) Isolation of a cDNA clone derived from a blood-borne non-A, non-B viral hepatitis genome. *Science* **244**, 359–362.
3. Bissell, D. M. (ed.) (1997) Management of hepatitis C. *Hepatology* **26 (Suppl. 1)**, 1S–156S.
4. Landro, J. A., Raybuck, S. A., Luong, Y. P. C., O'Malley, E. T., Harbeson, S. L., Morgenstern, K. A., et al. (1997) Mechanistic role of an NS4A peptide cofactor with the truncated NS3 protease of hepatitis C virus: elucidation of the NS4A stimulatory effect via kinetic analysis and inhibitor mapping. *Biochemistry* **36**, 9340–9348.
5. Behrens, S. E., Tomei, L., and DeFrancesco, R. (1996) Identification and properties of the RNA-dependent RNA polymerase of hepatitis C virus. *EMBO J.* **15**, 12–22.
6. Al, R. H., Xie, Y., Wang, Y., DeStaercke, C., van Beers, E. H., and Hagedorn, C. H. (1997) Expression of recombinant hepatitis C virus NS5B. *Nucleic Acids Symp.* **Series No. 36**, 197–199.
7. Lohmann, V., Korner, F., Herian, U., and Bartenschlager, R. (1997) Biochemical properties of hepatitis C virus NS5B RNA-dependent RNA polymerase and identification of amino acid sequence motifs essential for enzymatic activity. *J. Virol.* **71**, 8416–8428.
8. Al, R. H., Xie, Y., Wang, Y., and Hagedorn, C. H. (1998) Expression of recombinant hepatitis C virus NS5B in *E. coli. Virus Res.* **53**, 141–149.
9. Koonin, E. V. (1991) The phylogeny of RNA-dependent RNA polymerases of positive-strand RNA viruses. *J. Gen. Virol.* **72**, 2197–2206.
10. Strauss, E. G. and Strauss, J. H. (1986) Structure and replication of the alphavirus genome, in *The Togaviridae and Flaviviridae* (Schlesinger, S. S. and Schlesinger, M. J., eds.), Plenum, New York, pp. 35–90.
11. Westaway, E. G. (1987) Flavivirus replication strategy. *Adv. Virus Res.* **33**, 45–90.
12. Parsley, T. B., Towner, J. S., Blyn, L. B., Ehrenfeld, E., and Semler, B. L. (1997) Poly(rC) binding protein 2 forms a ternary complex with the 5'-terminal sequences of poliovirus RNA and the viral 3CD proteinase. *RNA* **3**, 1124–1134.
13. Richards, O. C. and Ehrenfeld, E. (1997) One of two NTP binding sites in polivirus RNA polymerase required for RNA replication. *J. Biol. Chem.* **272**, 23,261–23,264.
14. Pata, J. D., Schultz, S. C., and Kirkegaard, K. (1995) Functional oligomerization of poliovirus RNA-dependent RNA polymerase. *RNA* **1**, 466–477.
15. Xiang, W., Cuconati, A., Paul, A. V., Cao, X., and Wimmer, E. (1995) Molecular dissection of the multifunctional poliovirus RNA-binding protein 3AB. *RNA* **1**, 892–904.
16. Andino, R., Rieckhof, G. E., Achacoso, P. L., and Baltimore, D. (1993) Poliovirus RNA synthesis utilizes an RNP complex formed around the 5'-end of viral RNA. *EMBO J.* **12**, 3587–3598.

17. Hope, D. A., Diamond, S. E., and Kirkegard, K. (1997) Genetic dissection of interaction between poliovirus 3D polymerase and viral 3AB. *J. Virol.* **71,** 9490–9498.
18. Neufeld, K. L., Richards, O. C., and Ehrenfeld, E. (1991) Purification, characterization, and comparison of poliovirus RNA polymerase from native and recombinant sources. *J. Biol. Chem.* **266,** 24,212–24,219.
19. Hey, T. D., Richards, O. C., and Ehrenfeld, E. (1986) Synthesis of plus- and minus-strand RNA from poliovirion RNA template *in vitro*. *J. Virol.* **58,** 790–796.
20. Hagedorn, C. H., Spivak-Kroizman, T., Friedland, D. E., Goss, D. J., and Xie, Y. (1997) Expression of functional eIF-4E$_{human}$: purification, detailed characterization, and its use in isolating eIF-4E binding proteins. *Protein Expression Purif.* **9,** 53–60.
21. Tanaka, T., Kato, N., Cho, M. J., and Shimotohno, K. (1995) A novel sequence found at the 3' terminus of hepatitis C virus genome. *Biochem. Biophys. Res. Commun.* **215,** 744–749.
22. Kolykhalov, A. A., Feinstone, S. M., and Rice, C. M. (1996) Identification of a highly conserved sequence element at the 3' terminus of hepatitis C virus genome RNA. *J. Virol.* **70,** 3363–3371.

34

Detection and Molecular Cloning of the Extreme 3'-End of HCV

Torahiko Tanaka and Kunitada Shimotohno

1. Introduction

The 3'-end region of the HCV genome is composed of three characteristic elements: conventional 3'-untranslated region, subsequent poly (U) stretch, and a newly identified 3'-terminal sequence named the 3'X tail *(1,2)*. The 3'X tail is thought to be a common structure of the HCV genome, and should have important roles in initiation and regulation of the genomic replication of HCV.

The conventional 3'-untranslated region is a genotype-specific sequence of about 40 nucleotides downstream of the terminal codon. Nucleotide diversity in this region is about 10% within the same genotype. On the other hand, a high rate of diversity (up to 80%) is observed among different genotypes. The subsequent poly (U) stretch includes a small number of different nucleotides, mainly C and sometimes G or A, representing characteristic patterns for each isolate. The length of the poly (U) stretch differs among individual isolates ranging between 20 and 200 nucleotides. At the end of the poly U stretch, flanking the 3'X tail, there is a short highly heterogeneous region designated transitional region. Here, several C, CC, or CCC residues appear at intervals of 2–5 U residues, and sometimes A or G residues appear in this region.

The 3'X tail is a specific 98 nucleotide sequence, which starts with GGUGG motif and ends with UGU. The nucleotide sequence of the 3'X tail is highly conserved within the same genotype and even among distant genotypes. For instance, the type 1b and 2a HCVs are most genetically distant between each other, showing more than 35% of nucleotide difference. However, both types have very similar 98 nucleotide 3'X tail sequences downstream of the poly U stretch, and only four positions of nucleotide difference are seen between the two 3'X tail sequences *(2)*. The nucleotide changes among different genotypes seem to be concentrated in the 3'-half of the 3'X tail rather than in the 5'-half, and <5% in rate. The 3'X tail forms stable secondary structures by computer modeling, suggesting that the 3'X tail functionally interacts with some viral or cellular proteins. One stemloop has a long stem with 17 possible basepairings and may be very stable. The feature may be one of the reasons by which pioneers of molecular cloning of HCV genome failed to identify the 3'X tail.

The 3'X tail can easily be detected by conventional RT-PCR technique from HCV infected samples *(2)*. Until now, the 3'X tail sequences of types 1a, 1b, 2a, 2b, 3a, and 3b HCVs have been reported *(1–4)*. The information does not cover all the types of HCVs (more than 60 genotypes), but may be practical, because the clarified sequences are those of very distant HCV genotypes. Based on these reports, the 3'X tail sequence is roughly divided into two categories for convenience: type A, including 1a, 1b, and others; and type B, including 2a, 2b, and others. Therefore, we propose here two sets of primers for PCR amplification that are directed to the sequences of types A and B. Also we describe here the cloning methods of the 3'X tail by primer extension and RNA ligation experiments, for the sake of research groups analyzing new genotypes of HCVs.

2. Materials
2.1. RT-PCR

1. A 0.5-mL microtube of mineral oil.
2. Mineral oil (Sigma, St. Louis, MO).
3. RNA extraction kit for serum or tissue (RNAzol B, Biotecx Laboratories, or any other equivalents).
4. Reverse transcriptase (Superscript II, Gibco-BRL, or any other equivalents).
5. 5X concentrated 1st strand buffer: 0.25 M Tris-HCl, pH 8.3, 0.375 M KCl, 15 mM MgCl$_2$, supplied with the enzyme.
6. *Taq* polymerase (supplied from any company).
7. 10X PCR buffer (usually supplied with the enzyme).
8. dNTP mixture (2.5 mM each dATP, dGTP, dCTP, and dTTP).
9. 0.1 M dithiothreitol (DTT).
10. Water (nuclease-free).
11. Primers (10 μM each).

2.2. Primer Extension Experiment

1. 6 N NaOH, 6 N acetic acid, glycogen (20 μg/μL, Boehringer).
2. GENO-BIND silica matrix kit (Clontech).
3. Terminal deoxynucleotidyl transferase (TdT) (Toyobo or others) and 5X concentrated TdT buffer (0.5 M sodium cacodylate, pH 7.0, 10 mM MnCl$_2$, 0.5 mM DTT).
4. 2.5 mM dCTP.
5. 3 M sodium acetate (pH 5.2); 5 M ammonium acetate; ethanol.

2.3. RNA Ligation Experiment

1. Synthetic RNA (20–25-mer, any sequence, but it is recommended that the 5'-terminus be C and the 3'-terminus be U).
2. T4 polynucleotide kinase (Takara or others) and reaction buffer (usually supplied with the enzyme).
3. T4 RNA ligase (Takara or others).
4. 2X T4 ligase reaction buffer: 0.1 M Tris-HCl, pH 8.1, 40 mM MgCl$_2$, 20 mM DTT, 10 µM ATP, 0.2 mg/mL bovine serum albumin.
5. RNasin (Promega).
6. 3 M sodium acetate (pH 5.2), ethanol.

3. Methods

All steps of the experiment must be performed under nuclease-free manipulations.

3.1. Detection of the Extreme 3'-Terminal Structure of the HCV Genome, the 3'X Tail, by RT-Nested PCR

Primers used in this study are shown in **Fig. 1**.

1. The sample RNA is obtained from HCV-infected serum or liver by using a kit RNAzol B according to the manufacturer's protocol.
2. The RT reaction mixture (20 µL) consists of 4 µL of 5X concentrated first-strand buffer, 4 µL dNTP mixture, 1 µL DTT, 2 µL reverse primer, 1 µL of liver RNA (1 µg/µL) or serum RNA (derived from 50 µL of serum) and 7 µL water, and is overlaid by one drop of mineral oil.
3. The mixture is heated at 90°C for 3 min and rapidly cooled in ice water to denaturate RNA.
4. 1 µL of Superscript II is added to the reaction mixture, and then the mixture is incubated for 60 min at 50°C (high-stringency protocol) or 37°C (conventional protocol; *see* **Note 1**).
5. The mixture is incubated at 100°C for 30 min to inactivate Superscript II.
6. The reaction mixture for the first PCR (30 µL) is made with 3 µL of 10X concentrated PCR buffer (according to the manufacturer's protocol), 2.4 µL dNTP mixture, 2.4 µL each forward and reverse primers, 1.5 µL of the RT product, and 17.9 µL water and overlaid with one drop of mineral oil.
7. The mixture is heated for 2 min at 98°C and then held at 82°C, and 0.45 µL *Taq* polymerase (5 U/µL) is added to the mixture (*see* **Note 2**).
8. Thirty-four cycles of PCR (40 s at 93°C, 45 s at 55°C, and 2 min at 72°C) are performed.
9. The reaction mixture for the second PCR (50 µL) is made with 5 µL of 10X concentrated PCR buffer, 4 µL of dNTP mixture, 4 µL of each forward and reverse primers, 2 µL of the first PCR product, and 30.3 µL of water, and is overlaid with two drops of mineral oil.
10. PCR is done as in **steps 7** and **8** with 0.7 µL *Taq* polymerase.
11. Five to ten microliters of the PCR product are electrophoresed on 4.5% agarose gel (3:1 mixture of Nuesieve GTG and Seakem LE (FMC Bioproducts). The product size is 68 bp.

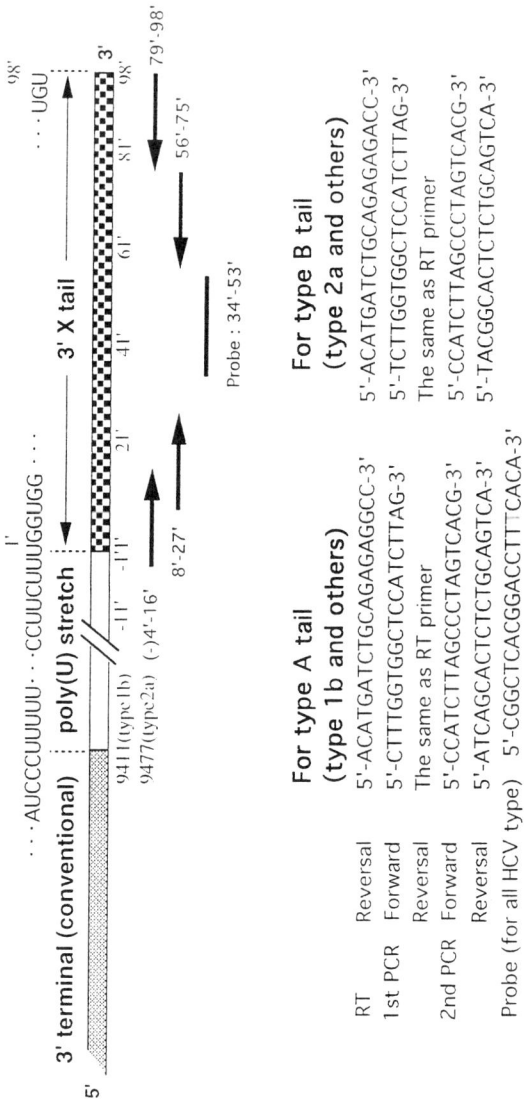

Fig. 1. Detection of the 3'X tail region of the positive-strand HCV genome.

12. If necessary, perform Southern blot analysis by using a probe shown in **Fig. 1** to confirm the 3'X tail sequence in the PCR product *(5)*.

3.2. Analysis of the 3'-Terminal Sequence by Primer Extension Experiment

Primer extension is performed on the 5'-terminal region of antigenomic strand of HCV present in infected liver, which should reflect the 3'-terminal sequence of the genomic strand of HCV. Arrangement of primers is shown in **Fig. 2**.

1. RT reaction mixture (5 tubes, 20 µL each) is made with 4 µL of 5X concentrated first-strand buffer, 4 µL dNTP mixture, 1 µL DTT, 2 µL forward primer, 1.5 µL liver RNA (1 µg/µL), and 6.5 µL water, and is overlaid with one drop of mineral oil.
2. The mixture is heated at 90°C for 3 min and rapidly cooled in ice water.
3. One microliter of Superscript II is added to each tube. Then the reaction is performed for 60 min at 50°C (primer extension).
4. 1.4 µL of 6 N NaOH is added to each tube, and the mixture is incubated at 65°C for 30 min to hydrolyze RNA.
5. The products are collected into one tube, and 7 µL of 6 N acetic acid are added to the mixture.
6. The cDNA is collected by ethanol precipitation with 2 µL acetic acid (6 N), 1 µL glycogen, and 200 µL ethanol.
7. The cDNA is purified by using GENOBIND silica matrix kit according to the manufacturer's protocol and dissolved in 8 µL water.
8. dC-tailing reaction mixture is made with 6 µL of 5X concentrated TdT buffer, 6 µL of 2.5 mM dCTP, 4 µL of cDNA fraction, and 12 µL water. The mixture is heated for 3 min at 98°C and rapidly cooled in ice water to denature the cDNA.
9. Two microliters of (50 U) TdT are added to the mixture, and incubation is performed at 37°C for 60 min.
10. The dC-tailed cDNA is collected by ethanol precipitation (two times), first with the aid of ammonium acetate and second with sodium acetate. The cDNA is dissolved in 8 µL water.
11. Nested PCR is performed as described in **Subheading 3.1., steps 6–10** with primers given in **Fig. 2**.
12. The second PCR primers have an *Xho*I site. Therefore, the PCR product can be subcloned in the *Xho*I site of vector plasmid, such as Bluescript KS, after *Xho*I digestion.
13. Positive clones are screened by colony hybridization technique *(5)* with a probe that hybridize the 3'-terminal region of the 3'X tail sequence (*see* **Fig. 2**).

3.3. Analysis of the 3'-Terminal Sequence by RNA Ligation Experiment

Synthetic RNA oligonucleotide is ligated to the 3'-terminus of the genomic strand of HCV RNA present in serum (*see* **Note 3**). Then, RT-PCR is performed between the oligomer sequence and internal region. Primers are shown in **Fig. 3**.

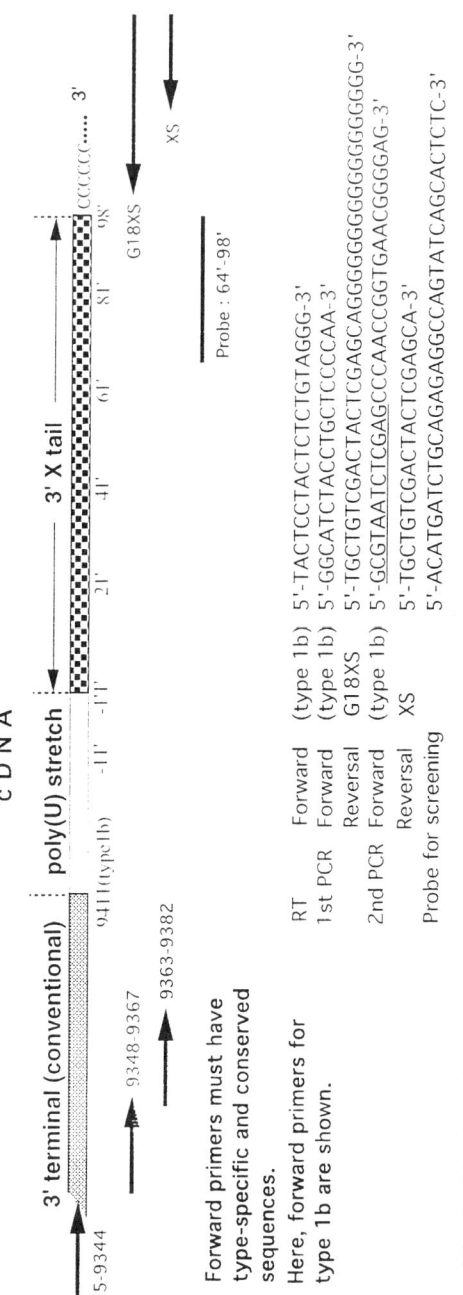

Fig. 2. Cloning of the 3'X tail sequence by primer extension. A tag sequence with an *XhoI* site is underlined.

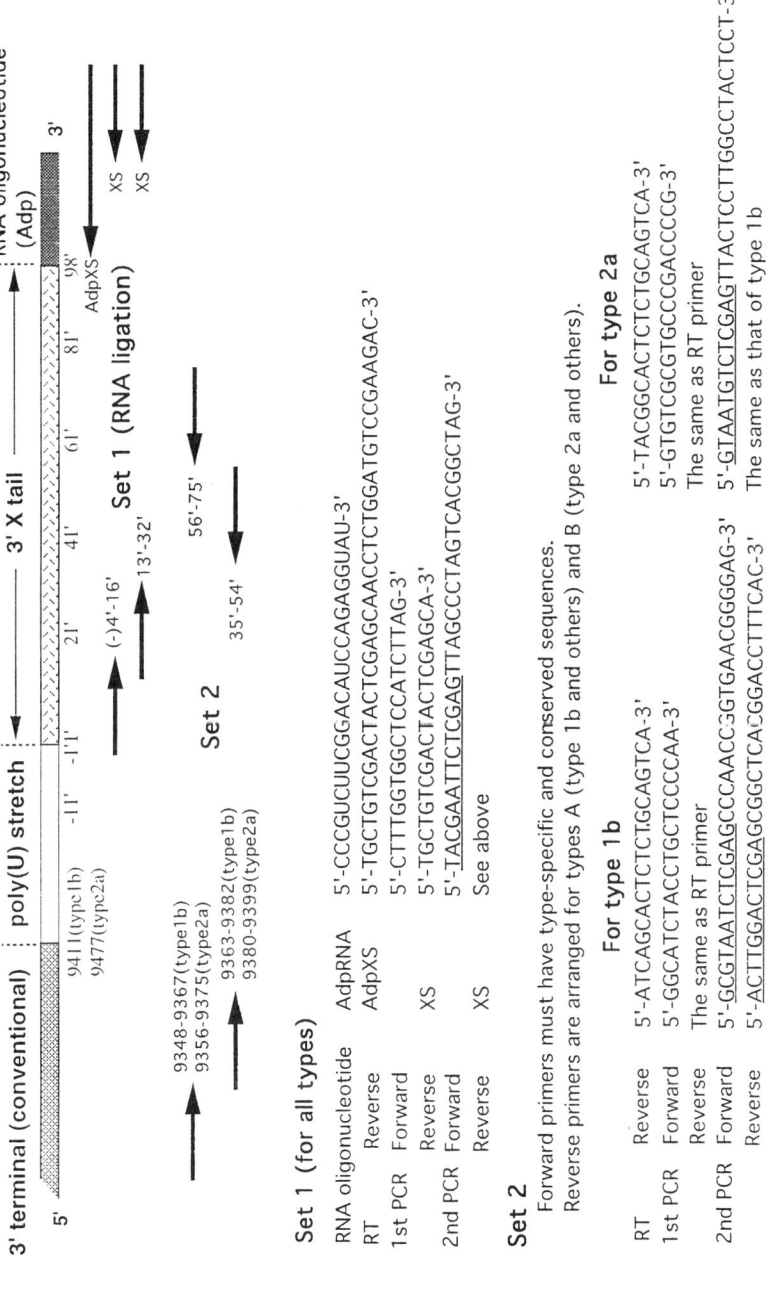

Fig. 3. Cloning of the 3'X tail by an RNA ligation experiment. Tag sequences with an *Xho*I site are underlined.

1. The 5'-terminus of the synthetic RNA oligonucleotide is phosphorylated by T4 polynucleotide kinase under standard protocols *(5)*.
2. The reaction mixture for RNA ligation is made with 10 μL of 2X T4 ligase reaction buffer, 4 μL RNA (derived from 100–200 μL serum), 5 μL of the 5'-phosphorylated RNA oligonucleotide (4 μ*M*), 1 μL RNasin, and 1 μL (50 U) T4 RNA ligase. The reaction is allowed to continue at 10°C for 12 h.
3. RNA is collected by ethanol precipitation with the aid of sodium acetate and dissolved in 8 μL water.
4. RT is done as described in **Subheading 3.1., steps 2–5** with one-half of the RNA fraction.
5. The nested PCR is performed as described in **Subheading 3.1., steps 6–10** (*see* **Note 4**).

4. Notes

1. Usual protocols for denaturing (70–80°C, slow cooling) and reaction (37°C) give higher efficiency but lower specificity than high-stringency protocol gives.
2. The PCR protocol described here is just a conventional hot-start technique. Advanced protocols using modified thermostable DNA polymerase, such as AmpliTaq Gold (Perkin Elmer) or other hot-start PCR kits are also available.
3. RNA oligonucleotide modified with an amino group at the 3'-end may be employed to avoid polymerization of the oligonucleotide during RNA ligation reaction *(4)*. However, this side reaction is less common under conditions described above.
4. Efficiency of RT-PCR with longer range, from the ligated oligoRNA sequence across the poly U stretch to conventional 3'-untranslated region, is lower than that of set 1 RT-PCR. However, when infected serum having a high titer of HCV (10^6/mL or more) was used, longer-range RT-PCR could be achieved using a combination of the reverse primer of set 1 and forward primer of set 2 (*see* **Fig. 3**).

References

1. Tanaka, T., Kato, N., Cho, M.-J., and Shimothono, K. (1995) A novel sequence found at the 3' terminus of hepatitis C virus genome. *Biochem. Biophys. Res. Commun.* **215,** 744–749.
2. Tanaka, T., Kato, N., Cho, M.-J., Sugiyama, K., and Shimotohno, K. (1996) Structure of the 3' terminus of the hepatitis C virus genome. *J. Virol.* **70,** 3307–3312.
3. Kolykhalov, A. A., Feinstone, S. M., and Rice, C. M. (1996) Identification of a highly conserved sequence element at the 3' terminus of hepatitis C virus genome RNA. *J. Virol.* **70,** 3363–3371.
4. Yamada, N., Tanihara, K., Takada, A., Yorihuzi, T., Tsutsumi, M., Shimomura, H., et al. (1996) Genetic organization and diversity of the 3' noncoding region of the hepatitis C virus genome. *Virology* **223,** 255–261.
5. Sambrook, J., Fritsch, E. F., and Maniatis, T. (1989) *Molecular Cloning: A Laboratory Manual.* Cold Spring Harbor Laboratory, Cold Spring Harbor, NY.

35

In Vitro Stability of Hepatitis C Virus RNA

Jane W. S. Fang

1. Introduction

Hepatitis C virus (HCV) is an encapsidated RNA virus, known to cause devastating liver diseases among the majority of infected individuals *(1–3)*. Latest breakthrough in molecular technology has greatly assisted the advancement in diagnostics and monitoring of virological response to therapy *(4)*. However, our understanding of the pathogenesis and replication of HCV has been impeded by the immense difficulty in culturing the virus in vitro and the lack of a small animal model. One of the possible explanations for this observation is the instability of the HCV RNA genome in vivo and in vitro. In 1996, two independent research teams described an extended 3' untranslated region (UTR) that is conserved among most HCV genotypes and had been missing in all published sequences prior to this discovery *(5,6)*. There has been speculation concerning its role in stabilizing the HCV RNA genome and in the initiation of the synthesis of the nascent minus RNA strand. In this chapter, a simple in vitro assay is used to analyze the stabilization effect of the various forms of the HCV 3' UTR that have been described in the literature.

Traditionally, microinjection of *Xenopus* oocytes used to take center stage for analyzing translation and degradation of RNA *(7–9)*. Nowadays, highly efficient in vitro translation systems using cell lysates from wheat germ, rabbit reticulocyte, and HeLa cells have replaced the role of *Xenopus*. These cell lysates of low nuclease activity offer the ease of technical application, dynamic manipulation of physical and biochemical conditions, and cost-effectiveness. The following protocol describes the use of an in vitro T7 transcription system to generate radiolabeled HCV RNA transcripts, purification of RNA transcripts, incubation in HeLa cytoplasmic extracts over time to assay for RNA stability, analysis of HCV RNA transcripts in a denaturing gel system, and quantification by phosphorimaging. Note that HeLa cytoplasmic extracts were chosen for its human origin and its relatively low nuclease activity. Parallel reactions using a liver-derived cell line, HepG2, was also tested.

2. Materials

1. HCV plasmids under T7 promoter.
2. T7 RNA polymerase (10–20 U/μL) and buffer (40 mM Tris-HCl, pH 7.9, 6 mM MgCl$_2$, 2 mM spermidine, 10 mM NaCl).
3. 10 μCi/μL α^{32}P-CTP, 1 mM ATP, UTP, GTP, CTP.
4. RNase inhibitor 40 U/μL.
5. 100 mM dithiothreitol.
6. 0.5% SDS buffer: 0.5% SDS, 100 mM NaCl, 10 mM Tris-HCl, pH 7.5, and 1 mM EDTA.
7. Mixed buffered phenol, pH 4.3, and chloroform/isoamyl alcohol (24:1 v/v) at 1:1 v/v.
8. Chloroform/isoamyl alcohol (24:1 v/v).
9. 3 M sodium acetate, pH 5.2.
10. 100% Ethanol.
11. 0.1% Diethylpyrocarbonate (DEPC) treated water.
12. Sephadex G50.
13. 10 mg/mL ycast transfer RNA.
14. TCA mix (7% trichloroacetic acid and 2% sodium pyrophosphate).
15. UV spectrophotometer.
16. HeLa cytoplasmic S10 extracts and translation buffer: 1 mM ATP, 1 mM GTP, 30 mM creatine phosphate, 0.4 mg/mL creatine kinase, 15.5 mM HEPES-KOH, pH 7.4, and 60 mM potassium acetate.
17. 1.1% Formaldehyde denaturing RNA gel electrophoresis.
18. Gel dryer.
19. Phosphorimager.
20. Scintillation counter.

3. Methods

1. In vitro T7 transcription: incubate 3 μg of linearized HCV plasmid, 10 mM DTT, 1X T7 buffer, 1 mM ATP, 1 mM GTP, 1 mM UTP, 1 mM CTP, 10 Ci α^{32}P-CTP, 20 U RNasin, and 3 μL T7 RNA polymerase in 100 μL total volume, at 37°C over 1 h (*see* **Note 1**). The reaction is terminated by adding 200 μL 0.5% SDS buffer.
2. Extract RNA transcripts with an equal volume of mixed buffered phenol, pH 4.3, and chloroform/isoamyl alcohol twice and chloroform/isoamyl alcohol once.
3. Precipitate RNA transcripts by adding 3 M sodium acetate, pH 5.2, to a final concentration of 0.2 M and 100% ethanol at three times the volume, at –20°C for 1 h.
4. Purify the RNA transcripts by gravitating through a 0.5-cm diameter × 8 cm length column of Sephadex G50/water. Collect 5 drops/fraction.
5. Dilute 5 μL/fraction into 500 μL water, and determine the RNA concentration by measuring absorbance at 260 nm. Select the RNA fractions with the initial

highest concentrations (*see* **Note 2**) and precipitate the purified RNA fractions as in **step 3**.
6. Pool the selected fractions into 30 µL water. Take 1 µL for TCA precipitation: mix this with 5 µL 10 mg/mL yeast transfer RNA and 3 mL of TCA mix. Incubate on ice for 15 min, and then filter through 0.2 µ of nitrocellulose. This is then read by the scintillation counter using the 0–1000 window. To quantify the pooled RNA concentration, 1 µL is diluted into 500 µL water and absorbance read at 260 nm. The specific radioactivity of the RNA transcripts can then be determined (*see* **Note 3**).
7. In vitro assay for RNA stability: incubate the radiolabeled RNA transcripts (about 1×10^6 cpm/30 µL reaction) in 50% (v/v) HeLa cytoplasmic S10 extracts and translation buffer in a total volume of 180 µL at 34°C over 0, 10, 20, 40, 60, and 120 min. At the end of each time interval, an aliquot of 30 µL is removed for analysis.
8. To the 30-µL reaction, add 270 µL 0.5% SDS buffer to stop the reaction. RNA is then extracted and ethanol-precipitated as in **steps 2** and **3**.
9. The entire RNA sample from each time-point is used in the denaturing 1.1% formaldehyde, 1% agarose electrophoresis gel. The gel is dried and exposed to autoradiograph as well as quantified by phosphorimaging.

4. Notes

1. To facilitate efficient T7 transcription, the DNA plasmids should be linearized downstream of the HCV 3'-UTR and gel-purified. Owing to the large size (9.6 kb) of the HCV cDNA, most gel-purification methods are inefficient. The author routinely uses the freeze-squeeze method for gel purification and has consistent high yield.
2. Note that there are usually two peaks of spectrophotometer detectable RNA as serially collected fractions are read after Sephadex G50 column. The initial peak contains most of the full-length RNA transcripts, whereas the second peak is generated by mostly unincorporated ribonucleotides and should be discarded as radioactive waste.
3. When comparing the stability of HCV RNA transcripts with different 3'-UTR, the same amount of radioactivity should be used in the in vitro RNA stability assay. The specific radioactivity per microgram of RNA should be very close for all of them owing to the similarity in genomic lengths. In so doing, the initial concentration of the RNA transcripts will be controlled and the degradation of both RNA transcripts will be comparable.
4. It is also important not to overwhelm the cell lysate system in its ability to degrade RNA or support translation. In anticipation of this possibility, it is prudent to titrate the initial amount of RNA to be used by analyzing the change in the RNA degradation profile. Based on previous titration experiments, the author uses 100–150 µg/mL RNA transcripts in in vitro translation and RNA stability assays.
5. Phosphorimaging of the full-length radiolabeled RNA transcripts over time after gel electrophoresis is more reflective of the RNA degradation profile than scintillation counting. The latter provides total radioactivity within the sample and not that of the full-length RNA transcript.

References

1. Alter, M. J., Margolis, H. S., Krawczynski, K., Judson, F. N., Mares, A., Alexander, W. J., et al. (1992) The natural history of community acquired hepatitis C in the United States. *N. Engl. J. Med.* **327,** 1899–1905.
2. Dienstag, J. L. (1997) The natural history of chronic hepatitis and what we should do about it. *Gastroenterology* **112,** 651–655.
3. Muller, R. (1996) The natural history of hepatitis C: clinical experiences. *J. Hepatol.* **24,** 52–54.
4. Davis, G. L. and Lau, J. Y. N. (1995) Choice of appropriate end points of response to interferon therapy in chronic hepatitis C virus infection. *J. Hepatol.* **22,** 110–114.
5. Kolykhalov, A. A., Feinstone, S. M., and Rice, C. M. (1996) Identification of a highly conserved sequence element at the 3' terminus of hepatitis C virus genome RNA. *J. Virol.* **70,** 3363–3371.
6. Tanaka, T., Kato, N., Cho, M. J., Sugiyama, K., and Shimotohno, K. (1996) Structure of the 3' terminus of the hepatitis C virus genome. *J. Virol.* **70,** 3307–3312.
7. Huez, G., Marbaix, G., Burny, A., Hubert, E., Leclercq, M., Cleuter, Y., et al. (1977) Degradation of deadenylated rabbit alpha-globin mRNA in *Xenopus* oocytes is associated with its translation. *Nature* **2266,** 473,474.
8. Drummond, D. R., Armstrong, J., and Colman, A. (1985) The effect of capping and polyadenylation on the stability, movement and translation of synthetic messenger RNAs in *Xenopus* oocytes. *Nucleic Acid Res.* **13,** 7375–7393.
9. Shennan, K. I. J. and Docherty, K. (1988) Expression of normal and human pre-pro-insulins in *Xenopus* oocytes. *Biochimie* **70,** 99–107.

36

Methods for the Study of Sequence-Specific Binding of Proteins to the HCV RNA Genome

Lee M. Kaplan and Raymond T. Chung

1. Introduction

The appropriate formation of specific RNA–protein complexes regulates the normal synthesis, trafficking, and metabolism of intracellular RNA. For RNA viruses, these interactions are essential for replication and translation of the viral genome, as well as packaging of progeny strands into mature virions. Sequence-specific RNA–protein interactions allow the replication and translation machinery to distinguish between viral and host-cell RNA species, thus insuring that the viral replicative apparatus acts on the appropriate RNA targets. Identifying these proteins and determining their biological activities provide important clues about the mechanisms of viral replication. Their physiological importance suggests that blocking these interactions may be effective means of inhibiting viral replication. Thus, the identification and characterization of sequence-specific RNA-binding proteins are valuable steps in the development of potent and selective antiviral agents.

Experience with several viruses has demonstrated that both viral and host cellular proteins participate in these specific RNA interactions *(1–10)*. Virus-encoded proteins are obvious candidates to recognize specific viral RNA sequences, since they are expressed only after viral infection. Since host cell proteins have presumably evolved to support normal cellular processes, their participation in viral replication reflects the ability of the virus to recruit them to its own purposes. Sequence-specific interaction between cellular proteins and viral RNAs reflects either the ability of the viral sequence to mimic the chemical structure of one or more cellular RNAs or the ability of the protein to adapt and recognize the viral RNA. Alteration of a protein's RNA-binding specificity may result from direct binding to a viral protein or sequestration of an interacting species by a viral protein. Alternatively, viral infection may affect the posttranslational modifications or subcellular localization of a host protein, in either case altering its binding characteristics and biologic properties.

The absence of an efficient system for replicating hepatitis C virus (HCV) in cell culture or in a small animal model has precluded many of the standard approaches to dissecting the viral lifecycle. In addition, the relatively low levels of viral RNA and proteins in infected cells has severely hampered direct analysis of changes in the structures and interactions of these molecules during normal replication. Much of our understanding of HCV replication has therefore been inferred by analogy with the lifecycle of other similar viruses, coupled with biochemical and cell biological studies of synthetic HCV RNA and expressed viral proteins. In the case of RNA–protein interactions, this biochemical approach has revealed that sequences at the 5' end of the viral genome can direct cap-independent RNA translation and that several host cellular proteins bind selectively to these sequences *(11–18)*. Although our understanding of the molecular regulation of HCV RNA translation remains incomplete, these studies provide early clues regarding mechanisms by which this virus alters cellular metabolism to favor its own replication.

Far less is known about the mechanisms of HCV genomic replication. The HCV genome is a single, linear, 9.5-kb RNA with positive polarity whose sequence and sequence organization are most similar to that of the pestiviruses *(11)*. There is no evidence for a DNA intermediate in the viral lifecycle, so the RNA genome appears to replicate by a direct RNA-to-RNA mechanism similar to that used by members of the picornavirus, flavivirus, and many other RNA virus families. By analogy with these other viruses, HCV RNA replication is thought to proceed in two phases. In the first, negative strand (antigenomic) RNA is synthesized using the genomic RNA as a template. This process likely initiates from the 3' end of the genomic RNA and extends continuously until the progeny strand is complete. In the second phase, genomic strand RNA is synthesized by replication of the negative strand intermediate, this process likely initiating at the 3' end of the template RNA. This process is shown schematically in **Fig. 1**, which depicts several rounds of RNA synthesis from a single negative strand intermediate (panel 5), a phenomenon that has been previously demonstrated during picornaviral RNA replication.

Replication of the viral RNA is likely catalyzed by the HCV NS5B protein, which has strong sequence homology to other viral RNA polymerases. Recombinant NS5B protein expressed in COS-7 cells or in baculovirus-infected insect cells has been shown to possess limited RNA-dependent RNA polymerase activity *(19–21)*. Replication of viral RNA in vivo likely requires the cooperative action of NS5B with several other viral and/or host proteins.

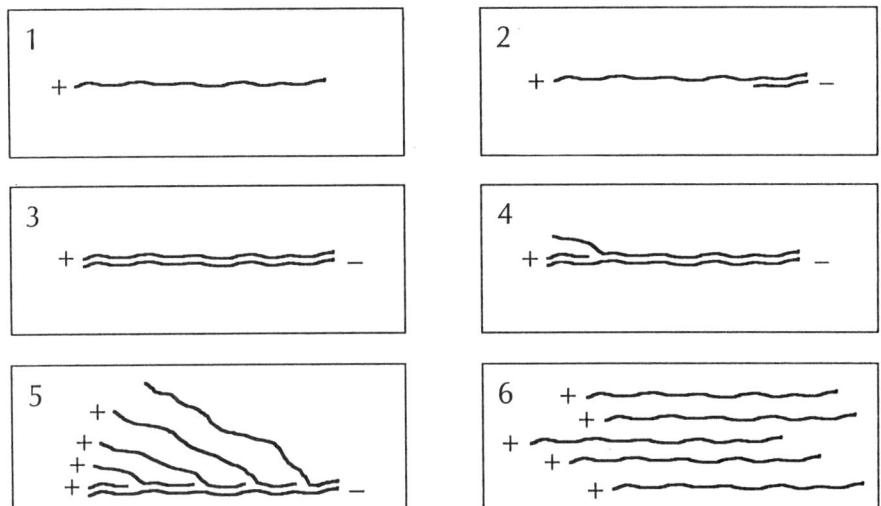

Fig. 1. Schematic model of HCV RNA replication.

Other than NS3, which possesses RNA unwinding (helicase) activity, the identity of these potential replicative proteins is currently unknown.

By analogy with other viruses, selectivity for viral RNA replication in infected cells is likely to occur at the initiation step in RNA synthesis. Although RNA strand *elongation* may also be viral sequence-specific, several features of the initiation reaction suggest its importance as a regulator of replication specificity. The sequences at both ends of the viral genome are extremely well conserved among different genotypes and viral isolates. This is particularly true of the stem-loop structure at the 3' end of the genome, parts of which are 100% conserved among all isolates reported to date *(22–24)*. Since this region likely serves as the site of initiation of negative strand synthesis, the high sequence conservation suggests the need for a specific RNA structure on which to assemble a functional replication complex. The initial stages of complex assembly likely involve specific interactions between one or more replicative proteins and the conserved RNA.

Similarly, the conserved sequence at the 5' end of the genome suggests that specific RNA–protein interactions are required for initiation of positive strand RNA synthesis. Since the 5' end of the genomic RNA is complementary to the 3' end of the negative strand, conservation of sequence suggests structural constraints on RNA–protein interactions in this region as well. As shown in **Fig. 2**, the predicted secondary structures differ considerably between the 3' ends of the positive and negative strands, respectively. These differences suggest that distinct initiation complexes may independently regulate replication of the two

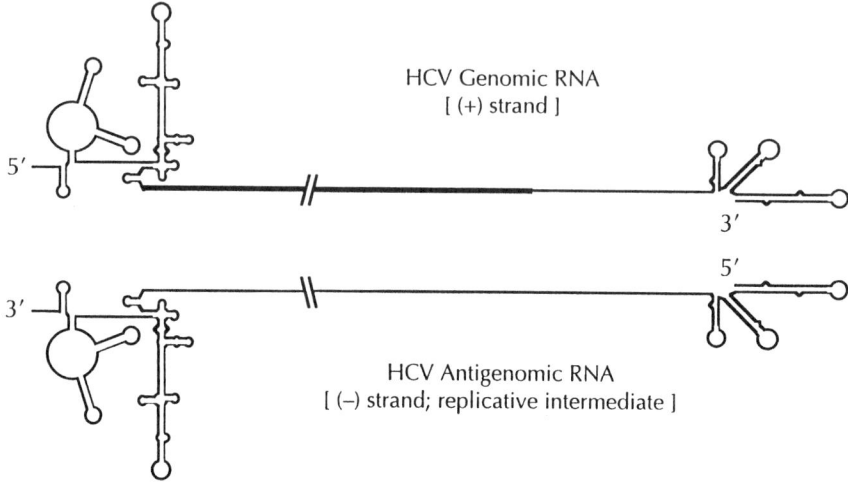

Fig. 2. Predicted structural elements at the ends of the HCV genome and negative strand RNAs.

strands. Such differential regulation might underlie the greater prevalence of positive strand RNA in HCV-infected liver cells. In addition, it provides an opportunity to differentially regulate the packaging or recurrent replication of nascent RNA strands.

Because of the apparent importance of protein complex assembly at the 3' ends of HCV genomic and negative strand RNAs, we sought to identify proteins that recognize these RNA structures specifically. For these studies, we used a variety of biochemical techniques to investigate RNA–protein interactions. The remainder of this chapter describes several methods that allow examination of the specific interaction between heterogeneous nuclear ribonucleoprotein I (hnRNP-I) and the conserved 3' terminus of HCV genomic RNA *(25)*. In keeping with the objectives of this text, the chapter is divided by techniques. As will be apparent, each technique permits investigation of selected aspects of RNA–protein interactions. They provide complementary information and are therefore used most effectively in concert.

hnRNP-I is a 57–62-kDa protein, widely expressed in eukaryotic cells, that regulates pre-mRNA splicing. Located primarily (but not exclusively) in the cell nucleus, this protein binds selectively to polypyrimidine tracts upstream of pre-mRNA splice acceptor sites *(26,27)*. As a result of its binding specificity, hnRNP-I has also been termed polypyrimidine tract-binding protein (PTB). Studies of tropomyosin I pre-mRNA splicing suggest that differential binding of hnRNP-I to the polypyrimidine tracts of different introns contributes to the

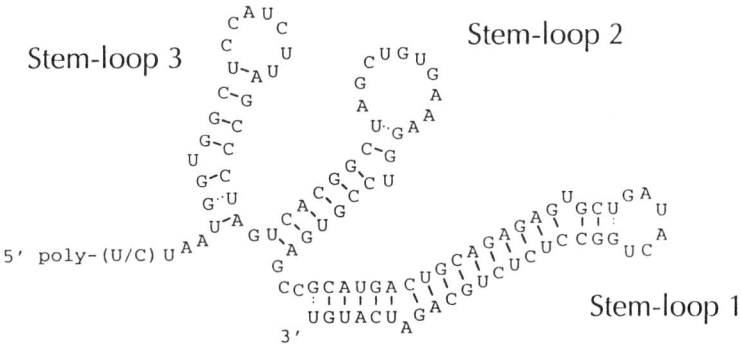

Fig. 3. Structure of the HCV 3'-terminal RNA.

control of splice site selection, although the precise mechanism of this regulation is not known *(28)*.

hnRNP-I/PTB has also been found to bind to the internal ribosome entry site (IRES) of several picornaviruses, including polio, encephalomyocarditis (ECMV), and hepatitis A, where it appears to be essential for IRES-dependent translation *(12–16)*. hnRNP-I/PTB has recently been shown to bind to HCV IRES sequences, although the functional significance of this observation is less clear *(17,29)*.

2. Use and Preparation of Radiolabeled RNA Probes

Each of the techniques described below depends on specific binding of one or more proteins to a defined RNA structure. For our studies of proteins that bind to the 3' terminus of the HCV genome, we examined protein binding to radiolabeled, synthetic RNAs corresponding to this region. **Figure 3** shows the structure of the 3'-terminus of genomic RNA. It includes three stem-loops (SL), each containing a 7- to 10-nucleotide loop sequence and one or two unpaired nucleotides in the stem portion. Experimental support for this structure, predicted to be the most energetically favorable RNA conformation, has come from nuclease sensitivity and primer extension analyses *(22,24,30)*. Sequences within SL2 and SL3 are extremely well-conserved among independent HCV RNAs isolated from patient samples. To date, no variation has been reported in this region *(22–24)*.

In selected cases, we examined protein binding to radiolabeled RNAs corresponding to other viral or unrelated sequences. Comparison of protein binding to various labeled probe RNAs is a valuable means of determining sequence or structural specificity of binding. Proteins that bind RNA nonspecifically will bind to many different labeled probes. Since sequence-specific RNA-binding proteins are more likely to regulate the initiation of viral replication and are better targets for antiviral development, we aimed to identify proteins that differentiate among labeled probe RNAs.

2.1. Method for Generating ^{32}P-Labeled HCV RNA Probes

A double-stranded oligonucleotide fragment containing the HCV 3'-terminal RNA sequence described by Kolykhalov et al. *(22)* was the gift of David Wong and Harry Greenberg. We amplified this sequence by PCR, using primers with upstream *Eco*RI and downstream *Xba*I adapters, respectively. The amplified product was cloned into the corresponding sites of plasmid pSP72 (Promega, Madison, WI), generating pHCV-3'T. The HCV sequence of pHCV-3'T was confirmed by automated fluorescent dideoxynucleotide sequencing (ABI Model 377, Applied Biosystems, Foster City, CA), according to protocols provided by the manufacturer. A second plasmid, pHCV-3'T+, was prepared by inserting sequences from the 3' end of the HCV coding sequence (nucleotides 9218–9389 of HCV-1). This 172-nucleotide sequence was amplified using primers containing upstream *Bgl*II and downstream *Eco*RI adapters, respectively, and ligated into the corresponding sites in pHCV-3'T. Synthetic RNAs were transcribed from linearized, plasmid DNA using T7 RNA polymerase (Ambion, Austin, TX) in reactions containing 5.6 µM [α-^{32}P]UTP (440 Ci/mmol; Dupont NEN, Boston, MA) and 0.25 mM each of ATP, GTP, and CTP. After transcription, template DNA was digested with 12.5 U RNase-free DNase I (Ambion) and the product RNA purified by two cycles of phenol-chloroform extraction, followed by precipitation with ammonium acetate. The size, integrity, and quantity of the synthesized RNA was determined by formaldehyde-agarose electrophoresis and ethidium bromide staining. For RNA corresponding to other regions of HCV genomic and negative strands, those sequences were amplified by RT-PCR and cloned into appropriate vectors. RNA was transcribed from linearized vectors using either T7 or SP6 RNA polymerase (Ambion).

3. Use of Unlabeled Competitor RNAs

Although protein binding to different labeled probe RNAs can demonstrate sequence specificity and provide some information about relative binding avidity, a more efficient and quantitative approach is to examine the ability of various unlabeled RNAs to compete for protein binding to the labeled probe. For these studies, the ability of unlabeled *homologous* RNA to reduce protein binding to the labeled probe is compared with the ability of *heterologous* (unrelated, or modified) RNA to compete for binding. Competition curves allow sensitive determination of the relative affinity of protein binding to different substrate RNAs. For example, a protein that binds weakly to a specific

RNA sequence may nonetheless generate RNA–protein complexes if it is present in sufficient concentration. Competition studies using the higher affinity RNA as labeled probe will reveal that homologous unlabeled RNA will compete for protein binding at a lower concentration than the heterologous (lower affinity) species. Conversely, if the lower affinity RNA is used as the labeled probe, higher concentrations of unlabeled homologous RNA will be required to achieve the same levels of competition as the heterologous (higher affinity) RNA.

Competition experiments examine the ability of various concentrations of competitor RNA to inhibit protein binding to the labeled probe. The concentration of competitor RNA is often defined in terms of the molar excess over probe RNA. The concentration (molar excess) of competitor required to inhibit protein binding to the labeled probe is dependent on the relative concentrations of RNA and protein in the reaction, as well as the strength of binding. In reactions in which the probe and competitor have the same structure (homologous competition), the strength of protein binding to the labeled and unlabeled RNAs is identical. Under these conditions, the molar excess of competitor RNA required to inhibit binding to labeled probe depends solely on the relative concentrations of protein and probe RNA. When RNA and protein are present in approximately equimolar concentrations, addition of a 10-fold excess of unlabeled competitor will reduce binding to the labeled RNA by approx 90%. However, when the protein concentration substantially exceeds the RNA concentration, addition of a 10-fold excess of homologous competitor may have minimal effect on protein binding to the labeled RNA. The added competitor RNA simply binds the excess unbound protein already present in the extracts. Only when the amount of competitor RNA exceeds the concentration of available protein will it appreciably decrease the concentration of labeled RNA–protein complexes.

Despite these limitations, competition studies provide an accurate estimate of the *relative* strength of protein binding to various competitor RNAs. They are the most rapid and effective means of demonstrating sequence specificity of protein binding and assessing the quantitative effects of RNA sequence changes on protein binding. Because synthetic, unlabeled RNAs are stable at –80°C for several months, it is often easier to examine the ability of several different competitor RNAs to inhibit binding to a single labeled probe than to radiolabel each of the RNAs to be studied. This is particularly true when examining protein binding to several different mutant sequences.

4. Protein Preparations

Not knowing the chemical properties or subcellular distribution of potential HCV RNA-binding proteins, we used crude cellular extracts for initial RNA-binding analysis. The source of protein can be an important determinant of the results of RNA-binding studies. Depending on the methods used for extraction, solubilization, and fractionation, crude preparations may contain widely different assortments of proteins. Examination of RNA–protein interactions with these different preparations can generate varied results. In addition, changes in pH and salt concentrations, and the inclusion of detergents, can alter the strength and specificity of RNA–protein binding. For our initial studies, we used low-salt cytoplasmic extracts prepared under conditions that tend to prevent contamination by nuclear extracts.

S10 cytoplasmic extracts were prepared from confluent cells using a modification of the procedure described by Yen et al. *(31)*. Cells were dislodged from culture plates with a cell scraper, washed twice in phosphate-buffered saline and resuspended in two packed cell volumes of lysis buffer (10 mM KCl, 1.5 mM MgAc$_2$, 20 mM N-2-hydroxyethylpiperazine-N'-2-ethanesulfonic acid [HEPES], pH 7.5, 1 mM dithiothreitol), and disrupted by 20 strokes with a B pestle in a Dounce homogenizer. Following the addition of 0.3 packed cell volumes of buffer B (0.2 M HEPES, pH 7.5, 1.2 M KAc, 40 mM MgAc$_2$, 50 mM dithiothreitol), the intact nuclei were removed by centrifugation at 2500g for 5 min. The supernatant was further centrifuged at 10,000 rpm for 15 min in a Sorvall SS34 rotor, and the supernatant saved as the S10 extract.

4.1. Methods for Preparing Proteins Used in RNA-Binding Studies

Recombinant hnRNP-I/PTB was expressed in *Escherichia coli*, using a plasmid (pETPTB) encoding hexahistidine-tagged PTB-1 under the control of the *E. coli lac*Z promoter (the gift of James Patton). Following induction with isopropyl-1-thio-β-galactoside (IPTG), mid-log phase bacteria transformed with this plasmid were isolated and extracts prepared as described by Patton *(32)*. hnRNP-I/PTB was purified from these lysates by affinity chromatography on a Ni-NTA column (Qiagen, Chatsworth, CA) eluted with a step gradient of imidazole (25–500 mM, pH 6.0). Fractions containing hnRNP-I/PTB were identified by Coomassie staining and Western blotting with an anti-(His)$_6$ antibody (Clontech, Palo Alto, CA) after separation by SDS-PAGE. Antibody bound to Western blots was detected with the ECL Western Detection System (Amersham, Arlington Heights, IL), according to the protocol provided by the manufacturer.

5. Electrophoretic Mobility Shift Assay (EMSA)

EMSA is a sensitive means of detecting protein binding to a labeled RNA probe. The RNA-binding protein(s) are incubated with the probe and the resulting mixture is separated by polyacrylamide gel electrophoresis under nondenaturing conditions. The conditions of electrophoresis allow the RNA–

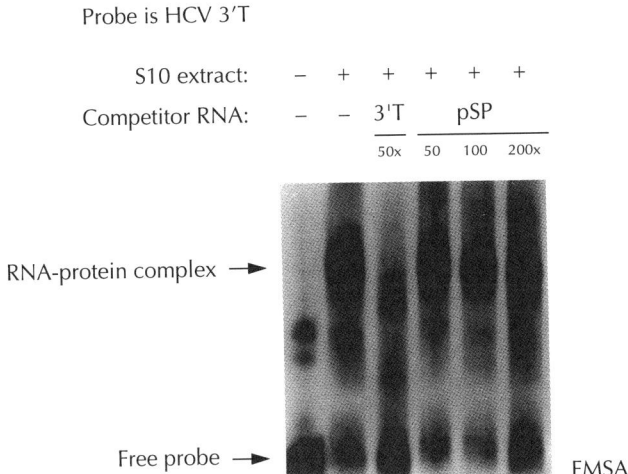

Fig. 4. EMSA analysis reveals cellular proteins binding specifically to the 3' terminus of HCV RNA.

protein complexes to remain intact. Protein binding slows the migration of the RNA probe leading to an upward shift of the labeled band. Retarded complexes detected by EMSA with crude protein preparations usually contain multiple proteins. These proteins can bind in varying combinations, leading to a large number of discrete bands, or a smear of retarded, labeled RNA. Special caution must be taken when performing EMSA (and other RNA–protein binding assays) with crude protein extracts to avoid degradation of the RNA probe. Ribonuclease inhibitors should be included in the incubation mixture. Incubations should be for as short a period as feasible, and when possible, should be performed at 0–4°C. EMSA, like other RNA–protein binding assays, reflects protein binding under the conditions studied. Variation of pH, salt conditions, detergents, and protein concentration can strongly affect the components and stability of the resulting complexes. Preliminary assays should therefore be performed under a variety of conditions to identify the most appropriate protocol for each application.

We used EMSA in initial experiments to determine whether cellular proteins recognize the 3' terminus of the HCV genome. As shown in **Fig. 4**, cytoplasmic S10 extracts prepared from either COS-7 cell retarded the migration of the probe RNA, leading to the formation of a single dominant RNA–protein complex. Formation of this labeled complex was inhibited by inclusion of as little as a 10-fold molar excess of homologous, unlabeled competitor RNA. In contrast, an unrelated competitor RNA sequence failed to inhibit complex formation at 100-fold molar excess and inhibited only minimally at 200-fold excess

(**Fig. 4**). These observations demonstrate that proteins present in uninfected cells bind specifically to the 3'-terminal region of the HCV RNA genome.

5.1. Method for Electrophoretic Mobility Shift Assay

EMSA was performed using a modification of the method described by Konarska and Sharp *(33)*. ^{32}P-labeled RNA (2 fmol/reaction) was incubated with cellular extracts containing a total of 4 µg protein at 30°C for 30 min in reactions containing 10 mM HEPES, pH 7.6, 0.3 mM MgCl$_2$, 40 mM KCl, 5% glycerol, 20 U/mL RNasin (Promega), 1 mM dithiothreitol, and 2 mg/mL yeast tRNA (Boehringer Mannheim, Indianapolis, IN). The reaction mixtures were separated by electrophoresis in nondenaturing, 5% polyacrylamide gels in 0.5X TBE (1X TBE = 89 mM Tris base, 89 mM boric acid, 2 mM EDTA). For competition experiments, unlabeled competitor RNA was added to the reaction mixtures just prior to addition of the labeled probe RNA. Labeled RNA–protein complexes were visualized by autoradiography.

6. UV-Crosslinking of RNA–Protein Complexes

One of the problems with EMSA using crude protein preparations is that the resulting complexes are composed of several different proteins. As a result, their rate of migration cannot be used to predict the size of individual binding proteins. (This is not the case for EMSA with purified proteins, which is a valuable method for detecting oligomerization of RNA-binding proteins). UV-crosslinking (UVC) is a valuable method for determining the size of specific RNA-binding proteins within a crude cellular extract. When multiple proteins bind a target RNA, UVC can frequently distinguish among them, allowing the detection of different binding affinities, specificities, or optimal conditions for binding. For UVC, RNA–protein complexes are formed as for EMSA. They are then subjected to UV irradiation, which covalently crosslinks one or more proteins in the complex to the labeled RNA. Since the complex is stably crosslinked, the RNA can subsequently be hydrolyzed with ribonuclease or alkali, leaving only a short, labeled oligonucleotide crosslinked to the protein. Because only a short RNA sequence remains, it is essential that the RNA probe be labeled internally (i.e., synthesized with radiolabeled nucleotides) rather than labeled by 5' or 3' end-phosphorylation. The oligonucleotide-tagged protein is then subjected to SDS-PAGE which allows separation on the basis of size. The short oligonucleotide label adds only 1–2 kDa to the protein, allowing for a reasonably accurate estimate of the protein size. Like EMSA, detection of RNA-binding proteins by UVC strongly depends on the conditions in which the RNA and protein are incubated. Even when these conditions favor the binding of multiple proteins in the complex, only a fraction of them is likely to be crosslinked to the RNA. UV crosslinking requires that the proteins be in close proximity to the RNA. Although increased duration of UV exposure can increase the number of crosslinked proteins, extensive irradiation may cause protein–protein crosslinks that confound the analysis. As with EMSA, preliminary assays should therefore be performed under a variety of conditions to identify the most appropriate protocol for each application. When necessary, several approaches can be used to increase the sensitivity of UV-crosslinking, including incorporating BrU or thioU residues in the RNA, increasing the power (decreasing the wavelength) of the UV light, or increasing its duration. Most important, however, is identifying incubation conditions that favor stable RNA–protein interactions.

To identify the cellular protein(s) that contribute to the observed RNA–protein complex, we attempted to crosslink one or more of these proteins to the 3'-terminal region of the HCV genome. UV-crosslinking of S10 cytoplasmic extracts to labeled HCV 3'-terminal RNA generated a single major band migrating as an approx 60 kDa species (**Fig. 5A**). Inclusion of a 50-fold molar excess of unlabeled, homologous competitor RNA inhibited formation of the labeled protein-RNA complex. In contrast, a 100-fold molar excess of unrelated RNA sequences exhibited little or no competition for protein binding. An identical labeled band was formed using RNA transcribed from pHCV-3'T+, which includes approx 175 nucleotides of NS5b-coding sequence immediately upstream of the 3'-terminal RNA (data not shown). These observations demonstrate that an approx 60 kDa protein binds selectively to the 3'-terminal region of the HCV genome. Since electrophoresis was performed in the presence of SDS and dithiothreitol, the 60 kDa species appears to represent a single polypeptide chain, which we now know to be hnRNP-I/PTB. This protein likely contributes to the specific RNA–protein complexes observed by EMSA, which may also include one or more additional proteins not detectable by our UV-crosslinking strategy. Demonstration that the RNA–protein complexes detected by EMSA include hnRNP-I/PTB can be achieved with antibody-mediated supershift analysis, as described below.

To examine the RNA binding of hnRNP-I/PTB directly, we expressed recombinant, histidine-tagged protein in *E. coli* and used an affinity-purified preparation in UV crosslinking. As with the native protein in crude S10 extracts, recombinant hnRNP-I/PTB could be competed by unlabeled, homologous competitor RNA, but not by unrelated sequences (**Fig. 5B**).

6.1. Method for UV-Crosslinking

UV-crosslinking experiments were performed by incubating ^{32}P-labeled RNA (10 fmol/reaction) with either S10 extracts or purified, recombinant hnRNP-I/PTB, under the same conditions used for EMSA. For experiments with recombinant hnRNP-I/PTB, 0.6 µg of protein was included in each reac-

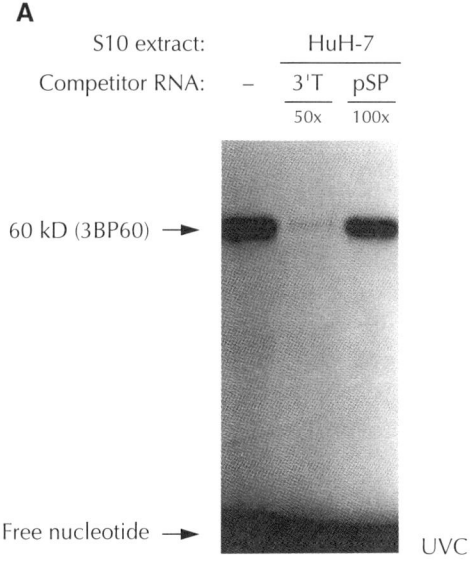

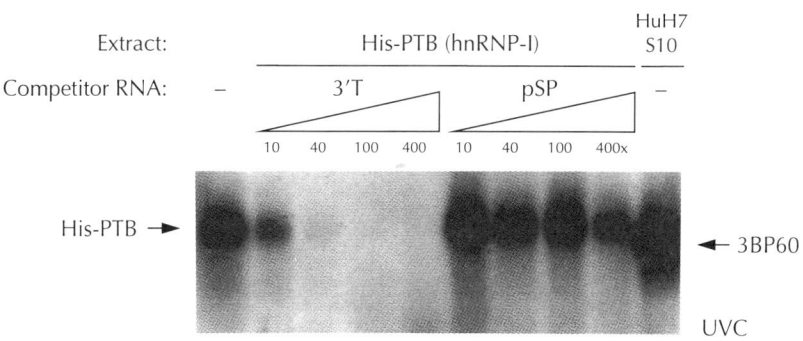

Fig. 5. **(A)** UV crosslinking analysis reveals binding of a 60 kDa protein to the 3' terminus of HCV RNA. **(B)** Recombinant hnRNP-I/PTB selectively binds the 3' terminus of HCV RNA.

tion. Reaction mixtures were then spotted onto Saran Wrap placed directly on a UV transilluminator (312 nm; Fisher Scientific) and irradiated at full power for 15 min at room temperature. Incubated reaction mixtures were recovered and incubated in the presence of either 0.1 N NaOH or a mixture of 500 U/mL RNase A and 20,000 U/mL RNase T1 at 37°C for 30 min. Reactions were then incubated at 100°C for 3 min and separated by electrophoresis through 12%

HCV-Specific RNA-Binding Proteins

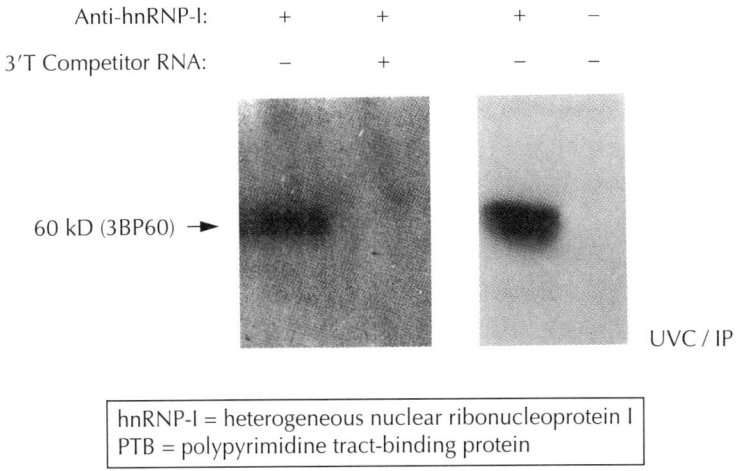

Fig. 6. Immunoprecipitation studies with specific antibodies reveal that the 60 kDa protein is hnRNP-I/PTB.

polyacrylamide gels containing sodium dodecyl sulfate (12% SDS-PAGE). The radiolabeled products, including proteins covalently bound to labeled oligonucleotides, were visualized by autoradiography and quantitated by computer densitometry (Molecular Dynamics, Sunnyvale, CA). For competition experiments, unlabeled competitor RNA was added to the incubation mixtures just prior to the addition of labeled probe RNA.

7. Immunoprecipitation of Protein Crosslinked to RNA

Based on size and its ability to bind poly(U) RNA (not shown), we initially postulated that the 60 kDa protein might be hnRNP-I/PTB. To test this hypothesis, we immunoprecipitated hnRNP-I/PTB from S10 extracts after UV-crosslinking to labeled HCV 3'-terminal RNA. As shown in **Fig. 6**, 7G12 MAb to hnRNP-I/PTB precipitated the 60 kDa protein radiolabeled in the crosslinking reaction. Precipitation of labeled 60 kDa protein depended on the 7G12 antibody and could be inhibited by inclusion of excess unlabeled 3'-terminal RNA in the initial UV-crosslinking reaction. For these experiments, the products of UV-crosslinking were digested with RNase A before immunoprecipitation to decrease the likelihood that adventitious binding of hnRNP-I/PTB to the covalent complexes might allow immunoprecipitation of the labeled protein. In separate experiments, addition of 7G12 to intact complexes (before RNase treatment) or in the presence of 1% Empigen BB, an ionic detergent that disrupts noncovalent protein–protein interactions also precipitated the labeled 60 kDa protein (data not shown). These experiments demonstrate that hnRNP-I/PTB in cellular extracts binds specifically to the 3'-terminal sequences of the HCV genome.

7.1. Method for Immunoprecipitation of UV-Crosslinked Products

Covalent RNA–protein complexes were prepared with radiolabeled HCV 3'-terminal RNA and S10 cytoplasmic extracts as described above. Following UV-crosslinking and RNase treatment in 10 μL reactions, samples were diluted to 500 μL in IP buffer (50 mM Tris-HCl, pH 7.4, 5 mM EDTA, 1 mM dithiothreitol, 100 mM NaCl, 0.05% NP-40). 7G12 antibody to hnRNP-I/PTB (5 μL of mouse ascites) was added, and the mixture was incubated at 4°C for 60 min. After addition of 10 μg of antibodies to mouse immunoglobulin G (Sigma, St. Louis, MO), the resulting immune complexes were immobilized on protein A-agarose beads (Pharmacia, Piscataway, NJ) and washed four times with IP buffer. The radiolabeled, immunoprecipitated proteins were separated by 12% SDS-PAGE and visualized by autoradiography.

8. Antibody-Mediated Supershift Analysis

A major difference between EMSA and UV-crosslinking studies is that with EMSA, the RNA–protein complexes are maintained relatively intact during electrophoretic separation. For EMSA with crude cellular extracts, the retarded bands may include a heterogeneous collection of RNA–protein complexes, each containing several proteins bound to the labeled RNA probe. Once having identified hnRNP-I/PTB as a 3'-terminal RNA-binding protein, we wished to determine whether this protein is a component of one or more of the retarded complexes observed by EMSA. Supershift analysis is an effective means of making this assessment. Supershift analysis detects a change in electrophoretic mobility of RNA–protein complexes as a result of the binding of an additional protein. For antibody-mediated supershift analysis, the bound protein is an antibody that binds to a protein presumed to be present in the complex. As shown in **Fig. 7** (lane 6), inclusion of 7G12 antibody to hnRNP-I/PTB generates an additional retarded band, demonstrating the presence of hnRNP-I/PTB in the RNA–protein complexes detected by EMSA (lanes 2 and 3).

8.1. Method for Antibody-Mediated Supershift Analysis

For antibody-mediated supershift analysis, dilutions of 7G12 (specific for hnRNP-I/PTB) or control antibodies were added to aliquots of recombinant hnRNP-I/PTB (0.6 μg/reaction) and incubated for 30 min at room temperature. The incubation products were then added to RNA-binding reactions containing 10 mM HEPES, pH 7.6, 0.3 mM MgCl$_2$, 40 mM KCl, 5% glycerol, 20 U/mL RNasin (Promega), 1 mM dithiothreitol, 2 mg/mL yeast tRNA (Boehringer

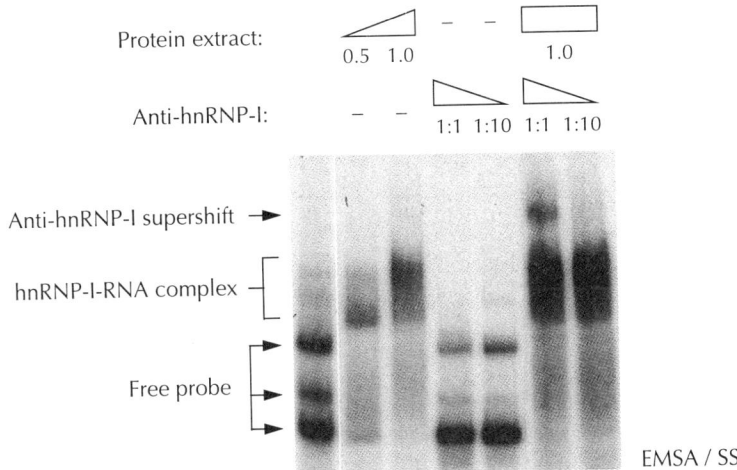

Fig. 7. Antibody-mediated supershift analysis reveals that hnRNP-I/PTB is a component of the RNA–protein complexes detected by EMSA.

Mannheim, Indianapolis, IN) and ^{32}P-labeled HCV 3'-terminal RNA. These reactions were incubated at 30°C for 30 min and then separated by electrophoresis in nondenaturing, 5% polyacrylamide gels in 0.5X TBE. The labeled products were detected by autoradiography of the vacuum-dried gel.

9. Use and Preparation of Mutant RNAs

The structural and sequence requirements for protein binding to a target RNA can be determined by examining the binding properties of RNAs containing specific mutations. We used three mutagenesis strategies to examine the requirements for hnRNP-I/PTB binding to the HCV 3'-terminal RNA. To determine the gross structural requirements for protein binding, we prepared RNAs in which stem-loop 1, 2, or 3 was deleted, respectively (**Fig. 8A**). In addition, we prepared a mutant RNA containing stem-loop 1 alone (i.e., with both stem-loops 2 and 3 deleted). For finer structure mapping, we prepared mutants with several bases deleted from one of the loop sequences and others in which we removed one of the unpaired uridines in the stem structures (**Fig. 8B**). Finally, to examine the sequence specificity of protein binding, we prepared RNAs with compensatory changes in one of the stem sequences (**Fig. 8C**). These mutations altered primary base sequence while preserving the stem structure itself. Such mutations can be valuable for differentiating structural from sequence-specific requirements for protein binding. In most cases, mutants were examined for their ability to *compete* for protein binding to labeled, wild-type RNA. In selected cases, we

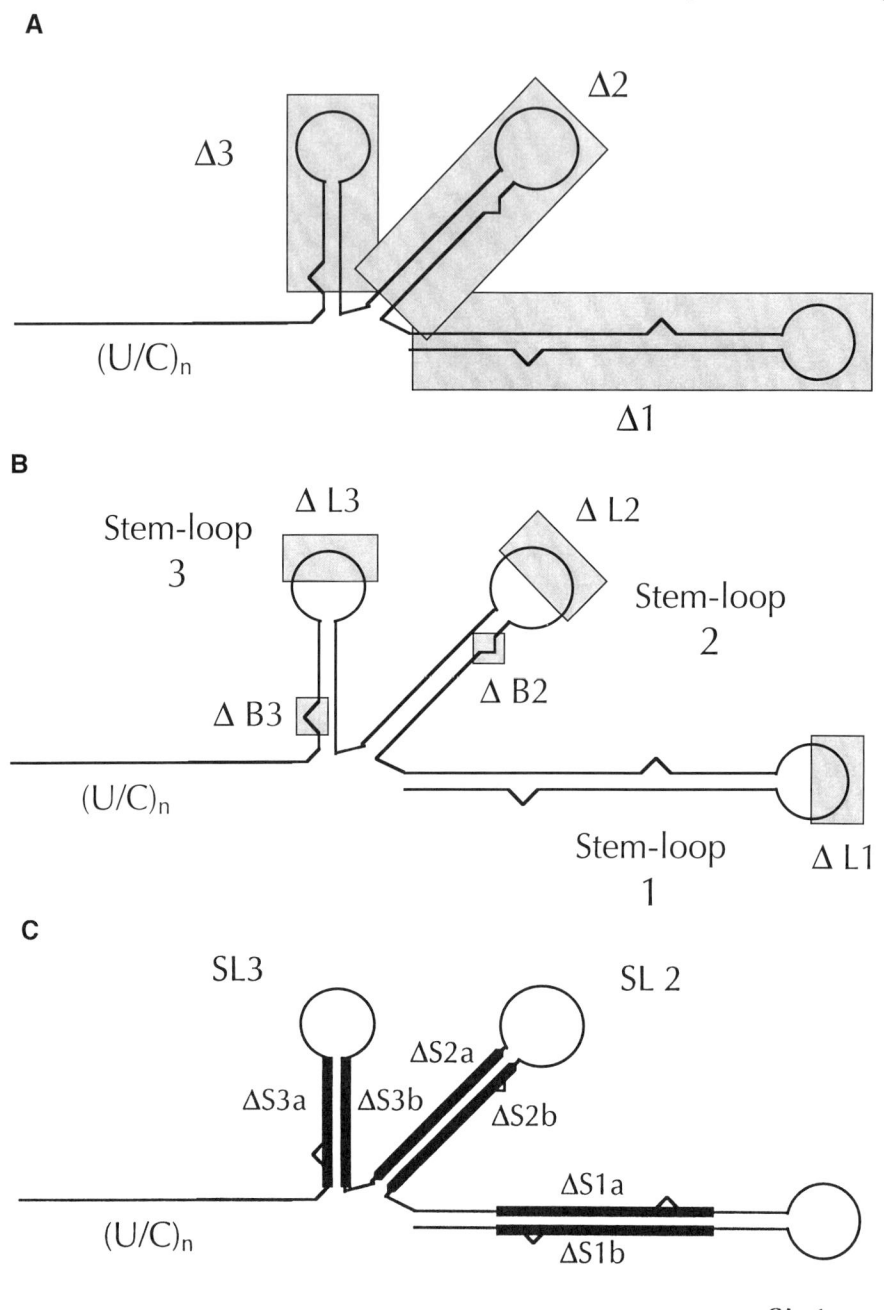

Fig. 8. **(A)** Gross deletion mutagenesis, **(B)** fine deletion mutagenesis, and **(C)** compensatory mutations of the HCV 3'-terminal RNA.

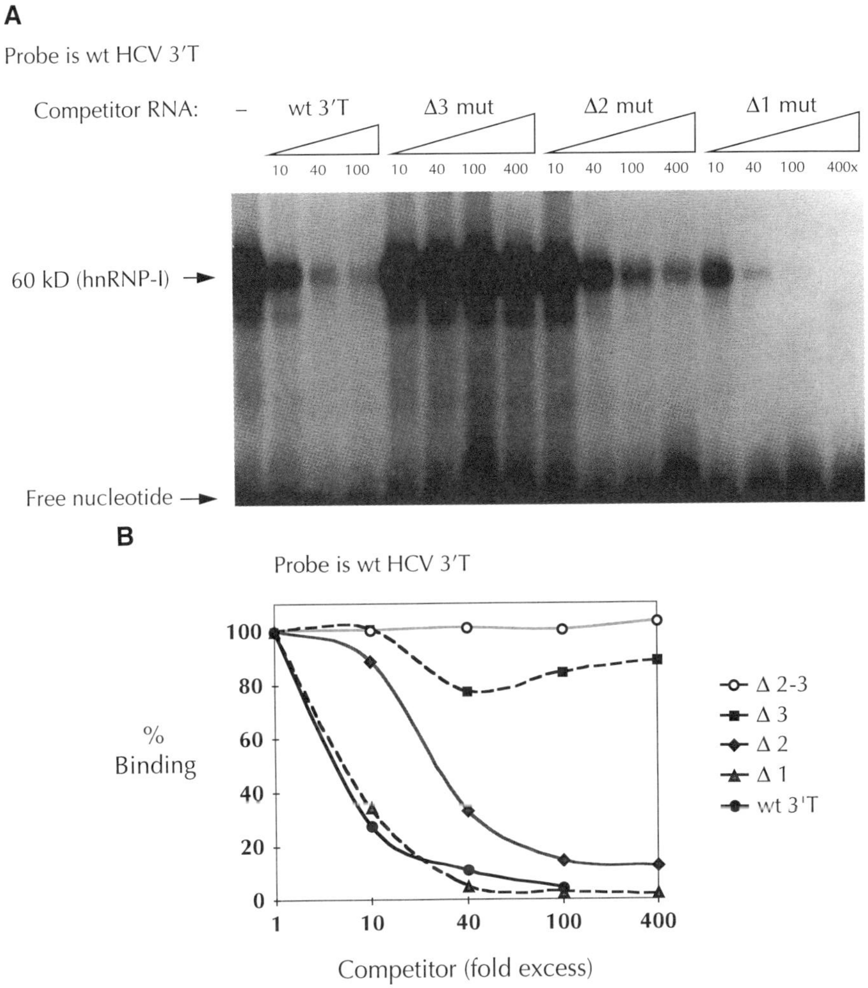

HCV-Specific RNA-Binding Proteins

Fig. 9. **(A)** Mutational analysis reveals the hnRNP-I/PTB binds selectively to stem-loops 2 and 3. **(B)** Quantitative analysis of UV-crosslinking-based mutational analysis shown in (A).

examined the binding of hnRNP-I/PTB to labeled mutant sequences. Both approaches revealed the same structural requirements for protein binding, although as noted above, subtle differences in binding avidity were more easily discernible in competition studies (**Fig. 9A, B**).

References

1. Blackwell, J. L. and Brinton, M. A. (1995) BHK cell proteins that bind to the 3' stem-loop structure of the West Nile virus genome RNA. *J. Virol.* **69,** 5650–5658.

2. Del Angel, R. M., Papavassiliou, A. G., Fernandez-Tomas, C., Silverstein, S. J., and Racaniello, V. R. (1989) Cell proteins bind to multiple sites within the 5' untranslated region of poliovirus RNA. *Proc. Natl. Acad. Sci. USA* **86,** 8299–8303.
3. Haller, A. A. and Semler, B. L. (1995) Stem-loop structure synergy in binding cellular proteins to the 5' noncoding region of poliovirus RNA. *Virology* **206,** 923–934.
4. Leopardi, R., Hukkanen, V., Vainionpaa, R., and Salmi, A. A. (1993) Cell proteins bind to sites within the 3' noncoding region and the positive-strand leader sequence of measles virus RNA. *J. Virol.* **67,** 785–790.
5. Liu, Q., Yu, W., and Leibowitz, J. L. (1997) A specific host cellular protein binding element near the 3' end of mouse hepatitis virus genomic RNA. *Virology* **232,** 74–85.
6. Nakhasi, H. L., Cao, X-Q., Rouault, T. A., and Liu, T-Y. (1991) Specific binding of host cell proteins to the 3'-terminal stem-loop structure of rubella virus negative-strand RNA. *J. Virol.* **65,** 5961–5967.
7. Pardigon, N. and Strauss, J. H. (1992) Cellular proteins bind to the 3' end of Sindbis virus minus-strand RNA. *J. Virol.* **66,** 1007–1015.
8. Pardigon, N., Lenches, E., and Strauss, J. H. (1993) Multiple binding sites for cellular proteins in the 3' end of Sindbis alphavirus minus-sense RNA. *J. Virol.* **67,** 5003–5011.
9. Quadt, R., Kao, C. C., Browning, K. S., Hershberger, R. P., and Ahlquist, P. (1993) Characterization of a host protein associated with brome mosaic virus RNA-dependent RNA polymerase. *Proc. Natl. Acad. Sci. USA* **90,** 1498–1502.
10. Todd, S., Nguyen, J. H. C., and Semler, B. L. (1995) RNA–protein interactions directed by the 3' end of human rhinovirus genomic RNA. *J. Virol.* **69,** 3605–3614.
11. Major, M. E. and Feinstone, S. M. (1997) The molecular virology of hepatitis C. *Hepatology* **25,** 1527–1538.
12. Chang, K. H., Brown, E. A., and Lemon, S. M. (1993) Cell type-specific proteins which interact with the 5' nontranslated region of hepatitis A virus RNA. *J. Virol.* **67,** 6716–6725.
13. Hellen, C. U. T., Witherell, G. W., Schmid, M., Shin, S. H., Pestova, T. V., Gil, A. M., and Wimmer, E. (1993) A cytoplasmic 57-kD protein that is required for translation of picornavirus RNA by internal ribosomal entry is identical to the nuclear pyrimidine tract-binding protein. *Proc. Natl. Acad. Sci. USA* **90,** 7642–7646.
14. Hellen, C. U. T., Pestova, T. V., Litterst, M., and Wimmer, E. (1994) The cellular polypeptide p57 (pyrimidine tract-binding protein) binds to multiple sites in the poliovirus 5' nontranslated region. *J. Virol.* **68,** 941–950.
15. Niepmann, M. (1996) Porcine polypyrimidine tract-binding protein stimulates translation initiation at the internal ribosome entry site of foot-and-mouth-disease virus. *FEBS Lett.* **388,** 39–42.
16. Witherell, G. W. and Wimmer, E. (1994) Encephalomyocarditis virus internal ribosomal entry site RNA–protein interactions. *J. Virol.* **68,** 3183–3192.

17. Ali, N. and Siddiqui, A. (1995) Interaction of polypyrimidine tract-binding protein with the 5' noncoding region of the hepatitis C virus RNA genome and its functional requirement in internal initiation of translation. *J. Virol.* **69**, 6367–6375.
18. Ali, N. and Siddiqui, A. (1997) The La antigen binds 5' noncoding region of the hepatitis C virus RNA in the context of the initiator AUG codon and stimulates internal ribosome entry site-mediated translation. *Proc. Natl. Acad. Sci. USA* **94**, 2249–2254.
19. Chung, R. T., Kawashima, T., and Kaplan, L. M. (1996) Expressed HCV NS5B polymerase catalyzes primer-dependent elongation. *Gastroenterology* **110**, A1172.
20. Lohmann, V., Korner, F., Herian, U., and Bartenschlager, R. (1997) Biochemical properties of hepatitis C virus NS5B RNA-dependent RNA polymerase and identification of amino acid sequence motifs essential for enzymatic activity. *J. Virol.* **71**, 8416–8428.
21. Behrens, S. E., Tomei, L., and De Francesco, R. (1996) Identification and properties of the RNA-dependent RNA polymerase of hepatitis C virus. *EMBO J.* **15**, 12–22.
22. Kolykhalov, A. A., Feinstone, S. M., and Rice, C. M. (1996) Identification of a highly conserved sequence element at the 3' terminus of hepatitis C virus genome RNA. *J. Virol.* **70**, 3363–3371.
23. Tanaka, T., Kato, N., Cho, M. J., and Shimotohno, K. (1995) A novel sequence found at the 3' terminus of hepatitis C virus genome. *Biochem. Biophys. Res. Commun.* **215**, 744–749.
24. Tanaka, T., Kato, N., Cho, M. J., Sugiyama, K., and Shimotohno, K. (1996) Structure of the 3' terminus of hepatitis C virus genome. *J. Virol.* **70**, 3307–3312.
25. Chung, R. T. and Kaplan, L. M. (1998) Heterogeneous nuclear ribonucleoprotein I (hnRNP-I/PTB) selectively binds the conserved 3' terminus of the hepatitis C virus genome. Submitted for publication.
26. Garcia-Blanco, M. A., Jamison, S. F., and Sharp, P. A. (1989) Identification and purification of a 62,000-dalton protein that binds specifically to the polypyrimidine tract of introns. *Genes Dev.* **3**, 1874–1886.
27. Ghetti, Z., Pinol-Roma, S., Michael, W. M., Morandi, C., and Dreyfuss, G. (1992) hnRNP I, the polypyrimidine tract-binding protein: distinct nuclear localization with hnRNAs. *Nucleic Acids Res.* **20**, 3671–3678.
28. Patton, J. G., Mayer, S. A., Tempst, P., and Nadal-Ginard, B. (1991) Characterization and cloning of polypyrimidine tract-binding protein: a component of a complex necessary for pre-mRNA splicing. *Genes Dev.* **5**, 1237–1251.
29. Reynolds, J. E., Kaminski, A., Kettinen, H. J., Grace, K., Clarke, B. E., Carroll, A. R., Rowlands, D. J., and Jackson, R. J. (1995) Unique features of internal initiation of hepatitis C virus RNA translation. *EMBO J.* **14**, 6010–6020.
30. Ito, T. and Lai, M. M. (1997) Determination of the secondary structure of and cellular protein binding to the 3'-untranslated region of the hepatitis C virus genome. *J. Virol.* **71**, 8698–8706.

31. Yen, J.-H., Chang, S. C., Hu, C.-R., Chu, S.-C., Lin, S.-S., Hsieh, S.-S., and Chang, M.-F. (1995) Cellular proteins specifically bind to the 5' noncoding region of hepatitis C virus RNA. *Virology* **208,** 723–732.
32. Lin, C. H. and Patton, J. G. (1995) Regulation of alternative 3' splice site selection by constitutive splicing factors. *RNA* **1,** 234–245.
33. Konarska, M. M. and Sharp, P. A. (1986) Electrophoretic separation of complexes involved in the splicing of precursors to mRNAs. *Cell* **46,** 845–855.

VII

HCV-Specific Immunologic Response

37

Role of Immune Response in HCV

Marion Peters

1. Introduction

The liver cell response to hepatitis C, a positive-strand RNA virus of the flaviviridiae, varies considerably from acute disease to chronic hepatitis, and from inapparent infection to cirrhosis. The cellular injury to the host depends on host–viral interactions (**Table 1**): in general, the more active the immune response, the greater the cellular injury. If viral infection leads to cell lysis, then the organism dies as is seen in fulminant hepatitis, a relatively rare event (<1% response seen after hepatotrophic viral infection and rare in HCV infection). If cellular dysfunction occurs, then clinical disease results. If viral replication occurs without cellular damage, then inapparent infection results. If the individual is exposed without attachment to the host, then no infection occurs.

Hepatotrophic viruses are not generally cytopathic, and the necroinflammatory disease seen in viral hepatitis results from the immune response. The incidence of exposure to HCV that does not result in disease is unknown. Acute self-limiting infection is uncommon (<15%), as is generally true of many viral infections. Once virus is resident in the liver, the majority of patients appear to have clinical disease of varying severities, with chronicity occuring in >90%. Chronic infection ranges from viremia and normal markers of liver inflammation (serum aminotransferases) to severe inflammation and scarring of the liver. Although the heterogeneity of HCV genotypes play a role (*see* Chapter 11), it is the host response and the host–viral interactions that determine the level of inflammation. This chapter will discuss how the immune response is important in producing chronic HCV infection.

2. Stages in Viral Pathogenesis

These are outlined in **Table 2**. The mechanism of viral entry into cells is well known for many viruses, but not identified for HCV. The prototype virus

Table 1
Host-Cell Response: Outcome of HCV Infection

Cellular response	Host response	HCV
Cell lysis	Death of organism	Fulminant failure rare
Viral multiplication without cell damage	Asymptomatic infection	Inapparent disease <15%
Cell dysfunction	Clinical disease	Common
Exposure without attachment	Exposure, no infection	Unknown

Table 2
Stages in Viral Pathogenesis

Entry into cell	Absorption of HCV parenteral
Primary replication	Penetration
Spread through host	Uncoating
Cell and tissue tropism	Transcription in liver, PBMC
Host immune response	Translation of host proteins
Secondary replication	Replication
Cell injury	Assembly
Persistence	Release to serum

will gain entry into the organism, utilize host machinery, and become persistent with or without major organ damage, and spread throughout the organism to avoid eradication. Viral damage occurs owing to interference with cellular mechanisms, alteration of cell membrane function, or damage via viral products. Viral infection in naive individuals induces an immune response that is rapid and nonspecific in the first few days. Viral titers are measurable in serum with similar kinetics to induction of interferons and natural killer (NK) cells. After days, delayed and specific cytolytic T-cell and neutralizing B-cell responses are induced.

3. Nonspecific Immune Responses

Nonspecific responses include complement, interferons, natural antibody, and NK cells. Most acute viral infections induce interferons: there is evidence that patients with chronic hepatitis C do not induce comparable amounts of interferons in vitro, but no studies have been undertaken in those few patients who clear HCV (<10%). Viral titers are detectable in serum in the first few days of most infections, and interferons (α and β), and NK activity are detectable with similar kinetics. Interferons are rarely detectable in serum in patients with any chronic disease. Interferons not only aid in control of viral entry and replication in the cells, but also induce NK cells, cytokines, and upregulate many cell membrane proteins essential for immune recognition *(1)*. NK cells are induced by cytokines, including interferon-α (IFN-α). They nonspecifically kill target cells by cell–cell contact, and release of perforins and granzymes. Killer cells lyse virally infected targets via their Fc receptor and preformed antibody, which recognizes viral antigen on the target cell. Cells are lysed via cell-to-cell contact and soluble mediators. Nonspecific immune events may control viremia but cannot eradicate it entirely.

4. Specific Immune Responses

It is the immunological memory and induction of specific cytotoxic T-cells and neutralizing antibody that eradicate viremia and abrogate recurrent viremia. In prototypic viral infections, individuals who do not develop neutralizing antibodies have recurrent bursts of viremia similar to primary infection, although cytotoxic T-cells will be activated to clear viremia with each burst of infection. Although cytotoxic T-lymphocytes (CTL) clear virus, neutralizing antibody provides protection from reinfection and/or spread of virus through serum. The host response is also determined by viral cytopathicity. For cytopathic viruses, inadequate or delayed CTL responses lead to death of the organism with high-titer viremia. For noncytopathic viruses, rapid CTL response leads to clearance of virus (unusual in HCV). Inadequate CTL responses cause higher titers of virus in blood with recurrent burst of CTL activity (to clear viremia) or no CTL activity, asymptomatic infection, or carrier state. The virus has an advantage over the host in that it has an extremely short generation time, multiplying frequently with numerous mutations. Lymphocytes are the answer to this problem: they have a short generation time with multiple numbers and are capable of great diversity.

In spite of an exquisitely responsive immune system, viruses have developed mechanism to evade the host immune response *(2)*. They can be hidden within the cell and not recognized; they can mutate and not be recognized; they can mutate, be recognized, but not induce a positive immune response; or they alter the effectors of the immune response. If virus is not multiplying, it may lay dormant in the cell and not induce an immune response unless reactiviated, as is seen with hepatitis B virus (HBV). HCV frequently mutates and may produce altered peptides, which can bind CTL via human lymphocyte antigen-T-cell reactivity (HLA-TCR), but do not activate the T-cell. These altered peptide ligands have been elegantly shown with HBV *(3)*. Many viruses encode host proteins or inhibitors of host proteins, which lead to weak or ineffective host defense. These include proteins that mimic cytokines or cytokine receptors inhibit cytokine signaling inhibit interferon-inducible proteins, or inhibit gene expression *(2)*.

5. Immune Response to HCV

There is an active immunological reaction to HCV in most individuals. This is evident by serum autoantibodies, extrahepatic manifestations of autoimmune disease, T- and B-cell responses and pathology *(4)*. Autoantibodies are common, although usually in low titer. There does appear to be some correlation between adequacy of rapid early T-cell response and possible clearance of acute infection. The liver pathology shows portal lymphocytic infiltrate with plasma cells; there are prominent lymphoid follicles with germinal centers; and there may bile duct lesions with intraepithelial lymphocytes *(5)*. The association between level of inflammation (ALT) and liver pathology is not absolute: recent data show that there are a percentage of patients who have normal ALT with ongoing infection *(6)*. The extrahepatic autoimmune manifestations are extensive, including cryoglobulins with vasculitis and glomerulonephritis, thyroiditis, sialadinitis, and autoantibodies. Although cryoglobulins are frequently found in the serum, with positive rheumatoid factor (60%), true disease from cryoglobulins is less common.

6. Cellular Immune Responses

T-cells' responses to viral infection are predominantly $CD8^+$ cytotoxic (CTL) lymphocytes, which recognize viral peptides (10–12 amino acids) in the context of HLA Class I. The peptide has HLA binding sites and T-cell receptor (TCR) binding sites. CTL are protective against some viral infections, but individuals chronically infected with HCV demonstrate specific HCV CTL activity. Multiple epitopes have been identified in the core and envelope regions of HCV and in nonstructural regions *(7–10)*. Some studies have used peripheral blood mononuclear cell (PBMC) and others liver lymphocytes. The peripheral blood may not reflect what is occurring in the liver with different cellular and cytokine responses *(11)*. In addition, most studies have found a low precursor frequency in HCV-specific CTLs in PBMC. HCV-specific CTL appear to be localized to the liver, the site of virally infected host cells. Studies have varied depending on the source of CTLs and the method of in vitro expansion (Chapters 39–41).

$CD4^+$ responses are essential for T-helper cell activity for antibody production. Proliferative responses are seen in individuals with acute and chronic infection and differ in those who have active inflammation and those with mild disease. This may relate to the ability of the immune response to drive a predominantly TH1 phenotype, i.e., IL-2 and IFN-γ production with T cell response or a TH2 phenotype (IL-4 and IL-10 production) with predominantly antibody responses *(12,13* and Chapter 38).

7. B-Cell Responses

Antibody responses are noted in patients with persisten infection and are not protective in chimpanzee studies *(14)*. Antibodies are used for diagnosis of HCV infection (Chapters 2 and 55) and immunodominant epitopes are found in core, envelope, and non-structural regions of the virus *(4,15)*.

Viral clearance is thus a balance between the host immune response and viral replication. That balance is achieved by host factors (CTL, B-cells, HLA, and nonspecific responses) and viral factors (viral load, viral genotype, and quasispecies). The balance is altered by immunosuppression, antiviral drugs, and drugs that activate the immune response. Thus, to clear HCV from the liver and extrahepatic sites, a number of factors may have to act in concert. These include lowering viral load, and activating nonspecific responses (NK cells, interferon, complement) and specific CTL responses. The host immune response is responsible for both viral clearance and cellular injury. The following chapters will outline how to assess T- and B-cell response to HCV. Since T-cell responses are seen in recovered patients as well as those with chronic HCV infection, is the difference that of specific epitope recognition? Are there differences in TH1/ Th2 ratios or between in vivo and in vitro responses? Elegant work has shown CTL responses in HCV infection, and some correlation between stages of infection and response to treatment *(16,17)*. Antibodies are noted but rarely shown to be protective *(14)*. There may be differences in various HLA disparate individuals. There is some suggestion that HLA plays a role in clearance of virus and response to treatment.

In summary, the cellular injury resulting from HCV infection appears not to be cytopathic. It results from interference with cellular functions and damage from the host immune response. Tumorigenesis occurs, but not from integration into the host genome. Fruitful areas for research will expand our knowledge about the kinetics of CTL and B-cell responses in HCV infection, the trafficking between PBMC and liver lymphocytes, the kinetics of neutralizing antibodies, and the proteins induced by the virus to evade the host immune response.

References

1. Peters, M., Davis, G. L., Dooley, J. S., and Hoofnagle, J. H. (1986) The interferon system in acute and chronic viral hepatitis. *Prog. Liver Dis.* **89**, 453–468.
2. Peters, M. (1996) Actions of cytokines on the immune response and viral interactions: an overview. *Hepatology* **23**, 909–916.
3. Carli, M., Fiaccadori, F., and Ferrari, C. (1994) Natural variants of cytotoxic epitopes are T-cell receptor antagonists for antiviral cytotoxic T cells. *Nature* **369**, 407–410.

4. Koziel, M. J. (1996) Immunology of viral hepatitis. *Am. J. Med.* **100,** 98–109.
5. Scheuer, P. J., Ashrafzadeh, P., Sherlock, S., et al. (1992) The pathology of hepatitis C. *Hepatology* **15,** 567–571.
6. Mondelli, M. U., Cerino, A., Bellotti, V., and de Koning, A. (1993) Immunobiology and pathogenesis of Hepatitis C virus infection. *Res. Virol.* **144,** 269–274.
7. Nelson, D. R., Marousis, C. G., Davis, G. L., et al. (1997). The role of hepatitis C virus-specific cytotoxic T lymphocytes in chronic hepatitis C. *J. Immunol.* **158,** 1473–1481.
8. Koziel, M. J., Dudley, D., Wong, J. T., et al. (1992) Intrahepatic cytotoxic T lymphocytes specific for hepatitis C virus in person with chronic hepatitis. *J. Immunol.* **149,** 3339–3344.
9. Koziel, M. J., Dudley, D., Afdhal, N., et al. (1993) Hepatitis C virus specific cytotoxic T lymphocytes recognize epitopes in the core and envelope proteins of HCV. *J. Virol.* **67,** 7522–7532.
10. Kaneko, T., Nakamura, I., Kita, H., et al. (1996) Three new cytotoxic T cell epitopes identified within the hepatitis C virus nucleoprotein *J. Gen. Virol.* **77,** 1305–1309.
11. Minutello, M. A., Pileri, P., Unutmaz, D., et al. (1993) Compartmentalization of T lymphocytes to the site of disease: intrahepatic CD4+ T cells specific for the protein NS4 of hepatitis C virus in patients with chronic hepatitis C. *J. Exp. Med.* **178,** 17–25.
12. Diepolder, H. M., Zachoval, R., Hoffmann, R. M., et al. (1995) The role of hepatitis C virus specific CD4+ T lymphocytes in acute and chronic hepatitis C. *J. Mol. Med.* **74,** 583–588.
13. Hoffmann, R. M., Diepolder, H. M., Zachoval, R., et al. (1995) Mapping of immunodominant CD4+ T lymphocyte epitopes of hepatitis C virus antigens and their relevance during the course of chronic infection. *Hepatology* **21,** 632–638.
14. Farci, P., Alter, H. J., Govindarajan, S., et al. (1992) Lack of protective immunity against reinfection with Hepatitis C virus. *Science* **258,** 135–140.
15. Mondelli, M. U., Cividini, A., and Cerino, A. (1997) Role of humoral immune responses in hepatitis B and C virus infections. *Eur. J. Clin. Invest.* **25,** 543–547.
16. Diepolder, H. M., Zachoval, R., Hoffmann, R. M., et al. (1995). Possible mechanism involving T-lymphocyte response to non-structural protein 3 in viral clearance in acute hepatitis C virus infection. *Lancet* **14,** 1006,1007.
17. Nelson, D. R., Gray, A. H., Kolberg, J. A., et al. (1995) Variations of hepatitis C virus NS5B sequence (nucleotides 8261–8566) do not correlate with response to interferon-alpha therapy. *J. Viral. Hepatol.* **2,** 285–292.

38

Determination of Hepatitis C Virus-Specific CD4+ T-Cell Activity in PBMC

J. Tilman Gerlach, Helmut Diepolder, and Gerd R. Pape

1. Introduction

T-cells are the key players in the field on which the virus and the immune response try to defeat or at least control each other. Two categories of T-cells are involved: $CD4^+$ and $CD8^+$ T-cells. $CD4^+$ and $CD8^+$ T-cells have different characteristics and functions and different roles in the immune response to viruses. This chapter discusses methods to determine the $CD4^+$ T-cell activity.

In order to activate a $CD4^+$ T-cell, its T-cell receptor (TCR) has to form a complex with a peptide presented in the context of major histocompatibility complex (MHC) class II antigens at the surface of antigen-presenting cells (APC: mainly dendritic cells, macrophages, and B-cells). In addition, for full activation of a T-cell, further activation signals delivered by the APC are required. These consist of specialized molecules on the surface of the APC and certain lymphokines secreted by the APC. The peptide binding site of Class II molecules is a groove with an eight-stranded β-pleated sheet forming its floor and two α-helical regions forming its walls. The presented class II peptides are approx 12 amino acids long. Extensive polymorphism within these pockets accounts for the allele specificity of peptide binding. The pathways by which class II molecules acquire peptides are sophisticated.

Determination of $CD4^+$ T-cell activity is performed by measuring proliferation of $CD4^+$ T-cells after stimulation with viral proteins or viral peptides. To analyze the T-cell response in detail, the cells have to be cloned. Isolation of the T-cells from peripheral blood, their proliferation to virus-specific proteins and peptides, the procedures to establish T-cell clones, the phenotypic characterization, and the MHC class II restriction of the T-cells are discussed in this chapter.

CD4+ T-cells excert their regulatory role mainly by the release of cytokines. Since the majority of CD4+ T-cells unlike CD8+ T-cells have only small amounts of lymphokines in storage, they produce and secrete these substances after activation. The cytokine pattern released from the cells is divided into two categories, the TH1 and the TH2 profile, where TH1 cytokines are mainly interferon-γ (IFN-γ), interleukin 2 (IL-2), and tumor necrosing factor (TNF)-β, whereas TH2 cytokines are IL-4, IL-5, IL-6, and IL-10. Many of the T-cells can produce cytokines of both categories in varying amounts and different ratios, and are referred to as TH0 cells. A complex and not very well-known interplay of TH1 cytokines favors a so-called TH1 response, a cellular immune response that results from activation of macrophages, NK cells, cytolytic T killer cells, and the DTH reaction, whereas TH2 cytokines favor antibody production by B-cells.

The determination of this key function of CD4+ T-cells by measuring different lymphokines produced by these cells after activation would be beyond the scope of this chapter.

2. Materials

1. Peripheral blood mononuclear cells (PBMC) are isolated from heparinized (Heparin Novo Nordisk Pharma, Germany) blood on Ficoll-isopaque gradients (Pharmacia, Uppsala, Sweden; density of Ficoll 1.077, stable at 4°C). PBMC are cultured and stimulated with antigens in 96-well round-bottom plates (Costar, Cambridge, MA).
2. Phosphate-buffered saline (PBS) with calcium and magnesium is used for washing procedures.
3. Medium A for stimulation and culturing of PBMC: RPMI 1640 (Gibco, Grand Island, NY) + 10% human AB serum + 100 U/mL penicillin and 100 µg/mL streptomycin. Medium for T-cell cloning and for T-cell cultivation contains additionally 15 U/mL IL-2 (IL-2 from Boehringer, Mannheim, Germany). Restimulation and expansion are performed with medium A + 15 U/mL IL-2 + 2 µg/mL phytohemagglutinin (HA16; Murex Diagnostics, Dartford, UK). All media are stable at 4°C for at least 1 wk and should be filtered through 0.2-µm filters (Nalgen, Rochester, NY) prior to use.
4. HCV antigens: Recombinant viral antigens (Microgen, Munich, Germany and Chiron, Emeryville, CA; **Fig. 1**) of at least 90% purity (HPLC-purified) are synthesized as (a) fusion proteins (gluthation-S-transferase [GST] fusion protein or C-terminal superoxide dismutase [SOD] fusion protein) or (b) with free carboxy- and amino-terminal end. Antigen-specific stimulation is performed with HCV proteins covering overlapping sequences within the virus. Fine specificity of clone cells is determined with 20-mer synthetic peptides (Chiron Mimotopes, Victoria, Australia) with 10 amino acid overlap that were purified by HPLC. Final protein and peptide concentration for T-cell stimulation is 1 µg/mL (stock solution with 100 µg/mL in PBS and 10% DMSO stable at –80°C).

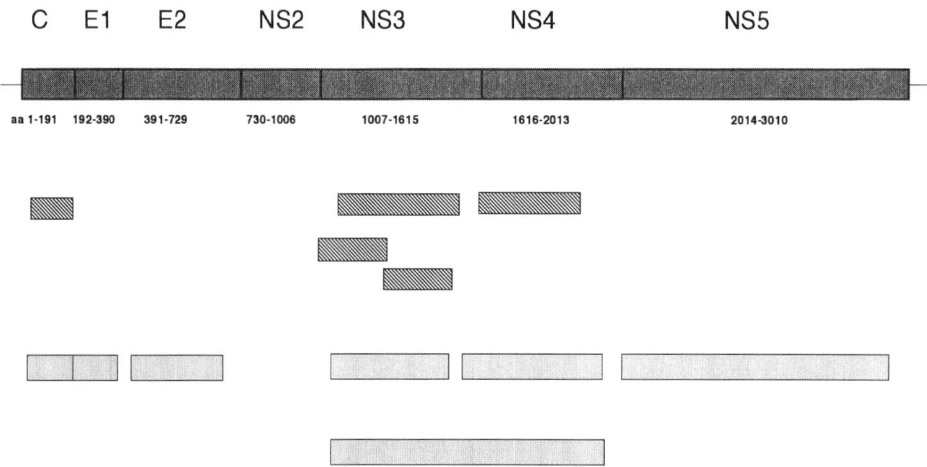

Fig. 1. Recombinant proteins covering overlapping regions within the HCV for antigen-specific stimulation of T-lymphocytes. (▨, Mikrogen; ▬, Chiron)

5. After antigen-specific stimulation, T-cell proliferation is measured by incorporation of ^{3}H-thymidin (Amersham; SA, 80 mCi/mmol).
6. Detection of radiolabled DNA: Labeled cells are collected with a cell harvester (Skatron, Sterling, VA) and are washed on filters (Dunn, Asbach, Germany). The amount of radiolable incorporated into DNA was determined by a β-counter (LKB/Pharmacia, Uppsala, Sweden).
7. Phenotypic characterization is determined by triple fluorescence staining with monoclonal antibodies (MAbs): anti-CD3 (FITC, Coulter-Immunotech, Hamburg, Germany), anti-CD4 (Leu-3a-PE, Becton Dickinson, Hamburg, Germany), anti-CD8 (3B5-TRIcolor; Medac, Hamburg, Germany) and CD25 (IL-2R, Becton Dickinson, Hamburg, Germany). Stained cells are analyzed with a FACScan (Becton Dickinson).
8. For assessment of MHC (MHC Class II, DR, DP, DQ) and the exact HLA class II molecule restriction, T-cell clones are cultured together with a panel of B-lymphoblastoid cell lines of different well-characterized HLA genotypes (according to the 10th International Histocompatibility Workshop) as APC. The following homozygous B-lymphoblastoid cell lines are used: Jesthom (DRA*0101, DRB1*0101, DRB6*0101, DQA1*0101, DQB1*0501, DPA1*01, DPB1*0401), Schu (DRA*0102, DRB1*1501, DRB5*0101, DRB6*0201, DQA1*0102, DQB1*0602, DPA1*01, DPB1*0402), KAS011 (DRA*0101, DRB1*1601, DRB5*02, DRB6*0202, DQA1*0102, DQB1*0502, DPA1*01/0201, DPB1*0401/1401), BOLETH (DRA*0101, DRB1*0401, DRB4*0101, DQA1*03, DQB1*0302, DPA1*01, DPB1*0401), SPO010 (DRA*0101, DRB1*1101, DRB3*0202, DQA1*0102, DQB1*0502, DPA1*01, DPB1*02012), CB6B (DRA*0101, DRB1*1301, DRB3*0202, DQA1*0103, DQB1*0603, DPA1*02021, DPB1*1901),

TEM (DRA*0101, DRB1*1401 , DRB3*0201, DQA1*0101, DQB1*05031, DPA1*01, DPB1*0401), DBB (DRA*0101, DRB1*07, DRB4*0101, DQA1*0201, DQB1*03032, DPA1*01, DPB1*0401), LUY (DRA*0102, DRB1*08032, DQA1*0601, DQB1*0301, DPA1*01/0201, DPB1*0101/0401).

3. Methods

3.1. Proliferation Assay

1. PBMC are isolated from freshly taken heparinized blood by Ficoll-isopaque gradients through centrifugation at 1000g and are washed four times in PBS subsequently (see **Note 1**).
2. Viable cells are counted microscopically by exclusion of trypan blue-stained cells and are adjusted at 5×10^5 cells/mL medium A (see **Note 2**).
3. 100 µL (5×10^4 cells) of this suspension are added to each well of a 96-well tissue-culture plate; individual antigens and controls are assayed as triplicate cultures. The final volume in each well is 150 µL (100 µL cell suspension + 50 µL antigen or control). Overlapping antigens and peptides help to confine the specific epitope (**Fig. 2**).
4. Routinely, basic proliferation is monitored by addition of 50 µL medium A without antigen. Maximal stimulation is achieved by addition of PHA to a final concentration of 2 µg/mL (see **Note 3**).
5. The stock solution of viral antigens is diluted with 50 µL medium A and is added to the cells leading to a final antigen concentration of 1 µg/mL (see **Note 4**).
6. 96-round well-cultured plates are cultured for 5 d at 37°C and 5% CO_2 (see **Note 5**).
7. On d 5, 2 µCi ^{3}H-thymidine in 10 µL medium A are added. After 16 h of incubation at 37°C and 5% CO_2, cells are collected with a cell harvester and are washed on filters (Dunn, Asbach, Germany) for subsequent analysis of counts per minute in a β-counter.
8. The stimulation index (SI) is calculated as the ratio of counts per minute of PBMC cultured in the presence of antigen divided by those incubated and counted without antigen (see **Note 7**).

3.2. Cloning of CD4⁺ T Lymphocytes

1. 2×10^6 PBMC in 4 mL medium A are plated in 40 wells of a 96-well, round-bottom plate. Simultaneously, the proliferation assay is performed as described above.
2. Generation of HCV-specific T-cell clones is achieved by stimulation of PBMCs with the recombinant HCV antigen for 10 d in medium A. The final concentration of the antigen is 1 µg/mL.
3. On d 6, IL-2 is added to a final concentration of 15 U/mL, and PBMC are cultured for 3 d in the presence of IL-2.
4. Stimulated cells are collected on d 10, and the cell number is counted if a significant SI was detected in the proliferation assay on d 6 of the same patient's sample (see **Note 8**).

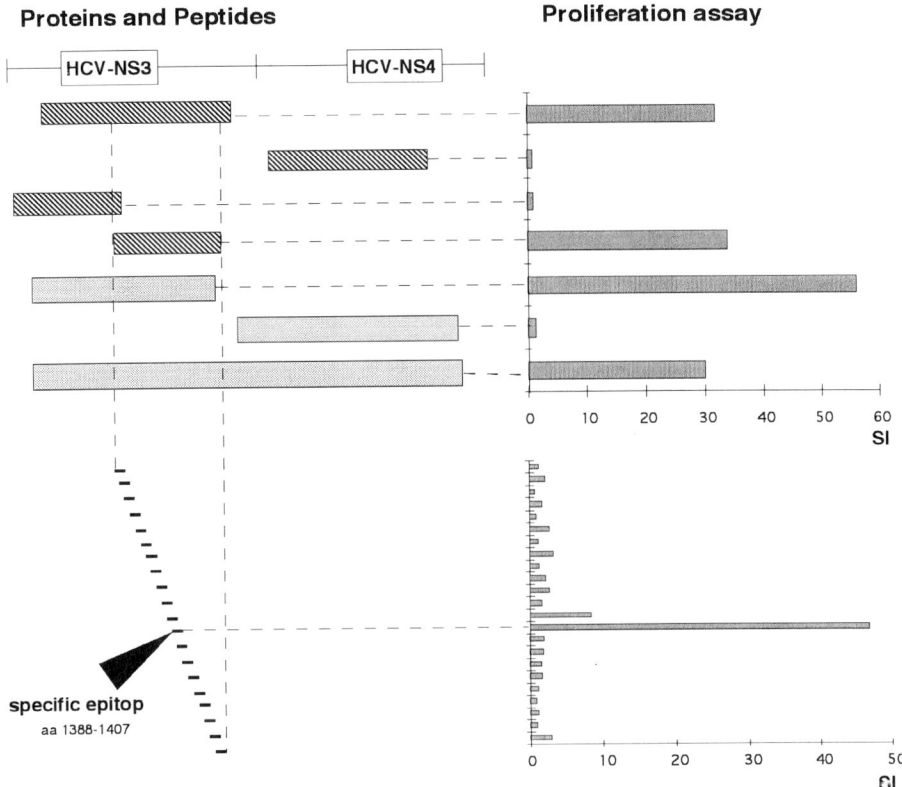

Fig. 2. The HCV specificity of a CD4+ T-cell clone is determined by stimulation with overlapping recombinant HCV proteins and synthetic 20-mer peptides (left). Antigen-specific stimulation leads to an uptake of ^{3}H thymidin in the corresponding proliferation assay (right). According to the proliferative response of the clone, SI is increased. Stimulation with overlapping HCV proteins (upper left) narrows the specific epitope down to 260 amino acids (aa). Synthetic 20-mer peptides with 10-aa overlap (lower left) identify the epitope specifically recognized by the CD4+ T-cell clone. The minimal epitope can then be determined by carboxy- and amino-terminal aa truncation.

5. Cells are diluted and plated at 75, 150, and 225 cells/well in a 96-well, round-bottom plate. After 4 h of sedimentation, the cell number of individual wells is counted under the microscope and a well containing approx 150 cells is choosen for limiting dilution (see **Note 9**).
6. These 150 cells are diluted in medium A + 15U/mL IL-2 and are distributed at 0.5 cells/well (50 µL/well). To each well, 50 µL of 3×10^4 autologous irradiated PBMC (3000 rad) and 50 µL PHA (final concentration 2 µg/mL) are added, and cells are cultured for 3–5 wk (see **Note 10**).

7. From d 10 after initial cloning, growing clone cells can be expanded from one to several wells. About 5 wk after cloning, 1×10^4 grown clone cells are tested for HCV antigen specificity by culturing 3×10^4 autologous, irradiated PBMC with and without the respective antigen for 5 d.
8. The proliferation assay is performed as described above (*see* **Note 11**).
9. Expansion of T-cell clones is performed every 3–5 wk with irradiated autologous or allogenic PBMC in medium A + 15 U/mL IL-2 and 2 µg/mL phytohemagglutinin. From the second week after PHA stimulation culture medium of clone cells is replaced twice a week by medium A + 15 U/mL IL-2.

3.3. Phenotypic Characterization and MHC—Restriction

1. HCV-specific T-cell clones are tested for their antigenic phenotype ($CD4^+$/$CD8^+$) by triple immunofluorescence staining; 2×10^4 T-cells are incubated at 4°C with the antibodies anti-CD3, anti-CD4, and anti-CD8 (10 µg/mL) for 45 min.
2. After staining, T-cells are washed twice with PBS and are adjusted in 50 µL PBS + 1% formaldehyde for subsequent analysis in a FACScan flowcytometer from Becton Dickinson. At least 5×10^3 $CD4^+$ lymphocytes are analyzed (*see* **Note 13**).
3. MHC restriction and exact HLA class II molecule restriction are determined in parallel to the proliferation assay. $1-2 \times 10^4$ specific clone cells are incubated for 20 h at 37°C and 5% CO_2 with 3×10^4 cells of various strains of homozygous B-lymphoblastoid cells matching one of the patients' HLA class II alleles together with the corresponding specific antigen (final concentration 1 µg/mL). Antigen-specific T-cell activation is detected as increased CD25 expression on $CD4^+$ clone cells by FACS analysis. Blocking of antigen presentation is achieved by addition of 10 µL (10 µg/mL) anti-DR antibodies, anti-DP antibodies, or anti-DQ antibodies. Staining of specific T-cells is performed as described above (**Fig. 3**) (*see* **Note 14**).

4. Notes

1. Since the best results in proliferative response of $CD4^+$ T-cells are achieved with PBMC of freshly drawn heparinized blood, we recommend the use of freshly isolated PBMC. PBMC may be stored on ice for up to 24 h. Twenty to 40 mL of heparinized blood give sufficient recovery of PBMC to carry out all the experiments mentioned above. Wash isolated PBMC after separation immediately three to four times to avoid a cytotoxic influence of Ficoll.
2. Cell number may be adjusted to $0.5-2 \times 10^5$ cells/well. Cultivation of T-cells should be performed in round-bottom well plates for cell numbers lower than 1×10^5 since close contact of cells is required for delivery of costimulatory signals.
3. Background or basic proliferation is detected by simply adding medium instead of antigen to the cell suspension. Background proliferation and mitogenic stimulation set up the frame in which the antigen-specific stimulation takes place. With the help of these limits, the strength of the antigen-specific stimulation can be estimated. Antigen-specific proliferation can also be compared with a standarized specific antigen, i.e., tetanus toxoid, which gives positive proliferative responses in about 80% of the normal population.

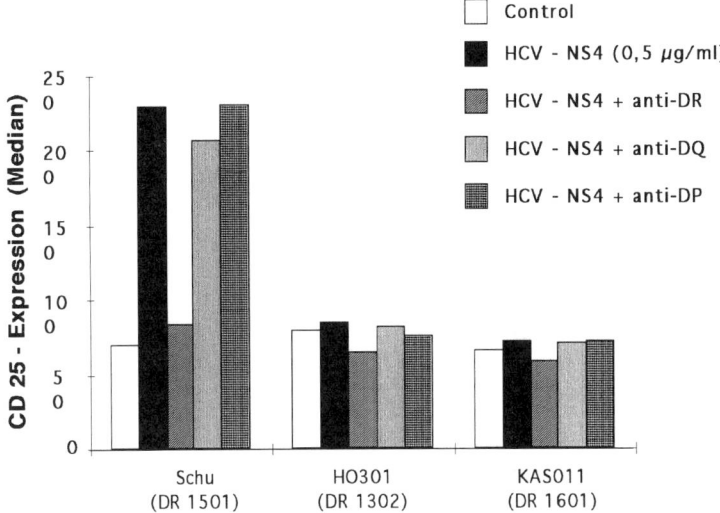

Fig. 3. Assessment of HLA class II restriction of CD4+ T-cell clones. Coculturing of an HCV-NS4 specific CD4+ T-cell clone with different homozygous B-lymphoblastoid cell lines (i.e., Schu, HO301 and Kas 011) as APCs together with the specific antigen results in a specific activation of clone cells. Activation can be monitored flowcytometrically by increased expression of CD25 (IL-2-receptor) on the clone cells. Recognition of the antigen by clone cells is restricted by HLA-DR 15, but not by DR13 or DR16. Addition of anti-DR antibodies, but not anti-DP or anti-DQ-antibodies inhibits the antigen-specific activation of clone cells.

4. For better stability, proteins and peptides should be stored lyophilized or at high concentration (stock solution at least 1 mg/mL) in 100% DMSO. Repeated thawing leads to degradation of proteins and peptides. Diluted proteins should be stored only for a few days at 4°C and should be used as soon as possible. For stimulation of PBMC, final antigen concentration of 1–10 µg/mL is recommended. T-cell clones recognize their specific antigen even at nanomolar concentrations.
5. Cultivation of PBMC in the presence of antigen may be performed every 4–7 d.
6. 2 µCi of ^{3}H-thymidin contains sufficient radiolabel for 0.5×10^5 PBMC, but may not be enough for 2×10^5 cells. Incubation with 2 µCi for longer than 16 h does not change the results for uptake significantly. After incubation, labeled cells can be stored at 4°C for several days for subsequent analysis.
7. Uptake of ^{3}H-labeled thymidin is closely correlated with the proliferation over a wide range of cell numbers in a linear fashion. Although the counts directly reflect the strength of proliferative responses, the SI (ratio of antigen-stimulated PBMC divided by the background control) takes into account the differences of background proliferation and delivers comparable results in multiple testing. The cut-

off of SI >3 for specific stimulation is calculated (mean + 2 × SD = 3) and has turned out to be a reliable value.

8. In order to increase the chance of cloning HCV-specific $CD4^+$ T-cells the cloning procedure should only be performed with PBMC of patients who have a proven strong proliferative response (i.e., antigen-specific $CD4^+$ T-cell precursors). Taking into account a relatively low precursor frequency of HCV-specific $CD4^+$ T-cells, the number of HCV specifically stimulated wells (5×10^5 PBMC) should not be <20–30. After the results of the proliferation assay confirm a strong proliferative response to HCV antigens, the supernatant of the bulk culture is removed, and 100 µL medium A + 15 U/mL IL-2 are added to each well. The IL-2 is supposed to support the growth of $CD25^+$ T-cells (i.e., antigen-specific stimulated T-cells). It is favorable to leave two wells without addition of antigen as controls. On d 10, those wells containing the most stimulated cells (i.e., clot forming cells) are chosen microscopically and are counted for limiting dilution.

9. Cells have to be accurately diluted with medium A + 15 U/mL IL-2 and are carefully plated in triplicate with increasing numbers (75, 150, and 225 cells/well in a final volume of 100 µL). The exacT-cell number can rather be counted in round-bottom well plates than in flat-bottom well plates, where 150 cells get lost. After sedimentation, which can be accelerated by careful centrifugation (800 U/min for 10 min), the cell number of each well is counted under a microscope. The well that contains close to 150 cells is choosen and diluted.

10. First the clone cells are plated very carefully at 0.5 cells/well in 300 wells. Afterwards 3×10^4 autologous irradiated PBMC are added, and finally mitogenic stimulation with PHA supports the growth of the clone cells. Do not mix PHA with cells before distribution, because PHA leads to clotting and prevents homogenous distribution of clone cells and feeder cells. Since only one cell is supposed to be in every other well, you have to add PBMC and PHA very carefully. Vigorous addition of PBMC may lead to dislocation of clone cells and may hamper the growth of the clone. Irradiated PBMC deliver the costimulatory signals, which are essential for mitogenic growth.

11. About 9–10 d after cloning, T-cells start to grow out of the central clot, but irradiated PBMC die. As soon as the clone grows continuously and exceeds the number of about $2-3 \times 10^4$ cells/well, you may expand the clone step by step. Clones should be monitored microscopically. Do not expand clone cells too fast. Otherwise, they will undergo apoptosis. When the clone stops growing 3–4 wk after cloning, it enters the resting phase for a limited time period. At this time it can be tested for antigen specificity. Too early testing for specificity may lead to exaggerated unspecific background proliferation. Proliferation assay for specificity is performed with $1-10 \times 10^3$ clone cells together with 3×10^4 autologous, irradiated PBMC that are needed for antigen presentation.

12. After 3 wk of growth, clones should be carefully observed under the microscope for cell death, which becomes evident by cell debris in the periphery of the well. As soon as the cell numbers decrease, for clonal expansion, the clone has to be restimulated unspecifically. For this purpose 3×10^3 clone cells are incubated

with 3×10^4 autologous PBMC in medium A + IL-2 and 2 µg/mL PHA. This expansion can be repeated every 3–5 wk.
13. Although the described cloning procedure is designed to generate CD4+ T-cell clones, the presence of CD4+ T-cells should be confirmed by flowcytometric analysis. Moreover, flowcytometry offers a wide field for further characterization of clone cells.
14. The usage of a panel of homozygous B lymphoblastoid cell lines as APCs proves the restriction of antigen presentation to the MHC. Recognition of the antigen in context with the autologous HLA receptor delivers the proliferative signal to the T-cell. This activation of the specific T-cell can be inhibited with MAbs against the class II receptor (i.e., HLA-DR, DP, or DQ). Instead of ^{3}H-thymidin uptake, the activation of T-lymphocytes can be detected already after 1 d of coculturing by flowcytometric assessment of CD25 expression (IL-2 receptor) on CD4+ T-cells. This increased CD25 expression (i.e., more than two times of control fluorescence intensity) on stimulated clone cells allows the determination of the exact HLA class II restriction element of the clone (**Fig. 3**) by comparison of various B-lymphoblastoid cell lines.

Suggested Reading

1. Diepolder, H. M., Jung, M. C., Albert, E., Hoffmann, R. M., Zachoval, R., and Pape, G. R. (1994) HLA and hepatitis B infection [Letter; comment]. *Lancet* **344,** 1772,1773.
2. Diepolder, H. M., Zachoval, R., Hoffmann, R. M., Wierenga, E. A., Santantonio, T., Jung, M. C., et al. (1995) Possible mechanism involving T-lymphocyte response to non-structural protein 3 in viral clearance in acute hepatitis C virus infection. *Lancet* **346,** 1006,1007.
3. Diepolder, H. M., Zachoval, R., Hoffmann, R. M., Jung, M. C., Gerlach, T., and Pape, G. R. (1996) The role of hepatitis C virus specific CD4+ T lymphocytes in acute and chronic hepatitis C. *J. Mol. Med.* **74,** 583–588.
4. Diepolder, H. M., Jung, M. C., Wierenga, E., Hoffmann, R. M., Zachoval, R., Gerlach, T. J., et al. (1996) Anergic TH1 clones specific for hepatitis B virus (HBV) core peptides are inhibitory to other HBV core-specific CD4+ T-cells in vitro. *J. Virol.* **70,** 7540–7548.
5. Ferrari, C., Valli, A., Galati, L., Penna, A., Scaccaglia, P., Giuberti, T., et al. (1994) T-cell response to structural and nonstructural hepatitis C virus antigens in persistent and self-limited hepatitis C virus infections. *Hepatology* **19,** 286–295.
6. Hoffmann, R. M., Diepolder, H. M., Zachoval, R., Zwiebel, F. M., Jung, M. C., Scholz, S., Nitschko, H., Riethmuller, G., and Pape, G. R. (1995) Mapping of immunodominant CD4+ T lymphocyte epitopes of hepatitis C virus antigens and their relevance during the course of chronic infection. *Hepatology* **21,** 632–638.
7. Jung, M. C., Diepolder, H. M., and Pape, G. R. (1994) T-cell recognition of hepatitis B and C viral antigens. *Eur. J. Clin. Invest.* **24,** 641–650.
8. Leroux Roels, G., Esquivel, C. A., DeLeys, R., Stuyver, L., Elewaut, A., Philippe, J., et al. (1996) Lymphoproliferative responses to hepatitis C virus core, E1, E2,

and NS3 in patients with chronic hepatitis C infection treated with interferon alfa. *Hepatology* **23,** 8–16.
9. Minutello, M. A., Pileri, P., Unutmaz, D., Censini, S., Kuo, G., Houghton, M., et al. (1993) Compartmentalization of T lymphocytes to the site of disease: intrahepatic CD4+ T-cells specific for the protein NS4 of hepatitis C virus in patients with chronic hepatitis C. *J. Exp. Med.* **178,** 17–25.
10. Missale, G., Bertoni, R., Lamonaca, V., Valli, A., Massari, M., Mori, C., et al. (1996) Different clinical behaviors of acute hepatitis C virus infection are associated with different vigor of the anti-viral cell-mediated immune response. *J. Clin. Invest.* **98,** 706–714.

39

Measurement of HCV-Specific CD8⁺ Cytotoxic T-Cell Activities in the Peripheral Blood by Europium Release Assay

Michio Imawari

1. Introduction

Peripheral blood mononuclear cells (PBMC) contain NK cells, cytotoxic T-lymphocytes (CTL), helper T-cells, and B-cells that respond to viral infection and act to eliminate the virus from infected individuals. CTLs are not only thought to be a major host defense against viral infection, but are also implicated in the immunopathogenesis. Classical CTLs are $CD8^+$ and recognize endogenously synthesized and processed antigen in association with a human leukocyte antigen (HLA) class I molecule. The antigens are usually 8–10 amino acids long. HCV-specific CTLs have been demonstrated in the peripheral blood of some of patients with HCV infection by stimulating PBMC with the HCV synthetic peptides *(1)*. The peptides were synthesized as overlapping peptides to encompass a certain region of the HCV antigen *(1)*, on the basis of antigenicity prediction from the amino acid composition of HCV *(2)*, or on the basis of the HLA binding motifs in the HCV antigen *(3)*. Several minimal and optimal epitopes in the HCV antigen and their HLA restriction of recognition by CTLs have been defined. Recently, it has been reported that HCV-specific CTLs may suppress the outgrowth of HCV *(4)*. In this chapter, methods will be discussed that demonstrate HCV-specific CTLs in the peripheral blood of patients with HCV infection. We use nonradioisotope europium (Eu) for assay of CTL activities.

The method described here assumes that HCV proteins contain CTL epitopes and that memory cytotoxic T-cells primed by the CTL epitopes within HCV exist in the peripheral blood of patients with HCV infection. Since the frequency of the memory HCV-specific CTLs may be low in the peripheral blood, the demonstration of the CTLs would require expansion of HCV-specific CTLs before assay. The demonstration of HCV-specific CTLs in the peripheral blood of patients with HCV infection and the identification of the CTL epitopes would contribute to the elucidation of the immunopathogenesis of HCV infection and the design of HCV T-cell vaccine.

2. Materials

1. Human AB serum, heat-inactivated at 56°C for 30 min.
2. RPMI medium 1640 (Gibco [Grand Island, NY] #31800-071).
3. Penicillin-streptomycin-glutamine (Gibco #10378-016).
4. MEM sodium pyruvate solution (Gibco #11360-13).
5. Anti-PPLO agent (Gibco #15220-015).
6. Hank's balanced salt solution (HBSS), powder (Gibco #61200-069).
7. Heparin (conservative-free), 1000 U/mL.
8. Ficoll-Paque (Pharmacia, Uppsala, Sweden).
9. Recombinant human interleukin-2 (rIL-2) (Boehringer-Mannheim, Mannheim, Germany).
10. Europium (Eu) atomic absorption standard solution (Aldrich [Milwaukee, WI] #20712-8).
11. Dietylenetriaminopenta-acetic acid (DTPA) (Triplex® GR, Merck #8426, Darmstadt, Germany).
12. DELFIA enhancement solution (Wallac Oy, Turku, Finland), obtainable through Pharmacia Biotech.
13. DELFIA research fluorometer (Wallac Oy), obtainable through Pharmacia Biotech.
14. Complete RPMI-1640 medium: RPMI medium 1640 supplemented with 2 mM L-glutamine, 100 U of penicillin G, and 100 µg of streptomycin/mL, 1 mM pyruvate, 0.22% sodium bicarbonate, 15 mM HEPES, anti-PPLO, and 5 × 10^{-5} M 2-mercaptoethanol. Store at 4°C.
15. 3.RPMI-10AB: complete RPMI-1640 medium supplemented with 10% human AB serum.
16. RPMI-10FCS: complete RPMI-1640 medium supplemented with 10% FCS.
17. HBSS-2: HBSS medium supplemented with 2% FCS.
18. HCV synthetic peptides–synthesized based on the reported HCV-specific CTL epitopes (**Table 1**), and are used to stimulate the effector cells in the peripheral blood and to sensitize the target cells. The >90% pure peptides can be synthesized commercially, and are dissolved in 100% DMSO at a concentration of 10 mg/mL, followed by diluting with an equal volume of Milli-Q water to a final concentration of 5 mg/mL. Aliquots are stored at –30°C. An aliquot is stored at 4°C as a working solution, and is discarded after 6 mo *(5–10)*.
19. Epstein-Barr virus-transformed B-cells (BCL). Autologous B-cells transformed by Epstein-Barr virus or HLA-compatible allogeneic BCLs are used as target cells for CTLs. The method to establish BCLs is beyond the scope of this chapter. BCLs are maintained by culturing them in RPMI-10FCS.

Table 1
Peptide Used for Simulation of CD8⁺ HCV-Specific CTLs

HLA restriction	HCV type	Amino acid residues	Region	Sequence	Reference
B44	1b, 2a	88–96	Core	NEGLGWAGW	*5*
	1b	88–96	Core	NEGMGWAGW	*4*
	1a, 2b	88–96	Core	NEGCGWAGW	*4*
	2a, 2b	2095–2103	NS5	AEVTQHGSY	*4*
B60	1a, 1b, 2a, 2b	27–28	Core	GQIVGGVYL	*6*
B35	1a	235–242	E1	ASRCWVAM	*7*
B50	1a	569–578	E2	CVIGGAGNNT	*8*
B51	1a	489–496	E2	YPPKPCGI	*8*
B53	1a	460–469	E2	RPLTDFDQGW	*9*
B7	1a, 1b, 2a, 2b	41–49	Core	GPRLGVRAT	*9*
B8	1a, 1b, 2a, 2b	1395–1403	NS3	HSKKKCDEL	*9*
A29	1a	826–838	NS2	LMALTLSPYYKRY	*7*
A11	1a	2–9	Core	STNPKPQK	*8*
	1a	621–628	E1	TINYTIFK	*9*
A23	1a	838–845	NS2	YISWCLWW	*9*
A3	1a	2588–2596	NS5	RVCEKMALY	*9*
A2	1a, 1b, 2a, 2b	35–44	Core	YLLPRRGPRL	*3,10*
	1a, 1b	132–140	Core	DLMGYIPLV	*2,10*
	1a	178–187	Core	LLALLSCLTV	*3,10*
	1a	1073–1081	NS3	CINGVCWTV	*3,9*
	1a	1169–1177	NS3	LLCPAGHAV	*3*
	1a	1406–1415	NS3	KLVALGINAV	*3*
	1a	1789–1797	NS4	SLMAFTAAV	*3*
	1a, 1b	1807–1816	NS4	LLFNILGGWV	*3,10*
	1a, 1b	1851–1859	NS4	ILAGYGAGV	*10*
	1a	2252–2260	NS5	ILDSFDPLV	*3*
	1a	2727–2735	NS5	GLQDCTMLV	*10*

20. Recombinant vaccinia virus expressing HCV antigens in infected cells: Recombinant vaccinia virus is used to infect target cells and express the HCV antigens endogenously. The method to construct a recombinant vaccinia virus is described elsewhere in this volume.
21. Buffer A: 50 mM HEPES, 93 mM NaCl, 5 mM KCl, 2 mM MgCl$_2$, adjusted to pH 7.4 with 1 N NaOH and sterilized by filtration. Store at 4°C.
22. Buffer B: 50 mM HEPES, 93 mM NaCl, 5 mM KCl, 2 mM MgCl$_2$, 2 mM CaCl$_2$, 10 mM glucose, adjusted to pH 7.4 with 1 N NaOH and sterilized by filtration. Store at 4°C.
23. 100 mM DTPA in 1 N NaOH. Store at 4°C.

24. 1 mM Eu–5 mM DTPA solution: mix 1.52 mL of Eu atomic absorption standard solution, 0.5 mL of 100 mM DTPA solution, and 7.98 mL of buffer A, and adjust pH to 7.4 with 1 N HCl. Store at 4°C.
25. 0.5% Dextran sulfate solution: dissolve 5 mg of dextran sulfate in 1 mL of buffer A. Prepare freshly each time.
26. Labeling buffer (x μM Eu): mix $(900-x)$ L of buffer A, 100 L of 0.5% dextran sulfate, and x μL of Eu-DTPA solution. Prepare freshly. Usually we use 80 μM labeling buffer.

3. Methods

3.1. Generation of HCV-Specific CTLs

1. Thirty-eight milliliters of peripheral venous blood are drawn into a syringe containing 2 mL of conservative-free heparin, and diluted with 20 mL of HBSS-2. Thirty milliliter-aliquots are layered carefully onto 15 mL of Ficoll-Paque in 50-mL tissue-culture tubes, and centrifuged for 30 min at 600 g at room temperature. Buffy coats are carefully collected and transferred to a 50-mL culture tube containing 20 mL of HBSS-2. The tube is centrifuged for 10 min at 800g at 4°C. The supernatant is removed by suction, and the cell pellet is suspended in 10 mL of HBSS-2. The tube is centrifuged for 10 min at 300g at 4°C. The procedure is repeated once. Finally, the cell pellet is suspended in 10 mL of RPMI-10FCS, and the cell number is counted. An aliquot is centrifuged for 10 min at 300g at 4°C, and the cell pellet is suspended with RPMI-10AB to a cell density of 2×10^6 cells/mL. One milliliter of PBMC suspension is necessary for each stimulator peptide. The rest of the PBMCs are centrifuged for 10 min at 300g, and the cell pellet is suspended in chilled complete RPMI-1640 medium supplemented with 50% FCS and 10% DMSO at a cell density of 5×10^6 to 1×10^7 cells/mL, is divided into 1-mL-aliquots, and stored in a liquid nitrogen for later use as feeder cells.
2. Stimulator synthetic peptide is added to 1 mL of PBMC suspension in each well of 24-well flat-bottom plates to a final concentration of 10 μg/mL on d 0. The cells are incubated at 37°C in a humidified 5% CO_2 atmosphere.
3. On d 2, rIL-2 is added to a final concentration of 50 U/mL (*see* **Note 1**).
4. On d 7–9, the cells in each well are suspended with a Pasteur pipet and transferred into a tube containing 10 mL of cold HBSS-2. The tube is centrifuged for 5 min at 300g at 4°C, and the cell pellet is resuspended in 10 mL of cold HBSS-2. The cell number is counted, and the tube is centrifuged again. The cell pellet is resuspended to a cell density of $1.2–1.6 \times 10^6$ cells/mL with RPMI-10AB, and a 500-μL portion is transferred to each well of 24-well flat-bottom plates.
5. PBMC stock (5×10^6 to 1×10^7 cells) is defrosted quickly in a 37°C water bath, and the cell suspension is transferred into a tube containing 10 mL of warm RPMI-10FCS. The tube is centrifuged for 5 min at 300g at room temperature. The washing is repeated once, the cell pellet is resuspended in 10 mL of RPMI-10FCS, and the cell number is counted. After the cells are irradiated at 30 yr, they are centrifuged for 5 min at 300g at room temperature, and the cells are resus-

pended in RPMI-10AB at a cell density of 2×10^6 cells/mL. A 500-μL portion of the irradiated PBMC is added to each well prepared in **step 4**. IL-2 and stimulator peptide are also added to final concentrations of 50 U/mL and 10 μg/mL, respectively.
6. Two days after **steps 4** and **5**, 1 mL of RPMI-10AB is overlaid in each well, and the cells are incubated further for 5 d.
7. On d 13–16, the cells in each well of 24-well plates are transferred into 15-mL tissue-culture tubes containing 10 mL of RPMI-10FCS, and are centrifuged for 10 min at 300g at room temperature. The cell pellets are suspended in 10 mL of RPMI-10FCS, and the cell suspension is re-centrifuged for 10 min at 300g at room temperature. The cell pellets are suspended in 10 mL of RPMI-10FCS, and the cell numbers are counted. The cells are centrifuged again for 10 min at 300g at room temperature. The cells are resuspended in RPMI-10FCS to give an appropriate effector to target (E/T) ratio in an Eu-release assay. We usually dilute the effector cells to 2×10^6 cells/mL, which give an E/T ratio of 40 in a Eu-release assay.

3.2. Preparation of HCV Peptide-Sensitized Target Cells

1. On the day before the assay, 5×10^6 autologous or HLA-matched allogeneic BCLs are harvested in a 15-mL culture tube, resuspended in 5 mL of chilled buffer A, and are centrifuged for 5 min at 200g at 4°C. Repeat once (*see* **Note 2**).
2. Resuspend the washed BCLs in 1 mL of labeling buffer. Incubate the tube on ice for 15–20 min by suspending the cells every 5 min by a Pasteur pipet.
3. Add 3 mL of chilled buffer B to the cell suspension, and incubate further for 5 min on ice.
4. After incubation, the tube is centrifuged for 5 min at 200g at 4°C. The cell pellets are washed with 5 mL of chilled buffer B twice.
5. The washed cell pellets in **step 4** are washed with 5 mL of RPMI-10FCS at room temperature once, and are resuspended in 1 mL of RPMI-10FCS. The cell number is counted, and the cell density is adjusted to $0.5–1 \times 10^6$ cells/mL with RPMI-10FCS in a new culture tube.
6. A 1-mL aliquot is transferred to each well of a 24-well plate, and HCV peptides are added to a final concentration of 10 μg/mL. No peptide is added to a well of nonsensitized target cells.
7. After overnight incubation at 37°C, the cells in wells are transferred into 1.5-mL Eppendorf tubes, and the tubes are centrifuged for 20 s at 8000g at room temperature.
8. The cell pellets are washed with 1 mL of RPMI-10FCS by suspending with Pasteur pipets and centrifuging for 20 s at 8000g at room temperature. Use new Pasteur pipets in each washing.
9. The precipitates are resuspended in 1 mL of RPMI-10FCS, and the cell number is counted.
10. Adjust the target cell density to 5×10^4/mL with RPMI-10FCS.

3.3. Cytotoxicity Assay

1. Target cells in 0.1 mL of RPMI-10FCS are plated into each well of 96-well, round-bottom plates. Three wells are prepared for each effector cell preparation. Wells for determining spontaneous release of Eu and maximum release of Eu from target cells are also prepared (three wells for each).
2. Add 0.1 mL of effector cells to the wells containing target cells in triplicate. Add 0.1 mL of RPMI-10FCS to the wells for determining spontaneous Eu release and 0.1 mL of 1% Triton X-100 to the wells for determining maximum Eu release.
3. Incubate the plates for 4 h at 37°C in a humidified 5% atmosphere.
4. After 4 h-incubation, 20 µL of supernatants are transferred to each well of 12-well strips in a holder.
5. One hundred microliters of DELFIA enhancement solution are added to each well.
6. Mix them briefly on a shaker, and incubate for 5 min at room temperature.
7. Measure the released Eu with a DELFIA research fluorometer.
8. Percentage of cytotoxicity is determined with the formula (*see* **Note 4**):

$$100 \times (\text{release in assay} - \text{spontaneous release}) / (\text{maximum release} - \text{spontaneous release}) \quad (1)$$

4. Notes

1. Adding rIL-2 on d 2 instead of on d 0 is important to minimize the nonspecific killing activities of effector cells.
2. Labeling of target cells and cytotoxicity assay should be done in a clean condition. Eu is contained in a dust, and the Eu may contaminate the solutions used in labeling and cytotoxicity assay, leading to falsely high counts.
3. Overnight culture after labeling target cells is important to reduce spontaneous release of Eu from target cells and to minimize nonspecific killing by effector cells.
4. As an alternative method for measuring cytotoxic activities, radioactive ^{51}Cr can be used for labeling target cells. The method for labeling target cells with ^{51}Cr are described in detail in *Current Protocols in Immunology (11)*. The current non-RI cytotoxicity assay gives results comparable to those obtained by ^{51}Cr release assay.

References

1. Kita, H., Moriyama, T., Kaneko, T., Harase, I., Nomura, M., Miura, H., et al. (1993) HLA B44-restricted cytotoxic T-lymphocytes recognizing an epitope on hepatitis C virus nucleocapsid protein. *Hepatology* **18,** 1039–1044.
2. Shirai, M., Okada, H., Nisioka, M., Akatsuka, T., Wychowski, C., Houghten, R., et al. (1994) An epitope in hepatitis C virus core region recognized by cytotoxic T cells in mice and humans. *J. Virol.* **68,** 3334–3342.
3. Cerny, A., McHutchinson, J. G., Pasquinelli, C., Brown, M. E., Brothers, M. A., Grabscheid, B., et al. (1995) Cytotoxic T lymphocyte response to hepatitis C-derived peptides containing the HLA A2.1 motif. *J. Clin. Invest.* **95,** 521–530.

4. Hiroishi, K., Kita, H., Kojima, M., Okamoto, H., Moriyama, T., Kaneko, T., et al. (1997) Cytotoxic T lymphocyte response and viral load in hepatitis C virus infection. *Hepatology* **25,** 705–712.
5. Kita, H., Hiroishi, K., Moriyama, T., Kaneko, T., Ohnishi, S., Yazaki, Y., et al. (1995) A minimal and optimal cytotoxic T-cell epitope within hepatitis C virus nucleoprotein. *J. Gen. Virol.* **76,** 3189–3193.
6. Kaneko, T., Nakamura, I., Kita, H., Hiroishi, K., Moriyama, T., and Imawari, M., (1996) Three new cytotoxic T cell epitopes identified within the hepatitis C virus nucleoprotein. *J. Gen. Virol.* **77,** 1305–1309.
7. Koziel, M. J., Dudley, D., Wong, J. T., Dienstag, J., Houghton, M., Ralston, R., et al. (1992) Intrahepatic cytotoxic T lymphocytes specific for hepatitis C virus in persons with chronic hepatitis. *J. Immunol.* **149,** 3339–3344.
8. Koziel, M. J., Dudley, D., Afdhal, N., Choo, Q.-L., Houghton, M., Ralston, R., et al. (1993) Hepatits C virus (HCV)-specific cytotoxic T-lymphocytes recognize epitopes in the core and envelope proteins of HCV. *J. Virol.* **67,** 7522–7532.
9. Koziel, M. J., Dudley, D., Afdhal, N., Grakoui, A., Rice, C. M., Choo, Q.-L., et al. (1995) HLA class I-restricted cytotoxic T lymphocytes specific for hepatitis C virus. Identification of multiple epitopes and characterization of patterns of cytokine release. *J. Clin. Invest.* **96,** 2311–2321.
10. Battegay, M., Fikes, J., Di Bisceglie, A. M., Wentworth, P. A., Sette, A., Celis, E., et al. (1995) Patients with chronic hepatits C have circulating cytotoxic T cells which recognize hepatitis C virus-encoded peptides binding to HLA-A2.1 molecules. *J. Virol.* **69,** 2462–2470.
11. Bidinson, W. E. (1996) Measurement of polyclonal and antigen-specific cytotoxic T cell function, in *Current Protocols in Immunology*, vol. 2 (Caligan, J. E., Kriusbeck, A. M., Margulies, D. H., Shevach, E. M., and Strober, W., eds.), Wiley, Philadelphia, PA, pp. 7.17.1–7.17.14.

40

Determination of HCV-Specific Bulk CD8⁺ Activity in Liver

David R. Nelson

1. Introduction

The host immune response to hepatitis C virus (HCV) infection comprises both humoral and cellular components, which accompany all viral infections. The cellular immune response involves both nonspecific and antigen-specific phases, with recovery thought to be largely dependent on classical $CD4^+$ and $CD8^+$ cytotoxic T-lymphocytes (CTLs). Intracellular and extracellular antigens present quite different challenges to the immune system, both in terms of recognition and appropriate response. In general, T-cells do not recognize native antigen; rather, they recognize short antigenic peptides that have been processed and presented on the cell surface. For an appropriate response, it is necessary that the T-cell receptor recognize a ligand composed of processed viral immunogenic peptide bound to a major histocompatibility complex (MHC) molecule on the surface of an antigen-presenting cell or target cell. Processed peptides are generally presented to $CD8^+$ cells by MHC class I molecules, which are expressed on virtually all cells.

CTLs have been found to offer protection in vivo against a number of viral infections (1,2), and in their attempt to control viral infection by eliminating viral infected cells, tissue damage may occur. The mechanisms by which $CD8^+$ effector cells resolve viral infection in HCV remain to be elucidated, but there is evidence for direct cytolysis as well as secreted antiviral factors (tumor necrosis factor and interferon-γ) (3,4). Our laboratory has recently demonstrated that the intrahepatic HCV-specific CTL response is playing a role in the control of viral replication and is contributing to hepatocellular damage (5). The $CD8^+$ CTL arm of the cellular immune system may therefore be important in the pathogenesis and control of HCV infection. The further characterization of this CTL response will have important implications for the future design of therapeutic strategies and the understanding of the pathophysiology of chronic HCV infection.

HCV-specific CTLs have been isolated from the liver *(6,7)* and peripheral blood mononuclear cells (PBMC) in a number of patients with chronic HCV infection *(8,9)*. One drawback to the study of T-cell response in the peripheral blood is that it may not necessarily reflect the pattern of T-cell responses in the liver. Studying the $CD8^+$ cell response in the liver has the advantage of analyzing the cell population that is functioning at the site of HCV infection.

In this chapter, methods will be described that allow for the development of an in vitro system to study intrahepatic CTLs and their recognition patterns. This model has several fundamental requirements. First, because of the HLA restriction of CTLs, a suitable HLA-restricted Target cell is required. Accordingly, Epstein-Barr virus (EBV) transformed B-lymphoblastoid cell lines (B-LCL) are generated from each patient's PBMC to serve as autologous target cells. Second, it is necessary for high-level transduction and expression of HCV antigens in the Target cell line in order to assess confidently the presence of HCV-specific CTLs. Since B-LCLs are permissive to vaccinia, recombinant vaccinia containing HCV genes derived from various HCV genotypes can be employed for efficient transfection and expression of the HCV antigens. Synthetic peptides can also be used to label Target cells. Third, sufficient numbers of CTLs must be available for study. This is accomplished from bulk T-cell selection and expansion using monoclonal antibodies (MAbs) and interleukin-2 (IL-2).

Two general methods can be employed for the selection of $CD8^+$ cells. One is by the positive selection of $CD8^+$ cells (Dynabeads), and the other is through negative selection and expansion (MAb CD3,4b). Both options will be described.

2. Materials

2.1. Preparation of $CD8^+$ Cells

1. Tissue-culture medium consists of RPMI 1640 containing HEPES (Life Technologies, Grand Island, NY) supplemented with 2 mM L-glutamine (Irvine Scientific, Santa Ana, CA), 0.5 mM sodium pyruvate (Life Technologies), 100 U/100 µg/mL penicillin/streptomycin (Irvine), and 10% heat-inactivated fetal calf serum (cRPMI-10).
2. Dynabeads M-450 human CD8 and Detachabead 4/8 (Dynal, New Hyde Park, NY) or MAb CD3,4B (supplied by Johnson Wong MD, Massachusetts General, Boston, MA).
3. Human recombinant IL-2 (Hoffman-LaRoche).
4. MAb anti-CD3 (12F6) (Johnson Wong, MD).

2.2. Preparation of Autologous Target Cells

1. cRPMI (Life Technologies).
2. Cyclosporin A (1 µg/mL stock) (Sandoz, East Hanover, NJ).
3. Filtered EBV stock supernatant.
4. Ficoll-Hypaque (Sigma, St. Louis, MO).
5. 25-cm^2 tissue-culture flask.

2.3. Bulk-Expanded CTL Assay

1. Target cell preparation.
2. Recombinant vaccinia virus (wild-type and HCV constructs) at 10^8 PFU.
3. Vaccinia vector vTF73 (T7 requirement needed for certain vectors).
4. Target cells (B-LCL).
5. cRPMI-10 medium.

2.4. Chromium Release Assay

1. Bulk-expanded CD8$^+$ cells (effector cells).
2. Na(^{51}CrO$_4$) (New England Nuclear).
3. 5% (v/v) Triton X-100 in H$_2$O.
4. 96-Well, round-bottom microtiter plates with lids.
5. γ-counter.
6. Target cells.

3. Methods
3.1. Preparation of CD8$^+$ Cells

1. Under sterile conditions, immerse 0.5- to 1.5-cm liver biopsy material in cRPMI-10 medium, and release cells by gently teasing the biopsy with two 21-gage needles.
2. Take cell suspension and proceed with selection of CD8$^+$ cells via one of the following methods:
    a. Dynabead (*see* **Note 1**): cool suspension to 2–40°C. Add Dynabeads (5 × 10^6 beads/mL) directly to the cell sample and incubate at 2–40°C on an apparatus that provides bidirectional mixing. Incubate for 30 min. Isolate the rosetted cells by placing the tube in a magnetic particle concentrator (Dynal MPC) for 2–3 min. Pour or pipet the supernatant while the rosetted cells are kept on the wall of the test tube. Resuspend the Dynabeads rosetted cells in a washing buffer (PBS/FCS), and wash with gentle pipeting three to four times. Pour off supernatant. Detachment of Dynabeads from the positively isolated CD8$^+$ cells can be achieved by incubating with Detachabead, placing in magnetic concentrator, and collecting CD8$^+$ cells in the supernatant (*see* **Note 2**).
    b. MAb CD3,4B: plate cell suspension in cloning medium (cRPMI-10 + IL-2 100 U/mL) in one well of a 24-well plate. Add MAb CD3,4B (*see* **Note 3**) to achieve final concentration of 0.5 µg/mL. Cell growth should be visible within 7 d.

3. Refeed CD8⁺ cells with cRPMI-10 supplemented with 100 U/mL IL-2. Cells should be confluent (1–2 × 10^6 cells) within 14 d.
4. 1 × 10^6 bulk-expanded cells are restimulated with irradiated feeder cells (3–4 × 10^6 allogeneic PBMC, irradiated with 50 gy) in cloning medium in the presence of the CD3-specific MAb 12F6 (working concentration 0.1 µg/mL). This results in the polyclonal expansion of the CD8⁺ cells.
5. Feed cells on d 4 and 7 by aspirating half of the medium, and replacing with fresh IL-2 containing cRPMI-10. By d 10–14 cells should have expanded 10- to 15-fold, and can be used for the bulk assay (*see* **Note 4**).

3.2. Preparation of Autologous Target Cells

In this procedure, autologous Target cells are prepared from a PBMC preparation. In vitro, EBV can immortalize B-lymphocytes giving rise to long-term cell lines. These B-LCL express HLA class I antigens and are capable of "processing" soluble antigens and "presenting" them to T-lymphocytes in an antigen-specific, MHC-restricted manner. *(10)* Since these B-LCL are derived from autologous cells, they will have the proper HLA class I restriction necessary for CTL recognition.

1. Obtain 15–20 mL of anticoagulated whole blood, and isolate PBMC by the Ficoll gradient method.
2. Place 15 mL of Ficoll in a 50-mL conical tube. Tilt the tube at a 45° angle and slowly pipet 15–30 mL anticoagulated blood over this. Centrifuge for 30 min at 400*g* at room temperature. The lymphocyte band lies within the clear interface.
3. Collect lymphocyte band (aspirate interface) (*see* **Note 5**), and wash in warm RPMI two times (400*g* for 10 min).
4. Count the PBMC (*see* **Note 6**) and place 10^7 cells into 5 mL of cRPMI-10 (no NaOH and HEPES).
5. Add 0.1 mL of EBV supernatant: The EBV stock is prepared from EBV-producing cell line, MCUV5-10. Briefly, the MCUV5-10 cells are grown to confluence and for an additional 7 d with changing medium in cRPMI. The supernatant, which contains EBV, is then harvested and spun at 2000*g* for 5 min to remove cell debris. The virus stock is then concentrated by spinning at 18,000*g* (with a SW27 rotor, Beckman) for 2 h and resuspended in a small volume of RPMI-10. This is then filtered through a 0.8-µm filter, aliquoted, and stored in 0.1-mL aliquots at –70°C (*see* **Note 7**).
6. Inoculate at 37°C for 2 h.
7. Pellet the cells, and wash with cRPMI-10, and resuspend with 10 mL cRPMI-10 in an upright 25-cm² tissue-culture flask (vented).
8. Add 1 µg/mL cyclosporin A (*see* **Note 8**) and incubate at 37°C in a 5% CO_2 incubator.
9. It takes about 3 wk for the lymphoblastoid cells to grow out (*see* **Note 9**) (the media will turn yellow). Do not change media during this initial period.
10. The B-LCL can then be maintained indefinitely by weekly medium changes (aspirate and replace 5 mL of medium + cells).

3.3. Bulk Expanded CTL Assay

In this procedure, target cells (EBV-transformed lymphoblastoid cells) are transfected with recombinant vaccinia vectors containing various HCV genes. Wild-type vaccinia virus will serve as a control. A multiplicity of infection (MOI) of 10 PFU/cell is used. The cells and vaccinia vectors are then incubated overnight in the presence of ^{51}Cr. The cells are then washed and mixed with effector CTL at appropriate effector-to-target cell ratios. The amount of ^{51}Cr released into the supernatant by killed target cells is quantitated. By comparison with ^{51}Cr release of controls, the corrected percentage of lysis is calculated for each concentration of effector cells (CTL).

3.3.1. Target Cell Preparation

1. Aliquot 1×10^7 B-LCL. Wash in warm RPMI and centrifuge for 10 min (400g) at room temperature. Gently resuspend 1×10^6 B-LCL/well of a 24-well plate for each vector to be used.
2. Transduce Target cells with vaccinia-HCV construct using MOI 10 and incubate for 2 h at 37°C with 5% CO_2. Wash two times with RPMI (10 min at 400g).
3. Resuspend transduced B-LCL in cRPMI-5 (*see* **Note 10**). Add 100 µCi Na(^{51}CrO$_4$) per 24-well plate used, and incubate overnight in tissue culture incubator (37°C, 5% CO_2).
4. After 8–12 h transfer cells and wash in cold cRPMI-10 three times, aspirating down to the cell pellet between wash and collecting the supernatant in radioactive waste container. Resuspend labeled target cells in 2 mL cRPMI-10, and determine viable cell count by trypan blue exclusion (*see* **Note 11**).
5. Resuspend at 1×10^5 cells/mL, and then use as target cells for CTL assay.

3.3.2. Bulk CTL Assay

1. Aliquot and wash approx 1×10^7 bulk expanded T-cells in cRPMI two times.
2. Aliquot labeled B-LCL in 96-well culture plate for target cells at 5×10^3 cells/well for each vaccinia vector to be tested, as well as for a spontaneous and maximal release.
3. Add in bulk T-cells at effector-to-target ratios of 100:1, 50:1, 25:1, and 10:1. All assays should be run in duplicate to assure accuracy.
4. Centrifuge the plate at 200g for 1 min to promote contact between effector and target cells, and then incubate for 5 h (37°C, 5% CO_2).
5. Centrifuge plate for 10 min at 200g. Add 0.1 mL of 5% Triton X-100 (lysing agent) (*see* **Note 12**) to measure maximum releasable ^{51}Cr to a replicate set of empty wells with 5×10^3 target cells.
6. Harvest 100 µL of each supernatant into a plastic tube for counting.

3.3.3. Determine CTL Activity

1. Count ^{51}Cr in a γ-scintillation counter (1–2 min/sample).
2. Calculate corrected percent specific lysis for each concentration of effector cells, using the mean cpm for each replicate of wells.

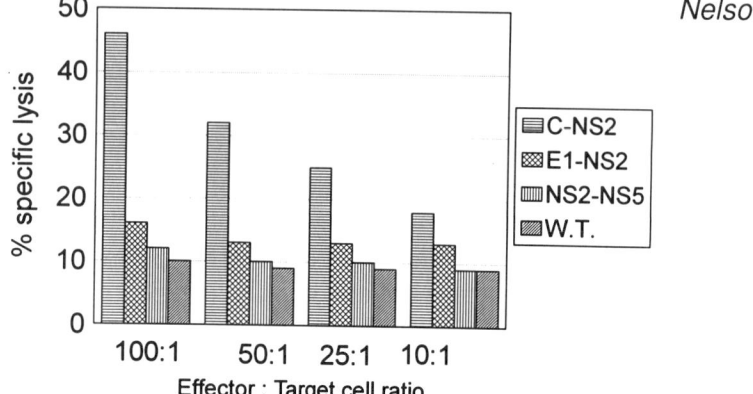

Fig. 1. CTL activity as determined using vaccinia/HCV-transduced B-LCL as target cells and intrahepatic CD8$^+$ lymphocytes as effector cells. Varying effector-to-target cell ratois are shown on the *X*-axis. Percent specific lysis is represented on the *Y*-axis. Three different recombinant vaccinia vectors expressing overlapping HCV genes were used and are represented by different bars. Wild-type vaccinia virus (strain WR) was used to determine the background lysis. Note that HCV specific activity is present against target cells expressing HCV core-NS2 genes (aa 1–967), but not E1-NS2 (aa 136–966) and NS3-NS5 (aa 827–3011). Thus, the major CTL activity is directed toward the core region.

$$\% \text{ Specific cytotoxicity} = \frac{(\text{Experimental release} - \text{spontaneous release})}{(\text{maximal release} - \text{spontaneous release})} \quad (1)$$

3. Determine bulk epitope regions: Assays should be excluded from analysis if spontaneous release is >25% (*see* **Note 13**). From our experience, a % lysis >30% with the bulk assay will usually lead to the detection of active clones on limiting dilution (*see* Chapter 41). Therefore by using three overlapping constructs (*see* **Note 14**) to cover the entire HCV genome, one can quickly screen for positive intrahepatic CTL activity. An example is shown in **Fig. 1**. Further fine mapping studies and cloning can then be performed as desired (*see* Chapter 41).
4. Confirm HLA restriction: To study the HLA restriction pattern, one can repeat the above CTL assay with different HLA Target cells (B-LCL that are matched and mismatched for different HLA class I loci). Another option is to add anti-HLA class I MAb to the CTL assays to block HLA I binding.

4. Notes

1. When isolating from high-viscosity cell suspensions, it is recommended that the sample be diluted with an equal volume of cold PBS immediately before the addition of Dynabeads. A bead-to-target cell ratio of 3:1 is recommended.
2. The isolated cells are pure (>99%), viable (>98%), and show unperturbed expression of CD3 and CD8.

3. This antibody has one arm that is specific for the cell-surface antigen CD3 and another for CD4, with a common Fc portion. In the presence of IL-2, selective expansion of $CD8^+$ cells and complement-mediated lysis of $CD4^+$ cells occur.
4. Cells should be tested for purity prior to further use by either fluorescent activated cell sorting (FACS) or by immunohistochemistry of cytospins.
5. Avoid aspiration of Ficoll (bottom layer), which is toxic to the cells.
6. Usual yield is $1-3 \times 10^6$ PBMC/mL of whole blood.
7. Viral infectivity declines if stored above $-70°C$. Also, repeat freezing and thawing inactivates the virus.
8. Cyclosporin A will inhibit T-cell proliferation, and prevent inhibition of B-cell growth by the EBV-specific T-cells.
9. Proliferating foci of B-cells are usually microscopically visible 1–2 wk after infection with EBV, and large clumps of cells are macroscopically visible after 3–4 wk.
10. We have found that chromium labeling of Target cells is optimized with a 5% fetal calf serum preparation, although you may need to optimize your own experimental conditions.
11. Target cells should have a high viability (>80%).
12. Triton X should cause lysis of all cells and give maximal chromium counts of 4000–6000 cpm/5000 target cells.
13. High spontaneous release is usually owing to either toxic effect of vaccinia (high MOI or long transfection time) or improper washing and preparation of target cells. Western reserve (WR)-labeled target cells serve as an important control in excluding the polyclonal expansion of CTL directed against EBV (particularly if one is studying PBMC-derived CTL). Our experience has shown that this is less a concern when starting from an intrahepatic source.
14. We use the following HCV/vaccinia constructs: (1) vv-core/E1/E2/NS2 aa 1–967 (2) vv-E1/E2/NS2 aa 136–966 (3) vv-NS2-NS5 aa 827–3011 (4) wild type vv (Western reserve strain).

References

1. Lukacher, A. E., Braciale, V. L., and Braciale, T. J. (1984) In vivo effector function of influenza virus-specific cytotoxic T lymphocyte clones is highly specific. *J. Exp. Med.* **160**, 814–826.
2. Robertson, M. (1992) Role of specificity of T-cell subsets in spontaneous recovery from Friend virus-induced leukemia in mice, *J. Virol.* **66**, 3271–3277.
3. Patel, T. and Gores, G. J. (1995) Apoptosis and hepatobiliary disease. *Hepatology* **21**, 1725–1741.
4. Nakamoto, Y., Guidotti, L. G., and Chisari, F. V. (1996) CTL-induced liver disease requires costimulation of both the fas ligand and perforin activated death pathways. *Hepatology* **24**, 351A.
5. Nelson, D. R., Marousis, C. G., Davis, G. L., Rice, C., Wong, J., Houghton M., et al. (1997) The role of hepatitis C virus-specific T lymphocytes in chronic hepatitis C. *J. Immunol.* **158**, 1473–1481.

6. Koziel, M. J., Dudley, D., Wong, J., Dienstag, J., Houghton, M., Ralston, R., et al. (1992) Intrahepatic cytotoxic T lymphocytes specific for hepatitis C virus in persons with chronic hepatitis. *J. Immunol.* **149,** 3339–3344.
7. Koziel, M., Dudley, D., Afdhal, N., Choo Q., Houghton, M., Ralston, R., et al. (1993) Hepatitis C virus (HCV)-specific cytotoxic T lymphocytes recognize the epitopes in the core and envelope proteins of HCV. *J. Virol.* **67,** 7522–7532.
8. Cerny, A., McHutchinson, J. G., Pasquinelli, C., Brown, M. E., Brothers, M. A., Grabsheild, B., et al. (1995) Cytotoxic T lymphocyte response to hepatitis C virus-derived peptides containing the HLA A2.1 binding motif. *J. Clin. Invest.* **95,** 521–530.
9. Kaneko, T., Nakamura, I., Kita, H., Hiroishi, K., Moriyama, T., and Imawari, M. (1996) Three new cytotoxic T-cell epitopes identified within the hepatitis C nucleoprotein. *J. Gen. Virol.,* **77,** 1305–1309.
10. Lanzaveccia, A. (1985) Antigen-specific interaction between T and B cells. *Nature* **314,** 537–539.

41

Characterization of HCV-Specific Cytotoxic T-Lymphocytes from Liver Tissue

Margaret James Koziel

1. Introduction

Cellular immune responses, especially those mediated by cytotoxic T-lymphocytes (CTLs), are an important component of the host immune response in many viral infections. For many years, it has been observed that $CD8^+$ cells were present in large numbers in the liver of patients with chronic HCV *(1)*, but it was unknown whether these cells represented virus-specific immune responses. In order to understand the potential role of these $CD8^+$ lymphocytes in the disease course, it is first necessary to define the functional characteristics of the cells, including a precise definition of the epitopes, which are recognized by these $CD8^+$ lymphocytes.

In order to characterize HCV-specific CTL responses, it is necessary to have methods of isolation of the lymphocytes and expression of viral antigens in a context that can be recognized by potential CTL. Following infection of a cell, viral proteins undergo proteolytic degradation into short peptides fragments, which are then complexed with nascent class I molecules and β-2 microglobulin. The resulting complex is sent to the cell surface, where it is recognized by the T-cell receptor of the $CD8^+$ CTL. In vivo, the major site of viral replication is the hepatocyte. Some investigators have demonstrated that liver-infiltrating lymphocytes from HCV-infected individuals with chronic hepatitis can lyse autologous hepatocytes *(2,3)*. However, use of autologous hepatocytes as target cells is limited by the small numbers of cells that can be isolated from clinical biopsy material as well as the inability to identify either the epitopes or restricting HLA types of the immune response. Therefore, alternate target cells that express class I on the cell surface are needed. Epstein-Barr virus-immortalized B-cells, also known as B-lymphoblastoid cell lines (B-LCL), have been used by a number of laboratories for this purpose. These cell lines can be readily established from nearly all individuals, are easy to maintain in culture for indefinite periods of time, and express high levels of class I and II antigens on the cell surface. In order to express HCV antigens, recombinant HCV–vaccinia viruses are used. Recombinant vaccinia viruses can infect B-LCL as well as other cell types, and the recombinant antigens produced after infection subsequently undergo normal processing and glycosylation *(4,5)*. The cells can be labeled with ^{51}Cr. When effector cells are added to these labeled B-LCL, if the CTL recognizes the peptide fragments expressed on the cell surface, the target cells are lysed and ^{51}Cr is released, providing an indirect assay for cell killing *(6)*. This methodology has been used to identify virus-specific CTL in a number of viral infections, including HBV, HIV-1, and dengue *(7–9)*.

Although CD4$^+$ CTL have been reported in a number of viral infections, as well as rejecting tissue allografts *(10)*, the hepatocyte itself expresses class I on the cell surface, and so our studies have focused on methods for isolation of CD8$^+$ lymphocytes. CD8$^+$ liver-infiltrating lymphocytes are first expanded using a polyclonal stimulus to CD8$^+$ cell proliferation *(11)*. After the liver-infiltrating lymphocytes are enriched for the presence of CD8$^+$ cells, they are cloned using anti-CD3 antibodies as a nonspecific source of T-cell stimulus *(8)*. Such clones can be maintained for long periods of time in culture, which facilitates the precise identification of immunogenic epitopes. The advantage of this nonspecific stimulation is that in the absence of exogenous antigenic stimulation, the fine specificities of CTLs likely represent epitopes recognized in natural infection. It is also not necessary to confine examination of CTL responses to those of a given HLA type or require *a priori* knowledge of the peptides that bind to a given HLA molecule. Although the peptides that bind to HLA A2.1 and a number of other human and murine histocompatability loci have been defined *(12)*, for other HLA molecules the binding motif is unknown, or the predicted epitopes do not conform to what is recognized by antigen-specific CTL *(13)*. Therefore, in order to characterize a polyclonal immune response potentially restricted by the full range of HLA types present in infected humans, it is necessary to adopt a broad approach.

Historically, in most chronic viral infections, CTLs cannot be detected in freshly isolated peripheral blood mononuclear cells (PBMC) in the absence of specific antigenic stimulation. Certainly in hepatitis B virus infection (HBV), virus-specific CTL are present in the blood of acutely infected individuals, but cannot be readily detected in the blood of chronically infected individuals *(14)*. However, when the liver-infiltrating lymphocytes were examined for the presence of HBV-specific CTL, these cells were present even in chronically infected individuals *(15)*. By analogy, therefore, HCV-specific CTL are likely to be concentrated in the liver. The reasons for this tissue specificity are not entirely clear, although it is likely that the concentration of antigen expressed on cells plays a major role. Liver has a 100-fold higher concentration of virus than serum *(16)* and, although other cell types can be infected, is likely to be the principal site of viral replication. This is indeed the case, as in the absence of specific antigenic stimulation, our laboratory was unable to identify HCV-specific CTL within PBMC, whereas they were present within the $CD8^+$ liver-infiltrating lymphocytes of chronically infected individuals *(17,18)*. Using this methodology, it is possible to identify individual clones of CTLs that recognize distinct epitopes within HCV in the context of multiple HLA types *(19)*. In a given individual, the CTL response to HCV can be broadly directed at multiple HLA types; even with the constraints imposed by a number of technical factors, it is possible to demonstrate that as many as five different epitopes may be targeted in a single individual *(20)*. Synthetic peptides that span the protein of interest can be used to identify the fine specificity of the clones.

2. Materials

2.1. Isolation of Intrahepatic T-Lymphocytes from Liver Biopsy Specimens

1. RPMI 1640 medium, supplemented with 100 U/mL of penicillin, 100 μg/mL of streptomycin, 2 mM L-glutamine, and 10 nM HEPES buffer, at 37°C.
2. Fetal calf serum (FCS), heat inactivated at 55°C for 45 min.
3. Human recombinant interleukin 2 (rIL-2; Hoffman-LaRoche).
4. CD3,4B or CD3,8 MAb (Johnson Wong, Massachusetts General Hospital, Boston, MA).
5. Anti-CD3 MAb (12F6, Johnson Wong, Massachusetts General Hospital).

2.2. Epstein-Barr Virus Transformation of B-Lymphocytes for B-Lymphoblastoid Cell Lines (B-LCL)

1. Cyclosporine A, 1 μg/mL stock stored at –70°C.
2. Ficoll-Hypaque, warmed to 37°C prior to use.
3. Filtered supernatant from B95-8 cells.
4. Trypan blue.

2.3. Preparation of Target Cells for Screening of Cells

1. Recombinant vaccinia-HCV at 10^8–10^{10} PFU/mL.
2. Autologous B-LCL.
3. $Na_2^{51}CrO_4$ in normal saline (1 mCi/mL, New England Nuclear).
4. 5% Triton X-100.

2.4. Fine Mapping of Epitopes Recognized by HCV-Specific CTL

Use synthetic peptides spanning the HCV region of interest, reconstituted at 2 mg/mL in sterile distilled water with 10% sterile dimethyl sulfoxide (DMSO) and 1 mM dithiothreitol. Stock solutions are stored at –70°C until use.

3. Methods

3.1. Isolation of Intrahepatic T-Lymphocytes from Liver Biopsy Specimens

1. To obtain $CD8^+$ lymphocytes, place a 4–6 mm × 1.5 mm diameter liver biopsy specimen in RPMI 1640 medium supplemented with 10% heat-inactivated FCS plus 100 U/mL of rIL-2, in one well of a 24-well plate (*see* **Note 1**).
2. To this well, add the bispecific MAb CD3,4B at 0.5 µg/mL. In the first week, there will be visible outgrowth of cells from the margins of the liver biopsy (*see* **Notes 2–4**).
3. On d 5–7, aspirate the medium, and refeed with fresh RPMI 1640 medium supplemented with 10% heat-inactivated FCS medium supplemented with 100 U/mL of recombinant IL-2.
4. When the cells in the well are confluent ($2–5 \times 10^6$ cells), which usually occurs in 2–3 wk, they can either be further expanded in bulk or cloned at limiting dilution.
5. For polyclonal bulk expansion of T-lymphocytes, 1×10^6 cells are stimulated with 4×10^6 feeder cell suspension (*see* **Note 5**). The feeder cell suspension consists of 10^6 cells/mL of irradiated (3000 rad) allogeneic PBMC in RPMI 1640 medium supplemented with 10% heat-inactivated FCS media supplemented with 100 U/mL of rIL-2. The CD3-specific MAb 12F6 is added at 0.1 µg/mL as a polyclonal stimulus to T-cell proliferation (*see* **Note 4**).
6. Ten to 14 d after restimulation, there will have been a polyclonal expansion of the $CD8^+$ T-lymphocytes. There should be approx $10–20 \times 10^6$ cells. These can be tested for purity by fluorescent activated cell sorting (FACS). The remainder can be used as effector cells in a cytotoxicity assay (*see* **Subheading 3.3.**).
7. For limiting dilution cloning of T-lymphocytes, serial dilutions of cells are suspended in feeder cell suspension plus 12F6 to give final concentrations of 50, 25, 10, and 5 cells/well when plated in a final volume of 200 µL (*see* **Note 6**). For convenience, 50 mL of a 250 cells/mL cell suspension is made, and then 30 mL are diluted with 30 mL of the feeder cell suspension plus 12F6. This is continued until a final concentration of 25 cells/mL is made. For each dilution, 200 µL of the cell suspension are plated in a single well of a 96-well, round-bottom, tissue-culture plate.
8. Seven days after cloning, 100 µL of medium are aspirated from the top of the wells and are replaced with fresh RPMI 1640 medium supplemented with 10% heat-inactivated FCS medium plus 100 U/mL of recombinant IL-2. This is repeated twice a week until the cells are confluent. In the round-bottom wells, this can also easily be assessed by looking for alkalization (yellowing) of the media in the wells with growing colonies.
9. When the colony is confluent, the entire contents of the 96-well plate is removed and placed into a single well of a 24-well plate, containing fresh feeder cell suspension plus 12F6 (*see* **Note 7**). When the cells in the well are confluent (usually at d 7–10 after restimulation), they can be used as effectors in a cytotoxicity assay.
10. $CD4^+$ lymphocytes can be expanded using the bispecific antibody CD3,8 (**step 2**), with antigen-nonspecific stimulation for subsequent expansions (**step 4**).

3.2. Epstein-Barr Virus Transformation of B-Lymphocytes for B-Lymphoblastoid Cell Lines (B-LCL) (see Note 8)

1. Obtain 15–30 mL of anticoagulated blood. Preservative-free heparin is preferred as an anticoagulant but virtually any commercially available collection device for whole blood can be used. The typical yield for healthy individuals is $1-4 \times 10^6$ PBMC/mL of whole blood.
2. Mix 1:1 with warmed RPMI. Mix thoroughly to break up any clumps of cells.
3. Place 15 mL of Ficoll into a 50-mL conical. Tilt the tube to about at a 45° angle, and very slowly pipet 30 mL of the blood–RPMI mixture over this. At the end, there should be a clear interface between the Ficoll on the bottom and the blood on the top.
4. Centrifuge at 400g for 30 min at room temperature. The brake on the centrifuge should be "off" during this step in order to avoid disturbance of the monolayers at the end of the run (*see* **Note 9**).
5. Carefully collect the lymphocyte band, which is at the interface of the RPMI and the Ficoll. Place this volume (about 5–10 mL) in a fresh 50-mL conical (*see* **Note 9**).
6. Wash two times with 35 mL RPMI (400g for 10 min).
7. Resuspend the final cell pellets in RPMI medium, using 1 mL for every 5 mL of whole blood. Determine cell viability and number by trypan blue exclusion.
8. Resuspend cells in RPMI medium supplemented with 20% heat-inactivated FCS (R-20) at 5×10^6 per mL. Place into one well of a 24-well plate:
   - 1.6 mL of cell suspension.
   - 0.2 mL of filtered B95-8 supernatant (*see* **Note 8**).
   - 0.2 mL of cyclosporine A, for a final concentration of 100 ng/mL.
9. Place the flask into a humidified incubator at 37°C with 5% CO_2 (*see* **Note 10**).
10. Seven days later, remove the top layer of medium by aspiration, leaving about 0.75 mL in the well. Feed with fresh R-20. Repeat this process 1–2 times/wk, observing for visible growth of transformed cells. These will be apparent after 2–4 wk in culture as clumps of cells that progressively increase in size.
11. When B-LCL reach a density of $2-3 \times 10^6$ (a confluent well in the plate), they can be split into a 25-cm^2 vented tissue-culture flask (*see* **Note 11**). Split once to twice weekly to maintain the cells at about 2×10^6/mL (*see* **Notes 12 and 13**).

3.3. Cytotoxicity Assay

1. Aliquot $5-10 \times 10^6$ B-LCL into a 15-mL conical for each target, and centrifuge at 400g for 10 min (*see* **Notes 14 and 15**).
2. Aspirate supernatant. Add 300 µL of RPMI containing $5-50 \times 10^6$ PFU (a multiplicity of infection [MOI] of 1–5 is usually used) (*see* **Notes 16 and 17**).
3. Vortex gently to disrupt the pellet.
4. Incubate in the conicals, with caps loosened for venting, at 37°C in a humidified tissue-culture incubator with 5% CO_2 for 90 min.
5. Wash two times with 10 mL RPMI (400g for 10 min).
6. Resuspend at $2-4 \times 10^6$ cells/mL in RPMI supplemented with 20% FCS (R-20).
7. Add 100 µCi $Na_2{}^{51}CrO_4$ (*see* **Note 18**).

8. Incubate cells overnight at 37°C in a humidified tissue-culture incubator with 5% CO_2.
9. In the morning, transfer cells to a 15-mL conical.
10. Wash three times with ice-cold RPMI 1640 medium supplemented with 10% heat-inactivated FCS, centrifuging at 200g for 7 min with each wash.
11. Resuspend cells in 2 mL cold RPMI 1640 medium supplemented with 10% heat-inactivated FCS and count by trypan blue exclusion.
12. Resuspend cells at 1×10^5 cells/mL and keep on ice for use as targets in the cytotoxicity assay (*see* **Note 19**).
13. For the cytotoxicity assay, effector cells (bulk polyclonal lymphocytes or clones) are added at varying effector:target cell ratios to a constant number of target cells (*see* **Note 20**). For bulk assays, E:T are generally 100:1, 50:1, and 25:1. For cloned cells, E:T range from 10:1–1:1 (*see* **Table 1**).

    A convenient way to set up a plate for multiple targets is shown in **Fig. 1**.
14. Incubate the plate for 4–6 h at 37°C in a humidified tissue-culture incubator with 5% CO_2 (clones, 4 h; bulk, 6 h).
15. Centrifuge the plate at 200g for 5 min at 4°C to spin down cells into the bottom of the wells.
16. Carefully aspirate 100 µL from each well to a separate plastic counting tube, and then add 100 µL of 5% Triton X-100 to inactivate the vaccinia virus.
17. Count the tubes in a γ-counter.
18. Calculate the percent specific cytotoxicity by the following formula (*see* **Note 21**):

$$\% \text{ Specific cytotoxicity} = \frac{\text{Experimental release} - \text{spontaneous release}}{\text{Maximal release} - \text{spontaneous release}} \times 100 \quad (1)$$

3.4. Fine Mapping of Epitopes Recognized by HCV-Specific CTL

This is based on a protocol originally described by Townsend et al. *(19)*. Short synthetic peptides can form a complex with HLA class I molecules on the cell surface and, thus, sensitize these target cells for lysis by CTL.

1. Pellet 2×10^6 B-LCL and resuspend in 2 mL fresh R-20.
2. Label overnight with 100 µCi of $Na_2^{51}CrO_4$ as described in **steps 7** and **8** in **Subheading 3.3.**
3. Following an overnight incubation, pellet the cells at 400g, and resuspend in 150 µL of fresh R-20.
4. Add peptide at the desired concentration (*see* **Note 22**). For screening studies to map an epitope, overlapping 20 amino acid (aa) peptides that span the entire region of interest are used (*see* **Notes 23** and **24**). The concentration of the peptides is 100 µg/mL. For fine mapping of epitopes, lower concentrations of shorter peptides are used, generally 5–20 µg/mL. Peptide is added in a total volume of 50 µL (*see* **Note 25**).
5. Incubate the cells for 1 h at 37°C in a humidified tissue culture incubator with 5% CO_2.
6. After a 1 h incubation, wash the cells three times and use as targets in a standard cytotoxicity assay (**steps 10–18** in **Subheading 3.3.**). For determining the mini-

**Table 1
Determination of Amounts of Reagents Needed
for the Cytotoxicity Assay**[a]

E:T	Target cells, 1×10^5/mL	Effector cells, 10×10^6/mL	R-10	Triton X-100, 5%
100:1	100	100	0	0
50:1	100	50	50	0
25:1	100	25	75	0
Spon	100	0	100	0
Max	100	0	0	100

[a]Add R-10 to each well, then effector cells. Add C_r-labeled targets last. Final dilutions of effector cells can be adjusted to give a desired E:T. All conditions are plated in triplicate. All values are µL/well of a round bottom 96-well plate. A convenient way to set up the 96-well plate is shown in **Fig. 1**.

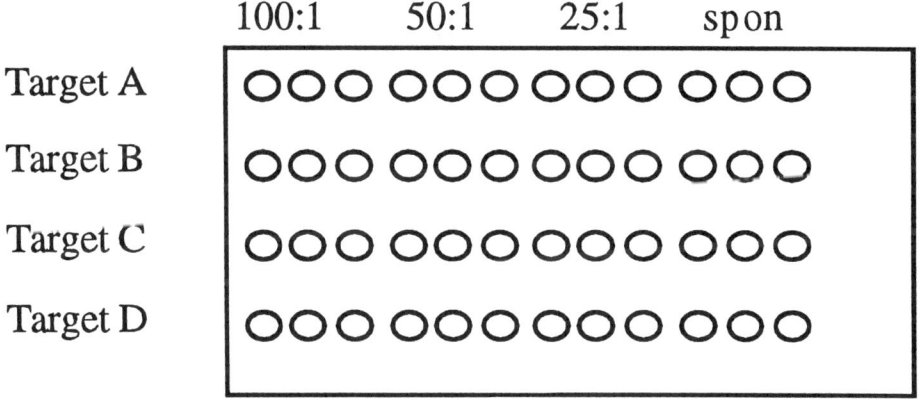

Fig. 1. Diagram of the setup of a chromium release assay. Max release wells are on a separate 96-well plate.

mal epitope of a cloned cell, a final E:T of 1:1–5:1 and a 4 h incubation are usually sufficient.

Alternate protocol: For fine mapping studies and serial dilution studies to determine the optimal minimal epitope recognized by HCV-specific CTL, preparation of individual target cells with each separate peptide or dilution would result in a cumbersome number of targets. As an alternate method, peptides can be incubated with the targets in the plates *(18)*.

1. Label B-LCL with 100 µCi of $Na_2{}^{51}CrO_4$ as described above.
2. Wash the cells three times with cold RPMI 1640 medium supplemented with 10% heat-inactivated FCS, and determine viable cell number.
3. Resuspend the cells at 2×10^5 cells/mL in cold RPMI 1640 medium supplemented with 10% heat-inactivated FCS, and keep on ice.
4. While cells are washing, add 50 µL of RPMI 1640 medium supplemented with 10% heat-inactivated FCS containing two times the desired final concentration of peptide into the well of a round-bottom, 96-well plate. All conditions are in triplicate.
5. Add 50 µL of the ^{51}Cr-labeled target cells to the wells, being careful prevent crosscontamination of the wells.
6. Incubate for 1 h at 37°C in a humidified tissue-culture incubator with 5% CO_2.
7. Add 100 µL of the effector cell at the desired E:T ratio.
8. Incubate for 4–6 h at 37°C in a humidified tissue-culture incubator with 5% CO_2.
9. Spin plates, and harvest supernatant as in **steps 14–18** in **Subheading 3.3.**

4. Notes

4.1. Isolation of Intrahepatic T-Lymphocytes from Liver Biopsy Specimens

1. Liver biopsy material is collected by a standard procedure. After the biopsy, the entire contents of the needle is deposited onto a sterile surface (the top of a sterile urine container is often suitable). Four- to 6-mm sections are then placed into sterile RPMI 1640 medium supplemented with 10% heat-inactivated FCS medium in a 50-mL conical. This tissue can be removed from the conical using a 10-mL sterile pipet in a minimal volume of fluid.
2. CD3,4B and CD3,8 antibodies have been supplied by Johnson Wong (Massachusetts General Hospital, Boston, MA). The CD3,4B antibody has one arm that is specific for the CD3 cell-surface antigen, and one arm specific for the CD4 cell-surface antigen, with a common Fc portion *(21)*. When added to lymphocytes in the presence of IL-2, this antibody results in the expansion of the CD8 lymphocytes fraction and depletion of the CD4-bearing fraction of lymphocytes. This is thought to occur because the CD3 arm stimulates all the CD3-expressing cells to proliferate, whereas the CD4 arm provides bridging between CD3-expressing and CD4-expressing cells, with resultant lysis of the CD4-expressing cells *(11)*. FACS analysis demonstrates that the lymphocytes stimulated in this manner are 95–98% $CD8^+$ (data not shown). The CD3,8 antibody works in a similar manner to expand $CD4^+$ lymphocytes.
3. If bispecific MAbs are not available, polyclonal nonspecific stimulation using anti-CD3 alone was also successful in the isolation of HCV-specific CTL. The liver biopsy is placed in RPMI 1640 medium supplemented with 10% heat-inactivated FCS medium supplemented with 100 U/mL of recombinant IL-2 and 12F6, and restimulated as with $CD8^+$ cell lines. The disadvantage of this procedure is that $CD4^+$ cells seem to expand more readily than $CD8^+$ cells, thus diluting

the HCV-specific CD8+ cells. However, in some subjects with high frequencies of HCV-specific cells present within the liver biopsies, this method has yielded comparable numbers of antigen-specific clones when done in parallel with CD3,4B stimulation.
4. Commercially available anti-CD3 antibodies have been used by other laboratories with equivalent success *(22)*.
5. Allogeneic feeder cells are prepared from freshly drawn blood, as in the EBV transformation protocol. It is not necessary to use autologous feeder cells.
6. In the absence of antigenic stimulation, it is usually necessary to clone cells at relatively high numbers of cells per well in order to obtain sufficient numbers of cell lines for screening. In our experience, cell lines selected from plates in which there is 25% or less growth in the wells maintain fine specificity over long periods of time. In addition, when these cell lines are subcultured at 0.3 and 1 cell/well, the subclones have the same specificity as the parental cell line. However, the subclones generally are less viable. Therefore, the parental cell lines are referred to functionally as clones.
7. It is best to keep the developing cells at relatively high density ($2–3 \times 10^6$ cell/mL).

4.2. Epstein-Barr Virus Transformation of B-Lymphocytes for B-Lymphoblastoid Cell Lines (B-LCL)

8. The B95-8 cell line can be obtained from the American Type Tissue collection (ATCC; 12301 Parklawn Drive, Rockville MD 20852). This cell line is grown in R-20. It is best to obtain early passage cultures if possible. The supernatant, which contains EBV particles, is harvested when the cells are in log-phase growth, generally 1–2 d after a split. The supernatant is then filtered through a 0.45-μm filter, and stored in aliquots at $-70°C$ until use. Once thawed, the stock should not be refrozen, so generally, it is best to store in 0.5-mL aliquots.
9. When performing the lymphocyte separation, it is important to minimize shaking of the conical, which might disturb the monolayer. When aspirating the monolayer, avoid aspiration of the Ficoll, which is toxic to cells.
10. If there is an usually good yield of PBMC, the entire process can be scaled up and performed in 25-cm^2 tissue-culture flasks.
11. It is important not to oversplit the cell lines at any point, since they prefer to be kept above 1×10^6 cells/mL. Cells are ready to be split when the media spontaneously turn yellow after 2 d in culture.
12. Occasionally a subject will be encountered where it appears there is good growth of the cells initially, only to have the cell line die off after 3–4 wk in culture. This is likely owing to the persistence of EBV-specific T-cells. In these cases, it is sometimes helpful to repeat the addition of cyclosporine to the cell culture at wk 2 in order to kill any remaining T-cells.
13. Once the cell line is established, it is best quickly to grow up a large number of cells for frozen storage. Although many B-LCL grow for months in culture, some lines will only grow for a limited number of passages.

4.3. Preparation of Target Cells for Screening of Cells

14. Viability of the B-LCL should be >85% prior to vaccinia virus infection in order to maximize antigen expression and minimize spontaneous release of chromium.
15. For studies of the HLA restriction pattern of cloned cells, different B-LCL matched and mismatched across different HLA loci can be used as target cells.
16. The MOI of the vaccinia virus infection is variable. Generally good results are obtained with an MOI of 1–5, although in selected circumstances, an MOI of 10 may be necessary. Higher MOIs do not necessarily result in increased antigenic expression, since vaccinia virus is so efficient at infecting cells, and may result in increased cellular toxicity, resulting in increased spontaneous release values because of vaccinia-induced lysis of the target cells.
17. Vaccinia virus stocks should be stored in small aliquots at $-70°C$ to avoid repeated freeze–thaw cycles, which diminish the effective titer of the virus stock.
18. Cells can also be labeled with $Na_2^{51}CrO_4$ for 1 h on the day of the assay, although in that case, it is often preferable to use slightly larger amounts of chromium (150 µCi).
19. The target cells should be handled gently and kept cold at each step in order to minimize spontaneous release of chromium.
20. Generally it is easiest to add the effectors into the 96-well plate while the targets are washing. The targets are then added to the effectors, with care taken to avoid crosscontamination of wells.
21. If the spontaneous release is >30%, this indicates that either the MOI of the vaccinia virus was too high, the B-LCL were not in log-phase growth, or the cells were not handled properly during the multiple washes. Washes are best done using simple inversion of tightly sealed conicals rather than vigorous pipeting. Care should also be taken in the pipeting of the target cells into the wells.

4.4. Fine Mapping of Epitopes Recognized by HCV-Specific CTL

22. All peptide stock solutions should be frozen in small aliquots in order to avoid repeated freeze–thaw cycles.
23. For mapping studies using peptides that are longer than the minimal epitope, it is occasionally necessary to use high concentrations of peptide *(23)* or overnight incubation of the peptide with the cells *(24)*.
24. When mapping studies are performed using large numbers of peptides, it is possible to incubate target cells with two noncontiguous peptides to reduce the total numbers of target cells.
25. It is very important when incubations are done in the 96-well plates to avoid crosscontamination when adding the labeled target cells of the effector cells. This can be accomplished by working from low to high concentrations of peptides when adding the labeled target cells, as well as changing pipet tips when adding effector cells to different peptides.

References

1. Dienes, H., Hutteroth, T., Hess, G., and Meuer, S. (1987) Immunoelectron microscopic observations on the inflammatory infiltrates and HLA antigens in hepatitis B and non-A, non-B. *Hepatology* **7**, 1317–1325.

2. Imawari, M., Nomura, M., and Kaieda, T. (1989) Establishment of a human T cell clone cytotoxic for both autologous and allogeneic hepatocytes from chronic hepatitis patients with type non-A, non-B virus. *Proc. Natl. Acad. Sci. USA* **86**, 2883–2887.
3. Liaw, Y. F., Lee, C. S., Tsai, S. L., Liaw, B. W., Chen, T. C., Sheen, I. S., and Chu, C. M. (1995) T-cell-mediated autologous hepatocytotoxicity in patients with chronic hepatitis C virus infection. *Hepatology* **22**, 1368–1373.
4. Chakrabati, S., Robert-Guroff, M., Wong-Staal, F., Gallo, R. C., and Moss, B. (1986) Expression of the HTLV-III envelope gene by a recombinant vaccinia. *Nature* **320**, 535–537.
5. Grakoui, A., Wychowski, C., Lin, C., Feinstone, S., and Rice, C. (1993) Expression and identification of hepatitis C virus polyprotein cleavage products. *J. Virol.* **67**, 1385–1395.
6. Brunner, K. T., Mauel, J., Cerottini, J. C., and Chapuis, B. (1968) Quantitative assay of the lytic action of immune lymphoid cells on 51-Cr-labelled allogeneic target cells in vitro; inhibition by isoantibody and by drugs. *Immunology* **14**, 181–196.
7. Bertoletti, A., Ferrari, C., Fiaccadori, F., Penna, A., Margolskee, R., Schlicht, H. J., Fowler, P., Guilhot, S., and Chisari, F. V. (1991) HLA class I-restricted human cytotoxic T cells recognize endogenously synthesized hepatitis B virus nucleocapsid antigen. *Proc. Natl. Acad. Sci. USA* **88**, 10,445–10,449.
8. Walker, B. D., Flexner, C., Birch-Limberger, K., Fisher, L., Paradis, T. J., Aldovini, A., Young, R., Moss, B., and Schooley, R. T. (1989) Long-term, culture and fine specificity of human cytotoxic T lymphocyte clones reactive with human immunodeficiency virus type 1. *Proc. Natl. Acad. Sci. USA* **86**, 9514–9518.
9. Livingston, P. G., Kurane, I., Dai, L.C., Okamoto, Y., Lai, C. J., Men, R., Karaki, S., Takiguchi, M., and Ennis, F. A. (1995) Dengue virus-specific, E-ILA-B3 5-restricted, human CD 8+ cytotoxic T lymphocyte (CTL) clones. Recognition of NS3 amino acids 500 to 508 by CTL clones of two different serotype specificities. *J. Immunol.* **154**, 1287–1295.
10. Hahn, S., Gehri, R., and Erb, P. (1995) Mechanism and biological significance of CD4-mediated cytotoxicity. *Immunol. Rev.* **146**, 57–59.
11. Wong, J. T., Pinto, C., Gifford, J., Kurnick, J., and Kradin, R. (1989) Characterization of the CD4+ and CD8+ tumor infiltrating lymphocytes propagated with bispecific monoclonal antibodies. *J. Immunol.* **143**, 3403–3411.
12. Falk, K., Rotzschke, O., Stevanovic, S., Jung, G., and Rammensee, H.-G. (1991) Allele-specific motifs revealed by sequencing of self-peptides eluted from MHC molecules. *Nature* **351**, 290–296.
13. Sadovnikova, E., Zhu, X., Collins, S. M., Zhou, J., Vousden, K., Crawford, L., Beverley, P., and Stauss, H. J. (1994) Limitations of predictive motifs revealed by cytotoxic T lymphocyte epitope mapping of the human papilloma virus E,7 protein. *Intl. Immunol.* **6**, 289–296.
14. Penna, A., Chisari, F. V., Bertoletti, A., Missale, G., Fowler, P., Giuberti, T., Fiaccadori, F., and Ferrari, C. (1991) Cytotoxic T lymphocytes recognize an HLA-A2-restricted epitope within the hepatitis B virus nucleocapsid antigen. *J. Exp. Med.* **174**, 1565–1570.

15. Barnaba, V., Franco, A., Alberti, A., Balsano, C., Benvenuto, R., and Balsano, F. (1989) Recognition of hepatitis B virus envelope proteins by liver-infiltrating lymphocytes in chronic HBV infection. *J. Immunol.* **143,** 2650–2655.
16. Nakagawa, H., Shimomura, H., Hasui, T., Tsuji, H., and Tsuji, T. (1994) Quantitative detection of hepatitis C virus genome in liver tissue and circulation by competitive reverse transcriptionpolymerase chain reaction. *Digest. Dis. Sci.* **39,** 225–233.
17. Koziel, M. J., Dudley, D., Wong, J., Dienstarg, J., Houghton, M., Ralston, R., and Walker, B. D. (1992) Intrahepatic cytotoxic T lymphocytes specific for hepatitis C virus in persons with chronic hepatitis. *J. Immunol.* **149,** 3339–3344.
18. Koziel, M., Dudley, D., Afdhal, N., Choo, Q.-L., Houghton, M., Ralston, R., and Walker, B. (1993) Hepatitis C virus-specific cytotoxic T lymphocytes recognize epitopes in the core and envelope proteins of HCV. *J. Virol.* **61,** 7522–7532.
19. Townsend, A. R., Rothbard, J., Gotch, F. M., Bahadur, G., Wraith, D., and McMichael, A. J. (1986) The epitopes of influenza nucleoprotein recognized by cytotoxic T lymphocytes can be defined with short synthetic peptides. *Cell* **44,** 959–968.
20. Koziel, M. J., Dudley, D., Afdhal, N., Grakoui, A., Rice, C. M., Choo, Q.-L., Houghton, M., and Walker, B. D. (1995) HLA class I-restricted cytotoxic 1 lymphocytes specific for hepatitis C virus. Identification of multiple epitopes and characterization of patterns of cytokine release. *J. Clin. Invest.* **96,** 2311–2321.
21. Wong, J. T. and Colvin, R. (1987) Bispecific monoclonal antibodies: selective binding and complement fixation to cells that express two different surface antigens. *J. Immunol.* **139,** 1369–1374.
22. Erickson, A. L., Houghton, M., Choo, Q.-L., Weiner, A. J., Ralston, R., Muchmore, E., and Walker, C. (1993) Hepatitis C virus-specific CTL responses in the liver of chimpanzees with acute and chronic hepatitis C. *J. Immunol.* **151,** 4189–4199.
23. Johnson, R. P., Trocha, A., Yang, L., Mazzara, G. P., Panicali, D. L., Buchanan, T. M., and Walker, B. D. (1991) HIV-1 gag-specific cytotoxic T lymphocytes recognize multiple highly conserved epitopes. Fine specificity of the gag-specific response defined by using unstimulated peripheral blood mononuclear cells and cloned effector cells. *J. Immunol.* **147,** 1512–1521.
24. Hogan, K. T., Shimojo, N., Walk, S. F., Engelhard, V. H., Maloy, W. L., Coligan, J. E., and Biddison, W. E. (1988) Mutations in the alpha 2 helix of HLA-A2 affect presentation but do not inhibit binding of influenza virus matrix peptide. *J. Exp. Med.* **168,** 725–736.

42

Production of Human Monoclonal Antibodies to Hepatitis C Virus and Their Characterization

Mario U. Mondelli and Antonella Cerino

1. Introduction

Human monoclonal antibodies (hMAb) provide novel ways to probe the B-cell repertoire in health and disease. However, the development of hMAb technology has met with several difficulties owing to the instability of the cell lines, the low level of specific antibody secretion, and the poor cloning efficiency, particularly when using lymphoblastoid cells *(1,2)*. In order to overcome these problems, some investigators have fused human B lymphocytes with human/mouse myeloma heterohybrids. However, in such systems, human chromosomes are unstable and may occasionally be deleted. Despite the potential emergence of technical pitfalls, B-cell immortalization with EBV has been extensively used for hMAb production, because of its simplicity and because EBV can bind to and penetrate in virtually all B lymphocytes, theoretically allowing the exploration of the whole B-cell repertoire. The most recent protocols have made use of techniques aimed at expanding the population of antigen-specific B-cell precursors and improving the capacity of B-cells to grow at low density. These methods will be discussed below.

Antibody phage-display technology *(3)* has been widely applied in recent years to the study of humoral immune responses in several diseases, particularly those of viral origin *(4–8)*. Although recombinant antibodies obtained from random combinatorial libraries can be very useful as molecular tools for research, and diagnostic and therapeutic purposes, they can only provide presumptive information on the features of the humoral immune response during the course of a specific disease. In fact, despite some indirect evidence *(5,9)* there is no definite proof that the original light- and heavy-chain pairing is maintained in the recombinant construct. At the present time, the only possibilities of characterizing an antibody that undoubtedly corresponds to the one originally produced in vivo are either to use techniques that preserve the original chain pairing, even when a mixed population of B-cells is used as in the cell PCR methodology *(10)* or to clone the antibody from single cell lines *(11–14)*. Other important limitations of combinatorial libraries are that they are usually unsuitable to fish out B-cells that are present at very low frequency and they tend to generate low-affinity ($K_a = 10^5$–10^6 M) antibodies.

To circumvent problems related to low B-cell precursor frequencies, techniques have been proposed to enrich the initial population of Ag-specific B-lymphocytes by panning or sorting B-cells binding to specified antigens *(15)*. However, such methodologies have been abandoned because of technical difficulties and unreproducibility. To expand the population of Ag-specific B-cells, in vitro immunization or restimulation techniques have been devised, which result in a significant improvement in the retrieval of Ag-specific B-cell clones (*see* **step 14, Subheading 3.**).

2. Materials

1. (2-Aminoethyl)-isothiouronium bromide hydrobromide-(AET, Sigma Chemical Co., St. Louis, MO) activated sheep red blood cells (SRBC).
2. Standard culture medium (M): RPMI-1640 Dutch Modification with 1 g/L NaHCO$_3$ and 20 mM HEPES (Sigma Chemical Co.), containing 10% fetal calf serum (FCS, HyClone Laboratories, Inc., Logan, UT), 4 mM L-glutamine (ICN Flow, Costa Mesa, CA), 1 mM sodium pyruvate (ICN Flow, Costa Mesa, CA), 1% nonessential amino acids (ICN Flow), 100 U/mL penicillin, 100 µg/mL streptomicin (ICN Flow).
3. EBV-productive B95-8 marmoset cells (ATCC CRL 1612)—available through American Type Culture Collection (Rockville, MD).
4. Supplemented medium (SM): standard culture medium supplemented with 20 U/mL recombinant IL-6 and 10% human endothelial cell-culture supernatant (HECS).
5. IL-6 (Novartis, Basel, Switzerland).
6. HECS (*see* **Note 2**).
7. Coating buffer: bicarbonate buffer 0.01 M, pH 9.6.
8. Washing buffer: Phosphate-buffered saline (PBS) 0.1 M, pH 7.2, + 0.05% Tween 20.
9. PBT buffer (blocking buffer): PBS containing 2% bovine serum albumin (BSA fraction V, Sigma Chemical Co.) and 0.1% Tween 20.
10. Horseradish peroxidase (HRP)-conjugated rabbit antihuman IgG (DAKO A/S, Glostrup, Denmark).
11. HRP-conjugated rabbit antihuman IgM (DAKO A/S).
12. Mouse monoclonal antihuman IgG subclasses (Sigma Chemical Co.).
13. HRP-conjugated rabbit antimouse Ig (DAKO A/S).
14. HRP-conjugated rabbit antihuman or light chains (DAKO A/S).
15. *Ortho*-phenylenediamine 2 HCl (OPD): dissolve 1 OPD tablet and 1 urea hydrogen peroxide-buffer tablet in 20 mL of deionized water (Sigma Chemical Co.).

16. Rabbit antihuman Ig (DAKO A/S) is utilized to capture hMAb on solid phase.
17. DNase I (Worthington Biochemicals, Freehold, NJ).
18. Dulbecco's Modified Minimum Essential Medium (DMEM, Sigma Chemical Co.).
19. Protein G-Sepharose columns (HiTrap Protein G, Pharmacia LKB Biotechnology, Uppsala, Sweden).
20. Glycine buffer: 0.1 M glycine–HCl, pH 2.7; PBS; Tris-HCl 0.02 M pH 8.0.

3. Methods

The following technique, summarized in **Fig. 1**, had been initially reported in **ref. *16*** with subsequent minor modifications *(17,18)*.

1. Preparation of AET-activated SRBC: Dissolve 1 g of crystalline AET in 21 mL distilled water, add approx 2 mL of 2 N NaOH to bring the pH to 8.5, add distilled water to a final volume of 24 mL and filter solution through a 0.22-μm pore filter (Nalgene, Nalge Co., Rochester, NY). Add 4 vol of AET to 1 vol of pelleted SRBC previously washed in normal saline. Resuspend gently and incubate at 37°C for 12–13 min. Wash five times in normal saline and resuspend at the concentration of 2% in RPMI-1640 without FCS.
2. Prepare EBV-containing supernatant: Thaw out B95-8 cells, wash, and resuspend in RPMI-1640 medium supplemented with 2 mM L-glutamine, 5% FCS, and antibiotics. Culture at 37°C in an atmosphere of 5% CO_2 in air at ≈3 × 10^5 cells/mL in 25 cm^2 standing tissue-culture flasks (Corning, NY). Split cultures by adding RPMI-1640 without serum (v/v) to the supernatant to reach a final FCS concentration of <1%. Culture cells until color of supernatant turns yellow, centrifuge, filter, and store at –80°C indefinitely until use.
3. Prepare HECS: HECS is prepared from a 24- to 48-h culture of human endothelial cells isolated from the umbilical vein as described *(19)*. Briefly, obtain a fragment (at least 20 cm) of freshly cut umbilical cord, and place it in a sterile container. Flush vein with sterile saline to remove blood, and fill vessel with approx 20 mL of warm sterile saline containing 200 mg collagenase type IA (Sigma Chemical Co.). Incubate at 37°C for 10 min while gently manipulating the umbilical cord. Collect effluent, wash 1X at 200g with M (*see* **Subheading 2.2.**), and culture in six-well plates (Costar, Cambridge, MA) in an atmosphere of 5% CO_2 in air. Harvest supernatants after 24–48 h, centrifuge at 1200g, filter through a 0.22-μm pore filter, and store at –80°C until use (*see* **Note 2**).
4. Obtain peripheral blood mononuclear cells (PBMC) by Ficoll-Hypaque gradient centrifugation from subjects with chronic HCV infection and high-titer circulating antibodies to the recombinant HCV protein against which you plan to produce hMAb. PBMC are enriched in B lymphocytes by removing T cells with AET-treated SRBC and subsequent centrifugation over a Ficoll-Hypaque gradient (*see* **Note 1**).
5. After washing, resuspend cells at 1.5 × 10^6/mL in M containing 50% cell-free supernatant from the B95-8 cell line, and incubate overnight at 37°C in an atmosphere of 5% CO_2 in air.

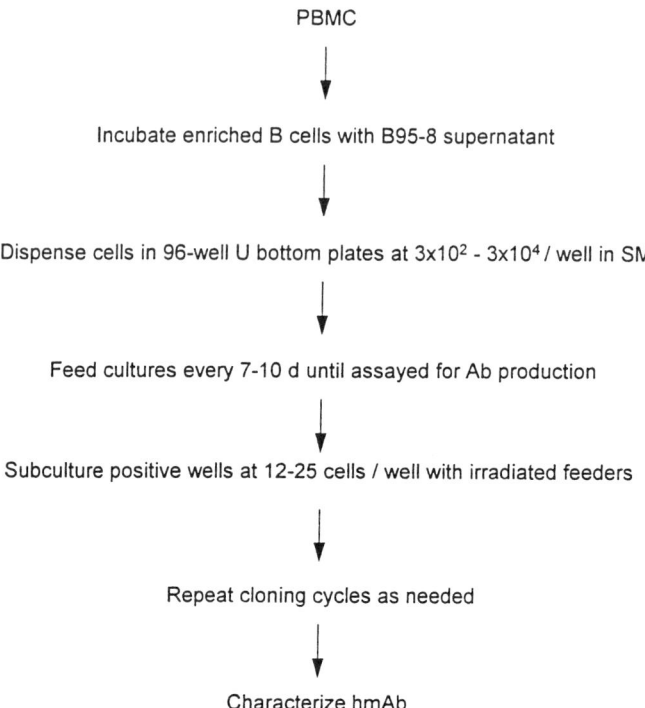

Fig. 1. Flowchart of B-cell cloning procedure from anti-HCV-positive patients.

6. After extensive washing, resuspend cells in SM and seed them in 96-well U-bottom plates at densities ranging from 3×10^4 to 3×10^2 cells/well. Incubate at 37°C in a humidified atmosphere of 5% CO_2 in air.
7. Replenish half the volume of spent medium with fresh SM every 7–10 d until cultures are assayed for specific antibody production (usually after 3–4 wk).
8. Subculture positive wells with supernatants showing absorbance values >2 at 12–25 cells/well in U-bottom wells with 3000 R-irradiated allogeneic PBMC as feeder cells in SM. Repeat cloning cycles as needed until criteria for mono–clonality are satisfied (*see* **Notes 3** and **4**).
9. Determine Ig isotype: Incubate B-cell clone supernatants on Ag-coated wells for 1 h at 37°C, and after washing, add HRP-conjugated rabbit antihuman IgM or IgG for 1 h. IgG subclass-specific murine MAbs are employed as in the first step to identify the MAb IgG subclass. To determine Ig light chains, HRP-conjugated rabbit antihuman light chain is used in a direct assay. The reaction is developed with OPD 2 HCl as substrate, and read at 492 nm (*see* **Note 5**).
10. Determine Ig production by quantitative ELISA: Coat ELISA microplate wells overnight at 4°C with rabbit antihuman Ig appropriately diluted in coating buffer. Ig preparations purified from patients with multiple myeloma are used as standards. Incubate appropriately diluted B-cell clone supernatants for 1 h at 37°C

and, after washing, add HRP-conjugated rabbit antihuman IgG or IgM to the wells for 1 h. Develop with OPD as above (*see* **Note 6**).

11. Determine hMAb affinity: Determine the K_d of the hMAb as described by Friguet et al. *(20)* modified in our laboratory *(21)* (*see* **Note 7**). The procedure is based on competitive inhibition exerted by soluble Ag on binding to the same Ag on the solid phase essentially as described in **Note 8**.

12. Estabilish hMAb fine specificity: Fine specificity of hMAb can be determined by coating Ag onto the solid phase in a standard direct ELISA. Overlapping synthetic oligopeptides covering the immunoreactive region of interest are normally used for this purpose. Reactivity is usually stronger if relatively long (15–20-mer) peptides are used as Ag. Recognition can also be significantly improved by using biotinilated peptides bound to streptavidin-coated plates. This can result in significant savings, since as little as 3 pmol of peptide can be used/well. Peptides should be preferably purified by HPLC to approx 90% purity and lyophilized. They can then be dissolved in 0.1% TFA, 30% acetonitryl in water, and stored at a concentration of 1 mg/mL at $-70°C$ until use. This solution is usually adequate to dissolve most peptides, including those rich in hydrophobic residues. However, in some cases, it may be helpful to add 2% DMSO or 10–20 µL glacial acetic acid and sonicate at 37°C. Peptides are then further diluted in coating buffer and used in a standard ELISA as extensively described above (*see* **Notes 8–10**).

13. Purify hMAb (the following technique has been developed for purification of IgG): Harvest supernatants when cell density reaches $0.8–1.2 \times 10^6$ cells/mL. Apply supernatant containing IgG to a protein G-Sepharose column. Elute with 0.1 M glycine-HCl, pH 2.7, and dialyze against PBS. HMAb can be further purified by anion-exchange HPLC equilibrated with 20 mM Tris-HCl buffer, pH 8.0, using a linear gradient from 0 to 1 M NaCl. Fractions containing the hMAb are pooled, dialyzed against PBS, and stored at $-20°C$ until use. Although protein G can bind bovine IgG, contamination of human IgG with bovine IgG present in the FCS is irrelevant for most purposes. If high-purity hMAb is required, supplemented media containing no serum are suggested for culture of stable B-cell cloned lines. Antibodies should be store at $-20°C$ until use.

14. (Additional information 1): For the situation in which the specific B-cell precursor frequency is low, isolation of Ag-specific B-cell lines can be difficult. In order to maximize generation of Ag-specific B-cell clones, in vitro stimulation protocols are currently used *(22)*. PBMC, 4×10^6/mL, are cultured for 6 d at 37%C in 5% CO_2 in 25-cm^2 standing flasks in RPMI-1640 medium containing 20 mM HEPES, 4 mM L-glutamine, 1 mM sodium pyruvate, 1% nonessential amino acids supplemented with 10% heat-inactivated AB+ human serum, 5 U recombinant IL-2, and 25% (v/v) of supernatant from human T lymphocytes stimulated for 24 h with 10 µg/mL pokeweed mitogen (PWM, Sigma Chemical Co.), in the presence of different Ag concentrations (we normally use 25, 125, 625 ng/mL). B-cells are subsequently enriched by removing T-cells by AET-rosetting on a Ficoll-Hypaque gradient or by incubation with anti-CD2-coated Dynabeads. T-cell depletion with consequent removal of EBV-specific cytotoxic T-cells is important to optimize B-cell immortalization by EBV.

15. (Additional information 2): To maximize growth of Ab-secreting B-cells, clones can be stabilized by fusion with mouse-human heteromyelomas. Cells are transferred to a 24-well plate and expanded; hybridomas are obtained by fusing B-cells with K6H6/B5 *(23)* or F3B6 (ATCC HB 8785) heterohybrid partners using polyethylenglycol, PEG 4000 (Merck, Darmstadt, Germany) or by electro–fusion *(23)* as follows. Heteromyeloma cells are added to EBV-transformed B-cell clones at a ratio of 2:1. The cell mixture containing 6.5×10^5 B-cells is placed in a cuvet equipped with an electrode connected to an electroporator. Cells are aligned for 30 s at 200 V/cm and then treated for 15 µs at 1500 V/cm. After resting for 30 min, cells are resuspended in M. After 24 h, 100 µM hypoxantine, 0.4 µM aminopterine, 16 µM thymidine, and 1 µM oubain are added. After fusion, hybridomas are cloned at a density of 1–3 cells/well and tested for specific Ab production as described above.
16. Further characterization of the use of the monoclonals in detecting the corresponding antigens in a cell-expression system and for the use in Western blotting is described in **Notes 11** and **12**.

4. Notes

1. Although purification of lymphocyte subsets is now efficiently achieved with magnetic beads (Dynabeads, Dynal A. S., Oslo, Norway) coated with murine MAbs specific for cluster differentiation antigens, AET-treated SRBC are equally adequate for the purpose of depleting T-cells from the PBMC preparation prior to EBV exposure and are significantly cheaper than MAb-coated magnetic beads.
2. This is an important, though ill-defined mixture of B-cell growth factors, which includes IL-6.
3. The following criteria are routinely considered as indicative of monoclonality:
    a. Stability of Ab secretion as a function of time in culture (>6 mo).
    b. Secretion of only one Ig isotype (*see* **Subheading 3., step 9**).
    c. Typically restricted Ig banding pattern on isoelectrofocusing (**Fig. 2**).
    d. 100% of wells secreting specific Ab following at least two subcloning cycles at 12 cells/well.
4. Assay for specific Ab production at least 1 wk after changing medium to avoid untoward dilution of secreted Ab.
5. The technique employed in our laboratory tends to select for B-cell clones secreting high-affinity IgG, rather than IgM class hMAb. All the clones isolated so far produced IgG1, similarly to findings obtained by others *(1)*.
6. Typical hMAb concentrations in supernatants after 6–8 d in culture are 8–20 µg/mL of culture medium.
7. Typical K_d for human IgG range from 10^{-7} to 10^{-9} M *(23)*.
8. Fine specificity of hMAb can also be determined by competitive inhibition in which soluble peptides derived from the region of interest are incubated with hMAb prior to transfer to ELISA plates coated with purified recombinant protein *(17,23)*. This protocol may occasionally give some problems. The following conditions have been found to yield reproducible results in our laboratory. Aliquots

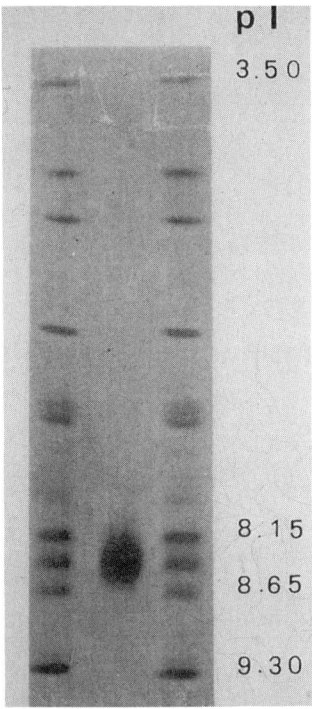

Fig. 2. Isoelectrofocusing of hMAb specific for the HCV NS4 protein shown in the central lane. Side lanes indicate pI standards.

of PBT buffer (60 µL) containing 0.3 µg of hMAb are mixed with aliquots of PBT buffer (60 µL) containing increasing amounts (0.01–50 µg) of peptide. After and 18-h incubation at room temperature, mixtures are transferred to ELISA wells precoated with recombinant protein (2.5 µg/mL). After a 1-h incubation at 37°C and subsequent washing with PBT buffer, the hMAb bound to the solid-phase Ag is measured. Ag binding activity of hMAb in the presence of soluble ligand is expressed as the percentage of its binding activity measured under identical conditions, but in the absence of any soluble ligand.

9. Sequential epitopes can be most efficiently identified at a resolution of a single amino acid residue by PEPSCAN *(24)*. This method consists of chemically coupling short peptides (usually 6–12-mer) to solid supports assembled in a format and spacing of a microtiter plate. Hundreds of peptides encompassing an entire protein region and overlapping by one residue can be synthesized and coupled to polyethylene pins arranged to fit in a 96-well ELISA plate. The assay is then essentially carried out by a standard methodology. Solid-phase bound MAb can also be chemically eluted from the peptides and the pins recycled. A representative example of a PEPSCAN analysis of a linear epitope in the HCV NS4 region

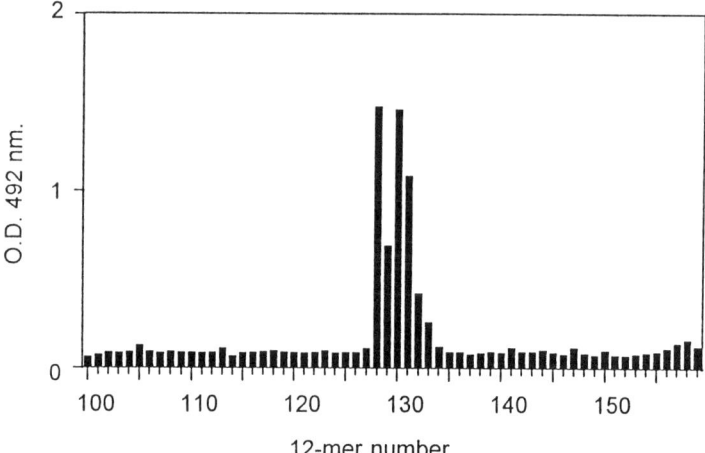

Fig. 3. Fine specificity of an hMAb recognizing a linear epitope within the HCV NS4 protein determined by PEPSCAN analysis. The MAb was tested on pin-bound 12-mer, scaled by one amino acid residue, covering the entire NS4 region sequence. Shown here is the critical region recognized by the MAb. 12-mer 130, DREVLYREFDEM, contains the minimal B-cell epitope.

is given in **Fig. 3**. Custom-made pin-bound oligopeptides can be purchased from Chiron Mimotopes (San Diego, CA).

10. An alternative technique to define the specificity of an MAb is recombinant epitope mapping. This method is particularly recommended when attempting to identify conformational or discontinuous B-cell epitopes that cannot be defined by peptides *(25,26)*. This is the case, for instance, in the HCV helicase domain, which displays a complex antigenic structure *(18)*. The sequence encoding for the protein is amplified using specific primers by polymerase chain reaction (PCR) from an HCV cDNA clone. PCR products are isolated from Tris borate EDTA-polyacrylamide gel (8% PAGE) by electroelution. Aliquots of the PCR-amplified material are digested under controlled conditions: 25°C, 10–60 min, in a final volume of 25 µL containing 1 mM MnCl$_2$, 20 mM Tris-HCl (pH 7.5), and 0.6 U DNase I *(25,26)*. The digestions are stopped by addition of phenol-chloroform-isoamyl alcohol (v/v), and extracted. DNAase digestions are controlled by nick translation. Fragments with a length of approx 50–200 bp are isolated by diffusion following fractionation on 8% PAGE *(27)*. Parts of these fractions are subsequently tailed with oligo(-dG) according to the manufacturer's recommendations (Gibco-BRL, Gaithersburg, MD). PCR is then performed on the tailed product using poly-C as primer attached to a terminal *Eco*RI site. After *Eco*RI digestion and phenol extraction, the products are cloned in λgt11 arms and transfected into *Escherichia coli* as detailed by the manufacturer (Promega, Madison, WI). PCR on libraries using λgt11 primers reveals smears with lengths concordant with those of the inserted fragments. The libraries are

screened on duplo filters using standard procedures with the human MAb and representative human sera at a dilution of 1:50 for comparison. The reaction is detected using alkaline phosphatase-conjungated goat antihuman IgG (Sigma Chemical Co.). Positive phages are rescreened to identify positively their contents and their inserts subsequently transferred to the vector pGEM7Zf(+) (Promega). The inserts in this vector are sequenced using commercial kits (i.e., Pharmacia T7-sequencing kit, Pharmacia LKB Biotechnology, Uppsala, Sweden) as suggested by the manufacturer.

11. To test the capacity of HCV-specific hMAbs to bind to the corresponding cell-associated antigen, the vaccinia virus T7 transient expression system has been used in a transfection assay as described (27). HeLa cell monolayers are seeded on glass cover slips and infected with vaccinia virus vTF7-3 at a multiplicity of 5. After adsorption for 30 min at 37°C, 3 mL of DMEM supplemented with 10% FCS are added. Cells are incubated for an additional 30 min at 37%C. Twenty micrograms of plasmid DNA expressing a full-length HCV construct (nt 1–9416) or subgenomic fragments, are precipitated in calcium phosphate and added directly to each plate. At 6 h posttransfection, cells are fixed with methanol for 4 min at –20°C, rehydrated in PBS, and incubated with culture supernatant from an HCV-specific B-cell clone diluted 1:20 in PBS containing 5% BSA. Cells are then labeled with FITC-conjugated goat antihuman Ig (Sigma Chemical Co.), mounted in 90% glycerol, 10% PBS 10X, and photographed by epifluorescence with a 100× planar objective. Nontransfected or mock-transfected HeLa cells are used as control substrate.

12. HMAb should also be assayed for their capacity to recognize HCV proteins on Western blot, since some Ab only recognize conformation-dependent epitopes. Fifty nanograms of purified HCV protein or a similar quantity of a control protein are separated on 10% SDS-PAGE, and after transfer to nitrocellulose, strips are immersed in 1% skimmed milk in TBS (20 mM Tris-HCl, 500 mM NaCl, pH 7.5) (blocking buffer) for 20 min at room temperature. The appropriate primary antibody diluted in blocking buffer is then applied to nitrocellulose strips and incubated for 1 h at room temperature. Typical dilutions are 1:50 for hMAb supernatants, 1:2000 for animal polyclonal antisera, and 1:200 for anti-HCV positive or negative control human sera. After three 10-min washings in blocking buffer, antihuman or antirabbit Ig conjugated with alkaline phosphatase is applied at a 1:2000 dilution in blocking buffer. After 1 h of incubation at room temperature, membranes are washed thrice for 10 min and developed with 100 mM Tris-HCl buffer, pH 9.5, containing 100 mM NaCl, 5 mM MgCl$_2$, 0.33 mg/mL p-nitro-blue-tetrazolium-chloride, and 0.165 mg/mL 5-bromo-4-chloro-3-indolyl-phosphate.

References

1. James, K. and Bell, G. T. (1987) Human monoclonal antibody production. Current status and future prospects. *J. Immunol. Methods* **100**, 5–40.
2. Pistillo, M. P., Mazzoleni, O., Tanigaki, N., Hammerling, U., Longo, A., Frumento, G., et al. (1988) Human anti-HLA monoclonal antibodies: production, characterization and application. *Hum. Immunol.* **21**, 265–278.

3. Winter, G., Griffiths, A. D., Hawkins, R. E., and Hoogenboom, H. R. (1994) Making antibodies by phage display technology. *Annu. Rev. Immunol.* **12,** 433–455.
4. Zebedee, S. L., Barbas, C. F. III, Hom, Y.-L., Caothien, R. H., Graff, R., DeGraw, J., et al. (1992) Huma combinatorial antibody libraries to hepatitis B surface antigen. *Proc. Natl. Acad. Sci. USA* **89,** 3175–3179.
5. Williamson, R. A., Burioni, R., Sanna, P. P., Partridge, L. J., Barbas, C. F. III, and Burton, D. R. (1993) Human monoclonal antibodies against a plethora of viral patogens from single combinatorial libraries. *Proc. Natl. Acad. Sci. USA* **90,** 4141–4145.
6. Burioni, R., Williamson, R. A., Sanna, P. P., Bloom, F. E., and Burton, D. R. (1994) Recombinant human Fab to glycoprotein D neutralizes infectivity and prevent cell-to-cell transmission of herpex simplex viruses 1 and 2 *in vitro. Proc. Natl. Acad. Sci. USA* **91,** 355–359.
7. Crowe, J. E., Murphy, B. R., Chanock, R. M., Williamson, R. A., Barbas, C. F. III, and Burton, D. R. (1994) Recombinant human respiratory syncytial virus (RSV) monoclonal antibody Fab is effective therapeutically when introduced directly into the lungs of RSV-infected mice. *Proc. Natl. Acad. Sci. USA* **91,** 1386–1390.
8. Barbas, C. F. III, Hu, D., Dunlop, N., Sawyer, L., Cababa, D., Hendry, R. M., et al. (1994) In vitro evolution of a neutralizing human antibody to human immunodeficiency virus type 1 to enhance affinity and broaden strain cross reactivity. *Proc. Natl. Acad. Sci. USA* **91,** 3809–3813.
9. Caton, A. J. and Koprowski, H. (1990) Influenza virus hemagglutinin-specific antibodies isolated from a combinatorial expression library are closely related to the immune response of the donor. *Proc. Natl. Acad. Sci. USA* **87,** 6450–6454.
10. Embleton, M. J., Gorochov, G., Jones, P. T., and Winter, G. (1992) In-cell PCR from mRNA: amplifying and linking the rearranged immunoglobulin heavy and light chain V-genes within single cells. *Nucleic Acids Res.* **20,** 3831–3837.
11. Mullinax, R. L., Gross, E. A., Hay, B. N., Amberg, J. R., Kubitz, M. M., and Sorge, J. A. (1992) Expression of a heterodimeric Fab antibody protein in one cloning step. *BioTechniques* **12,** 864–867.
12. Esposito, G., Scarselli, E., and Traboni, C. (1994) Phage display of a human antibody against Clostridium tetani toxin. *Gene* **148,** 167,168.
13. Esposito, G., Scarselli, E., Cerino, A., Mondelli, M. U., La Monica, N., and Traboni, C. (1995) A human antibody specific for hepatitis C virus core protein: synthesis in a bacterial system and characterization. *Gene* **164,** 203–209.
14. Jiang, W., Bonnert, T. P., Venugopal, K., and Gould, E. A. (1994) A single chain antibody fragment expressed in bacteria neutralizes Tick-borne flavivirus. *Virology* **200,** 21–28.
15. Casali, P., Inghirami, G., Nakamura, M., Davies, T. F., and Notkins, A. L. (1986) Human monoclonals from antigen-specific selection of B lymphocytes and transformation by EBV. *Science* **234 (4775),** 476–479.
16. Cerino, A. and Mondelli, M. U. (1991) Identification of an immunodominant B-cell epitope on the hepatitis C virus non structural region defined by human monoclonal antibodies. *J. Immunol.* **147,** 2692–2696.

17. Cerino, A., Boender, P., Rosa, C., La Monica, N., Habets, W., and Mondelli, M. U. (1993) A human monoclonal antibody specific for the N-terminus of hepatitis C virus nucleocapsid protein. *J. Immunol.* **151,** 7005–7015.
18. Mondelli, M. U., Cerino, A., Boender, P., Oudshoorn, P., Middeldorp, J., Fipaldini, C., et al. (1994) Significance of the immune response to a major, conformational B cell epitope on the hepatitis C virus NS3 region defined by a human monoclonal antibody. *J. Virol.* **68,** 4829–4836.
19. Astaldi, G. C., Janssen, M. C., Lansdorp, P., Willems, C., Zeijlemaker, W. P., and Oosterhof, F. (1980) Human endothelial culture supernatant (HECS): a growth factor for hybridomas. *J. Immunol.* **125 (4),** 1411–1414.
20. Friguet, B., Chaffotte, A. F., Djavandi-Ohanaiance, L., and Goldberg, M. E. (1985) Measurement of the true affinity constant in solution of antigen-antibody complexes by enzyme-linked immunosorbent assay. *J. Immunol. Methods* **77,** 305–319.
21. De Lalla, C., Cerino, A., Rosa, C., Griva, S., Bonelli, F., and Mondelli, M. U. (1993) Properties of human monoclonal antibody specific for the NS4 region of hepatitis C virus. *J. Hepatol.* **18,** 163–167.
22. Ohlin, M. and Borrebaeck, C. A. K. (1993) Production of human monoclonal antibodies, in *Methods of Immunological Analysis* (Masseyeff, R. F., Albert, W. H. W., and Staines, N. A., eds.), VCH Verlagsgesellschaft mbH, Weinheim, pp. 298–235.
23. Carroll, W. L., Thielemans, K., Dilley, J., and Levy, R. (1986) Mouse x human heterohybridomas as fusion partners with human B cell tumors. *J. Immunol. Methods* **89,** 61–72.
24. Geysen, H. M., Meloen, R. H., and Barteling, S. J. (1984) Use of peptide synthesis to probe viral antigens for epitopes to a resolution of a single amino acid. *Proc. Natl. Acad. Sci. USA* **81,** 3998–4002.
25. Mehra, V., Sweetser, D., and Young, R. A. (1986) Efficient mapping of protein antigenic determinants. *Proc. Natl. Acad. Sci. USA* **83,** 7013–7017.
26. Habets, W. J., Sillekens, P. T. G., Hoet, M. H., McAllister, G., Lerner, M. R., and van Venrooij, W. J. (1989) Small nuclear RNA-associated proteins are immunologically related as revealed by mapping of autoimmune reactive B-cell epitopes. *Proc. Natl. Acad. Sci. USA* **86,** 4674–4678.
27. Tomei, L., Failla, C., Santolini, E., De Francesco, R., and La Monica, N. (1993) NS3 is a serine protease required for processing of the hepatitis C virus polyprotein. *J. Virol.* **67,** 4017–4026.

VIII

IN VITRO CULTURE MODEL

43

Specific Detection of Negative Strand RNA of Hepatitis C Virus Using Chemical RNA Modification

Toshiaki Gunji and Kunitada Shimotohno

1. Introduction

Hepatitis C virus (HCV), the genome of which was molecularly cloned in the US and Japan, causes most, if not all, cases of posttransfusional non-A, non-B hepatitis (NANBH) and nearly half those of sporadic hepatitis. Prospective and retrospective studies revealed that nearly half of patients with acute infection develop a chronic state of HCV infection, and half of them develop to liver cirrhosis and hepatocellular carcinoma.

HCV is a positive-stranded RNA virus 9.8 kb in length distantly related to human flaviviruses and animal pestiviruses. This sequence contains a single open reading frame capable of encoding a 3010 amino acid polyprotein precursor from which individual structural and nonstructural proteins are processed by cellular and viral proteases.

Two major techniques are currently available to detect HCV infection. The first technique is an immunoassay system for detecting circulating antibodies to a recombinant HCV fusion protein expressed in yeast, and the importance of this test has been established by sero-epidemiologic studies on patients with NANBH. The presence of anti-HCV antibodies, however, does not necessarily imply ongoing viral replication or the existence of the viral genome itself in the serum, since the appearance of the antibodies in serum depends on the immune response of the host. Moreover, the low sensitivity in the serological test and a time lag between infection and seroconversion occasionally result in false-negative results. Therefore, direct estimation of viral RNA seems more suitable than assay of the antibodies for evaluation of the biological events involved in HCV infection and replication. The second technique detects HCV

From: *Methods in Molecular Medicine, Vol. 19: Hepatitis C Protocols*
Edited by: J. Y. N. Lau © Humana Press Inc., Totowa, NJ

RNA itself directly through a reverse transcriptase followed by polymerase chain reaction method (RT-PCR). Because of the relatively small amounts of HCV RNA present in clinical specimens from patients with HCV infection, HCV RNA cannnot be reliably detected by standard molecular hybridization techniques, and it can usually be detected only by using the PCR, which is an extremely sensitive technique capable of detecting several hundreds of copies of HCV genomes.

Although molecular aspects of HCV have been studied intensively, the precise strategy involved in viral replication in infected individuals still remains to be determined. Since HCV is distantly related to the flaviviruses, it is assumed that replication of HCV involves the production of a complementary genomic-length negative RNA strand through RNA synthesis using the positive-strand RNA as a template. Positive-strand RNAs are then amplified using the negative strand as a template. Thus, the negative strand of HCV RNA is referred to as " replicative intermediate." In other words, negative strand should be detected in the sites where HCV is actually replicating. From these points of view, to obtain a deeper insight into the virological events involved in HCV infection and replication, it is important to clarify the accurate distributions of negative-strand RNA in the infected hosts with HCV. In addition, establishment of a method for detecting the positive and negative strand of HCV RNA specifically is also crucial to development of an in vitro culture system of HCV.

To detect each RNA strand of HCV separately, a modification of PCR which is called "strand-specific RT-PCR," has been widely employed in recent investigations. In these lines of studies, cDNAs for the positive and negative strand of HCV RNA are synthesized with an antisense and sense primer, respectively, for reverse transcription, followed by PCR. Even though this conventional strand specific RT-PCR method has been commonly applied in analysis of distributions of positive and negative strands, the specificity of this strategy indistinguishing between the two RNA strands has not been confirmed so far. To determine the validity of this method, we conducted the control experiments using positive and negative strands of HCV RNA purified separately by in vitro transcription, which were subsequently mixed with hepatic cellular RNA from normal liver to mimic clinical specimens, and found that such conventional strategy as used in most studies of negative strand cannot detect positive and negative strand separately due to primer-independent cDNA synthesis during reverse transcription *(1)*. Although we do not know why primer-independent cDNA synthesis took place, it might be possible that fragmented cellular and/or viral RNAs could possibly serve as nonspecific primers for reverse transcription. To prevent fragmented RNAs from acting as nonspecific primers, we adopted the strategy of modifying RNA samples at the 3'-end with

RNA Extraction from Serum, Liver Tissues and PBMCs by Acid Guanidium / Phenol / Chloroform Method

Chemical Modification of RNA Molecules at Their 3' End

[1] Denaturation of RNA sample

[2] Oxidation with NaIO$_4$

[3] Reduction with NaBH$_4$

cDNA Synthesis in RT mixture Containing Specific Primer for Positive or Negative Strand of HCV RNA

1st PCR Amplification Using External Primers Derived from 5' Noncoding Region or Core Region of HCV Genome

2nd PCR Amplification Using Internal Primers instead of External Ones

Electrophoresis of PCR Products on 1% -2% Agarose Gel

Fig. 1. Flowchart of strand-specific RT-PCR associated with chemical RNA modification.

chemical agents prior to reverse transcription, since RNAs with a modified 3'-end are expected to be no longer able to act as primers (*see* **Note 1**).

This chapter describes a novel strand-specific RT-PCR strategy combined with chemical modification of RNA samples at their 3'-end, which was primarily done by periodate oxidation followed by reduction with sodium tetrahydroborate. Since the specificity of our strategy was verified by appropriate control experiments using synthetic positive and negative strands of HCV RNA, detection of the negative strand by the current method would probably represent the most accurate sites and mode of HCV replication. A flowchart of this strategy is shown in **Fig. 1**.

2. Materials

1. Clinical specimens, such as sera, liver tissues, and PBMCs, collected from infected patients with HCV. Store these samples at –70°C until use, and avoid repeated freeze and thaw.
2. Sodium periodate solution, $NaIO_4$: Prepare 20 mM of $NaIO_4$ solution freshly as required.
3. Sodium acetate solution: 50 mM NaOAc, pH 5.0.
4. Sodium tetrahydroborate solution, $NaBH_4$: Prepare 0.1 M $NaBH_4$ solution dissolved in 0.01 M NaOH. Stable at –20°C for up to 1 wk.
5. Ethylene glycol: Prepare 10% w/w solution. Stable for several months at room temperature.
6. Moloney murine leukemia virus (M-MLV) RT for cDNA synthesis (Bethesda Research Laboratories, Gaithersburg, MD).
7. RT Buffer: 50 mM Tris-HCl, 75 mM KCl, 3 mM $MgCl_2$, pH 8.3.
8. *Taq* DNA polymerase for DNA amplification (Perkin-Elmer-Cetus, Norwalk, CT).
9. PCR buffer: 10 mM $(NH_4)_2 SO_4$, 70 mM Tris-HCl, 2 mM $MgCl_2$, 1 mM DTT, bovine serum albumin (BSA) at 100 mg/mL, 0.1% Triton X-100, pH 8.8.

3. Methods

1. RNA extraction: Extract RNAs from clinical specimens of 100–200 µL of serum, 50–100 µg of liver biopy specimens, and 10^6 cells of PBMC by the acid guanidium thiocyanate/phenol/chloroform extraction method. Suspend the extracted RNAs in 20 mL of sterile water and store at –70°C.
2. Chemical modification of 3' end of RNA molecules:
   a. Denature RNA samples at 80°C for 10 min, chill on ice and suspend in 200 µL of 50 mM NaOAc (pH 5.0) (*see* **Note 2**). Incubate with 50 µL of 20 mM $NaIO_4$ at 30°C for 12 h in the dark (*see* **Notes 3** and **4**).
   b. Stop the reaction by adding 60 µL of 10% ethylene glycol, and leave it for 10 min at room temperature, followed by ethanol precipitation.
   c. Suspend the resulting pellet in 300 µL of DEPC-treated water, and incubate with 100 mL of 0.1 M $NaBH_4$ at 0°C for 1 h in the dark (*see* **Note 5**).
   d. Stop the reaction by adding 20 µL of ice-cold acetic acid, followed by ethanol precipitation. Suspend the pellet in 20 µL of water, and subject to RT-PCR assay as described below.
3. cDNA synthesis: After denaturation of RNA samples at 80°C for 10 min, synthesize cDNA in 10 µL of reaction mixture containing 4 µL of RNA samples modified at their 3'-end, 1X RT buffer, 500 mM of each dNTP, 200 U of M-MLV-RT, and 1 mM of either sense or antisense primer for negative or positive strand HCV RNA, respectively. Incubate the reaction mixture at 42°C for 1 h. After RT reation, boil the mixture at 100°C for 30 min to inactivate RT, chill on ice, and then incubate with 1 µg of RNase A at 37°C for 90 min to degrade residual RNA templates (*see* **Note 6**).
4. DNA amplification: Carry out the first PCR amplification of the cDNAs by addition of 40 µL of reaction mixture containing 1X PCR buffer, 1 mM of each sense

and antisense primer, 200 mM of each dNTP, and 3 U of *Taq* polymerase for 40 cycles. Each cycle consists of annealing at 55°C for 45 s, primer extension at 72°C for 2 min, and denaturation at 94°C for 1 min, followed by a final extension at 72°C for 8 min. Subject a 1 µL aliquot of the first amplification product to the second PCR for 34 cycles in the same conditions as for the first PCR, except using the internal primers instead of the external ones. The amplified products were electrophoresed in 2% agarose gel and visualized with ethidium bromide staining under UV light (*see* **Note 7**).

4. Notes

1. In our previous control experiments using synthetic positive- and negative-strand HCV RNA that were mixed with hepatic cellular RNA from normal liver to mimic clinical specimens, we demonstrated that amplification of each strand by conventional strand-specific RT-PCR occurred irrespective of the primer for reverse transcription *(1)*. Surprisingly, both RNA strands were also amplified by RT-PCR without any primer during RT step. The evidence presented by us implies that conventional RT-PCR strategy is not suitable for specific detection of negative strand. Subsequently, several different investigators also reported the amplification of HCV RNA in an independent manner with respect to the primer used for reverse transcription *(2–4)*, which are consistent with our previous observations. All these lines of studies suggest primer-independent cDNA synthesis during the RT step, probably owing to random priming of cullular and/or viral RNAs, self-priming within HCV RNA molecules, or mispriming. We speculated that these nonspecific priming events might be overcome if the 3'-ends of RNAs were modified prior to the addition of the specific primer for the RT step, and proved the nonspecific priming to be made strand-specific by treatment of RNA samples with $NaOI_4$ and $NaBH_4$, a procedure that is known to convert the 3'-end terminal nucleotide of RNA to a di-alcohol.
2. Heat-denaturing of RNA samples prior to chemical modification is important, because unfolded RNA molecules are expected to be more susceptible to oxidation with $NaOI_4$.
3. Since $NaOI_4$ is light-sensitive, it should be freshly prepared, and reaction with $NaOI_4$ should be done in the dark.
4. Since $NaBH_4$ is unstable in acidic solution, it should be dissolved in alkaline solution (0.05 M NaOH). $NaBH_4$ as well as $NaOI_4$ is also light-sensitive, and reduction with $NaBH_4$ must be done in the dark. It might be possible that prolonged incubation of RNA samples with NaBH4 in alkaline solution degrades RNA molecules. Therefore, reduction with $NaBH_4$ should be completed in no more than 1–2 h.
5. When an excess amount of $NaBH_4$ was degraded with ice-cold acetic acid, $^3H_2$ gas appeared in the reaction mixture. If a large number of samples were treated simultaneously, it was better to do it in a draft chamber.
6. Treatment of cDNA mixture with RNase A is to digest RNA molecules that might possibly act as a template for cDNA synthesis by residual RT or possible RTase

activity of *Taq* polymerase during PCR reaction, which would lead to false-positive detection of a negative strand. An alternative to RNase treatment is alkaline inactivation of RNA with 0.1–0.4 N NaOH *(5)*.
7. The current RT-PCR can detect 100 copies of HCV RNA molecules present in 1 mg cellular RNAs of liver, which is sensitive enough to analyze a positive or negative strand of HCV RNA in biological samples from infected patients with HCV.

References

1. Gunji, T., Kato, N., Hijikata, M., Hayashi, K., Saitoh, S., and Shimotohno, K. (1994) Specific detection of positive and negative stranded hepatitis C viral RNA using chemical RNA modification. *Arch. Virol.* **134,** 293–302.
2. Mcguinness, P. H., Bishop, G. A., McCaughan, G. W., Trowbridge, R., and Gowans, E. J. (1994) False detection of negative-strand hepatitis C virus RNA. *Lancet* **343,** 551,552.
3. Lanford, R. E., Sureau, C., Jacob, J. R., White, R., and Fuerst, T. R. (1994) Demonstration of in vitro infection of chimpanzee hepatocytes with hepatitis C virus using strand-specific RT/PCR. *Virology* **202,** 606–614.
4. Lerat, H., Berby, F., Trabaud, M. A., Vidalin, O., Major, M., Trepo, C., et al. (1996) Specific detection of hepatitis C virus minus strand RNA in hematopoietic cells. *J. Clin. Invest.* **97,** 845–851.
5. Tanaka, T., Kato, N., Cho, M. J., and Shimotohno, K. (1995) A novel sequence found at the 3' terminus of hepatitis C virus genome. *Biochem. Biophys. Res. Commun.* **215,** 744–749.

44

Strand-Specific rTth RT-PCR for the Analysis of HCV Replication

Robert E. Lanford and Deborah Chavez

1. Introduction

Because of the very low level of HCV present in the serum of infected individuals, as well as the low level of replication in the host, reverse transcription-polymerase chain reaction (RT-PCR) assays are the only method suitable for the routine detection of HCV RNA. The use of RT-PCR to monitor HCV replication in vivo as well as the in vitro inoculation of cultured cells presents unique problems. The extreme sensitivity of PCR permits the detection of HCV RNA in tissues not permissive for replication of the virus, and following in vitro infections, the residual inoculum can be detected for extended time periods depending on the sensitivity of the PCR procedure. Since HCV is a positive-stranded RNA virus, the detection of negative-strand RNA should be indicative of active viral RNA replication, assuming that the inoculum contains primarily positive-strand RNA. Early attempts to detect negative-strand RNA employed a strand-specific PCR technique that utilized only one primer during cDNA synthesis, followed by inactivation of the RT and amplification of the cDNA by PCR. During the course of our studies, we found this technique to lack significant strand specificity using synthetic RNA. A series of experiments suggested that the lack of specificity was probably owing to a combination of factors, including false priming of the incorrect strand (e.g., the positive strand in a negative-strand assay) by the cDNA primer, self-priming of the RNA, and random priming by extraneous nucleic acids (illustrated in **Fig. 1A**). As long as the falsely primed cDNA spans the area encompassed by the two PCR primers, a product indistinguishable from the correctly primed product will result. This finding has been supported by publications from four laboratories *(1–4)* and should not be surprising, since it is

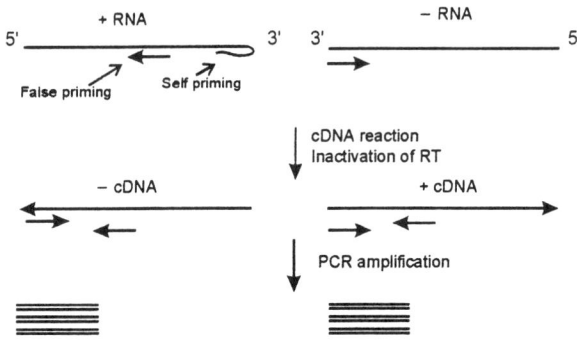

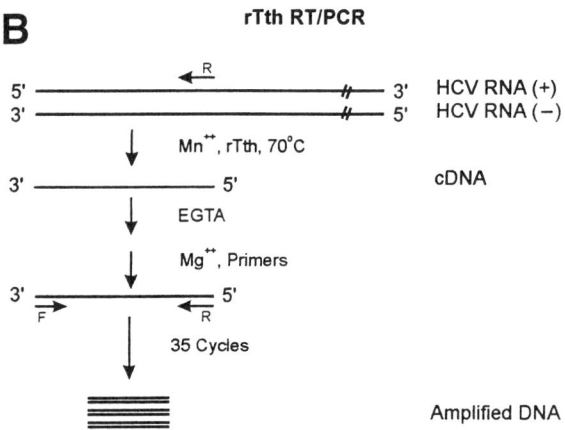

Fig. 1. Schematic diagram of conventional strand-specific RT-PCR and rTth RT-PCR procedures. **(A)** The amplification of HCV negative-strand RNA using conventional strand-specific RT-PCR and the false amplification of the HCV positive-strand RNA by the same procedure. A cDNA copy of the RNA is made with primer complementary to negative-strand RNA. At the reduced temperatures used for cDNA synthesis, this primer can misanneal at sites on the positive-strand RNA with partial homology to the primer. cDNA synthesis can also be primed by contaminating nucleic acids and by terminal hairpin structures that can occur anywhere in genome if the RNA is partially degraded. Following cDNA synthesis, the RT activity is inactivated and PCR amplification is performed with *Taq*. False-primed positive-strand RNA yields the same product as negative-strand RNA provided that the cDNA produce from false priming spans the sequence encompassed by the PCR primers. **(B)** The amplification of HCV negative-strand RNA by rTth RT-PCR is depicted. A cDNA

well appreciated in molecular biology techniques that at reduced temperatures (37–42°C), primers anneal to sites with low levels of homology. To circumvent this problem, we developed two modified RT-PCR assays capable of accurately discrimnating between positive- and negative-strand RNA *(1)*. To demonstrate the utility of both assays, our initial studies utilized one method for the detection of negative strand RNA, whereas the other was used for detection of positive-strand RNA.

A procedure referred to as tagged RT-PCR was designed to overcome detection of falsely primed cDNA products and was chosen as the assay for negative-strand RNA. This method relies on the use of a primer during cDNA synthesis that contains non-HCV sequences at the 5'-end (the tag). PCR amplification of the tagged cDNA is performed using only the tag portion of the cDNA primer as one of the primers and an HCV-specific oligonucleotide for the opposing primer *(1)*. This method yields much greater strand specificity, because it prevents the production of a correct-sized product from falsely primed cDNA, since falsely primed cDNA will have variable ends, which contain the tag primer site. Thus, falsely primed products in theory create a smear that in practice is not detected using Southern hybridization to detect the first-round PCR product. When properly utilized, this assay can yield up to four logs of differential between detection of the correct and incorrect strand of RNA. One limitation of this method that is not widely appreciated is the requirement for the cDNA primer to be exhausted during the cDNA step. If excess cDNA primer remains during PCR amplification, the degree of strand specificity will be compromised. Determination of the optimum level of cDNA primer requires titration experiments with synthetic RNAs. The method also requires that all RT activity be inactivated prior to PCR by heating to 100°C for 1 h. For these reasons, we now use the rTth RT-PCR method to detect both strands of HCV RNA.

In the rTth assay, false priming is prevented by conducting the cDNA reaction at an elevated temperature (70°C) using the rTth reverse transcriptase (**Fig. 1B**). The cDNA products are amplified by a conventional PCR reaction, except that rTth is used as the thermostable DNA polymerase instead of *Taq* polymerase. This method requires that following cDNA synthesis, the reverse transcriptase activity of rTth is inactivated by chelation of the Mn^{2+} and the DNA polymerase activity of rTth is activated by addition of Mg^{2+}. The RT activity of this

---

copy of the RNA is made with a primer complementary to the negative strand of RNA using the rTth thermostable reverse transcriptase at 70°C. The RT activity of rTth is inactivated by chelation of Mn^{2+} with EGTA. Following the addition of Mg^{2+} and the reverse primer, PCR is conducted using the thermostable DNA polymerase activity of rTth.

enzyme appears to have an absolute specificity for Mn^{2+}. Analysis of synthetic RNA using this assay yielded four logs of differential between the correct and incorrect strands of RNA. We have used this assay to detect HCV negative-strand RNA routinely in HCV-infected primary hepatocytes *(1)* and to evaluate extrahepatic tissues for indications of HCV replication *(5)*. The assay has also been adapted to monitor the replication of HEV in primary cultures of cynomolgus monkey hepatocytes *(6)*.

2. Materials
2.1. PCR Reagents

1. rTth DNA polymerase with buffer pack (Perkin Elmer, Foster City, CA).
2. Prime RNase inhibitor (5'-3', Boulder, CO).
3. RNAzol B (Biotecx, Houston, TX).
4. Oligonucleotide primers (Genosys Biotechnologies, Inc., The Woodlands, TX): Resuspended in nuclease-free water to a concentration of 1 μg/μL and stored at –20°C. A working stock of 50 ng/mL is prepared from this stock.
5. Nuclease-free water (Promega, Madison, WI).
6. Ultrapure deoxynucleotide triphosphates (dNTPs) (Pharmacia Biotech, Piscataway, NJ). Each nucleotide is provided separately as a 100-mM solution. Equal volumes of each dNTP are mixed to provided a 25-mM stock solution of all four dNTPs.
7. DNA thermal cycler 480 (Perkin Elmer).
8. Thin-walled PCR reaction tubes, 600-μL vol (Perkin Elmer).

2.2. RNA Synthesis

1. RNase-free DNase (Promega).
2. Megascript In Vitro Transcription Kit (Ambion, Austin, TX).

2.3. Gel and Hybridization Reagents

1. Ultrapure agarose (Gibco-BRL, Grand Island, NY).
2. TAE: 40 mM Tris, pH to 7.4 with acetic acid, 1 mM EDTA.
3. GeneScreen Plus Hybridization Transfer Membranes (Dupont/NEN, Boston, MA).
4. Turboblotter Rapid Downward Transfer Systems (Schleicher and Schuell, Keene, NH).
5. Prime It II Random Primer Labeling Kit (Stratagene, La Jolla, CA).
6. Hybridization solution: 50% formamide, 7% SDS, 0.25 M sodium phosphate buffer (mono- and dibasic mixture to obtain pH 7.2), 0.25 M NaCl, 1 mM EDTA.
7. 20X SSPE: 3 M NaCl, 0.2 M NaH$_2$PO$_4$, 20 mM EDTA, pH to 7.4 with 1 M NaOH, and sterilize by autoclaving.
8. 20X SSC: 3 M NaCl, 0.3 M sodium citrate, pH to 7.0 with 1 M NaOH, and sterilize by autoclaving.

3. Methods
3.1. Production and Purification of Synthetic RNA Standards

1. RNA is produced using the pSP73/2 T7 transcriptional vectors (Promega) containing an HCV insert of nucleotides 1–582. The insertion has been cloned in both orientations, such that positive and negative strands can be obtained using T7. The plasmid is linearized using the restriction enzyme *Nde*I followed by a phenol/chloroform extraction and ethanol precipitation. The final DNA is resuspended in water to a final volume of 1 mg/mL.
2. Use 1 µg of linear DNA to synthesize RNA using Ambion's T7 Megascript InVitro Transcription Kit following the protocol provided by the manufacturer.
3. Digest with DNase for 1 h at 37°C using the RNase-free DNase supplied with the Ambion kit.
4. Purify the RNA by RNAzol extraction and ethanol precipitation. Adjust the volume to 100 µL with nuclease-free water, and add 900 µL RNAzol B. Add 100 µL of chloroform, and mix by rotating the tube for about 15 s. Incubate on ice for 5 min, and separate the phases by spinning in a microfuge at top speed for 15 min. Transfer the upper aqueous phase to a new microfuge tube, and add 1 vol of cold isopropanol. Incubate on ice for at least 15 min, and pellet the RNA at top speed in a microfuge for 15 min. Wash the pellet twice with 75% ethanol, and pellet for 8 min in the microfuge. After removing the ethanol, perform one final quick spin to remove residual ethanol. Resuspend the pellet in 25 µL of nuclease-free water containing a 1/200 dilution of Prime RNAse Inhibitor.
5. Add 2 U of RNase-free DNase and 4 µL of 25 mM MnCl$_2$, and incubate for 1 h at 37°C. Add 900 µL RNAzol B, and repeat **step 4** above. Resuspend the final RNA in 50 µL of nuclease-free water containing a 1/200 dilution of Prime RNase Inhibitor.
6. Determine the RNA concentration and purity by reading a 1/100 dilution of the RNA in a spectrophotometer at 260 and 280 nm. Run 5 µg of RNA on a 1% agarose gel along with a known quantity of a similar-sized standard RNA to evaluate the integrity of the RNA and confirm the concentration.
7. Make 10-fold dilutions of the RNA such that 10-µL aliquots contain 100 pg to 0.1 fg for testing in the strand-specific RT-PCR assays. The dilutions should be made in a 100 µg/mL total cellular RNA pool. The total cellular RNA should be obtained from a mammalian cell line by RNAzol extraction and ethanol precipitation.

3.2. Purification of RNA

1. This protocol has been optimized for the purification of total cellular RNA from a monolayer of primary hepatocytes growing in a well of a six-well dish, or purification of RNA from 100 µL of serum. When purifying RNA from serum, tRNA is added at 1 µg/mL to serve as a carrier.
2. Add 900 µL RNAzol B to the tissue-culture well or to the 100 µL of serum. To solubilize the hepatocytes better, scrape the cells into the RNAzol and pipet the suspension up and down several times.

3. Transfer the RNAzol cell suspension to a 1.5-mL microfuge tube.
4. Purify the RNA as described in **Subheading 3.1, step 4**.
5. Resuspend the pellet in 25 μL of nuclease-free water containing a 1/200 dilution of Prime RNase Inhibitor for the total cellular RNA, or in 100 μL of water plus RNase inhibitor for serum.

3.3. rTth RT-PCR Protocol

1. Add total cellular RNA (2 μL contains approx 2 μg of total cellular RNA), or dilution of synthetic or serum RNA (10 μL) adjusted to a total volume of 10 μL with nuclease-free water in a PCR reaction tube. Layer mineral oil over the RNA solution, and place the tubes in a thermocycler set at 4°C. All subsequent steps are performed on the thermocycler to maintain the appropriate temperature.
2. Denature the RNA using a 1-min cycle at 95°C, and then cycle to 70°C and hold.
3. Prepare cDNA master mix (10 μL/reaction):

Volume	Final concentration of 1X reaction
2 μL 10x rTth buffer	10 mM Tris, pH 8.3, 90 mM KCl
2 μL 10 mM MnCl$_2$	1 mM MnCl$_2$
0.16 μL 25 mM dNTP mix	200 μM of each dNTP
1 μL cDNA primer (50 ng)	
2.84 μL H$_2$O	
2 μL (5 U) rTth	

    The cDNA primer for negative strand (forward primer) = 5'GGGGGC–GACACTCCACCA3'.
    The cDNA primer for positive strand (reverse primer) = 5'TCGCGAC–CCAACACTACTC3'.

4. Heat the cDNA master mix to 70°C for 1.5 min on the thermocycler prior to use. Add 10 μL of preheated cDNA master mix to each tube, while the tubes are at 70°C in the thermocycler.
5. Cycle at 60°C for 2 min and 70°C for 15 min for the cDNA reaction, and then to hold, at 70°C. The time on hold at 70°C is kept to a minimum so as not to extend the cDNA reaction time.
6. Prepare the chelating buffer by 1:5 dilution in nuclease-free water. Warm to 70°C on the thermocycler for a few minutes before use. Add 40 μL of chelating buffer to each tube at the completion of the cDNA reaction.
7. Prepare the PCR master mix (40 μL/tube): 6 μL 25 mM MgCl$_2$, 1 μL PCR primer (50 ng of the cDNA primer for the opposite strand), and 33 μL water. Warm the PCR master mix to 70°C for a few minutes prior to use, and add 40 μL to each tube.
8. Initiate the PCR cycles as follows:
    a. 94°C, 3 min.
    b. 94°C, 1 min.
    c. 60°C, 2 min.
    d. 72°C, 3 min.

e. Cycle 44 more times to **step b**.
f. 72°C, 7 min.
g. 4°C and hold.

3.4. Hybridization

1. Run 20 µL of the first-round PCR products on a 1% agarose gel in TAE buffer. Electrophorese at 80 V for 1 h, stain the gel with ethidium bromide, and photograph.
2. Treat the gel in 0.25 M HCl for 10 min at room temperature on a gentle shaker. Equilibrate the membrane in 0.4 N NaOH for 30 min at room temperature on a gentle shaker.
3. Cut a piece of GeneScreen Plus membrane to the same size as the gel. Rinse the membrane in hot water, and equilibrate in 0.4 N NaOH for 15 min at room temperature on a gentle shaker.
4. Assemble the transfer apparatus using a Schleicher and Schuell Turboblotter following their downward transfer protocol. Transfer for 1 h at room temperature in 0.4 N NaOH.
5. Following the transfer, rinse the membrane for a few minutes in 2X SSPE.
6. Prehybridize the membrane at 42°C for 4 h in a hybridization bag containing 10 mL of hybridization solution.
7. Prepare a labeled DNA probe. The DNA for the probe is a gel-purified RT-PCR product of HCV spanning nucleotides 1–582. The probe is labeled with ^{32}P-dCTP using the Prime It II Random Prime Labeling Kit following the protocol of the manufacturer.
8. Mix the labeled probe (10^7 counts/min) with an equal volume of formamide, boil for 10 min, and cool on ice for 5 min.
9. Open a corner of the hybridization bag, inject the probe, and reseal the bag.
10. Hybridize for 16 h at 42°C.
11. Wash the membrane three times for 10 min with 2X SSC–0.1% SDS at 42°C, and then three times for 12 min with 0.1X SSC–0.1% SDS at 60°C.
12. Expose the membrane to X-ray film with one intensifying screen at –80°C.

4. Notes

1. A number of precautionary steps are taken to reduce and eliminate essentially contamination of samples with amplified or cloned HCV materials. All procedures prior to the amplification cycles are conducted in a room separate from the remainder of the laboratory. No reagent including water is obtained from the main laboratory. Water is purchased as nuclease-free water from Promega. Although nuclease-free water is probably not essential, the cost is low, and it provides an outside source of water for the PCR room. When possible, premade buffers are purchased for this room. All chemicals, buffers, enzymes, and reagents are purchased separately for this room and delivered directly to the room. Personnel do not wear lab coats from the main laboratory into this room. Each person using this room keeps a separate lab coat in the room.

2. The PCR room has several stations for conducting different steps of the procedure. Each station has its own set of micropipets, pipet tips, and gloves. The first station is for compiling the various master mixes required for the procedure. The second station is for the purification of RNA from biological samples and the addition of RNA to the PCR tubes. RNAzol extracts from biological samples are prepared under a laminar flow hood in a P2 facility. The extracts are transferred to the PCR room for purification. A third station is at the thermocycler. All steps including the amplification cycles are conducted at this station, but the tubes are never opened inside of this room after the amplification cycles have been conducted.

3. Strand-specific RT-PCR must be routinely validated for the level of sensitivity and specificity. Adherence to the protocols in the chapter should provide the desired level of specificity, but this should not be assumed without proper validation. The preferred method of validation is the production of highly purified, synthetic positive- and negative-strand HCV RNA, and the testing of dilutions of this RNA in both the positive- and negative-strand assays to determine the level of sensitivity and specificity. An example of this type of analysis is depicted in **Fig. 2**. The synthetic RNAs should be diluted in total cellular RNA to simulate better the conditions encountered in the use of this assay, since the presence of cellular RNA will affect both sensitivity and specificity. Once validation has been accomplished, it is preferable to run specific dilutions of RNA in each assay as controls for that assay. The correct strand of RNA should be run at the last positive and the first negative dilution to determine the sensitivity of the assay. The incorrect strand should also be run at the last positive and first negative dilution to confirm specificity. A differential of three to four logs should be obtained between detection of the correct and incorrect strands. Although these controls are preferably included in each assay, the problem of producing high-quality, intact synthetic RNA that is completely free of contamination from the transcriptional vector DNA is not trivial and sometimes appears impossible. Plasma with a high titer of HCV RNA can be used as an alternative control. Normally, a plasma that yields a positive-strand signal at a 10^4 dilution (this equals 10^6 PCR U/mL, since the RNA is from 10 μL of sera.) will have a weak negative-strand signal using undiluted plasma. We believe this signal to be owing to positive-strand RNA being detected in the negative-strand assay, rather that negative-strand RNA being present in the serum, but neither possibility can be entirely excluded. Nonetheless, serum RNA can be used to confrm 4 logs of differential between the positive- and negative-strand assays, and an example of such an assay is included in **Fig. 2**.

In the original description of the rTth RT-PCR method, we estimated that the level of sensitivity of the negative-strand assay was approx 3000 copies of RNA when that RNA was present in total cellular RNA and 300 copies in the absence of cellular RNA. This estimation was based on the use of synthetic RNA diluted to very low copy number. We now believe that this underestimated the sensitivity of the assay. In addition, several improvements in the assay procedure have

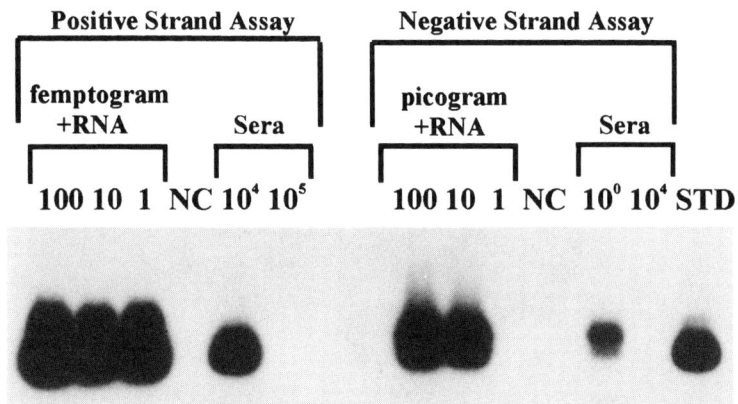

Fig. 2. Analysis of synthetic positive-strand HCV RNA and serum-derived HCV RNA using strand-specific rTth RT-PCR. Synthetic positive-strand RNA encompassing the 5'-untranslated region of HCV (nt 1–582) was prepared as described under **Subheading 3.1.** Dilutions of the RNA were made in total cellular RNA to mimic the conditions for analysis of hepatocyte cultures, and positive- and negative-strand RNA assays were conducted using the rTth RT-PCR assay. PCR was conducted for one round of 45 cycles followed by agarose-gel electrophoresis and Southern hybridization. A positive-strand assay was conducted on 1, 10, and 100 fg of positive-strand RNA and 10^4 and 10^5 dilutions of HCV positive serum, and a negative-strand assay was conducted on 1, 10, and 100 pg of positive-strand RNA and 10^0 and 10^4 dilutions of HCV positive serum. Negative controls (NC) contained water instead of an RNA sample. STD is a standard to control the sensitivity of the transfer and hybridization process; the same amount of a DNA fragment homologous to the probe is loaded on all gels. Comparison of the positive- and negative-strand assays demonstrates that the positive- and negative-strand assays exhibit 4 logs of differential in the detection of the same synthetic RNA as well as serum-derived RNA.

been made that are detailed in this chapter. The assay appears to be approx 10-fold more sensitive based on the use of RNA extracted from dilutions of an HCV positive serum that had been quantitated using the bDNA assay (Chiron Corp.). The sensitivity of the positive-strand assay was 40 copies; a 10-μL aliquot containing an estimated 40 copies of RNA was positive, whereas the 10-μL aliquot containing an estimated 4 copies was negative.

4. One of the important uses of strand-specific assay including rTth RT-PCR will be the analysis of cells transfected with full-length, synthetic HCV RNA in pursuit of an infectious clone. A highly sensitive method for detection of replication will be required unless a clone is anticipated that has much higher replicative capacity than HCV exhibits in vivo in the infected host. However, even the 4 logs of specificity observed with rTth RT-PCR may be insufficient to distinguish an infectious clone from an nonreplicating clone. A routine transfection uses 1 μg of

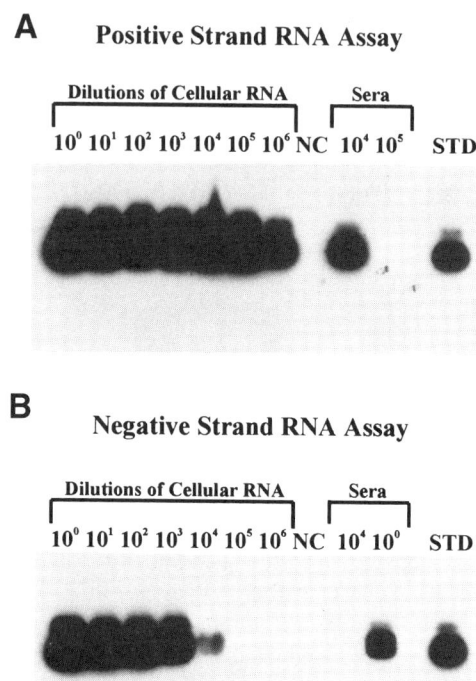

Fig. 3. Analysis of HCV RNA by rTth RT-PCR following transfection of cells with full-length HCV RNA. Huh7 cells were transfected with 1.5 μg of full-length, positive-stranded, replication-defective HCV RNA, and total cell RNA was harvested from the cultures 14 d after transfection. Dilutions of the total cell RNA were analyzed by positive- (**A**) and negative-strand (**B**) rTth RT-PCR assays. NC is a negative control in which water replaces the RNA in the PCR reaction. Dilutions of a high-titer HCV containing serum were used to confirm the sensitivity of the positive-strand assay and the specificity of the negative-strand assay as described in the legend to **Fig. 2**. Since the transfected positive-stranded RNA was replication-defective, the positive-strand RNA signal is owing to the input RNA. The negative-strand RNA signal is owing to detection of positive-strand RNA in this assay when it is present at very high levels. For discussion of this experiment, *see* **Note 3**.

RNA, and a 9600-nt RNA has 2×10^{11} mol/μg. This level of positive-strand RNA would yield a false signal in a negative-strand assay equivalent to approx 2×10^7 mol of negative-strand RNA. Even if the input positive-strand RNA is degraded to a significant degree over time, a nonreplicating positive-strand RNA may still yield results suggestive of replication. An example of such an assay is depicted in **Fig. 3**. Huh7 cells were transfected with 1.5 μg of a full-length HCV RNA with mutations to render the clone nonreplicative. The cellular RNA was harvested 14 d after transfection and was analyzed by rTth RT-PCR. The cellular RNA was still strongly positive in a positive-strand assay at a 10^6 dilution, but was negative at a

10^7 dilution (dilution not shown). In the negative-strand assay, the RNA was weakly positive at a 10^4 dilution and strongly positive at a 10^3 dilution. The inclusion of the same serum RNA controls as used in **Fig. 2** confirms that the assay was performing properly. Approximately 3–4 logs of differential were observed between the positive- and negative-strand assays. Thus, the detection of a negative-strand RNA signal in a highly specific assay is not sufficient to document that HCV replication is being detected. The persistence of nonreplicating input positive-strand RNA for considerable time periods will certainly confound efforts to isolate an infectious clone.

Acknowledgment

This work was supported by a grant from the National Institute of Allergy and Infectious Diseases (AI40035).

References

1. Lanford, R. E., Sureau, C., Jacob, J. R., White, R., and Fuerst, T. R. (1994) Demonstration of *in vitro* infection of chimpanzee hepatocytes with hepatitis C virus using strand-specific RT-PCR. *Virology* **202,** 606–614.
2. McGuinness, P. H., Bishop, G. A., McCaughan, G. W., Trowbridge, R., and Gowans, E. J. (1994) False detection of negative-strand hepatitis C virus RNA. *Lancet* **343,** 551,552.
3. Willems, M., Moshage, H., and Yap, S. H. (1993) PCR and detection of negative HCV RNA strands. *Hepatology* **17,** 526.
4. Gunji, T., Kato, N., Hijikata, M., Hayashi, K., Saitoh, S., and Shimotohno, K. (1994) Specific detection of positive and negative stranded hepatitis C viral RNA using chemical RNA modification. *Arch. Virol.* **134,** 293–302.
5. Lanford, R. E., Chavez, D., Chisari, F., and Sureau, C. (1995) Lack of detection of negative-strand hepatitis C virus RNA in peripheral blood mononuclear cells and other extrahepatic tissues by the highly strand-specific rTth reverse transcriptase PCR. *J. Virol.* **69,** 8079–8083.
6. Tam, A. W., White, R., Reed, E., Short, M., Zhang, Y. F., Fuerst, T. R., et al. (1996) *In vitro* propagation and production of hepatitis E virus from in vivo-infected primary macaque hepatocytes. *Virology* **215,** 1–9.

45

Cell Culture Systems for the Detection of HCV Infection

Yohko K. Shimizu and Hiroshi Yoshikura

1. Introduction

In spite of the recent progress in molecular biology of the hepatitis C virus (HCV) genome, the biological characteristics of this virus remain poorly known. This is primarily because biological assays for HCV have been limited to the experimental inoculation of chimpanzees. It is imperative to develop either a less expensive animal model or a cell-culture system for propagating HCV. Several studies, including ours, have provided evidence for replication of the HCV genome in cell cultures. Although the reported systems are not yet fully satisfactory for wide application to in vitro studies of HCV, they are useful at least for examining the infectivity of HCV materials.

We initially reported that the human T cell lines, Molt4Ma and HPBMa cells infected with amphotropic murine leukemia-sarcoma virus complex, were susceptible to HCV infection *(1,2)*. A clone (no. 10-2) of HPBMa cells was subsequently found to support the viral replication more consistently than Molt4Ma cells. The viral replication in this clone was productive for infectious HCV; multicycle transmission from infected cells to new cells was demonstrated by coculture with drug-resistant cells as recipients *(3)*. Using HPBMa10-2 cells, we tested HCV inocula for their infectivity; the in vitro titers obtained correlated with the reported infectivity titers of the inocula measured in chimpanzees *(2)*. We also developed an assay for neutralizing antibodies to HCV, antibodies that bind to virions and prevent adsorption to cells, and initiation of the replication cycle of the virus *(4)*. Recently, Daudi cells, a lymphoblastoid cell line, were found to be capable of supporting productive infection of HCV as well *(5)*. Virus-like particles, measuring approx 50 nm in diameter, were observed by electron microscopy in HPBMa10-2 and Daudi cells infected with

HCV *(6)*. Appearance of characteristic tubular structures, which we originally reported for chimpanzee hepatocytes in association with HCV infection, was also noted in the infected Daudi cells.

This chapter describes our experience with human lymphocyte cell lines, HPBMa10-2 and Daudi cells, for the detection of HCV infection.

2. Materials

1. Cell lines: Daudi lymphoblastoid cells were purchased from American Type Culture Collection. HPBMa cells were obtained by infecting HPB ALL cells with an amphotropic murine leukemia virus pseudotype of murine sarcoma virus *(7)*. Cloning of the cells was performed by limiting dilution, and clone 10-2 (HPBMa10-2), which was the most sensitive to HCV, infection was selected.
2. Culture medium: RPMI 1640 (Gibco, Grand Island, NY) containing 8% heat-inactivated fetal calf serum and antibiotics.
3. Inoculum: Plasma H77 was collected from a human patient during the early acute phase of hepatitis C (7 wk after transfusion). It contained $10^{6.5}$ 50% chimpanzee infectious doses of HCV/mL *(8)*. The viral genome titer of H77 was 10^7 RT-PCR units/mL by end-point dilution *(2)*. This plasma has been shown to be negative for antibodies to HCV by enzyme-linked immunoabsorbant assay, immunoprecipitation with antihuman immunoglobulin, and determination of buoyant density *(9,10)* (*see* **Note 1**).

3. Methods

1. Subculture cells 1 d before use.
2. Pellet cells by centrifugation and resuspend in the PRPMI1640 medium at a concentration of approx 5×10^5 cells/mL.
3. Transfer 1 mL of the cell suspension into a 50-mL plastic tube and mix with 100 µL of a 10^{-1} dilution of plasma H77.
4. After incubation at 37°C for 2 h with occasional hand-shaking of the tube, wash cells twice with 20 mL of the medium, resuspend in 5 mL, transfer into a 25-cm³ cuture bottle, and culture at 37°C in a CO_2 incubator.
5. Subculture at a 3 to 4-d interval.
6. Harvest cells and supernatants at intervals to test for the presence of HCV (*see* **Note 2**).

4. Notes

1. Choice of inoculum: The choice of the inoculum is crucial for the success of the infection experiment. The inoculum has to be highly infectious. Aiming to find useful markers for predicting infectivity of HCV, we investigated differences among inocula with high and low in vivo infectivity. **Table 1** summarizes the results. Measurement of the genomic RNA titer by RT-PCR alone was not sufficient. However, combining RT-PCR with differential floatation in the 1.063 g/mL NaCl solution, immunoprecipitation with antihuman immunoglobulin, as well as

Table 1
Differences Among Inocula Based on Infectivity

	Inocula			
Characteristics	Patient H acute H	Implicated donor no. 6	Patient F chronic F	Patient N chronic no. 4
Buoyant density flotation at 1.063 g/mL	Top	Top/Bottom	Bottom	Bottom
Immunoprecipitation with antihuman immunoglobulin	No	No	Yes	Yes
Rate of adsorption to cells	1:10	1:10	1:1000	1:1000
In vitro infectivity/mL	10^5	$10^{2.5}$	10	<10
In vivo infectivity in chimps CID/mL	$10^{6.5}$	$10^{5.5}$	<10^2	<10^2
Genome titer/mL by RT-PCR	10^7	10^5	10^5	10^4

adsorption to HPBMa10-2 cells appeared to have a high predictive value for estimating whether a sample will be highly infectious *(9,10)*. In the case of highly infectious sera, HCV virions were found in the low-density fractions (1.063 g/mL) and could not be immunoprecipitated, whereas in the case of noninfectious sera, HCV virions had a high density and could be immunoprecipitated.

2. Evaluation of HCV replication: Because HCV is a virus with a single-stranded positive-sense RNA genome, the presence of negative-strand RNA (which serves as a template for transcription of positive-sense RNA) in infected cells can be used as a marker of the viral infection. Since the quantity of HCV RNA is likely to be very small, RT-PCR is usually employed. However, the specificity of detection of the negative-strand HCV genome by conventional RT-PCR has recently been questioned, possibly because of false priming of the incorrect strand. Therefore, Gungi et al. developed a strand-specific RT-PCR strategy combined with modification of RNA samples at their 3' end *(11)* and Lanford et al. developed an rTth RT-PCR method using thermostable rTth RT *(12)*. Detection of the negative-strand of HCV RNA should be confirmed by employing such methods.

Another problem in this approach is the possibility that negative-sense HCV RNA in the infected blood of the original inoculum can itself be found in the cells tested, compromising interpretation of the data *(13)*. However, it was shown that adsorption of negative-strand HCV RNA to target cells was not detetcted in any of the inocula, suggesting that the probability of detecting carryover negative strands in the cells is negligible *(2,4)*.

To test for expression of virus-encoded proteins, we examined the cells for HCV core and envelope antigens by indirect immunofluorescent staining with monoclonal antibodies (MAbs). The anibodies were produced by immunizing

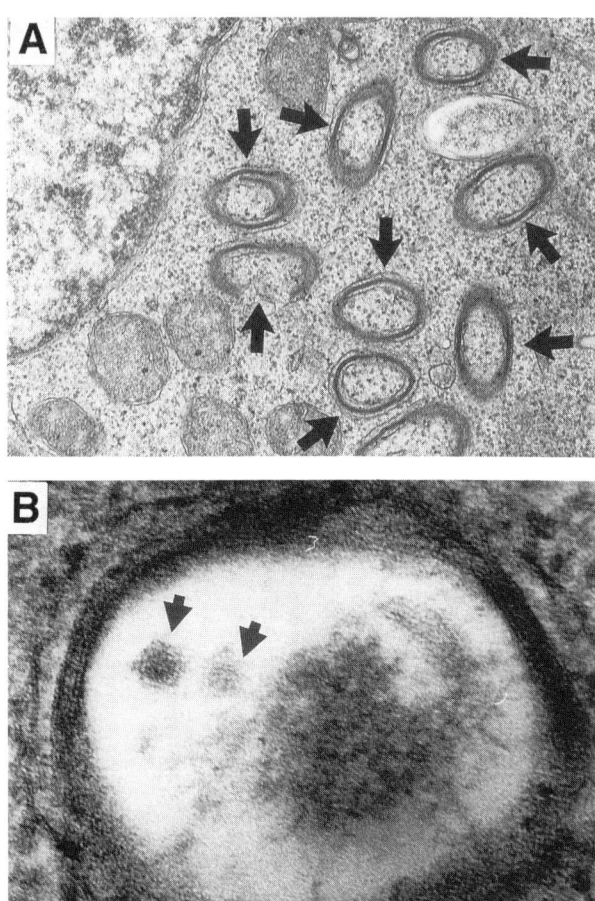

Fig. 1. Electron microscopy of Daudi cells harvested 15 d after HCV inoculation. **(A)** Tubular structures (arrows) in the cytoplasm. **(B)** Virus-like particles in a tubular structure.

mice with synthetic peptides based on the sequence of the HCV genome. Positive immunofluorescent staining was granular and located in the cytoplasms. The percentage of cells positive for HCV antigen never attained 100% of the cells even after repeated subcultures; it was usually a few percent and never exceeded 30%. The reason for this is not known at the moment.

As Daudi cells produce characteristic tubular structures on viral infection, a host response to the expression of interferon, detection of the structures by electron microscopy was also useful as an indirect marker of viral replication. **Figure 1A** shows a cluster of tubular structures in the Daudi cells harvested 15 d after HCV inoculation. Some of the structures contained virus-like particles with a diameter of approx 50 nm (**Fig. 1B**).

3. Infectivity of cell-culture-derived HCV: Infectivity of cell-culture-derived HCV has been demonstrated by three different methods: by cell–cell transmission and by infection of uninfected cells or a chimpanzee with the supernatant from the HCV-carrier cultures. To demonstrate cell–cell transmission of HCV, neomycine-resistant or hygromycin-B-resistant cells were constructed. HCV-infected drug-sensitive cells were cocultured with either of the drug-resistant cells for 5 d. The drug-resistant cells were then selected in the medium containing the appropriate drug. Transmission of HCV to the drug-resistant cells was demonstrated by RT-PCR amplification of the HCV genome. The presence of interferon-α or β prevented the replication of HCV, indicating that this system can be used for screening drugs for the treatment of HCV *(3)*. Infection of the cultured cells with the culture supernatants from the HCV-infected Daudi or HPBMa10-2 cells was also successful. The negative strand of HCV RNA appeared 7–8 d after inoculation, and the infectious titer of the culture supernatant to the cultured cells was around 10^2–10^3 infectious particles/mL. We also examined the in vivo infectivity of HCV grown in cell culture. The culture supernatant harvested from Daudi cells at 56 d of HCV infection was infectious in a chimpanzee; HCV RNA appeared in the serum and liver 5 wk after inoculation.

References

1. Shimizu, Y. K., Iwamoto, A., Hijikata, M., Purcell, R. H., and Yoshikura, H. (1992) Evidence for *in vitro* replication of hepatitis C virus genome in a human T cell line. *Proc. Natl. Acad. Sci. USA* **89,** 5477–5481.
2. Shimizu, Y. K., Purcell, R. H., and Yoshikura, H. (1993) Correlation between the infectivity of hepatitis C virus *in vitro* and its infectivity in *in vitro*. *Proc. Natl. Acad. Sci. USA* **90,** 6037–6041.
3. Shimizu, Y. K. and Yoshikura, H. (1994) Multicycle infection of hepatitis C virus in cell culture and inhibition by alpha and beta interferons. *J. Virol.* **68,** 8406–8408.
4. Shimizu, Y. K., Hijikata, M., Iwamoto, A., Alter, H. J., Purcell, R. H., and Yoshikura, H. (1994) Neutralizing antibodies against hepatitis C virus and the emergence of neutralization escape mutant viuses. *J. Virol.* **68,** 1494–1500.
5. Shimizu, Y. K. and Yoshikura, H. (1995) *In-vitro* systems for the detection of hepatitis C virus infection. *Viral Hepatitis Rev.* **1,** 59–65.
6. Shimizu, Y. K., Feinstone, S. M., Kohara, M., Purcell, R. H., and Yoshikura, H. (1996) Hepatitis C virus: detection of intracellular virus particles by electron microscopy. *Hepatology* **23,** 205–209.
7. Yoshikura, H. (1989) Thermostability of human immunodeficiency virus (HIV-1) in a liquid matriz is far higher than that of an ecotropic murine leukemia virus. *Jpn. J. Cancer Res.* **80,** 1–5.
8. Feinstone, S. M., Alter, H. J., Dienes, H., Shimizu, Y. K., Popper, H., Blackmore, D., et al. (1981) Non-A, non-B hepatitis in chimpanzees and marmosets. *J. Infect. Dis.* **144,** 588–598.
9. Shimizu, Y. K., Hijikata, M., Iwamoto, A., Purcell, R. H., and Yoshikura, H. (1994) Useful markers for predicting *in vivo* infectivity of hepatitis C virus. *Viral Hepatitis Liver Dis.* 115–117.

10. Hijikata, M., Shimizu, Y. K., Kato, H., Iwamoto, A., Shih, J. W., Alter, H. J., et al. (1993) Equilibrium centrifugation studies of hepatitis C virus: evidence for circulating immune complexes. *J. Virol.* **67,** 1953–1958.
11. Gungi, T., Kato, N., Hijikata, M., Hayashi, K., Saitho, S., and Shimotohno, K. (1994) Specific detection of positive and negative stranded hepatitis C viral RNA using chemical RNA modification. *Arch. Virol.* **134,** 293–302.
12. Landford, R., Chavez, E. F., Chisari, F. V., and Sureau, C. (1995) Lack of detection of negative-strand hepatitis C virus RNA in peripheral blood mononuclear cells and other extrahepatic tissues by the highly strand-specific rTth reverse transcriptase PCR. *J. Virol.* **69,** 8079–8083.
13. Shindo, M., Di Bisceglie, A. M., Akatsuka, T., Fong, T., Scaglione, L., Donets, M., et al. (1994) The physical state of the negative strand of hepatitis C virus RNA in serum of patients with chronic hepatitis C. *Proc. Natl. Acad. Sci. USA* **91,** 8719–8723.

46

Replication and Detection of Hepatitis C Virus in Liver-Derived Cell Lines

Regino P. González-Peralta

1. Introduction

A model of HCV replication has several potential important applications (**Table 1**). In addition to humans, the natural host for HCV, chimpanzees are the only other animals that have been shown to be permissive to HCV infection. However, the primate model for HCV infection presents several problems, namely, limited availability, cost, and different host response to HCV compared to humans.

It has been demonstrated that HCV may replicate in primary chimpanzee and human hepatocyte cultures, and established human lymphoblastoid cell lines *(1–7)*. However, primary hepatocytes are difficult to grow and maintain in culture, and have a limited viability. Establishing an in vitro cell-culture model of HCV infection using lymphoblastoid cell lines presents additional potential problems. Because HCV primarily infects liver cells in vivo, it may be more difficult to optimize HCV infection in lymphoblastoid cells. Further, results obtained in lymphoblastoid cells may be more difficult to correlate with in vivo HCV infection. For these reasons, our laboratory focused on developing an HCV replication model using established liver-derived cell lines *(8)*.

HCV replicates at a low rate, and therefore, its detection in cell culture requires reverse-transcriptase "nested" polymerase chain reaction (RT-PCR). Because of its extreme sensitivity, the use of RT-PCR for this purpose allows the detection of residual HCV RNA (from the inocula used to infect cell cultures) for an extended period of time. Accordingly, persistent detection of HCV (–) RNA (replicative intermediate) would be a better indicator of active viral replication in cell cultures.

Table 1
Potential Applications of a Model of HCV Replication

Study neutralizing antibodies
  Assist in vaccine development
Study viral replication
  Provide molecular basis for the design of novel therapies
Screen potential antiviral agents
Classify virus (serotype/phenotype)

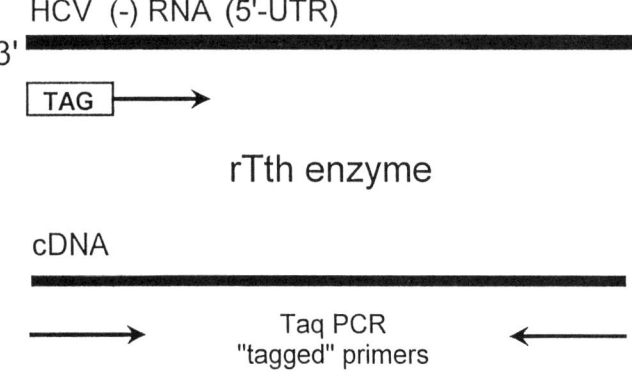

Fig. 1. Experimental outline of tail-PCR/rTth assay.

RT-PCR assays that use sense-specific primers to detect HCV (–) strand RNA have been shown to lack strand specificity *(2,9)*. However, the lack of specificity has recently been overcome by using primers with sequences unrelated to HCV during reverse transcription (tail-PCR) *(2)*, and performing cDNA synthesis at elevated temperatures (rTth assay) *(10)*. Our laboratory has also demonstrated enhanced specific detection of HCV (–) strand RNA by using a combined tail-PCR/rTth assay *(8)* (**Fig. 1**).

2. Materials

1. Serum samples, collected, spun, and frozen within 4 h of venesection (*see* **Note 1**).
2. Cell culture media (prepare using stringent sterile conditions): Add 100 mL of fetal bovine serum (FBS, Gibco-BRL, Grand Island, NY), 10 mL of 100X non-essential amino acids, 10 mL of 100 mM sodium pyruvate, 10 mL of 200 mM L-glutamine, and 10 mL of penicillin (5000 U/mL) and streptomycin (5000 µg/mL) solution to 1 L of minimum essential media (MEM, Cellgro, Mediatech, Washington, DC) (*see* **Note 2**).
3. Trypsin solution: 1X trypsin-EDTA solution (0.05% trypsin, 0.53 M EDTA) (Cellgro-Mediatech).

Replication of HCV

4. Liver-derived cell lines: WRL68 and HepG2 (American Type Cell Catalog, Rockville, MD).
5. rTth DNA polymerase (2.5 U/µL, Perkin-Elmer, Branchburg, NJ).
6. Chelating mix: Add 880 µL of 10X rTth chelating buffer (Perkin-Elmer) to 2970 µL of nuclease-free or diethylpyrocarbonate (DEPC)-treated water. Mix well and store at –20°C in 350 µL aliquots (10 reactions).
7. 10 mM MnCl$_2$ (Perkin-Elmer).
8. Ribonuclease inhibitor (RNasin, 40 U/µL, Promega, Madison, WI).
9. RT-PCR primers for detection of HCV (–) strand RNA: Store at –20°C.
   a. RT (REG6): **CTTGGGATTAGCGAGTATG**CTGTGAGGAACTACTGTCTT (Sequence unrelated to HCV RNA ["tag"] is shown in boldface.)
   b. First round PCR: REG7: **CTTGGGATTAGCGAGTATG** and REG8: GGTGCACGGTCTACGAGACCT.
   c. Second round "nested" PCR: *See* PCRb mix (Chapter 4).
10. RT mix (to make a total of 120 reactions): Add 240 µL of 10X rTth RT buffer (Perkin-Elmer), 240 µL of 10 mM MnCl$_2$ (Perkin-Elmer), 20 µL of a mixture of 25 mM each of dATP, dCTP, dGTP, dTTP (Pharmacia-Biotech, Piscataway, NJ), 4.5 µL (1.2 µmol) of primer REG6, and 700 µL of nuclease-free or DEPC-treated water. Mix well and store at –20°C in 100 µL aliquots (10 reactions). Before use, to each thawed 100 µL aliquot add 10 µL (400 U) RNasin (Promega) and 20 µL rTth DNA polymerase (50 U) (Perkin-Elmer).
11. First round PCR mix (to make a total of 120 reactions): Add 840 µL of 25 mM MgCl$_2$, 42 µL (2.8 µmol) of primer REG8, 48 µL (2.8 µmol) of primer REG7, and 3270 µL of nuclease-free or DEPC-treated water. Mix well and store at –20°C in 350 µL aliquots (10 reactions).
12. Second round "nested" PCR mix: *See* PCRb mix (Chapter 4).

3. Methods
3.1. Cell-Culture Infection (see Notes 3–7)

1. In 25-cm^2 culture flasks, grow WRL68 or HepG2 cells (American Type Cell Catalog) to 30% confluence (approx 1.2 million cells in 8 mL of MEM), and inoculate with 1 mL of freshly prepared HCV RNA-positive sera.
2. Incubate overnight (18–24 h), and replace media with fresh supplemented MEM. Afterward, change the media every 3 d (by which time cells have reached nearly 100% confluence and number approx 4 million cells in each flask).

3.2. Harvesting Cells on Days 3, 7, 10, and 14 Postinfection, and Weekly Thereafter

1. Remove media and wash cells (approx 3–4 million cells) with prewarmed (37°C) PBS three times. Add 1 mL of 1X trypsin (Gibco-BRL or Cellgro). Incubate for 45–60 s, gently rotating flask to cover the cell monolayer completely with solution.
2. Quickly detach monolayer by tapping firmly on the sides of the culture flask. The side of the flask to which cells are attached will become clear during this process.

3. Add 3 mL of supplemented MEM, and mix well. Transfer 1 mL of the cell suspension to a 25-cm^2 culture flask (approx 1 million cells), and extract total RNA from the remaining cells (approx 2–3 million cells), using the TRI- Reagent kit (Molecular Research Center, Cincinnati, OH). Dissolve RNA pellet in 20 µL of nuclease-free water and store at –70°C.

3.3. Detection of Total Cellular HCV RNA

Transfer 4 µL of cellular RNA solution (equivalent to approx 400,000 cells) to a microcentrifuge tube, and perform RT "nested" PCR (*see* Chapter 4).

3.4. Detection of HCV (–) Strand RNA Using Tail-PCR/rTth Assay (Fig. 1)

1. Dilute 5 µL of cellular RNA with 2 µL of DEPC-treated or nuclease-free water, and transfer to microcentrifuge tube containing 13 µL of RT mix. Vortex, place in thermal cycler (Perkin-Elmer), and heat at 70°C for 15 min (reverse transcription).
2. Remove from thermal cycler and transfer 10 µL of cDNA from above to microcentrifuge tube containing 35 µL of prewarmed chelating mix. Vortex, quick-spin, and add 35 µL of prewarmed first round PCR mix. Replace in cycler, and amplify as follows: 94°C for 4 min (denature), then 35 cycles of 94°C for 1 min (denature), 52°C for 1 min (anneal), and 72°C for 1 min.
3. Mix 4 µL of above solution with 40 µL of second-round PCR mix (*see* Chapter 4), and amplify as above except for performing a final extension at 72°C for 5 min.
4. Visualize 300 bp product using ethidium bromide-stained gel electrophoresis.

4. Notes

1. The method of serum preparation significantly affects HCV RNA levels. Thus, all serum samples are collected and used for infection within 4 h of venesection, conditions that our laboratory has previously shown by to preserve HCV RNA best *(11)*. HCV genotype of inoculating serum is determined by restriction fragment-length polymorphism (RFLP) based on the HCV 5'-untranslated region *(12)*, and HCV RNA levels are measured by bDNA (Chiron, Emeryville, CA).
2. Fetal bovine sera has been shown to be frequently contaminated with bovine viral diarrhea virus using RT-PCR with primers designed to detect HCV 5'-UTR *(13)*. To exclude this possibility, which would lead to "false" detection of HCV in cell cultures, all fetal bovine sera and cell-culture media used in our experiments have tested negative by the HCV RT-PCR assay described above.
3. Cells that have not been inoculated with serum or inoculated with serum from an HCV RNA-negative patient are used as controls for all infection experiments.
4. The effects of cell density on HCV infectivity are unknown, but enhanced in vitro viral infection has been observed when actively replicating cells are inoculated with human immunodeficiency virus and adenovirus (N. Muzyuski, University of Florida, personal communication). Based on this observation, the infections of liver-derived cells were grown to 30% confluence in 25-cm^2 cul-

ture flasks before inoculation with serum. Our laboratory is currently studying the effects of cell density on HCV replication.
5. Results of initial screening infections indicated that WRL68 and HepG2 cells (but not Alexander, Chang, HepG2, or Hep3B cells) supported HCV replication *(8)*. Subsequently, intermittent detection of total HCV RNA and HCV (-) strand RNA has occurred for up to 24 wk in 8 of 9 WRL 68 cell infections, and up to 16 wk in 4 of 5 HepG2 cell infections at the time of this writing.
6. Interestingly, we have observed limited viability in HCV-infected cells, but not in uninoculated cells or in those inoculated with HCV-negative serum. Similar reduced cellular viability in HCV-infected cells has been observed by others (*6*; L. Condreay et al., GlaxoWellcome, and G. Maarten, Innogenetics, personal communications). Although the mechanisms responsible for reduced viability of HCV-infected cells are unknown, it may be related to:
    a. The release of cytotoxic mediators by HCV-infected cells.
    b. The presence of cytotoxic factors in serum.
    c. Direct viral cytopathic effects.
7. At present, our laboratory is attempting to enhance HCV replication in WRL68 and HepG2 cells by systematically studying:
    a. Inoculation conditions (removing potential neutralizing antibodies from serum before inoculation, and using lipid-rich serum fraction for inoculation, and polyethylene glycol during inoculation.
    b. Nonspecific stimulation by inducers of differentiation and growth factors (sodium butyrate, dimethylsulfoxide, insulin, glucagon, epidermal and hepatocyte growth factors, and hydrocortisone).
    c. Induction of low density lipoprotein receptor expression in cells (using human growth hormone and phorbol myristate acetate).

Acknowledgments

The author would like to thank Wei-zhen Liu and Gang Guo for their excellent technical assistance, and my mentor, Johnson Y. N. Lau, for his continued guidance and support. These studies were supported in part by grants from the National Institutes of Health (KO8AI0148), the Blowitz-Ridgeway Foundation Health Scholar Award, the Children's Miracle Network Research Fund, and the Division of Sponsored Research of the University of Florida.

References

1. Iacovacci, S., Sargiacomo, M., Parolini, I., Ponzetto, A., Peschle, C., and Carloni, G. (1993) Replication and multiplication of hepatitis C virus in human fetal liver cells. *Res. Virol.* **144,** 275–279.
2. Lanford, R. E., Sureau, C., Jacob, J. R., White, R., and Fuerst, T. R. (1994) Demonstration of in vitro infection of chimpanzee hepatocytes with hepatitis C virus using strand-specific RT/PCR. *Virology* **202,** 606–614.
3. Ito, T., Mukaigawa, J., Zuo, J., Hirabayashi, Y., Mitamura, K., and Yasui, K. (1996) Cultivation of hepatitis C virus in primary hepatocyte culture from patients

with chronic hepatitis C virus results in release of high titer infectious virus. *J. Gen. Virol.* **77,** 1043–1054.
4. Kato, N., Ikeda, M., Mizutani, T., Sugiyama, K., Noguchi, M., Hirohashi, S., et al. (1996) Replication of hü atitis C virus in cultured non-neoplastic human hepatocytes. *Jpn. J. Cancer Res.* **87,** 787–792.
5. Shimizu, Y. K., Iwamoto, A., Hijikata, M., Purcell, R. H., and Yoshikura, H. (1992) Evidence for in vitro replication of hepatitis C virus genome in a human T-cell line. *Proc. Natl. Acad. Sci. USA* **89,** 5477–5481.
6. Shimizu, Y. K. and Yoshikura, H. (1994) Multicycle of infection of hepatitis C virus in cell culture and inhibition by alpha and beta interferons. *J. Virol.* **68,** 8406–8408.
7. Mizutani, T., Kato, N., Saito, S., Ikeda, M., Sugiyama, K., and Shimotohno, K. (1996) Characterization of hepatitis C virus replication in cloned cells obtained from a human T-cell leukemia virus type1-infected cell line, MT-2. *J. Virol.* **70,** 7219–7223.
8. González-Peralta, R. P., Liu, W., and Lau, J. Y. N. (1996) Identification of liver-derived cell lines that support low-level hepatitis C virus replication. [Abstract] *Hepatology* **24,** 217A.
9. McGuinness, P. H., Bishop, G. A., McCaughan, G. W., Trowbridge, R., and Gowans, E. J. (1994) False detection of negative-strand hepatitis C virus RNA. *Lancet* **343,** 551,552.
10. Lanford, R. E., Chavez, D., Chisari, F. V., and Sureau, C. (1996) Lack of detection of negative-strand hepatitis C virus RNA in peripheral blood mononuclear cells and other extrahepatic tissues by the highly strand-specific rTth reverse transcriptase PCR. *J. Virol.* **69,** 8079–8083.
11. Davis, G. L., Lau, J. Y. N., Urdea, M. S., Neuwald, P., Wilber, J. C., Lindsay, K., et al. (1994) Quantitative detection of hepatitis C virus RNA by solid phase branched DNA amplification method: definition and optimal conditions for specimen collection and clinical application in interferon-treated patients. *Hepatology* **19,** 1337–1341.
12. Lau, J. Y. N., Mizokami, M., Kolberg, J. A., Davis, G. L., Prescott, L. E., Ohno, T., et al. (1995) Application of six hepatitis C virus genotyping systems to sera from chronic hepatitis C patients in the United States. *J. Infect. Dis.* **171,** 281–289.
13. Yanagi, M., Bukh, J., Emerson, S. U., and Purcell, R. H. (1996) Contamination of commercially available fetal bovine sera with bovine diarrhea virus: implications for the study of hepatitis C virus in cell cultures. *J. Infect. Dis.,* in press.

47

Primary Human Hepatocyte Culture for the Study of HCV

John F. O'Connell, Stuart Cox, Peter Buontempo, Angela Skelton, Liubomir A. Pisarov, Kenneth Dorko, and Stephen C. Strom

1. Introduction

Research since 1983 has demonstrated that human hepatocytes can be isolated, cultured, and used for biological investigations, including studies of gene transcription and drug metabolism *(1,2)*. In addition, the ability to cyropreserve hepatocytes has facilitated clinical research of hepatitic cell transplantation *(3)*. We have used primary human heptocytes as host tissue for viral infection with hepatitis C. The availability of HCV-infected livers has also allowed for the culturing and analysis of HCV-positive cells. Our laboratory *(4)* and others *(5)* have confirmed the ability of these cells to display molecular markers of HCV replication. This chapter will review the basic steps of hepatocyte isolation and culturing and analysis for HCV by RT-PCR. We have also attempted to indicate alternative techniques that may be better suited to an individual investigator's needs.

Liver tissue that is infected with hepatitis C can be obtained from two different sources: (1) livers from organ donors, which are not suitable for transplantation owing to the presence of anti-HCV antibodies in the donor's serum and (2) livers from HCV-infected individuals that have been removed during orthotopic liver transplantation for end-stage liver disease. Generally, livers from organ donors provide the optimal source of viable cells. Normal livers (non-HBV/HCV) can be obtained from donor sources when the liver is not selected for transplantation owing to anatomic defects, the lack of suitable recipients, surgical errors in tissue harvest, cold ischemic time exceeding 20 h, micro- or macrosteatosis, and patient mortality prior to transplantation. Liver tissue from the resection of metastatic neoplasms is also available for research purposes.

2. Materials

1. Flasks: 25-cm^3 culture flasks (Corning).
2. Type 1 collagen (rat tail, Gibco, Gaithersburg, MD), 3.3 mg/mL in 0.1% acetic acid, diluted 1:100 in sterile water.
3. Catheter, 6-in. length of silicone tubing with polyethylene tubing connector (Masterflex, Cole Palmer Instruments Co., Chicago, IL).
4. Masterflex pump, 10-channel, model 7568-00 with pumpheads and silicone tubing.
5. Cell filters are made by attaching gauze sponges (Johnson & Johnson, 2 × 2, 8 ply) to polyethylene funnels with paper clips and autoclaving.
6. Perfusion buffer #1: 10 mM HEPES, 142 mM NaCl, 6.7 mM KCl, 1 mM EGTA, pH = 7.6.
7. Buffer #2: 100 mM HEPES, 67 mM NaCl, 0.67 KCl mM, 4.8 mM CaCl$_2$, 0.5% BSA, 200–400 mg/L Collagenase P, pH = 7.6.
8. Collagenase P from Boehringer Mannheim (Indianapolis, IN); all other reagents are from Gibco.
9. CDM media (a modification of media described by Isom and Georgoff, **ref. 6**) is a 1:1 mixture of Williams's Medium E and Ham's F12 Nutrient Mixture (both from Gibco), supplemented with 0.25% sodium bicarbonate, 0.08% fatty acid-free BSA, 65 µM ethanolamine, 7 µM linoleic acid in (0.08% BSA), 7 mM glucose, 0.4 mM sodium pyruvate, 0.1 mM ascorbic acid, 15 mM HEPES, 0.1 µM insulin, 0.1 µM dexamethasone (supplements from Sigma, St. Louis, MO).
10. TRI reagent RNA isolation kit (Molecular Research Center, Inc., Cincinnati, OH)
11. All PCR reagents (enzymes and buffers) are obtained from Perkin Elmer unless otherwise indicated.
12. Chelating buffer: 100 mM KCl, 10 mM Tris-HCl, pH 8.3, 0.75 mM EGTA, 0.05% Tween 20, 5% (v/v) glycerol.

3. Methods
3.1. Hepatocyte Isolation

Procedures for the isolation of hepatocytes from small wedges of hepatic tissue or whole livers are similar and involve collagenase perfusion *(1)*. Hepatocyte isolation from whole human livers is outlined below *(2)*. The two-step perfusion involves separating the intracellular junctions via a calcium-free step, followed by a collagenase digestion step.

1. Tissue from livers obtained at the time of orthotopic liver transplantation are placed directly in ice-cold University of Wisconsin solution (UW). UW is the liver transport media used to perfuse livers, *in situ* in preparation for whole-organ transplantation.
2. For convenience, the smaller, left hepatic lobe is usually chosen for perfusion. A right–left dissection is made by cutting along the falciform ligament. Purse-string sutures are tied around the large hepatic vein and all other major vessels on the

Primary Human Hepatocyte Culture

cut surface *(7)*. A single catheter is placed in the hepatic vein, and the sutures are drawn tight to prevent the efflux of perfusion buffer.
3. The lobe of liver with the catheter is placed in a sterile plastic bag, in a circulating water bath at 37°C, and connected to a perfusion pump. All tubing is sterilized by autoclaving.
4. Perfusion of the liver tissue (up to 300 g) proceeds with buffer #1 for 30 min at a rate of 35 mL/min. Perfusion is then continued for an additional 30 min with buffer #2. Larger pieces of tissue are perfused proportionally using more perfusion buffer and a greater flow rate attempting to maintain the exposure to collagenase containing buffer #2 for 30 min (*see* **Note 1**).
5. Following digestion with collagenase, the tissue is placed in a sterile beaker, covered in ice-cold buffer #1, and thoroughly chopped with a sterile scissors. When the capsule is cut, hepatocyes freed by the perfusion process are released into the buffer. Buffer and cells are decanted through sterile gauze-covered funnels.
6. Hepatocytes are enriched relative to nonparenchymal cells by three consecutive centrifugation steps at 100g for 4 min each. The cell pellet remaining after the three centrifugation steps is resuspended in culture media, and the viability is assessed by trypan blue exclusion. When performed correctly, visual inspection reveals parenchymal hepatocytes to be 95% of the cell population.

3.2. Plating and Monitoring of Hepatocytes

1. Coat flasks for 30 min (4–5 mL/T25 flask) with type 1 collagen. Collagen type 1 will support a culture for 4–6 wk. Other matrixes are discussed in **Note 3**.
2. Hepatocytes are added to the culture flasks in William's Medium E or CDM supplemented with 10% bovine calf serum.
3. Hepatocytes are allowed to attach for 4–16 h, and the flasks are washed in serum-free media to remove dead and unattached cells. Cultures are maintained by daily changes with serum-free CDM for the first week and three times weekly thereafter.
4. Cultures require careful monitoring to avoid overgrowth by fibroblasts. Choice of matrix and serum-free media (discussed below) also prevents fibroblast growth.
5. As previously published *(2,3)* monitoring of extracellular protein production by Western blot analysis is a quick and convenient method for assessing the cellular composition and metabolic activity of long-term hepatocyte cultures (**Note 4**).

3.3. Cryopreservation of Hepatocytes

1. To cryopreserve heptocytes, first plate them in serum-free media for 24 h, and then supplement the media with 2% dimethyl sulfoxide (DMSO) for an additional 24 h.
2. Hepatocytes are trypsinized and added to vials of media (CDM or UW solution) supplemented with 10% DMSO. Cells are frozen by placing the vials directly into a –80°C freezer, which results in a freeze rate of approx 5°C/min. Vials are transferred after 24 h into liquid nitrogen storage.

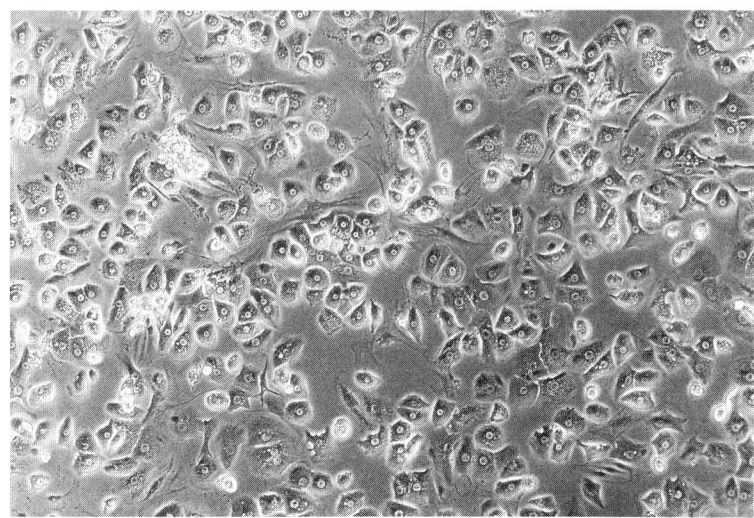

Fig. 1. HCV-positive hepatocytes 24 h after thawing from cyropreservation.

3. Hepatocytes are thawed by placing the freezer vials directly in a water bath (37°C) and decanting the thawed contents to 3 vol of warmed CDM plus 10% bovine calf serum. Cells are centrifuged at 100g for 4 min and resuspended in CDM plus 10% serum. Cells are plated as described above (**Note 5**). **Figure 1** shows HCV-positive hepatocytes 24 h after thawing.

3.4. Detection of HCV in Hepatocytes by RT-PCR

Analysis of samples for the presence of HCV RNA can be accomplished by a number of RT-PCR assays. The use of a strand-specific assay facilitates the accurate detection of positive- and negative-strand HCV RNA *(8)*. The procedure below outlines a nested assay for HCV positive strand with the RT and outer PCR steps being accomplished by the enzyme rtTh and the inner PCR step accomplished by *Taq* polymerase. The preparation of a master mix facilitates setup of multiple reactions.

1. RNA is isolated using the TRI Reagent Kit. The final pellet is resuspended in 300 μL of water and frozen at –70°C.
2. For the RT step, a single tube reaction (50 μL) contains 1/12 of RNA preparation, DEPC-treated water, 1X RT buffer (900 mM KCl, 100 mM Tris-HCl, pH 8.3), 0.4 mM MnCl$_2$, 1.0 μL of RNase inhibitor, 25 mM of each NTP (ATP, CTP, GTP, TTP), 2.5 U of rTth polymerase, and 50 pmol of RT primer. For the RT steps, use primer #1 (5'-TgC-ACg-gTC-TAC-gAg-ACC-TCC-Cg-3') for the positive strand assay. After preparation, samples are overlayed with 50 μL of mineral oil to prevent crosscontamination of the amplified DNA. The reaction

tubes are placed on a 9600 Perkin Elmer thermal cycler preheated to 94°C. The RT thermal profile is 94°C for 3 min, 70°C for 15 min, and then a 4°C soak.
3. After reverse transcription, the tubes are removed from the cycler, the lids are carefully opened, and primer-chelating mix is added so that each tube contains 1X chelating buffer primer (primer #1 and primer #2: 5'-gCC-ATg-gCg-TTA-gTA-TgA-gTg-TCg-3'). Tubes are placed back onto the preheated thermal cyler and subjected to the following thermal cycling: 94°C for 3 min, 25 cycles of 94°C for 30 s, 55°C for 30 s, and 72°C for 1 min, followed by an extension at 72°C for 10 min and a 4°C soak.
4. After cycling, the PCR tubes are carefully opened, and 5 µL of the reaction are removed and added to tubes for the nested PCR step. These PCR tubes contain 45 µL of a mixture of DEPC-treated water, 1X PCR buffer II, 25 mM of each dNTP, 2 mM MgCl$_2$, 1.25 U *Taq* polymerase, and 50 pmol of the inner primer pair (primer #3: 5'-gTg-CAg-CCT-CCA-ggA-CCC-C-3' and primer #4: 5'-ggg-CAC-TCg-CAA-gCA-CCC-TA-3'). The thermal cycling conditions are the same as those for the outer PCR reaction.
5. After cycling, 15 µL of inner reaction are loaded onto a 4% (3:1 Nuseive, FMC) agarose gel, and the appearance of a 211-bp band is indicative of the presence of HCV RNA. Confirmation of the band by sequencing should be performed.

4. Notes

1. Each lot of collagenase must be tested empirically for activity. Since collagenase requires 37°C for full activity, the perfusion buffer #1 must warm the liver from 4°C to 37°C.
2. The remaining nonparenchymal cells may be removed by further purification of parenchymal cells by Percol centrifugation *(9)*.
3. Isolated hepatocytes adhere to a variety of extracellular matrices including collagen I, collagen IV fibronectin, gelatin, and laminin. The choice of matrix influences the culture morphology and long-term viability. For example, Matrigel (Collaborative Research, MA) suppresses fibroblast replication and supports the propagation of hepatocytes to form a central lumen-like structure with proven sustained release of extracellular hepatocellular specific proteins. Differential quantitative expression of proteins has been noted on hepatocytes cultured on matrigel or collagen (for review, *see* **ref. 2**).
4. Antibody to liver-specific proteins (i.e., apolipoprotein E and α-fetoprotein) are commercially available (Chemicon, Temecula, CA) and sensitive detection can be observed using ^{125}I labeled protein G (ICN, Irvine, CA; *see* **ref. 9**).
5. Viability decreases approx 10% through the cryopreservation process. The plating efficiency of the cells following cryopreservation is approx 20–30%, but can be as high as 80–90% depending on initial health of the cells. In general, isolation of cells from a diseased liver leads to lower viability, poorer cultures, and less successful cultures after cyropreservation.
6. A number of controls are run with each sample in each assay. To ensure that the reaction with rtTh is strand-specific and that there is an absence of HCV self-

priming, each sample is subjected to an RT-PCR assay that lacks the RT primer. The presence of a band in these samples would indicate that the RT step was not primer-specific. To ensure that samples do not become contaminated with previously amplified DNA, each sample is subjected to a PCR assay that eliminates the RT step. In addition, the presence of water blanks positioned every sixth sample within the assay ensures that the spread of amplicon via aresoling is not occurring. DNA contamination is significantly reduced when separate preparation areas are used for each step of the assay. Serum and tissue samples from HCV-positive patients and negative controls are included in each assay.

References

1. Strom, S. C., Jirtle, R. L., Jones, R. S., Novicki, D. L., Rosenberg, M. R., Novotny, A., et al. (1982) Isolation, culture and transplantation of human hepatocytes. *J. Natl. Cancer Inst.* **68,** 771–778.
2. Strom, S. C., Pisarov, L. A., Dorko, K., Thompson, M. T., Schuetz, J. D., and Schuetz, E. G. (1996) Use of human hepatocytes to study P450 gene induction. *Methods Enzymol.* **272,** 388–401.
3. Strom, S. C., Fisher, R. A., Thompson, M. T., Sanyal, A. J., Cole, P. E., Ham, J. M., et al. (1998) *Transplantation,* in press.
4. Cox, S., Buontempo, P., Skelton, A., Pannucci, J., DeMartino, J., Albin, R., et al. (1985) Culturing of HCV- infected human adult hepatocytes to study the replication of HCV. Presented at 3rd International Hepatitis C Meeting, Australia.
5. Ito, T., Mukaigawa, J., Zuo, J., Hirabayaski, Y., Mitamura, K., and Yasui, K. (1996) Cultivation of hepatitis C virus in primary hepatocyte culture from patients with chronic hepatitis C results in release of high titre infectious virus. *J. Gen. Virol.* **77,** 1043–1054.
6. Isom, H. C. and Georgoff, I. (1984) Quantitative assay for albumin-producing liver cells after simian virus 40 transformation of rat hepatocytes maintained in chemically defined medium. *Proc. Natl. Acad. Sci. USA* **81,** 6378–6382.
7. Dorko, K., Freeswick, P. D., Bartoli, F., Cicalese, C., Bardsley, B. A., Tzakis, A., et al. (1994) A new technique for isolating and culturing human hepatocytes from whole or split livers not used for transplantation. *Cell Transplant.* **3,** 387–395.
8. Landford, R. E., Sureau, C., Jacob, J. R., White, R., and Fuerst, T. R. (1994) Demonstration of *in vitro* infection of chimpanzee hepatocytes with hepatitis C virus using strand specific RT/PCR. *Virology* **202,** 606–614.
9. Kreamer, B. L., Staecker, J. L., Sawada, N., Sattler, G. L., Hsia, M. T. S., and Pitot, H. C. (1986) Use of a low-speed, iso-density percoll centrifugation method to increase the viability of isolated rat hepatocyte preparations. *In Vitro Cell. Dev. Biol.* **22,** 201–211.

48

A Cultivation Method for Highly Differentiated Primary Chimpanzee Hepatocytes Permissive for Hepatitis C Virus Replication

Robert E. Lanford and Larry Estlack

1. Introduction

The liver performs a wide array of functions, a few of which include the synthesis and secretion of most of the plasma proteins, including the lipoproteins, cholesterol, and bile acid metabolism, and detoxification of the blood. In vitro analysis of most liver functions has been hampered by the difficulties encountered in isolating and maintaining functional cultures of primary hepatocytes. Although in vivo the liver has an amazing capacity for regeneration, hepatocytes in culture have limited proliferation capacity and are normally short-lived. We have developed methods for the isolation and cultivation of highly differentiated primate hepatocyte cultures that can be maintained for over 100 d without significant loss of differentiated function. This system has been used in our lab for the analysis of lipoprotein synthesis and hepatotropic virus replication. This chapter is designed to provide a detailed methodology of our approach. Numerous alternative hepatocyte cultivation systems have been described, but owing to space limitations, these systems will not be described here. A number of excellent reviews are dedicated to this subject, one of which is in a previous volume of this series (1), and another that is an entire book dedicated to the subject (2).

A brief overview of our prior work in the primate hepatocyte system is required to appreciate fully the power of the system for studies on hepatocyte functions and more specifically hepatitis C virus (HCV) replication. One prerequisite to our studies on in vitro cultivation of hepatitis viruses was the development of a culture system for highly differentiated primate hepatocytes. Cultivation of hepatocytes in conventional serum-supplemented media results in the rapid loss of differentiated functions and short-term viability. Our approach was to derive a serum-free medium supplemented with growth factors and hormones. The initial development of the serum-free medium was performed with baboon hepatocytes as part of our studies on genetic variations in lipoprotein metabolism. A liver wedge was obtained from baboons during a survival surgery, and hepatocytes were isolated by collagenase perfusion. During the development of media formulations, primary baboon hepatocyte cultures were analyzed for longevity, maintenance of morphology, and the secretion of stringent markers for hepatocyte differentiation. The current medium formulation is the result of several years of experimentation. Cultures have been maintained in this medium for over 100 d without the loss of differentiated function *(3)*. The synthesis and secretion of over 25 different liver-specific plasma proteins have been demonstrated in these cultures, and every liver specific marker that has been examined was expressed. This system was utilized to demonstrate the *de novo* synthesis of lipoprotein (a) by hepatocytes *(4)* and is still the only system amenable to study the effects of allelic variations on the biogenesis of lipoprotein (a) *(5–9)*.

This system was adapted for the culture of primary chimpanzee and human hepatocytes in order to develop systems for analysis of hepatotropic virus replication. The initial attempt to cultivate a hepatitis virus in our system utilized hepatocytes obtained from a chimpanzee chronically infected with HBV. The cultures were maintained for 27 d and were shown to secrete intact HBV virions that were positive in the endogenous polymerase assay *(10)*. In vitro infection with HBV has been more problematic, with our initial studies yielding no infection despite numerous attempts to infect normal hepatocytes with a variety of HBV inocula, including purified virions *(11)*. Recently, using high-titered, tissue-culture-derived inocula, we have succeeded in obtaining a low level of HBV infection in primary chimpanzee hepatocytes, but the system is far from optimal for this virus. A low level of HBV replication has also been observed in human hepatocytes by other investigators using our medium formulation *(12)*.

Although infections with HBV are marginal, this system is exceptionally well suited for the analysis of HDV replication. The infection of normal chimpanzee hepatocytes with an HDV inoculum that also contained high levels of HBV revealed that although the cells could not be infected with HBV, they were susceptible to infection with HDV *(11)*. This observation may indicate that HBV and HDV use different modes of entry into hepatocytes, despite the fact that HDV utilizes the HBV envelope proteins for virion formation. HDV RNA replicative forms were present for 42 d after infection, at which time the level of replication was still very high. Infection of hepatocytes obtained from an HBV chronically infected chimpanzee permitted a full replication cycle for

HDV with the appearance of virions in the culture medium *(11)*. An in vitro neutralization assay was developed for HDV and was used to map neutralization sites on the HBV envelope proteins *(13)*, and recombinant HDV particles assembled in hepatoma cell lines could be tested for infectivity in primary hepatocytes. This approach permitted analysis of the effect of mutations in the HBV envelope proteins on HDV infectivity *(14)*.

Recent studies have demonstrated that cynomolgus monkey hepatocytes cultivated in our SFM are highly permissive for HEV replication. Negative-strand RNA could easily be detected by rTth RT-PCR, sufficient virus was purified from the medium for EM analysis, and the virus could be passaged to fresh cultures *(15)*. An in vitro neutralization assay for HEV has been developed using this system that should be useful in vaccine development *(16)*.

In our initial studies on the replication of HCV (non-A, non-B hepatitis) in primary hepatocyte cultures, the hepatocytes were obtained from chimpanzees during the acute stage of infection. Since PCR was not available at that time, the active replication of HCV was demonstrated by the infection of a normal chimpanzee with tissue-culture medium. Increases in ALT and histopathological examination of liver biopsies (and retrospectively PCR) demonstrated an HCV infection in this animal *(17)*. The development of a well-documented system for the in vitro cultivation of HCV has been problematic. Owing to the very low levels of HCV replication both in vivo and in vitro, HCV RNA can be detected routinely only by RT-PCR. The extreme sensitivity of RT-PCR permits detection of residual inoculum for extended periods of time. This problem can be circumvented by the use of strand-specific RT-PCR to detect the replicative negative strand of HCV RNA; however, high levels of strand specificity for RT-PCR are not easily obtained. We developed two methods of strand-specific RT-PCR with sufficient specificity to document replication of HCV in our system *(18)* and to evaluate the potential for extrahepatic replication by HCV *(19)*. The tagged and rTth methods of RT/PCR are discussed in Chapter 44. Although positive-strand RNA was present from the time of inoculation because of residual inoculum, negative-strand RNA appeared on d 4 and remained at a fairly constant level throughout the infection. The ability to infect cultures of chimpanzee hepatocytes in vitro appears to vary from one experiment to the next, since the level of negative-strand RNA is near or below the level of detection in some experiments, despite the presence of abundant positive-strand RNA. Since positive-strand RNA cannot be taken as a direct indication of replication, in the absence of easily detected negative-strand RNA, we must assume that sufficient infection has not occurred. The variability would appear to be related to the inoculum or the susceptibility of the cells to infection, since cells obtained from an HCV-infected animal are invariably permissive for replication of HCV negative-strand RNA at high and very reproducible levels for long periods of time. The variability observed for susceptibility to in vitro infection places limitations on the use of the system for neutralization assays and other studies requiring a reproducible in vitro infection. However, the high level of permissiveness for HCV RNA replication makes primary chimpanzee hepatocytes obtained from HCV-infected animals highly desirable for the evaluation of antiviral drugs, and the normal hepatocyte cultures may be essential to the development of an infectious cDNA clone and a system for reverse genetics in HCV.

2. Materials
2.1. Hepatocyte Isolation
2.1.1. Buffers and Solutions

Unless noted all buffers are filtered through a 0.22-μm filter unit.

1. WME: William's Medium E-powder; Gibco-BRL (Grand Island, NY; cat. no. 31500-077). For 10 L of medium, add 2.2 g/L sodium bicarbonate and pH to 7.4 with 1 M HCl. Sterile-filter through a 0.22-μm Micro-Culture Capsule filter (Gelman Science, Ann Arbor, MI) into sterilized 500-mL Corning-Pyrex media bottles.
2. 500 mM EGTA in H_2O: ethylene gycol *bis* (β-aminoethyl ether)-N,N,N',N'-tetraacetic acid; Sigma Chemical Co. (St. Louis, MO; cat. no. E4378).
3. 1 M HEPES in H_2O, pH 7.4: 4-(2-hydroxyethyl) piperazine-2-ethanesulfonic acid; Calbiochem (La Jolla, CA; cat. no. 391338).
4. 1 M $CaCl_2$ in H_2O: Sigma (cat. no. C-3881).
5. 50 mg/mL gentamicin sulfate in H_2O: United States Biochemical Corp. (Cleveland, OH) (cat. no. 16051).
6. 200 mM L-glutamine in WME: Sigma (cat. no. G 5763).
7. WME basal: WME containing 10 mM HEPES and 50 (μg/mL gentamicin.
8. HBSS: Hank's Balanced Salt Solution without calcium and magnesium; Gibco-BRL (cat. no. 14170-112).
9. Washout buffer: HBSS containing 0.5 mM EGTA, 10 mM HEPES, pH 7.4, and 50 μg/mL gentamicin.
10. Collagenase solution: Prepared fresh the day of isolation. To 400 mL of HBSS, add 0.08–0.24 g of collagenase B (Boehringer Mannheim, Indianapolis, IN; cat. no. 1088 831) (final concentration; 0.02–0.06%; *see* **Note 1**). Shake gently for 15–30 min on a platform shaker to dissolve, and filter through a 0.45-μm filter unit followed by a 0.22-μm filter unit. Add 2 mL of 1 M $CaCl_2$ immediately prior to use.

2.1.2. Equipment and Supplies

Equipment sterilized by autoclaving. It is recommended that more than one of each item be available in case one should become contaminated.

1. Surgical instruments for handling liver tissue: A surgical instrument tray (VWR Scientific, WestChester, PA; cat. no 62687-027) containing one pair of $5^{1}/_{2}$ in. Rochester-Oshsner hemostatic forceps (VWR cat. no. 25607-380), one pair of 5-in. dissecting scissors (VWR cat. no. 25608-360), and one pair of very fine-point forceps (VWR cat. no. 25607-856).
2. Nalgene 1 L wide-mouth bottle for transport of liver tissue (VWR cat. no. 16125-118).
3. Pyrex 1-L beaker for waste liquids (VWR cat. no. 13912-604).
4. Gauze squares for filtration of hepatocytes (Professional Medical Products, Inc., Greenwood, SC; cat. no. 635).
5. Perfusion tubing: Norton-Tygon MicroBore tubing (VWR cat. no. 63018-088) connected to larger-diameter Nalgene tubing (1/8-in. id × 1/4-in. od × 1/16-in. wall; VWR cat. no. 8007-0020) using a male-to-male reduction adapter (Baxter Scientific, DeerField, IL).

Equipment that cannot be autoclaved:

1. Hospital bed heating pad (Duo-Therm Disposable Pad—18 × 24 in., Baxter Scientific; cat. no. 66N415CC) and water circulator (K-Module-Model K-20, American Pharmaseal Company, Valencia, CA).
2. Manostat varistaltic pump with a flow rate of 1–300 mL/min (VWR cat. no. 54847-113).
3. Water bath set at 42°C for maintaining collagenase solutions.
4. Corning sterile, disposable plastic Erlenmeyer flask: (VWR, cat. no. 29152-168).
5. Hemacytometer, Hausser (VWR cat. no. 15170-079).
6. Nalgene cryogenic vials, 2 mL (VWR cat. no. 66008-728).
7. Corning conical centrifuge tubes, 50 mL (VWR cat. no. 21008-714).
8. Corning filter units, 500 mL, 0.45 µm (VWR cat. no. 28199-836).
9. Corning filter units, 500 mL, 0.22 µm (VWR cat. no. 28199-803).

2.2. Hepatocyte Cultivation

2.2.1. Serum-Free Medium Components

1. WME basal: *see* **Subheading 2.1.**
2. Insulin-transferrin-selenium (ITS; Sigma-I 1884).
3. Insulin (Sigma-I 1882).
4. Glucagon-Pharmacy Emergency Kit for Diabetics (10 mg glucagon, no. 668; Eli Lilly and Co., Indianapolis, IN) or (Sigma-G3157).
5. Epidermal growth factor (EGF; Collaborative Biomedical, Bedford, MA- 4000 1B).
6. Linoleic acid/albumin (Sigma-L 8384).
7. Luteotropic hormone (prolactin; Sigma-L 6520).
8. Somatotropin (Sigma-S 4776).
9. Hydrocortisone (Collaborative Biomedical-40203).
10. Liver growth factor (GLY-HIS-LYS; Sigma-G 7387).
11. Ethanolamine (Sigma-E 9508).
12. Cholera toxin (ICN Biomedical, Costa Mesa, CA-150005).

2.2.2. Preparation of Reagent Stocks

1. 1 M HEPES in H_2O, pH 7.4: 100X.
2. Gentamicin sulfate, 50 mg/mL in H_2O: 1000X.
3. L-Glutamine, 200 mM in WME: 100X.
4. Linoleic acid/albumin, 500 mg in 10 mL of WME: 100X.
5. Glucagon, 10 mg (Eli Lilly) in 5 mL of 0.01 M HCl, freeze in 1-mL aliquots, or 2 mg (Sigma) in 1 mL of 0.01 M HCl: 1000X.
6. ITS, 1 vial (25 mg insulin, 25 mg transferrin, 25 µg sodium selinite) in 5 mL of H_2O, freeze in 1 mL aliquots: 1000X.
7. Insulin, 100 mg in 20 mL of H_2O, freeze in 1-mL aliquots: 1000X.
8. Hydrocortisone, 50 mg in 13.8 mL of absolute ethanol, freeze in 200-µL aliquots: 10,000X.
9. EGF, 100 µg in 1 mL of WME: 1000X.
10. LGF, 500 µg in 2.5 mL of 0.1 N acetic acid, freeze in 100-µL aliquots: 10,000X.
11. Cholera toxin, 1 mg in 5 mL of WME, filter through 0.22-µm low-protein binding syringe filter, and freeze in 100-µL aliquots: 100,000X.
12. Somatotropin, 1 vial (4 IU) in 4.0 mL of WME, freeze in 1-mL aliquots: 1000X.
13. Prolactin, 1 vial (250 IU) in 8.5 mL of WME, filter through 0.22-µm low-protein binding syringe filter, and freeze in 200-µL aliquots: 10,000X.
14. Ethanolamine, add 610 µL to 10 mL of H_2O, and then further dilute 100 µL with 10 mL of H_2O, filter through a 0.22-µm syringe filter, and freeze in 200-µL aliquots: 10,000X.

2.2.3. Coated Tissue-Culture Dishes

1. Falcon Primaria culture dishes (60 mm) (VWR cat. no. 25382-687) or six-well dishes (VWR cat. no. 62406-455).
2. Rat tail collagen (Collaborative Biomedical, cat. no. 40236).
3. Collagen coating of culture dishes: dilute collagen 1:5 in water, sterile filter through a 0.22-µm syringe filter, add sufficient collagen solution to each plate to cover the bottom of the plate, and then remove the excess solution. Dry plates with lids partially open overnight under a laminar flow hood with UV light.

3. Methods

3.1. Production of Serum-Free Medium (see Notes 2 and 3)

1. Warm 1 vial of linoleic acid/albumin and 1 vial of EGF.
2. Thaw 10 mL of 200 mM L-glutamine at 37°C.
3. Thaw frozen aliquots of other reagents on ice.
4. Place all thawed reagents under a laminar flow hood, and wipe vials with 70% ethanol.
5. Add 1000 mL of WME to a 1-L Corning sterile plastic disposable bottle.
6. Dissolve one vial of linoleic acid/albumin in 10 mL of WME.
7. Dissolve one vial of EGF in 1 mL of WME.

Table 1
Serum-Free Medium Supplements

Supplement	Stock	Volume/L	Final concentration
HEPES	100X	10 mL	10 mM
Gentamicin	1000X	1 mL	50 μg/mL
Glutamine	100X	10 mL	2 mM
Linoleic acid/BSA	100X	10 mL	5 μg; 500 μg /mL
EGF	1000X	1 mL	100 ng/mL
ITS	1000X	1 mL	5 μg, 5 μg, 5 ng /mL
Insulin	1000X	1 mL	5 μg/mL (final = 10 μg/mL)
Hydrocortisone	10,000X	0.1 mL	$1 \times 10^{-6}\ M$
Cholera toxin	100,000X	0.01 mL	2 ng/mL
Somatotropin	1000X	1 mL	1 mU/mL
Prolactin	10,000X	0.1 mL	3 mU/mL
Ethanolamine	10,000X	0.1 mL	$1 \times 10^{-6}\ M$
LGF	10,000X	0.1 mL	20 ng/mL
Glucagon	1000X	1 mL	2 μg/mL

8. To the 1000 mL of WME, add the following: 10 mL of 1 M HEPES, pH 7.4, 1 mL of 50 mg/mL gentamicin sulfate, 10 mL of 200 mM L-glutamine, 10 mL of linoleic acid/albumin, 1 mL of EGF, 1 mL of ITS, 1 mL of insulin, 100 μL of hydrocortisone, 10 μL of cholera toxin, 1 mL of somatotropin, 100 μL of prolactin, 100 μL of ethanolamine, 100 (l of LGF, and 1 mL of glucagon. *See* **Table 1**.
9. Swirl contents of bottle to mix SFM.
10. Filter through an Acro-Cap 0.22-μm filter unit (Gelman Sciences, Ann Arbor, MI; product no. 4480) using a peristaltic pump at a flow rate of 40 mL/min. Collect into Corning 50-mL conical centrifuge tubes (add 40 mL to each tube).
11. Tighten all caps firmly; label the tubes with SFM and the date, and store at −70°C.

3.2. Isolation of Hepatocytes

In our studies, hepatocytes are isolated by a two-step collagenase perfusion method *(20,21)*. Liver wedge surgeries are performed in accordance with procedures approved by the institutional animal research committee. Animals are immobilized with TELEZOL, and anesthesia is maintained using nonhepatotoxic pentobarbitol.

3.2.1. Preparations the Day Before Isolation

1. Prepare equipment: The following items should be autoclaved the day before isolation: two surgical stainless steel trays (VWR cat. no. 62687-049), two perfusion tubings with both ends wrapped in foil and autoclaved inside of self-seal

sterilization pouches (7.5-in. × 13-in., cat. no. 92713; American Hospital Supply Corp., Valencia, CA), one surgical instrument tray (with hemostats, scissors, and fine-point forceps), one container of gauze squares, one beaker for liquid wastes, one Nalge beaker for liver transport. After autoclaving, place the equipment in a laminar flow hood under UV light overnight.
2. Collagen-coat tissue-culture dishes.
3. Prepare solutions: The volume of solutions to be prepared will depend on the anticipated size of the liver wedge. For a 50–100 g piece of tissue, we prepare three 400-mL bottles each of WME Basal-5% FBS, washout buffer, and collagenase buffer (collagenase is prepared on the day of isolation).

3.2.2. Preparations on the Day of Isolation

1. Prepare three bottles of collagenase buffer.
2. Prepare the isolation hood. Wipe the inside of the hood with 70% ethanol. Connect the heating pad to the water circulator, set the water circulator to 43°C, and place one of the stainless-steel trays on the heating pad. Place the instrument tray and the gauze container in one corner of the hood, and place the liquid waste beaker at the back of the hood.
3. Place one bottle of washout buffer in a 42°C water bath inside of the hood.
4. Place the peristaltic pump inside of the hood, and insert the perfusion tubing into the pump. It is very important to use a sterile technique when setting up the tubing. Immediately prior to use, open the foil-wrapped ends, place the large end of the tubing inside of the bottle of washout buffer, and permit the individual holding the liver to grasp the microbore tubing without breaking sterile technique.

3.2.3. Hepatocyte Isolation

1. Take a 1-L Nalge bottle with 200 mL of washout buffer on ice to surgery to obtain the liver tissue. A piece of tissue is obtained with only one severed surface if at all possible.
2. All remaining procedures are performed under a laminar flow hood with absolute sterile technique. The procedure requires two people under the hood, such that the individual handling the liver tissue never touches a nonsterile surface. Until the perfusion steps are completed, the liver tissue is gently held by one individual. Carefully remove the liver tissue from the transport beaker by pouring off the excess buffer into the waste beaker and then carefully pouring the liver tissue into the hands of the individual who will hold the tissue throughout the perfusion. Open one of the sterile stainless-steel trays to catch the spent fluid during perfusion. We do not recirculate perfusion buffers in our procedure. During perfusion, spent fluid drains to the tray placed directly under the hands of the individual holding the liver tissue. The temperature is maintained by keeping the perfusion solutions in a water bath under the hood and using a rapid flow rate of the solutions. This obviates the need to monitor pH and oxygen level closely. Later when the tissue is placed in collagenase solution in one of the stainless-steel trays, the temperature is maintained by placing the stainless-steel tray on a hospital bed warming pad.

3. Carefully remove the small end of the perfusion tubing from its sterile package.
4. Using the flow of washout buffer from the perfusion tubing, rinse residual blood and clots from the liver tissue, and search for a good vessel for perfusion.
5. While holding the liver wedge between your thumb and forefinger, begin perfusion of a vessel with washout buffer. It is very important to find a good vessel for perfusion. When multiple vessels are exposed, the tubing can be moved periodically from one vessel to the next. In order to obtain some perfusion pressure, gentle pressure is applied across the severed end of the liver tissue with the thumb and forefinger. The liver tissue should become turgid owing to the fluid pressure, and blanching of the liver should become apparent.
6. Perfuse with washout buffer at a rate of 30 mL/min for at least 20 min. This minimal time is required for the desmosomes to disassociate. Complete blanching of the liver tissue should occur within this time period.
7. Add 2 mL of 1 M $CaCl_2$ to 400 mL of prewarmed collagenase solution and swirl to mix. Place the bottle inside of the water bath.
8. Switch the perfusion tubing to a bottle with collagenase solution, and continue to perfuse the liver tissue with collagenase at 30 mL/min for at least 20 min. This will require at least two bottles of collagenase solution. During collagenase perfusion, the outer capsule of the liver may become slippery. Wrapping the tissue with a thin layer of gauze will permit a gentle, yet secure grip on the tissue.
9. After approx 15–25 min, a decrease in the firmness of the liver tissue should become apparent, and the liver capsule may begin to disassociate from the tissue.
10. At the end of the perfusion period, a new sterile stainless-steel tray is opened, and the liver tissue is placed in the tray.
11. While holding the liver tissue by a vessel with hemostats, strip off the outer capsule with the fine-point tweezers, making sure that all of the capsule is removed from both sides of the tissue.
12. Add 100 mL of collagenase to the pan and gently shake the liver tissue by holding onto a vessel with the hemostats. Shake for 5–10 min. Cells should gradually detach from the tissue causing the collagenase solution to become very cloudy.
13. Gently pipet 25 mL of cellular suspension from the tray with a wide-tip 25-mL plastic pipet, and gently filter the cellular suspension through one-half thickness of a gauze square placed on the top of a 50-mL conical tube. The cells should gently run down the side of the tube rather than fall to the bottom. Add 25 mL of cold WME basal–5% FBS to each of the four tubes of cellular suspension. From this time forward, the tubes should be maintained on ice or in a 4°C centrifuge.
14. Pellet the cells (first pellet) for 5 min at 50g.
15. Pour off the supernatant and suspend the cells by gently shaking the tube. In order to prevent loosing a portion of the cell pellet, a small amount of supernatant will remain when the supernatant is poured off. The remaining supernatant is used to suspend the pellet by gentle shaking. Combine the pellets from all four tubes, and add WME basal–5% FBS to 50 mL. Maintain these cells on ice until the remainder of the liver has been processed to this point.
16. Repeat **steps 13–15** for a total of four to five "washes" of the liver tissue.

17. Pellet all individual washes (second pellet) for 5 min at 50g.
18. Pour off the supernatants, and resuspend the pellets as before. Combine the pellets into one or two tubes, depending on the volume of the cell pellets. No more than 10 mL of cell pellet should be combined into a single tube. Some isolations may yield more than 10 mL of cells. Add WME basal–5% FBS to 50 mL/tube.
19. Pellet the cells for a third and final time.
20. This time, carefully remove the supernatant with a pipet, such that all of the supernatant can be removed. Resuspend the cell pellets with WME basal–5% FBS.
21. Transfer the cells to a sterile 250-mL Erlenmeyer flask, and gently swirl to obtain a uniform cell suspension. Since hepatocytes will rapidly settle to the bottom of the flask, care must be exercised to obtain a uniform suspension any time that cells are being removed.
22. Count viable cells based on the exclusion of trypan blue stain.
23. Dilute cells in WME basal–5% FBS to 1×10^6 cells/mL.
24. Plate the cells in collagen-coated dishes at a density of 1×10^6 cells/well for six-well dishes and 3×10^6 cells for 60-mm plates (*see* **Note 4**). Allow the cells to attach at 37°C–5% CO_2 for 3–4 h. Replace the WME basal–5% FBS plating medium with SFM.
25. Change the medium every 2–3 d; usually on Monday, Wednesday, and Friday.
26. All experiments are performed using confluent cultures that have been maintained for 5–7 d (*see* **Notes 5** and **6**; **Figs. 1** and **2**).

4. Notes

1. The selection of a suitable lot of collagenase and the optimal collagenase concentration for that lot must be determined empirically. Lots of collagenase can be tested by perfusion of a rat liver, but we have found this to be a poor indicator of how well a specific lot of collagese will perform on primate or human liver. Primate liver is more difficult to disassociate than rodent tissue. Some ancillary protease activity (caseinase, neutral protease, and trypsin-like activity) is desirable. High levels, especially for trypsin, are detrimental. We have used collagenase from a number of different suppliers and have been able to select lots with satisfactory results. We currently use either collagenase A or B from Boehringer Mannheim. We have not found collagenase specifically designated for hepatocytes or human hepatocytes to be well suited to our procedure. A satisfactory lot of collagenase can be selected by first reviewing the available lots of these two types of collagenase and selecting a lot with moderate levels of ancillary protease activity. A few lots with appropriate values are then tested in hepatocyte isolations with primate or human tissue. The concentration of the chosen lot is then adjusted to yield the desired level of disassociation in 15–25 min. Most lots are used at a concentration near 0.06%.
2. Many different serum media formulations for liver cells have been described in the literature *(2,22–28)*. Each has been developed for specific purposes. A medium developed working with rodent tissue will not necessarily perform well on primate tissue. Our medium was developed empirically, in the beginning,

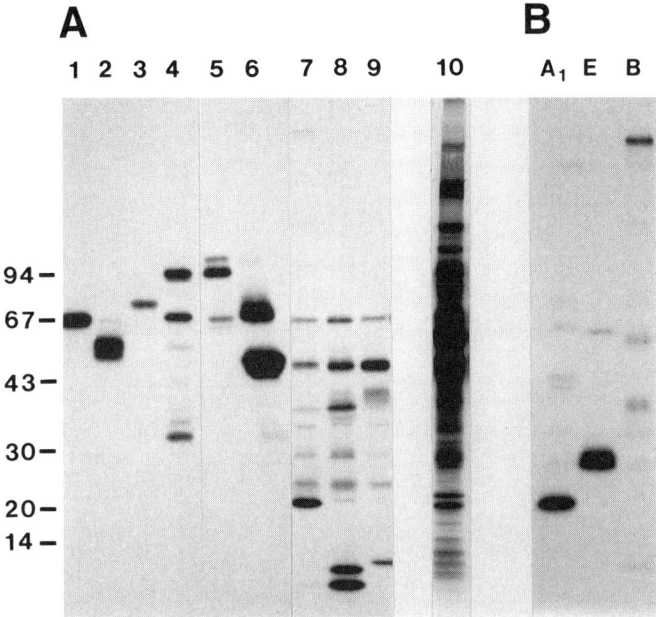

Fig. 1. Analysis of serum protein secretion by immunoprecipation. A primary baboon hepatocyte culture that had been maintained in SFM for 40 d was labeled for 16 h with [^{35}S]-methionine. The methods for immunoprecipitation analyses have been described in detail elsewhere (3,5–9). Briefly, the labeled culture medium was clarified and adjusted to contain 1% NP40. The various proteins were immunoprecipitated with specific antibodies bound to protein A agarose beads (Repligen Corporation, Cambridge, MA). The beads were washed three times, and proteins were eluted from the beads in SDS gel sample buffer. Samples were analyzed by 4–15% gradient polyacrylamide SDS gel electrophoresis followed by fluorography. **(A)** Lanes 1–9 represent immunoprecipitation of albumin; α 1-antitrypsin; transferrin; complement C4; plasminogen; fibrinogen; C-reactive protein; $β_2$-microglobulin; and prealbumin, respectively. The three proteins observed in lanes 4 and 6 represent the different chains of complement C4 and fibrinogen, respectively. Only the lower-most bands in lanes 7, 8, and 9 represent the specific immunoprecipitated proteins. Lane 10 demonstrates the complexity of the total proteins secreted by these cultures. **(B)** Immunoprecipitation of apolipoproteins A_1, E, and B. (This figure was reproduced from **ref. 3** with permission of the Society for In Vitro Biology).

relying on what had been reported in the literature. We then adopted the approach of evaluating various concentrations and combinations of growth factors and hormones on cultures of baboon hepatocytes. The cultures were monitored for the maintenance of hepatocyte morphology, longevity, and the continued expression of highly stringent markers of hepatocyte differentiation (3). We have continued

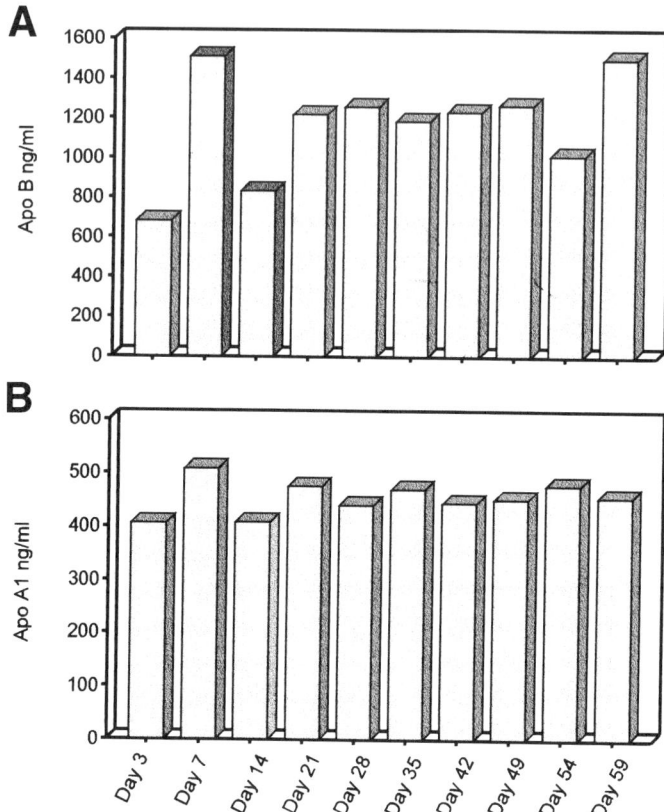

Fig. 2. Analysis of long-term lipoprotein secretion by ELISA. ELISA assays for apolipoprotein B (**A**) and apolipoprotein A1 (**B**) were performed as previously described *(9)* using medium from primary cultures of baboon hepatocytes grown in six-well dishes. Briefly, microtiter wells were coated with a polyclonal antibody specific for the individual apolipoprotein, and excess protein binding sites were blocked. The wells were incubated with 100 µL of culture medium followed by an alkaline phosphatase-conjugated antibody to the specific apolipoprotein and the substrate for alkaline phosphatase. Optical density values were analyzed using simple least-squares linear regression techniques. The estimates of sample concentrations (ng/mL) were calculated using a regression equation fitted to a standard curve based on log–log-transformed optical density data of five calibrators having known concentration. All ELISA data are the mean of four values.

to experiment with our formulation over the years. Changes in the formulation can be made to impact positively or negatively on the expression of a specific gene product, but such changes may have a very different influence on a different gene product. We have been pleased with the properties of hepatocytes grown in our medium, and thus rarely make permanent changes in the formulation.

3. We have evaluated a number of media formulations with respect to HCV replication in hepatocytes obtained from HCV-infected chimpanzees. These cultures replicate HCV RNA at very reproducible levels, thus allowing comparison of multiple media formulations by monitoring HCV negative-strand RNA using the rTth RT/PCR assay. Formulations that represented minor variations of our current formulation continued to support high levels of HCV RNA replication, whereas formulations very distant to our formulation resulted in the loss of HCV negative-strand RNA over a 14-d cultivation period. Specifically, formulations that included FBS and various growth factors and hormones with and without dimethyl sulfoxide failed to support HCV RNA replication. In addition, serum-free formulations that represented the minimal medium capable of supporting some degree of hepatocyte differentiation also failed to support HCV RNA replication. Owing to the restricted availability of chimpanzee hepatocytes and the limitations imposed by using RT-PCR to evaluate HCV replication, efforts to develop further the optimal medium for HCV replication are constrained.
4. We have examined numerous substrata for the growth of hepatocytes. Cells grown in our medium formulation rapidly establish a very thick and viscous extracellular matrix. We have not observed an advantage of providing a complex biological matrix in our system. Various growth factors and hormones present in our medium may supply signals to the hepatocyte receptors that eventually yield the same growth or differentiation response as obtained from a complex biological matrix. The thin collagen film utilized in our system is helpful in the initial attachment and establishment phase. Attachment factors are also present in the FBS used in the attachment medium.
5. Primate hepatocytes are difficult to freeze and revive with a high percentage of viability. We have evaluated numerous procedures over the years and have developed methods that work quite well with hepatoctyes from lower primates. Typically, we expect 80–90% viability from frozen baboon hepatocytes. However, the viability of chimpanzee and human hepatoctyes following freezing is still quite variable. We have found that UW solution containing 10% FBS and 10% DMSO is the preferred freezing fluid. UW solution or University of Wisconsin/Belzer's Solution is available commercially as Dupont Via Span Cold Storage Solution (DuPont Merck Pharmaceutical Co., Wilmington, DE; cat. no. 1000-46 06). In order to freeze cells, the cells are suspended in UW solution following the final pelleting. FBS is added to 10%, and then DMSO is added drop by drop while gently swirling the cells. The freezing density should not exceed 5×10^7 cells/mL. The vials are placed in open styrofoam racks and are frozen in a –70°C freezer overnight. We use the racks in which 15-mL conical tubes are sold. On the next day, the vials are transferred to a liquid nitrogen freezer.
6. We have used our cultivation system for the evaluation of numerous hepatocyte functions other than hepatotropic virus replication. Hepatocytes isolated and maintained using our procedures exhibit a high degree of differentiation over an extended cultivation period and appear to be suitable for studies of many liver-specific functions. **Figures 1** and **2** are examples of the continued synthesis and secretion of a number of hepatocyte-specific serum proteins.

Acknowledgments

This work was supported by grants from the National Institutes of Heart, Lung and Blood (HL28973) and Allergy and Infectious Diseases (AI40035).

References

1. Bayliss, M. K. and Skett, P. (1996) Isolation and culture of human hepatocytes, in *Methods in Molecular Medicine: Human Cell Culture Protocols* (Jones, E. J., ed.), Humana, Totowa, NJ, pp. 369–389.
2. Berry, M. N., Edwards, A. M., and Barritt, G. J. (1991) *Isolated Hepatocytes Preparation; Properties and Applications.* Elsevier, New York.
3. Lanford, R. E., Carey, K. D., Estlack, L. E., Smith, G. C., and Hay, R. V. (1989) Analysis of plasma protein and lipoprotein synthesis in long-term primary cultures of baboon hepatocytes maintained in serum-free medium. *In Vitro Cell. Dev. Biol.* **25,** 174–182.
4. Rainwater, D. L. and Lanford, R. E. (1989) Production of lipoprotein(a) by primary baboon hepatocytes. *Biochim. Biophys. Acta* **1003,** 30–35.
5. White, A. L., Rainwater, D. L., and Lanford, R. E. (1993) Intracellular maturation of apolipoprotein(a) and assembly of lipoprotein(a) in baboon hepatocytes. *J. Lipid Res.* **34,** 509–517.
6. White, A. L., Hixson, J. E., Rainwater, D. L., and Lanford, R. E. (1994) Molecular basis for "null" lipoprotein(a) phenotypes and the influence of apolipoprotein(a) size on plasma lipoprotein(a) level in the baboon. *J. Biol. Chem.* **269,** 9060–9066.
7. White, A. L. and Lanford, R. E. (1994) Cell surface assembly of lipoprotein(a) in primary cultures of baboon hepatocytes. *J. Biol. Chem.* **269,** 28,716–28,723.
8. White, A. L. and Lanford, R. E. (1995) Biosynthesis and metabolism of lipoprotein(a). *Curr. Opin. Lipidol.* **6,** 75–80.
9. Lanford, R. E., Estlack, L., and White, A. L. (1996) Neomycin inhibits secretion of apolipoprotein[a] by increasing retention on the hepatocyte cell surface. *J. Lipid Res.* **37,** 2055–2064.
10. Jacob, J. R., Eichberg, J. W., and Lanford, R. E. (1989) *In vitro* replication and expression of hepatitis B virus from chronically infected primary chimpanzee hepatocytes. *Hepatology* **10,** 921–927.
11. Sureau, C., Jacob, J. R., Eichberg, J. W., and Lanford, R. E. (1991) Tissue culture system for infection with human hepatitis delta virus. *J. Virol.* **65,** 3443–3450.
12. Condreay, L. D., Condreay, J. P., Jansen, R. W., Paff, M. T., and Averett, D. R. (1996) (–)-*Cis*-5-fluoro-1-[2-(hydroxymethyl)-1,3-oxathiolan-5-yl]cytosine (524W91) inhibits hepatitis B virus replication in primary human hepatocytes. *Antimicrob. Agents Chemother.* **40,** 520–523.
13. Sureau, C., Moriarty, A. M., Thornton, G. B., and Lanford, R. E. (1992) Production of infectious hepatitis delta virus *in vitro* and neutralization with antibodies directed against hepatitis B virus pre-S antigens. *J. Virol.* **66,** 1241–1245.

14. Sureau, C., Guerra, B., and Lanford, R. E. (1993) Role of the large hepatitis B virus surface envelope protein in infectivity of the hepatitis delta virion. *J. Virol.* **67**, 366–372.
15. Tam, A. W., White, R., Reed, E., Short, M., Zhang, Y. F., Fuerst, T. R., et al. (1996) In vitro propagation and production of hepatitis E virus from in vivo-infected primary macaque hepatocytes. *Virology* **215**, 1–9.
16. Tam, A. W., White, R., Yarbough, P. O., Lanford, R. E., and Fuerst, T. R. (1997) In vitro infection and replication of hepatitis E virus in primary cynomolgus macaque hepatocytes. *Virology* **238**, 94–102.
17. Jacob, J. R., Sureau, C., Burk, K. H., Eichberg, J. W., Dressman, G. R., and Lanford, R. E. (1991) In vitro replication of non-A, non-B hepatitis virus, in *Viral Hepatitis and Liver Disease* (Hollinger, F. B., Lemon, S. M., and Margolis, H. S., eds.), Williams and Wilkins, Baltimore, pp. 387–392.
18. Lanford, R. E., Sureau, C., Jacob, J. R., White, R., and Fuerst, T. R. (1994) Demonstration of *in vitro* infection of chimpanzee hepatocytes with hepatitis C virus using strand-specific RT/PCR. *Virology* **202**, 606–614.
19. Lanford, R. E., Chavez, D., Chisari, F., and Sureau, C. (1995) Lack of detection of negative-strand hepatitis C virus RNA in peripheral blood mononuclear cells and other extrahepatic tissues by the highly strand-specific rTth reverse transcriptase PCR. *J. Virol.* **69**, 8079–8083.
20. Berry, M. N. and Friend, D. S. (1969) High yield preparation of isolated rat liver parenchymal cells. *J. Cell Biol.* **43**, 506–520.
21. Seglen, P. O. (1973) Preparation of rat liver cells. II. Effects of ions and chelators on tissue dispersion. *Exp. Cell Res.* **76**, 25–30.
22. Edge, S. B., Hoeg, J. M., and Triche, T. (1986) Cultured human hepatocytes. Evidence for metabolism of low density lipoproteins by a pathway independent of the classical low density lipoprotein receptor. *J. Biol. Chem.* **261**, 3800–3806.
23. Enat, R., Jefferson, D. M., and Ruiz-Opazo, N. (1984) Hepatocyte proliferation in vitro: its dependence on the use of serum-free hormonally defined medium and substrata of extracellular matrix. *Proc. Natl. Acad. Sci.* **81**, 1411–1415.
24. Leffert, H. L. and Koch, K. S. (1982) Hepatocyte growth regulation by hormones in chemically defined media: a two-signal hypothesis, in *Growth of Cells in Hormonally Defined Media* (Sato, G. H. and Sirbasku, A. A., eds.), Cold Spring Harbor Laboratory, Cold Spring Harbor, NY, pp. 597–613.
25. Reid, L. M. and Jefferson, D. M. (1984) Culturing hepatocytes and other differentiated cells. *Histopathology* **4**, 548–559.
26. Salas-Prato, M. (1982) Growth of fetal mouse liver cells in hormone-supplemented serum-free medium, in *Growth of Cells in Hormonally Defined Media* (Sato, G. H. and Sirbasku, A. A., eds.), Cold Spring Harbor Laboratory, Cold Spring Harbor, NY, pp. 615–624.
27. Sells, M. A., Chernoff, J., and Cerda, A. (1985) Long-term culture and passage of human fetal liver cells that synthesize albumin. *In Vitro Cell. Dev. Biol.* **21**, 216–220.
28. Lippi, G., Lo Cascio, C., Ruzzenente, O., Poli, G., Brentegani, C., and Guidi, G. (1996) Simple and rapid procedure for the purification of lipoprotein(a). *J. Chromatogr. B Biomed. Appl.* **682**, 225–231.

IX

CONSTRUCTION OF RECOMBINANT VIRAL VECTORS FOR THE EXPRESSION OF HCV GENES

49

Construction of Recombinant Vaccinia Virus Expressing HCV Genes

Joyce A. Feller

1. Introduction

Hepatitis C virus (HCV) remains the leading cause of non-A, non-B hepatitis, and a major indicator for orthotopic liver transplantation. To date, finding a cure or even a commonly effective therapy for infection with HCV has proven to be an elusive goal. One major problem that has hampered attempts to develop antiviral agents is the ongoing inability to grow the virus in tissue culture. Without an efficient in vitro system for the propagation of HCV, it is difficult to generate the large amounts of viral protein needed for this sort of study; nor can the effects of known antiviral agents be assessed on the replication of HCV. Recently, some laboratories have reported preliminary evidence of HCV replication in cultured cells *(1,2)*, but even the best of these systems does not produce significant amounts of progeny virus. Although these methods may be applicable in the future, at present they are not yet practical.

Until an in vitro system is developed that can support the necessary high levels of HCV replication, alternate strategies must be employed for the dissection of viral replication and the investigation of antiviral agents. Many of these approaches involve artificially expressing large amounts of one or more HCV proteins and purifying them for biochemical study. This approach permits study of cleavage of the HCV polyprotein, testing of protease and RNA-dependent RNA polymerase inhibitors, and generation of anti-HCV antibodies. One simple way to express large amounts of HCV proteins for study is to construct a vaccinia virus (VV) recombinant which contains the desired HCV coding region, and thereby expresses the viral protein(s). Unlike HCV, VV grows well in tissue culture and is easy to manipulate.

From: *Methods in Molecular Medicine, Vol. 19: Hepatitis C Protocols*
Edited by: J. Y. N. Lau © Humana Press Inc., Totowa, NJ

VV, the prototype member of the genus *Orthopoxviridae*, is a large and complex virus. Its genome consists of a linear double-stranded DNA molecule of approx 180 kb pairs with covalently linked termini. The exact size of the viral genome is variable and quite flexible *(3)*; it is possible to insert at least 25 kb pairs of exogenous DNA into the viral genome without adverse effect *(4)*. Therefore, unlike most other virus vectors, size constraint on the amount of DNA packaged in a VV virion is not an obstacle. Furthermore, VV is a highly recombinogenic virus and can readily incorporate new DNA by site-specific recombination.

Poxviruses replicate in discrete viral factories located in the cytoplasm of the host cell, making them unique among DNA viruses, which typically replicate within the cell nucleus. As a consequence of this cytoplasmic site of replication, poxviruses must encode and package most of the components necessary for viral DNA replication and messenger RNA transcription. One significant result of this is that poxviruses have evolved distinctive promoters, which control transcription of their genes. These promoters are unique to poxviruses and are not recognized by the eukaryotic RNA polymerase II *(5)*. Therefore, any foreign coding region to be expressed in VV must be placed under the control of a poxvirus promoter. Fortunately, several highly efficient poxvirus promoters have been cloned and are available in plasmid cassettes.

Finally, unlike most eukaryotic genes, poxvirus genes do not contain any introns, so their transcripts do not undergo splicing, consistent with the cytoplasmic site of viral replication. This bypasses the potential dilemma of finding unexpected pseudosplicing sites within the foreign DNA insert, which is an inherent possibility when using DNA virus vectors that replicate in the nucleus of the host cell.

Thus, the advantages of expressing HCV genes in VV are based on the flexibility in the size of the VV genome, its highly recombinogenic nature, and the ability to have foreign coding sequence controlled by a VV promoter and expressed to a high level by the virus. To generate a VV/HCV recombinant, the cDNA from the desired HCV coding region is first cloned into a VV shuttle plasmid, placing it under the control of a VV promoter and translational start signal. The promoter and HCV cDNA insert are bilaterally flanked by left and right segments of VV sequence from a nonessential region (**Fig. 1**), that serves as the target site in the viral genome. The cassette containing the HCV coding region is then recombined into wild-type virus by transfection of the shuttle plasmid into VV-infected cells, leading to homologous recombination which results in stable recombinant virus *(6–8)* (**Fig. 2**). This process has been used extensively to create specific, defined recombinants where the interrupted copy of the viral gene precisely replaces the intact genomic locus. The recombinant viruses will both transcribe the inserted gene and synthesize the encoded pro-

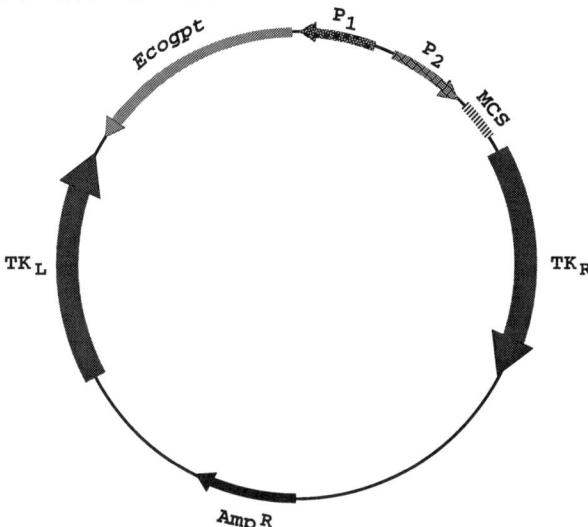

Fig. 1. Generalized structure of a VV insertion plasmid. TK_L and TK_R represent the left and right halves of a nonessential viral gene, in this case the TK gene. This is the site in the viral genome where the recombination will occur. P1 and P2 represent two independent poxvirus promoter elements required for expression of the foreign genes in the VV milieu. In this example, P1 provides expression of the *E. coli* (*Ecogpt*) gene, which confers resistance to mycophenolic acid and is the basis for selection. P2 directs expression of the HCV coding region, which would be cloned into the multicloning site (MCS). In practice, the identity of the target insertion site and promoters can vary from plasmid to plasmid, as can the orientation of the two promoter cassettes within the VV flanking sequence.

tein *(9,10)*. Furthermore, it has been demonstrated that a single shuttle plasmid may be used to integrate multiple independent foreign genes simultaneously into one genomic insertion site *(11)*. The resulting recombinant virus will express each of the encoded proteins provided that each inserted gene is controlled by a poxvirus promoter.

After the transfection, recombinant viruses are selected from the background of wild-type VV. There are several methods by which the recombinants may be identified. One frequently used method is to target the insertion into the viral thymidine kinase (TK) gene, and perform a functional assay for the insertional inactivation of the TK gene. The TK⁻ recombinant viruses are selected by passage of the total transfection progeny on a TK⁻ cell line in the presence of the inhibitor 5-bromo-2'-deoxyuridine. This compound inhibits the replication of wild-type virus, permitting only TK⁻ viruses to grow. Unfortunately, since the VV TK gene is nonessential for viral replication, it exhibits a fairly high rate of spontaneous mutation to an inactive phenotype. This necessitates

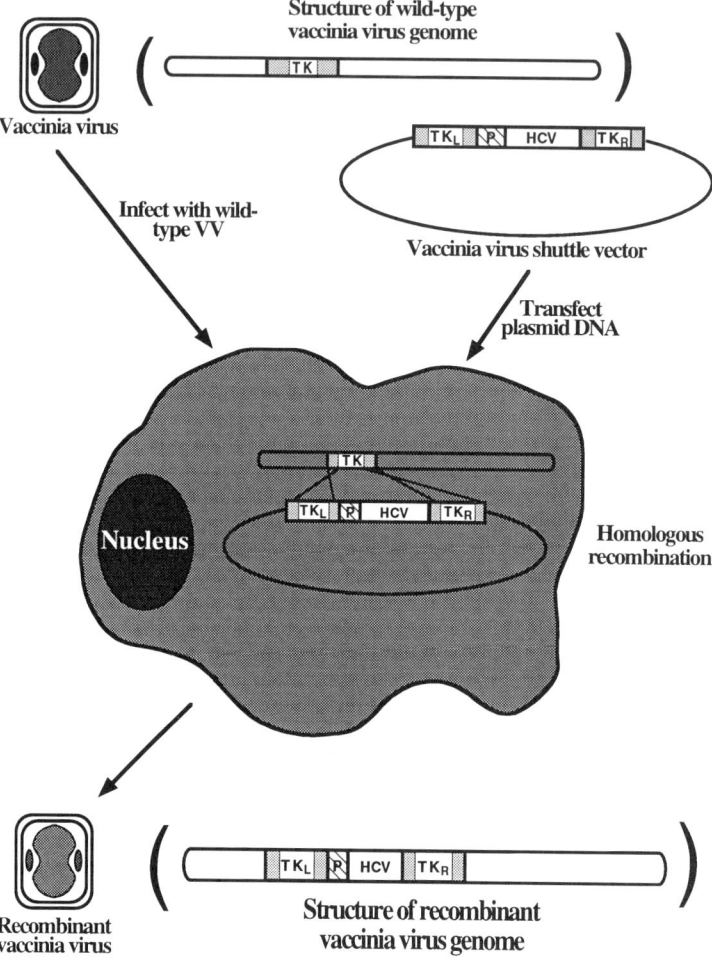

Fig. 2. Homologous recombination within a VV-infected and transfected cell. Tissue culture cells are first infected with wild-type VV. After viral adsorption, the cells are transfected with the VV shuttle plasmid, which contains the desired HCV coding region and the *E. coli gpt* cassette, each controlled by a poxvirus promoter element. A proportion of the cells will take up both the virus and the plasmid DNA. It is in the cytoplasm of these cells that homologous recombination occurs between the viral genome and the interrupted copy of the VV gene carried on the plasmid. This process neatly replaces the genomic copy of the gene with the engineered one. These genomes are then packaged into virions as recombinant virus, which can then be selected from the background of wild-type virus.

further differentiation of the desired recombinants from spontaneous TK$^-$ mutants, but this process is time-consuming and requires some expertise. Furthermore, this method of selection does not easily permit the placing of a second insertion into the recombinant virus. This would require the use of a second nonessential insertion site, and few nonessential VV genes have a convenient assay for their function. Therefore, although traditionally a widely used method, insertion into the VV TK gene and selection for TK⁻ progeny have some significant limitations.

A better, more flexible alternative is to have the shuttle plasmid contain a second, selectable marker gene under the control of a separate poxvirus promoter. Perhaps the simplest and most flexible of these is a dominant selectable marker from *Escherichia coli*, the xanthine-guanine phosphoribosyltransferase gene, or *gpt*. It encodes the enzyme XGPRT, which is involved in the salvage pathway of purine biosynthesis and catalyzes the phosphorylation of xanthine into xanthine monophosphate, a precursor of GTP (*see* **Fig. 3**). XGPRT utilizes xanthine considerably more efficiently than hypoxanthine as a substrate in nucleotide synthesis *(12)*. In contrast, the mammalian counterpart, hypoxanthine-guanine phosphoribosyltransferase (HGPRT) does not display any significant activity with xanthine *(13)*. Therefore, although both the mammalian and bacterial enzymes can support the salvage pathway of purine biosynthesis using hypoxanthine or guanine as substrate (*see* **Fig. 3**), only the bacterial enzyme is active on xanthine. This is the basis of *gpt* selection *(14,15)*.

Mycophenolic acid (MPA) is a mycotoxin that inhibits the enzyme inosine monophosphate dehydrogenase, an enzyme that converts inosine monophosphate (IMP) to xanthine monophosphate (XMP) (*see* **Fig. 3**), thus blocking *de novo* GMP synthesis *(15,16)*. In the presence of MPA, the intracellular GTP pools are depleted in the absence of guanine, the substrate necessary for the mammalian salvage pathway. MPA thereby also inhibits the growth of VV *(17,18)*. However, the *E. coli gpt* gene can alleviate this nucleotide shortage in the presence of xanthine, allowing the *gpt*-containing recombinant viruses to replicate. Viral recombinants expressing this gene will therefore have the unique ability to grow in the presence of the inhibitor MPA and xanthine. Because the eukaryotic enzyme cannot use this substrate, spontaneous MPA resistance is not possible. Using this selection, any nonessential VV region may be used as the target for insertion, and the recombinants selected simply by doing the transfection *(18)* and subsequent plaque purifications *(17,18)* in the presence of MPA and xanthine. Individual MPA-resistant plaques can be rapidly and easily isolated, expanded, and tested for expression of the HCV proteins (*see* **Note 1**).

Furthermore, several groups of researchers have devised methods by which this selection procedure can be made even more versatile and able to be used repeatedly to create sequential mutations within a virus clone. The first employs a simple reverse selection step using the purine analog 6-thioguanine in an HGPRT⁻ cell line to delete specifically the *gpt* gene from the recombinant virus so that it may be used again to generate a second insertion elsewhere in the

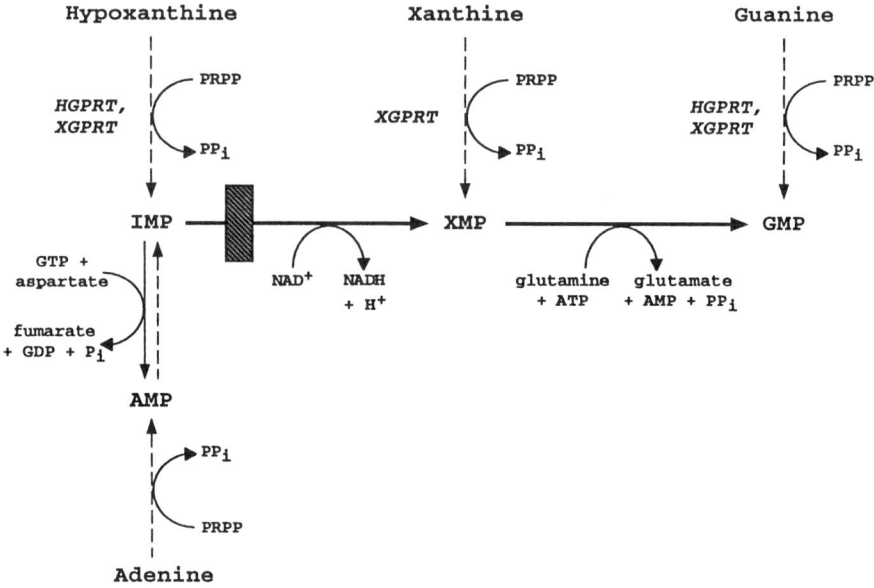

Fig. 3. The roles of the *E. coli gpt* protein and MPA in purine biosynthesis. Solid horizontal lines represent the *de novo* pathway of synthesis of guanosine monophosphate (GMP), whereas dashed vertical lines represent the salvage pathways of purine biosynthesis. The enzymes that catalyze the conversions in the salvage pathways are shown next to each reaction. MPA blocks *de novo* conversion of IMP to XMP, as represented by the hatched box on the diagram. This depletes the intracellular pool of GMP. This block may be bypassed by the salvage pathway using guanine in a mammalian cell, or guanine or xanthine in a cell containing the bacterial gene. Note that only the bacterial enzyme can convert xanthine into a precursor of GMP. This forms the basis of MPA/*gpt* selection. XGPRT, bacterial xanthine-guanine phosphoribosyltransferase (*gpt*); HGPRT, mammalian hypoxanthine-guanine phosphoribosyltransferase (adapted from **ref. 15**).

genome *(19)*. Others utilize transient selections, where the gpt gene is only temporarily *(20)* or never *(21)* actually incorporated into the genome of the recombinant viruses. These are all variations on the basic method. Therefore, this chapter focuses on the generation of VV/HCV recombinant viruses using the *E. coli gpt* gene as a dominant selectable marker (*see* **Note 2**).

2. Materials
2.1. Plasmid Construction

1. VV insertion plasmid containing both the *E. coli gpt* gene under a poxvirus promoter and a second promoter for control of the foreign gene insert (**Fig. 1**). There are several such plasmids available, providing the choice of promoters,

available restriction sites for cloning the foreign gene, and gene orientation within the VV flanking sequence. Examples include the pTKgpt-F1s, F2s and F3s series *(17)* and pTM3 *(22)*.
2. cDNA from the HCV coding region of interest.

2.2. Transfection and Generation of Recombinant Viruses

1. A high-titered stock of wild-type VV. Basically any strain of VV is acceptable, but the titer of the stock should be at least 1×10^8 PFU/mL. Virus stocks are best stored at $-70°C$ in aliquots.
2. A DNA stock of the completed VV shuttle plasmid containing the desired HCV coding region (*see* **Note 3**).
3. Sixty millimeter dishes containing monolayers of CV-1 (African green monkey kidney) cells (American Type Culture Collection, Rockville, MD). These cells are very easy to grow and maintain, and can remain as a fairly healthy monolayer even when confluent. For MPA selection, dishes at ~80% confluence should be pretreated with 1X selection medium from overnight to up to 24 h, to deplete the intracellular GTP pool.
4. Eagle's MEM with Earle's salts (e.g., Life Technologies, Gaithersburg, MD) supplemented with 5% FBS, 2 mM glutamine, 50 units penicillin, 50 µg streptomycin, 1 mM nonessential amino acids, and 1 mM pyruvate/mL (supplements are available as sterile 100X stocks from Life Technologies).
5. Virus diluent: Eagle's MEM with Earle's salts containing only the antibiotics and glutamine. This serum-free medium is for virus dilution and adsorption.
6. Phosphate-buffered saline (PBS), pH 7.2 (10 mM Na_2HPO_4, 10 mM NaH_2PO_4, 150 mM NaCl). (Unless otherwise indicated, chemicals were purchased from Fisher Scientific, Pittsburgh, PA.)

	1 L
Na_2HPO_4	1.42 g
NaH_2PO_4	1.38 g
NaCl	8.76 g

Dissolve the components in ~900 mL deionized water, pH to 7.2, and bring the volume to 1 L. After autoclaving, the solution may be stored at room temperature.
7. Lipofectin transfection reagent, a cationic lipid compound (Life Technologies) (*see* **Note 4**): This reagent should be stored at 4°C, where it has an extended shelf-life.
8. Small sterile polystyrene tubes. Four-milliliter snap-cap tubes work well for this purpose.

2.3. Selection of Recombinant Viruses

1. Confluent 60-mm dishes of CV-1 cells, also pretreated with 1X MPA selection medium. For each transfection, six to eight dishes will be used, plus one for an uninfected control. These need to be seeded 1 or 2 d prior to usage.
2. Hypoxanthine stock solution, 10 mg/mL: Dissolve 0.1 g hypoxanthine (6-hydroxypurine, Sigma Chemical Company, St. Louis, MO) in 10 mL deionized water, filter-sterilize with a 0.2-µm filter. Store at $-20°C$.

3. Xanthine stock solution, 5 mg/mL: Dissolve 0.5 g xanthine (2-6-Dihydroxypurine, Sigma Chemical Company) in ~90 mL 0.1 N NaOH. Adjust the pH of the solution to 10.5 using 0.1 N HCl, then bring the volume to 100 mL. Filter-sterilize with a 0.2-μm filter and store at room temperature in 10-mL aliquots.
4. Mycophenolic acid stock, 10 mg/mL: Dissolve 0.1 g MPA (6-[4-Hydroxy-6-meth-7-methyl-3-oxo-5-phthalanyl]-4-methyl-4-hexenoic acid, Sigma Chemical Company) in 10 mL of 95% EtOH. Filter-sterilize with a 0.2-μm filter and store at room temperature.
5. 2X MEM: Purchase a 1-L packet of powdered Eagle's MEM with Earle's salts, and make it into 500 mL of 2X medium. Dissolve the powder in ~475 mL of deionized water, and add 2.2 g $NaHCO_3$ (the solution will change from a yellowish to red color). Bring the volume to 500 mL, and pH to 7.1–7.2 with 1 N NaOH or 1 N HCl as necessary. Filter-sterilize through a 0.2-μm filter, and supplement with 4 mM glutamine, 100 units penicillin, 100 μg streptomycin, 2 mM nonessential amino acids and 2 mM pyruvate/mL (twice the usual concentrations) and 5% FBS. Store the completed medium at 4°C, where it will have the same shelf-life as standard 1X medium.
6. 1X MPA selection medium: (15 μg/mL hypoxanthine, 250 μg/mL xanthine, 25 μg/mL MPA):

	100 mL
1X MEM containing FBS and supplements	95 mL
10 mg/mL hypoxanthine solution	150 μL
5 mg/mL xanthine solution	5 mL
10 mg/mL mycophenolic acid solution	250 μL

For best results, this medium should be assembled immediately before use.
7. 2X MPA selection medium (30 μg/mL hypoxanthine, 500 μg/mL xanthine, 50 μg/mL MPA):

	50 mL
2X MEM containing FBS and supplements	45 mL
10 mg/mL hypoxanthine solution	150 μL
5 mg/mL xanthine solution	5 mL
10 mg/mL mycophenolic acid solution	250 μL

For best results, this medium should also be made fresh immediately before use.
8. 2% SeaKem LE agarose (FMC BioProducts, Rockland, ME): Measure out 2 g of agarose, and place it in an autoclavable bottle. Add 100 mL deionized water, and autoclave. This may be prepared ahead of time and stored capped for months at room temperature. To use, simply microwave the bottle to melt the agarose.
9. Neutral red solution (Life Technologies).

3. Methods

3.1. Plasmid Construction

The optimum method for cloning the desired HCV coding region into the VV shuttle plasmid will depend on the plasmid insertion vector chosen. Most likely the cloning will require amplification by polymerase chain reaction to place the required restriction sites at the termini; these will vary with the shuttle plasmid. Three important points to consider are:

1. Once cloned, any region generated by polymerase chain reaction should be either sequenced or tested for function to exclude the possibility of *Taq*-induced point mutations that may affect gene function.
2. If you are planning to clone the HCV coding region under the control an early temporal class poxvirus promoter (the original reference for your plasmid should contain this information), the HCV insert must be checked for TTTTTNT motifs. This is the signal for termination of transcription of early poxvirus messages *(23–25)*, and its presence may prohibit generation of full-length RNA from your HCV insert. If present, the motif may be removed by mutagenesis; otherwise a late promoter should be used. Late genes do not use a discrete termination signal.
3. If you are instead going to be cloning your fragment under the control of a promoter from the late temporal class, the reading frame must be in frame with the TAAATG motif of the promoter, since translation of the message will begin at this ATG *(26,27)*. (For further information, *see* **ref. 8**).

3.2. Transfection and Generation of Recombinant Viruses

1. One to 2 d prior to doing the transfection, prepare monolayers of CV-1 cells in 60-mm dishes. They will need to be ~80% confluent on the day of transfection (*see* **Note 5**). Once the cells are nearly to the proper density, remove the medium, and replace with 1X MPA selection medium and incubate from overnight to up to 24 h prior to transfection. This pretreatment step depletes the intracellular GTP pool, permitting the effect of the *gpt* gene to be observed. The addition of the selection medium will generally halt any significant further cell division. You will need only 1 dish/transfection, plus a dish for an uninfected control if desired.
2. Calculate the volume of wild-type VV stock that will be needed for each 60-mm dish, using a multiplicity of infection (MOI) of 0.05–0.1 plaque-forming units (PFU)/cell and an infection volume of 0.5 mL. Assuming ~5×10^6 cells for a confluent monolayer, this would mean 2×10^5 PFU at a MOI of 0.05 and 4×10^5 at 0.1. This will require making a dilution series of the virus stock in virus diluent.
3. Thaw the virus stock (brief thawing at 37°C is acceptable) and place it in ice. Sonicate the virus in a water bath sonicator for 30–60 s, then quickly return the tube to ice. After 4–5 minutes on ice, resonicate the virus. (*see* **Note 6**). The dilutions can now be made. Once diluted, the virus will not require resonication.
4. Label the dishes to be transfected, and rinse the monolayers once with warm PBS, using 2–3 mL/dish. Remove the PBS, and replace with the 0.5 mL of inoculum.
5. Allow the virus to adsorb to the cells by incubating at 37°C in a 5% CO_2 incubator for 1 h. Rock the dishes after 30 min both to evenly distribute the virus and to keep the cells moist.
6. During this adsorption period, separately dilute the DNA and Lipofectin reagent in polystyrene tubes (*see* **Note 7**). You may use either sterile water or virus diluent for this. For each 60-mm dish, dilute 10 µg of plasmid DNA to a volume

of 50 μL and 30 μg Lipofectin (30 μL) to 50 μL. Once the two components have been separately diluted, combine them into one tube, and mix by gently flicking the tube (vortexing is not recommended). Let the complex form for at least 15 min at room temperature (*see* **Note 8**).
7. Once the viral adsorption is complete, remove the inoculum, and rinse the monolayers twice with warm diluent. Place 3–4 mL of 1X MPA selection medium containing 5% FBS into each dish (*see* **Notes 9** and **10**).
8. Add the Lipofectin/DNA complex to the cells dropwise while gently swirling the dish. Incubate an additional 48 h at 37°C. After this time any attached cells remaining will be harvested by scraping them into the medium and collecting everything.

3.3. Selection of Recombinant Viruses

1. Lyse any intact cells in the transfection harvest by three rounds of freeze-thawing. For the sake of speed, it is easiest to freeze the tubes in a dry ice bath and thaw at 37°C.
2. Vortex the transfection harvest well, and prepare serial 10-fold dilutions in virus diluent, assuming 0.5 mL/dish. At least for the first use of this method, make dilutions from 10^{-1} to 10^{-5} (this may be cut back once the approximate efficiency of recombination has been determined). It is also a good idea to prepare duplicate plates of each dilution.
3. Label the pretreated 60-mm dishes, and wash the CV-1 monolayers once with PBS. Plate 0.5 mL of the dilutions on the rinsed dishes, and adsorb for 1 h with rocking, as done for the transfection.
4. During the adsorption, melt the 2% agarose solution, and place it in a 45°–50°C bath. Also warm the 2X selection medium in a 37°C bath to remove the refrigerator chill.
5. After the incubation period, remove the inoculum, and overlay the monolayers with 5 mL virus overlay/dish. The overlay is made by simply mixing equal proportions of warmed 2X selection medium with liquid 2% agarose (*see* **Notes 11** and **12**). Add the overlay to the plate by gently running it down the inside wall of the dish. Let the agarose overlay solidify in the hood and then place the dishes back in the incubator.
6. After 48 h of incubation, overlay the agarose with a solution of neutral red (Life Technologies) diluted 1:30 in 1X selection medium, and return the dishes to 37°C. The viral plaques should be visible after an overnight incubation. Staining with neutral red will not harm the virus.
7. Once plaques are visible (they will appear as colorless areas on a light red background), aspirate off the neutral red solution, and mark the locations of the plaques to be purified on the bottom of the dish. Use the wide end of a sterile Pasteur pipet to collect the agarose plug, and place it in a 1.5-mL microcentrifuge tube containing 0.5 mL 1X selection medium. Then use the tip of a 20λ pipet to scrape any cells remaining from the plaque off of the surface of the dish, and transfer them into the tube along with the agarose.

8. Freeze–thaw the purified plaques three times, and repeat the purification step. This time, dilutions of 10^{-1}–10^{-3} should cover the necessary range. After the second round, the plaques can be expanded and tested for expression of the desired HCV proteins (see **Note 1**).

4. Notes

1. Although it is not often noticed, there is one possible difficulty with this protocol: the selection is so powerful that it will select for all viral genomes that have incorporated the *gpt* gene. This means that the population of recombinants may contain both the desired virus with a stable integration resulting from a double-crossover event as well as those with unstable integrations subsequent to a single crossover. The latter set of viruses, though much less commonly seen, is highly volatile, since the single crossover leads to integration of the entire shuttle plasmid and a tandem repeat of the target gene. If selection pressure is removed, these will spontaneously resolve and may thereby delete the entire insertion, giving rise to wild-type virus. One round of plaque purification in the absence of MPA selection should permit these intermediates to resolve, so that only the stable *gpt*-containing recombinants will be able to form plaques. Even after this step, however, it is probably wise to confirm the structure of the recombinant viruses by polymerase chain reaction before generating any large stocks.
2. In 1995 there were two new methods described for making VV recombinants. The first, published by Blasco and Moss, uses a mutant virus having a deletion in the gene encoding vp37, a viral envelope protein *(29)*. This mutant is unable to form plaques on cell monolayers. It is used in conjunction with a shuttle plasmid that carries an intact copy of the VV vp37 gene as a marker, along with sites to clone in the desired foreign gene under the control of a VV promoter. After transfection, recombinants are simply isolated by their ability to form plaques. The second method, described by Pfleiderer et al, uses a specially modified virus genome, which contains two unique restriction sites engineered into its sequence *(30)*. The target gene of interest is amplified by polymerase chain reaction to be flanked by these two sites and is directionally cloned into the mutant genome, thereby placing it under the control of a VV promoter. This eliminates construction of plasmid intermediates and facilitates screening of the recombinants. Although both of these methods are simple and well-designed, they may not be as versatile as the *Eco gpt* method of selection described in this chapter. The first requires a special virus strain, which may be difficult for a novice to titer and work with, and the second requires the VV genomic clone generated by Pfleiderer et al. Although second-generation plasmids may be constructed for the Blasco and Moss method to target insertions into any desired site in the viral genome *(26)*, Pfleiderer et al.'s method can only target insertions to the one specific engineered site. In addition, neither of these methods allows the sequential insertion of a second foreign gene into an existing recombinant virus. In truth, each of these three basic methods for creation of VV recombinants has its own advantages and disadvantages. Therefore, individual investigators should choose the method that best suits the needs and technical expertise of their laboratory.

3. For this purpose, the DNA does not have to be exceptionally clean, so standard alkaline lysis protocols followed by phenol/chloroform/isoamyl alcohol (25:24:1) extraction and ethanol precipitation are sufficient. It is, however, prudent to prepare plasmid DNA from 100-mL rather than 1.5-mL cultures for two reasons. First, a fair amount of plasmid DNA (10 µg) is used for transfection of each 60-mm dish. Second, these larger cultures usually result in a higher final DNA concentration, so less of any possible contaminants in the DNA are taken with each 10-µg aliquot.
4. Transfection of VV-infected cells generally has an extremely high efficiency (at least 90%, using Lipofectin) as measured by production of a plasmid-encoded β-galactosidase reporter protein. Therefore, virtually any transfection product, from calcium chloride to the most expensive commercial compound, can be substituted.
5. Cells transfect more efficiently if actively growing, but the MPA treatment will prevent further cell division once it is put onto the cells. Therefore, 80% confluence is a compromise between the needs for active growth and for a sufficient number of cells to infect.
6. Since most crude stocks of VV contain large amounts of cellular debris, sonication is recommended to break up any large clumps of virus that may form. However, the cavitation produced by sonication generates localized heat, so the virus should be thoroughly chilled on ice. Sonication is generally believed to be effective for approx 1 h, after which it is recommended to repeat the procedure.
7. The reagents must be diluted in polystyrene tubes, because the Lipofectin reagent tends to stick to polypropylene.
8. Occasionally the Lipofectin/DNA mixture will become cloudy after combining the two solutions, but there should be no visible precipitate. If a precipitate does form, it will be necessary to reprepare the solution by separately diluting the same amount of Lipofectin and DNA in virus diluent, in double to triple the previous volume. For osmolality reasons, it is better to use virus diluent medium than water in this situation.
9. Gibco states that Lipofectin may increase the permeability of the cells to antibiotics, so the company suggests that the transfection be done in the absence of penicillin and streptomycin. However, the author has not personally found the presence of the antibiotics to be a problem and prefers to include them in her medium.
10. According to the manufacturer's recommendations, the transfection may be done in the presence of serum as long as the Lipofectin/DNA complexes are formed in its absence.
11. This step will involve purifying individual plaques. To maintain discrete, isolated plaques, the dishes are overlaid with a 1% final agarose solution, in selection medium. Because the medium cannot be boiled, the agarose and medium are made separately at 2X concentration and mixed together just prior to usage. By keeping the solution at an elevated temperature, the agarose can be kept liquid until it is applied to the dishes.

12. It is important that the overlay solution be at the correct temperature for this step to work. If the solution is too hot, it can kill the monolayer. However, if it is too cool, the agarose may solidify before the overlays are completed. It is therefore best to work only with a limited number of dishes at one time (≤10 as a start), leaving the rest at 37°C until the previous set is done. The temperature of the solution is acceptable if a drop of the overlay can be dripped onto your wrist without feeling noticeably warm.

References

1. Lanford, R. E., Sureau, C., Jacob, J. R., White, R., and Fuerst, T. R. (1994) Demonstration of in vitro infection of chimpanzee hepatocytes with hepatitis C virus using strand-specific RT/PCR. *Virology* **202,** 606–614.
2. Mizutani, T., Kato, N., Saito, S., Ikeda, M., Sugiyama, K., and Shimotohno, K. (1996) Characterization of hepatitis C virus replication in cloned cells obtained from a human T-cell leukemia virus type 1-infected cell line, MT-2. *J. Virol.* **70,** 7219–7223.
3. Moss, B., Winters, E., and Cooper, J. A. (1981) Deletion of a 9000 base pair segment of the vaccinia genome that codes for nonessential polypeptides. *J. Virol.* **40,** 387–395.
4. Smith, G. L. and Moss, B. (1983) Infectious poxvirus vectors have capacity for at least 25,000 base pairs of foreign DNA. *Gene* **25,** 21–28.
5. Puckett, C. and Moss, B. (1983) Selective transcription of vaccinia virus genes in template dependent soluble extracts of infected cells. *Cell* **35,** 441–448.
6. Nakano, E., Panicali, D., and Paoletti, E. (1982) Molecular genetics of vaccinia virus: demonstration of marker rescue. *Proc. Natl. Acad. Sci. USA* **79,** 1593–1596.
7. Smith, G. L. and Moss, B. (1984) Vaccinia virus expression vectors: construction, properties and applications. *Biotechniques* **2,** 306–312.
8. Mackett, M., Smith, G. L., and Moss, B. (1985) The construction and characterization of vaccinia virus recombinants expressing foreign genes, in *DNA Cloning: A Practical Approach* (Glover, D. M., ed.), IRL, Oxford, UK, pp. 191–211.
9. Mackett, M., Smith, G. L., and Moss, B. (1982) Vaccinia virus: a selectable eukaryotic cloning and expression vector. *Proc. Natl. Acad. Sci. USA* **79,** 7415–7419.
10. Panicali, D. and Paoletti, E. (1982) Construction of poxviruses as cloning vectors: insertion of the thymidine kinase gene from herpes simplex virus into the DNA of infectious vaccinia virus. *Proc. Natl. Acad. Sci. USA* **79,** 4927–4931.
11. Perkus, M. E., Piccini, A., Lipinskas, B. R., and Paoletti, E. (1985) Recombinant vaccinia virus: immunization against multiple pathogens. *Science* **229,** 981–984.
12. Miller, R. L., Ramsey, G. A., Krenitsky, T. H., and Elion, G. B. (1972) Guanine phosphoribosyltransferase from *Escherichia coli*, specificity and properties. *Biochemistry* **11,** 4723–4731.
13. Krenitsky, T. A., Papaioannou, R., and Elion, G. B. (1969) Human hypoxanthine phosphoribosyltransferase. I. Purification, properties, and specificity. *J. Biol. Chem.* **244,** 1263–1270.

14. Mulligan, R. C. and Berg, P. (1980) Expression of a bacterial gene in mammalian cells. *Science* **209**, 1422–1427.
15. Mulligan, R. C. and Berg, P. (1981) Selection for animal cells that express the *Escherichia coli* gene encoding for xanthine-guanine phosphoribosyltransferase. *Proc. Natl. Acad. Sci. USA* **78**, 2072–2076.
16. Franklin, T. J. and Cook, J. M. (1969) The inhibition of nucleic acid synthesis by mycophenolic acid. *Biochem. J.* **113**, 512–524.
17. Falkner, F. G. and Moss, B. (1988) *Escherichia coli gpt* gene provides dominant selection for vaccinia virus open reading frame expression vectors. *J. Virol.* **6**, 1849–1854.
18. Boyle, D. B. and Coupar, B. E. H. (1988) A dominant selectable marker for the construction of recombinant poxviruses. *Gene* **65**, 123–128.
19. Isaacs, S. N., Kotwal, G. J., and Moss, B. (1990) Reverse guanine phosphoribosyltransferase selection of recombinant vaccinia viruses. *Virology* **178**, 626–630.
20. Falkner, F. G. and Moss, B. (1990) Transient dominant selection of recombinant vaccinia viruses. *J. Virol.* **64**, 3108–3111.
21. Kurilla, M. G. (1997) Transient selection during vaccinia virus recombination with insertion vectors without selectable markers. *Biotechniques* **22**, 906–910.
22. Moss, B., Elroy-Stein, O., Mizukami, T., Alexander, A., and Fuerst, T. R. (1990) Product review. New mammalian expression vectors. *Nature* **348**, 91,92.
23. Yuen, L. and Moss, B. (1986) Multiple 3' ends of mRNA encoding vaccinia virus growth factor occur within a series of repeated sequences downstream of T clusters. *J. Virol.* **60**, 320–323.
24. Yuen, L. and Moss, B. (1987). Oligonucleotide sequence signaling transcriptional termination of vaccinia virus early genes. *Proc. Natl. Acad. Sci. USA* **84**, 6417–6421.
25. Upton, C., DeLange, A. M., and McFadden, G. (1987) Tumorigenic poxviruses: genomic organization and DNA sequence of the Shope fibroma virus genome. *Virology* **187**, 20–30.
26. Hänggi, M., Bannwarth, W., and Stunnenberg, H. G. (1986) Conserved TAAAT motif in vaccinia virus late promoters: overlapping TATA box and the site of transcription initiation. *EMBO J.* **5**, 1071–1076.
27. Rosel, J. L., Earl, P. L., Weir, J. P., and Moss, B. (1986) Conserved TAAATG sequence at the transcriptional and translational initiation sites of vaccinia virus late genes deduced by structural and functional analysis of the HindIII H genome fragment. *J. Virol.* **60**, 436–449.
28. Moss, B. (1990) Poxviridae and their replication, in *Virology* (Felds, B. N., Knipe, D. M., Chanock, R. M., Hirsch, M. S., Melnick, J. L., Monath, T. P., and Roizman, B., eds.), Raven, New York, pp. 2079–2111.
29. Blasco, R. and Moss, B. (1995) Selection of recombinant vaccinia viruses on the basis of plaque formation. *Gene* **158**, 157–162.
30. Pfleiderer, M., Falkner, F. G., and Dorner, F. (1995) A novel vaccinia virus expression system allowing construction of recombinants without the need for selection markers, plasmids and bacterial hosts. *J. Gen. Virol.* **76**, 2957–2962.

50

Construction of Recombinant Adeno-Associated Virus (AAV)

Markus Reiser and Sergei Zolotukhin

1. Introduction

Efficient and stable transfer of foreign DNA into cells both in vitro and in vivo has become a powerful tool in the study of the pathogeneses of various diseases, such as cancer and infectious diseases. The study of hepatitis C virus (HCV) pathogenesis has been hampered by the lack of an easily available animal model or in vitro replication system. A new approach to the establishment of an HCV model are cell-culture systems stably expressing viral genes.

Recombinant adeno-associated viral (rAAV) vectors are powerful gene delivery tools, which are capable of transducing a wide variety of human cells, including quiescent cells *(1,2)*. AAV is a single-stranded DNA virus that belongs to the family of parvoviridae. AAV is characterized by its high viability, the potential for site-specific intregration, and long-term expression of the delivered genes *(3–5)*. rAAVs are constructed by substituting the wild-type AAV genes with the target genes to be delivered (**Fig. 1**). Only the 145-bp-long noncoding AAV inverted-terminal repeats (iTR) flanking the construct originate from wild-type virus are necessary for replication, packaging, and integration of the delivered DNA construct (**Figs. 1** and **2**). Constructs with sizes close to that of wild-type genome (4.7 kb) are most efficiently packaged into viral particles. Smaller constructs can still be packaged with good efficiency, but genomes larger than 5.2 kb are not suitable for constructing rAAV *(6,7)*. Since the the AAV backbone we use for constructing rAAV already contains the neomycin resistance gene, which allows for the positive selection of stably transduced cells, target genes of up to 2 kb can be cloned into this construct (**Fig. 1**).

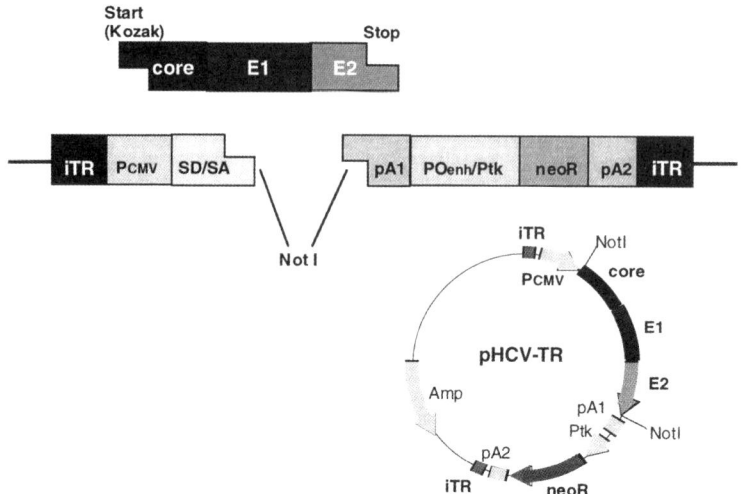

Fig. 1. Recombinant AAV expression cassette and plasmid-pHCV-TR. The target genes (HCV structural genes) were cloned into the *Not*I restriction site of the AAV expression cassette. iTR: adeno-associated virus (AAV) inverted terminal repeat; facilitates packaging and integration of recombinant AAV. PCMV: CMV early promoter/enhancer. pA1: SV40 polyadenylation signal. pTK: PYF441 polyoma enhancer/HSV-TK promotor. neoR: neomycin resistance gene. pA2: bovine growth hormon polyadenylation signal.

2. Materials
2.1. Plasmids and Cell Culture

1. Plasmid pTR-UF, used to clone the target gene into the AAV expression cassette (*see* **Fig. 1**), and plasmid pIM45, the AAV helper plasmid that contains the AAV genes, but no AAV iTRs (*see* **Note 1**).
2. Adenovirus Ad5 (as helper virus for packaging; *see* **Note 2**).
3. 293 cells (ATCC) of low passage number (<40).
4. Dulbecco's Modified Eagle's Medium, high glucose (Gibco-BRL) containing 25 mM HEPES pH 7.5, and pen/strep, supplemented with 10% bovine serum.
5. 0.05% Porcine trypsin/0.02% EDTA (for splitting cells).
6. Phosphate-buffered saline (PBS) w/o Mg^{2+} and Ca^{2+}.
7. 15-cm tissue-culture plates.
8. 2 M CaCl in H_2O, sterile filtered through a 0.22-μm filter, stored at –20°C.
9. 2X HEPES-buffered saline (HBS): 280 mM NaCl, 10 mM KCl, 1.5 mM Na_2HPO_4, 12 mM glucose, 50 mM HEPES, pH adjusted to 7.05 with 0.5 M NaOH; sterile filtered through a 0.22-μm filter, stored at –20°C.
10. 0.1X TE, pH 8.0: 1 mM Tris-HCl, 0.1 mM EDTA (pH 8.0); sterile filtered through a 0.22-μm filter, stored at 4°C.

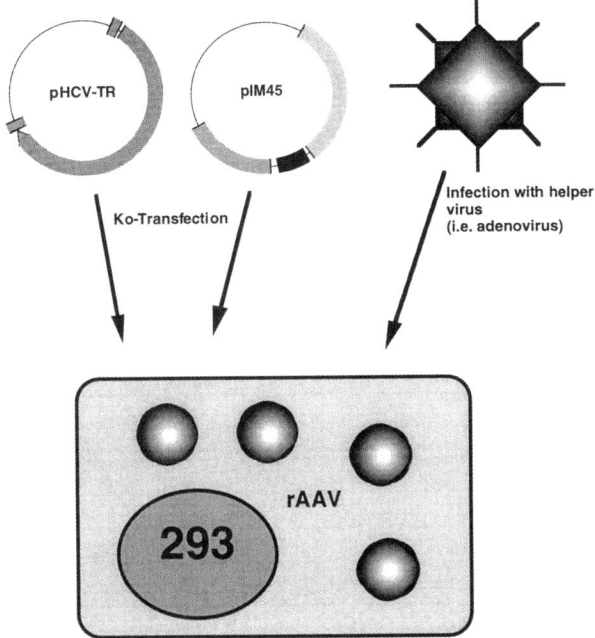

Fig. 2. Packaging of recombinant AAV expressing HCV structural genes. The recombinant AAV plasmid pHCV-TR containing AAV terminal repeats (*see* **Fig. 1**) and wild-type AAV plasmid pIM45 (no terminal repeats) are cotransfected into 293 cells. After infection with helper virus (adenovirus) the recombinant AAV cassette is rescued and packaged into AAV particles.

2.2. Purification of rAAV

1. Harvest buffer: 50 mM Tris-HCl, pH 8.4, 150 mM NaCl.
2. Ammonium sulfate ($[NH_4]_2SO_4$) solution, saturated at 4°C, pH 7.0.
3. CsCl 1.5 g/mL: 45.4 g CsCl in 54.6 mL PBS; sterile filtered through a 0.22-µm filter.
4. 15-mL and 50-mL sterile polypropylene tubes.
5. Ultracentrifuge: rotors SW28.1 and SW41 with tubes (Beckman) or equivalent.

2.3. Detection of rAAV

1. DNase I reaction mix: 50 mM Tris-HCl, pH 7.5, 10 mM MgCl$_2$, 0.1 U DNase I/µL.
2. PCR reaction mix: 10 mM Tris-HCl, pH 8.3; 50 mM KCl, 1.5 mM MgCl$_2$, 50 ng each of neoR specific primers: 5'-TATGGGATCGGCCATTGAAC-3'; 5'-CCTGATGCTCTTCGTCCAGA-3'; 1.25 U *Taq* polymerase.
3. Neutralization solution: 0.5 M Tris-HCl, pH 7.2, 1.5 M NaCl.
4. Church's hybridization buffer: 0.5 M NaHPO$_4$, pH 7.2, 7% SDS, 0.5 mM EDTA.
5. Proteinase K.
6. 10X proteinase K buffer: 100 mM Tris-HCl (pH 8.0), 100 mM EDTA (pH 8.0), 1% SDS.

7. 1X alkaline buffer: 0.4 M NaOH, 10 mM EDTA (pH 8.0).
8. Phenol/chloroform/isoamyl alcohol: 24:24:1 (pH 8.0).
9. 3 M Na-acetate, pH 7.0.
10. Glycogen (from mussels), 20 μg/μL.

3. Methods
3.1. Cell Culture and Transfection

1. At least 10 15-cm plates of 293 cells are needed for packaging AAV. Confluent 293 cells are split 1:3 to 1:4 the day before transfection. The cells should be healthy and 50–70% confluent for transfection.
2. Cells are transfected with a 1:2 ratio mixture of recombinant AAV/pIM45 plasmid (7 μg/15 μg of plasmid DNA/plate) by calcium phosphate coprecipitation.

    For 10 plates: 70 μg rAAV plasmid + 150 μg pIM45 helper plasmid are diluted into 8.8 mL (total volume) of 0.1X TE, pH 8.0, 10 mL of 2X HBS buffer are added. Under constant mixing (using air bubbled from an electric pipeting device) 1.25 mL of 2 M CaCl solution are added dropwise. A precipitate will form in 10–20 min (*see* **Note 2**). The precipitate is resuspended by pipeting up and down using a Pasteur pipet. Two milliliters of the DNA–calcium phosphate coprecipitate are added to each 15-cm dish of 293 cells.
3. Eight hours after transfection, the medium is replaced by fresh medium containing Ad5 at an MOI of 3 (*see* **Note 3**).

3.2. Purification of rAAV

1. CPE should develop in 3–4 d. Cells are harvested in media by washing the cells off the plate using an electic pipeting device. Cells are pelleted by spinning at 1000g at 4°C for 15 min, and the supernatant is discarded. The cell pellets can be stored at –20°C for up to 6 mo.
2. The cell pellet is resuspended in harvest buffer. Viral particles are released by freezing and thawing three times.
3. The cell debris is pelleted at 2000g at 4°C for 10 min, and the supernatant is saved.
4. The pellet is resuspended in 10 mL harvest buffer, and sonicated with 40 bursts at 50% duty, power 2 to release remaining virus.
5. The cell debris is pelleted again, and the supernatants are pooled (**steps 3** and **4**).
6. The adenovirus (helper virus) is inactivated at 56°C for 15 min (*see* **Note 4**). After cooling down on ice, the newly formed precipitate is pelleted at 2500g at 4°C for 10 min. The supernatant is saved for further processing.
7. One-third volume of ammonium sulfate solution is added dropwise to the supernatant. This solution is mixed and incubated on ice for 30 min.
8. The precipitated proteins are pelleted at 20,000 rpm at 4°C for 20 min in an SW 28.1 (Beckman) or equivalent swing-out rotor. The viral particles remain in the supernatant.
9. Two-thirds volume of ammonium sulfate solution is added to the supernatant. After mixing and incubating on ice for 30 min, the viral particles are pelleted by spinning as described in **step 8**.

10. The newly formed pellet is resuspended in 9 mL of PBS.
11. 5.5 g of solid CsCl are added and dissolved. The solution is transferred into an ultraclear centrifuge tube (Beckman or equivalent), underlaid with 1 mL CsCl solution of 1.5 g/mL density and centrifuged in a SW41 Beckman (or equivalent) rotor at 41,000 rpm at 18°C for 48 h.
12. A continuous gradient will form, which is fractionated by dripping approx 0.6 mL fractions from the bottom (*see* **Note 5**).

3.3. Detection of rAAV

1. One microliter of each fraction is transferred into a separate tube containing 100 µL of DNase I reaction mix. After incubating at 37°C for 1 h, 1 µL from each tube is transferred into a PCR reaction tube containing 50 µL of PCR reaction mix. Cycling conditions are: 92°C for 40 s; 60°C for 40 s; 72°C for 1 min, 30 s; 30 cycles. Fifteen microliters of amplified product are subjected to electrophoresis in a 1% agarose gel.
2. Positive fractions are pooled; the virus is concentrated by spinning in Centricon-30 at 4000g at 4°C for 30 min.
3. The concentrated viral stock is dialyzed by dilution with 5 vol of PBS and centrifugation as described in **step 2**. Several rounds of dilution–concentration are performed to eliminate the residual CsCl.
4. To estimate the functional titer of the rAAV stock, target cells can be infected in 3.5-cm dishes (20–30% confluent) with 0.001 µL–1 µL of virus stock (use serial dilutions). Cells are replated into a 10-cm dish when about 80% confluent, and selection is begun with geneticin (G418). Single G418 resistant cell clones will be visible within 2 wk of selection (*see* **Note 6**).

3.4. Quantitation of Total AAV Particles (i.e., Infectious and Defective Particles) Can Be Performed by PCR Assay (see Note 7)

1. One microliter virus sample is incubated in 100 µL DNase I reaction mix for 1 h at 37°C.
2. Ten microliters of 10X proteinase K buffer are added to inactivate DNase I. One microliter of proteinase K (18.6 g/L) is then added and the reaction is incubated for 1 h at 37°C.
3. The reaction mixture is extracted twice with 100 µL phenol/chloroform solution and once with 100 µL chloroform. The aqueous (upper) phase is transferred into a fresh Eppendorf tube.
4. The viral DNA is then precipitated with 10 µL of 3 M Na-acetate, 1 µL glycogen, and 250 µL EtOH at –80°C for 30 min.
5. The viral DNA is pelleted at 12,000g (table centrifuge, top speed), 4°C for 5 min. The pellet is washed with 70% EtOH, dried, and resuspended in 100 µL H_2O.
6. PCR is performed with serial dilutions of viral DNA (from previous step) side by side with serial dilutions of standard plasmid DNA template (rAAV plasmid used to package the virus) of known concentration. PCR conditions are as described in **Subheading 3.3.**

4. Notes

1. The AAV iTRs are unstable in recombination compentent *Escherichea coli* and can be deleted when constructs are grown in these cells. Use SURE cells (which are recombination defective) to grow rAAV plasmids. Highest transformation efficiencies are obtained with plasmid DNA purified by equilibrium centrifugation in CsCl-ethidium bromide density gradients.
2. The optimal time for the DNA coprecipitate to form will be different for each HBS buffer. Optimize by transfecting a reporter plasmid, e.g., pTR-UF, which contains the green fluorescence protein (gfp) gene. Expression of gfp can conveniently be monitored using a fluorescence cell microscope (excitation at 450 ± 25 nm[6]).
3. An MOI of 3 means that 3 infectious adenoviral particles are applied/cell. A 15-cm cell-culture dish, 50–70% confluent, contains approx 1.5–2.0×10^7 cells.
4. Heating will inactivate any contaminating adenovirus (helper virus). However, the rAAV titer will also decrease during this heating step.
5. This is best done by gently clamping the tube into a stand, sealing the tube with parafilm, and then carfully drilling a whole into the bottom of the tube using a 21-gage needle.
6. Selection for G418 resistant clones also gives information on the functional titer of the rAAV stock for the cell line used. Since the infective potential may vary between different cell lines, titers of different rAAV stocks can only be compared with regard to the particular cell line used.
7. One nanogram of DNA = 1×10^{12} DNA bases = 2×10^8 copies of 5 kb ssDNA.

References

1. Muzyczka, N. (1992) Use of adeno-associated virus as a general transduction vector for mammalian cells. *Curr. Topics Microbiol. Immunol.* **158,** 97–129.
2. Flotte, T. R. and Carter, B. J. (1995) Adeno-associated virus vectors for gene therapy. *Gene Ther.* **2,** 357–362.
3. Flotte, T. R., Afione, S. A., Conrad, C., McGrath, S. A., Solow, R., Oka, H., et al. (1993) Stable in vivo expression of the cystic fibrosis transmembrane conductance regulator with an adeno-associated virus vector. *Proc. Natl. Acad. Sci. USA* **90,** 10,613–10,617.
4. Kaplitt, M. G., Leone, P., Samulski, R. J., Xiao, X., Pfaff, D. W., O'Malley, K. L. et al. (1994) Long-term gene expression and phenotypic correction using adeno-associated virus vectors in the mammalian brain. *Nature Genet.* **8,** 148–154.
5. Urcelay, E., Ward, P., Wiener, S. M., Safer, B., and Kotin, R. M. (1995) Asymmetric replication in vitro from a human sequence element is dependent on adeno-associated viurs Rep protein. *J. Virol.* **69 (4),** 2038–2046.
6. Zolotukhin, S., Potter, M., Hauswirth, W. W., Guy, J., and Muzyczka, N. (1996) A "humanized" green fluorescent protein cDNA adapted for high-level expression in mammalian cells. *J. Virol.* **70 (7),** 4646–4654.
7. Reiser, M., Neumann, I., Schmiegel, W., and Lau, J. Y. N. (1997) Stable epression of hepatitis C viurs structural genes in mammalian cells—viral vs constitutional promoters [Abstract]. *Dig. Dis. Week* **5/97,** Washington, DC. *Gastroenterology* **112,** A1365.

51

Production of Replication-Deficient Adenovirus Recombinants

Gavin W. G. Wilkinson, Carole Rickards, and Berwyn E. Clarke

1. Introduction

In essence, replication-deficient (RD) adenovirus (Ad) vectors can be considered to function as an extremely efficient DNA transfection system capable of providing transgene expression in up to 100% of cells both in vitro or in vivo. As researchers continue to realize the full potential of this vector system, discover novel applications, and further develop and enhance systems, the use of this vector system has increased exponentially. The exploitation of Ad recombinants in HCV research is encouraged by demonstration that the virus will efficiently infect and express transgenes in hepatocytes and that following iv inoculation, transgene expression can readily be detected in hepatocytes in the liver *(1–5)*. A number of HCV proteins have now been expressed in Ad recombinants *(6–8)* whereas these vectors have also been used to deliver antisense and ribozyme molecules as prototype HCV therapeutics *(9)*.

RDAd vectors have a deletion in the E1 region of the viral genome. The E1 gene performs an essential function in that its expression is required to activate all early (E2-E4) and late-phase Ad transcription (**Fig. 1**). Although essential for virus replication, Ad E1 deletion mutants can be propagated on helper cell lines, which constitutively express an E1 helper function *in trans* (e.g., 293 cells). The principle behind the vector lies in the fact that when an RDAd vector infects a target cell (without the E1 helper function), the viral genome is delivered efficiently to the nucleus, but Ad gene expression is not activated. However, if a transgene is inserted into an Ad E1- vector under the control of a constitutive or inducible promoter, expression of the transgene alone will be achieved in the target cell. Thus, in the target cell, there can be efficient

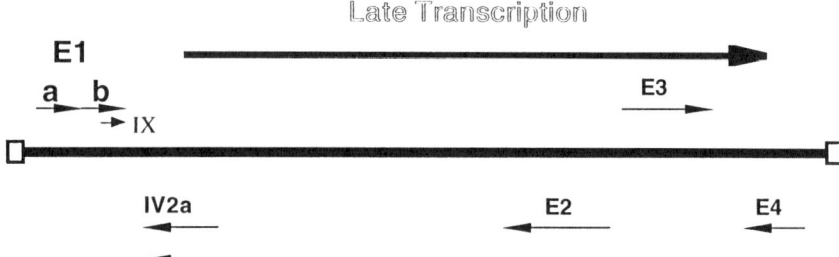

Fig. 1. Simplified transcriptional map of the adenovirus genome (~36 kbp). Each of the transcriptional units illustrated utilize alternative splicing to generate an extremely complex pattern of gene expression *(10)*. The E1 gene region is expressed immediately following infection and is responsible for activating further early phase transcription (E2-E4) with abundant late phase transcription from the major late promoter follows replication of the virus genome. Replication-deficient Ad vectors carry deletion in the E1 gene region of up to 3180bp. Original vectors based on Ad5 dl309 have a small deletion/substitution in the E3 gene region *(26)*. Deletion of the complete E3 gene region (up to 3132 bp) in recent vectors allows up to 8kb to be inserted into standard Ad5 vectors *(25)*.

expression of the transgene in the absence of any significant expression from the Ad genome.

Adenovirus is a relatively straightforward virus to work with in the laboratory and its molecular biology has been studied extensively (reviewed by Shenk *[10]*).The Ad replication cycle is <48 h with a single cell capable of yielding on the order of 10^5 virus particles. High-titer stocks of recombinant virus (10^8–10^{11} PFU/mL) can readily be produced from cell extracts, whereas further purification and concentration of virus can be achieved by CsCl gradient centrifugation. The level of transgene expression can be controlled by (1) gene dosage, i.e., the number of viruses infecting the target cell, and (2) promoter selection. When the strong constitutive CMV major IE promoter is used, transgene expression can constitute as much as 25% of total protein, i.e., levels of expression can rival those obtained using replication-competent baculovirus vectors *(11–13)*. The Rous sarcoma virus (RSV) LTR and the weaker SV40 promoters have also been used extensively in Ad vectors.

This chapter will describe a straightforward method for producing a first-generation RDAd recombinant, which involves two steps: (1) the cloning of a transgene into a transfer vector and (2) cotransfection of the transfer vector (containing appropriate insert) and a plasmid containing the entire Ad type 5 genome into 293 cells. Homologous recombination between the two plasmids results in the generation of the recombinant. This method was first described by McGrory et al. *(14)*, and has as a major advantage that the vectors are available from a commercial supplier (Microbix). These vectors permit insertions of DNA fragments up to ~8 kbp in either the E1 or E3 gene regions. The E3 region encode genes important for efficient Ad infection in vivo (e.g., down regulation of cellular MHC-I), but dispensable for replication in vitro and most Ad vectors have deletions of part, or all, of E3. However, when generating RDAd recombinants, insertion of the transgene at the E1 locus is considered preferable: (1) if recombination/rescue of the E1 deletion were to occur, then it would tend to eliminate the transgene and (2) it will avoid the transgene sequences being expressed as part Ad late transcriptional unit (**Fig. 1**).

Second-generation vectors have been constructed in which not only the E1 gene, but other regions of the virus (e.g., E2a, E4 protein IX) have been removed to make vectors more disabled and deletion of these additional sequences has been found to reduce the potential for breakthrough to Ad early/late-phase gene expression *(3,4,15)*. The ideal situation is to remove all potential Ad protein-coding sequences (third-generation vectors), and such strategies are being developed *(16)*. Additionally, it is possible to use cell-specific promoters to restrict the range of cells in which the transgene can be expressed *(17)* or, more recently, to modify the fiber protein to alter the virus tropism toward specific cell types *(18,19)*. For most purposes, however, the first-generation vectors are adequate and are certainly the most straightforward.

A variety of alternative technologies have been developed to facilitate the generation of Ad recombinants in addition to the method described here, e.g.:

1. By homologous recombination with DNA purified from virus particles *(20,21)*.
2. By homologous recombination in *Escherichia coli (22)*.
3. The exploitation of Cre-mediated excision to deplete Ad helper virus in a helper-dependent Ad vector system *(16)*.

Great care should be taken before construction of a recombinant virus to anticipate and avoid potential hazards to health and the environment and many countries have a statutory obligation for researchers to carry out this analysis. Adenoviruses are seldom associated with clinically important disease in immunocompetent individuals. There are at least 47 Ad serotypes that have been associated primarily with upper respiratory tract infection (a significant cause of the common cold) and keratinoconjunctivitis, although certain serotypes are associated with enteric infection and can be a significant cause of gastroenteritis. The serotypes most commonly used in vector construction (Ad2 and Ad5) are associated with upper respiratory tract infections, predominantly in childhood. Although deletion of the E1 gene region does disable the vector, the potential still exists for the deletion to be rescued from the helper cell line *(23)* or from wt Ad in the environment. To avoid the former possibility, vector systems/helper cell lines are being designed to minimize the potential for rescue *(24)*. The fact that RDAd vectors are so powerful, particularly as vehicles for in vivo gene delivery, does have safety implications. Virus stocks are typically of extremely high titer and can efficiently infect human cells following direct contact or by aerosol transmission. Levels of expression in vivo can be extremely high. The biological consequences of in vivo expression of the cloned transgene should be assessed in advance so that appropriate precautions can be taken. Although RDAd vectors are normally associated with transient expression, the virus genome is known to integrate into the target cell genome, although at low efficiency, and may thus be maintained in daughter cells. This aspect is a particular problem when considering the insertion of potential oncogenes into an RD Ad vector. Although there is currently no direct evidence for any oncogenic potential from HCV, the lack of an efficient in vitro culture system to prove this unequivocally means that the generation of AdHCV should be approached with caution.

2. Materials

1. Plasmids: Plasmids for the construction of adenovirus recombinants can be obtained from: Microbix Biosystems Inc., 341 Bering Avenue, Toronto, Ontario, Canada. Tel: 416-234-1624; Fax: 416-234-1626.

    Clearly, the range of plasmids available is liable to change with time. Currently, Kit A is designed for the insertion of plasmids into the E1 gene region of Ad5 and contains the plasmids: pΔE1sp1A, pΔE1sp1B, pFG140, and pJM17 (*see* **Notes 1–3**). The gene of interest must first be inserted into the transfer vector pΔE1sp1A. pΔE1sp1A is a prokaryotic vector containing Ad 5 sequences 1–341, a polylinker with potential cloning sites to insert the transgene followed by Ad sequences 3524–3520. Insertion into pΔE1sp1A is designed to flank the transgene with Ad 5 sequences from upstream and downstream of the E1 gene region, similar to the construct pMV79 (**Fig. 2**). pΔE1sp1B is identical pΔE1sp1A, except the polylinker is in the opposite orientation *(25)*. Additional transfer vectors are available that allow transgenes to be inserted under the control of the HCMV major IE promoter (e.g., pCA3, pCA4) *(25)*. The plasmid pJM17 contains the entire genome of Ad5*dl*1309 with the prokaryotic vector pBRX inserted in the E1 gene region. region. Ad5*dl*1309 also has a small characterized deletion in E3 gene region *(26)*. In order to express transgenes larger than 5 kb it is necessary to recombine into a recipient Ad genome in which both the E1 and E3 genes are deleted, provided by the bacterial plasmids pBHG11 *(25)*. Microbix also provides an infectious Ad5 plasmid (pFG140) as a positive control for transfection.

2. Cells: RDAd recombinants must be generated and propagated on a cell line expressing an E1 gene helper function. Two hundred ninety-three cells were generated from human embryo kidney cells transformed with sonicated Ad5 DNA *(27)* and are available from Microbix Biosystems Inc. (cat. no. PD-02-01), the European Centre for Animal Cell Cultures (ECACC cat. no. 92052131), or ATCC

(cat. no. CRL 2573). Two hundred ninety-three cells grow rapidly in Minimal Eagle's Medium (MEM) supplemented with 8% fetal calf sera, and monolayers can be split routinely at ratios up to 1:10. Two hundred ninety-three cells do not adhere strongly to surfaces and are very sensitive to overtrypsinization. Monolayers will tend to form clumps, which are difficult to disperse if allowed to overgrow.

3. TEP buffer: DNA is dissolved in a very dilute buffer (TEP), so that its pH does not unduly affect that of the final transfection mix. TEP buffer is generated by adding 100 µL of 1 M Tris-HCl, pH 7.5, and 10 µL of 0.5 M EDTA, pH 8.0, and making up to a final volume of 100 mL with autoclaved deionized H_2O.
4. 2 M $CaCl_2$ (Analar grade, BDH).
5. 2X HBS buffer (5.6 mL 5 M NaCl; 50 mM HEPES; 0.75 mL 0.2 M Na_2HPO_4 made up to ~80 mL with H_2O, adjusted to pH 7.12 with 1 M NaOH before being made up to a final volume of 100 mL). The pH of the 2X HBS buffer is critical for efficient transfection. Additionally, the pH electrode must be washed well before use, especially if held in phosphate buffer. All transfection buffers should be made from the best-quality reagents available and filter-sterilized, rather than autoclaved, before use. Aliquots should be stored frozen at –70°C. Even then, the transfection efficiency will decrease gradually with time and fresh buffers should be made up at regular intervals—approx every 6 mo.
6. Trifluorocarbon Arklone P: this reagent is becoming more difficult to obtain, but is currently still available from the Basic Chemical Company, High Wycombe, UK (Manufacturer ICI).
7. CsCl solutions: 1.45 g/mL in 5 mM Tris-HCl, pH 7.8, 133 g/mL in 1 mM EDTA, and 5 mM Tris-HCl, pH 7.8.
8. 10 mM Tris-HCl, pH 7.8.

3. Methods
3.1. Cloning into Transfer Vector

In the initial cloning step, the transgene must be inserted into the transfer vector under the control of an appropriate promoter (*see* **Note 4**). In most instances, transgenes are expressed using their own start and stop codons. However, the expression of HCV-encoded using the Ad vector requires appropriate translational signals to be incorporated with the transgene. **Figure 2** describes the construction of RAd79, am RDAd recombinant encoding the HCVE2 gene. The E2 gene was initially generated by PCR so that it included an ATG start codon (added in the sense PCR primer), the E2 leader sequence (required for transport to the protein to the endoplasmic reticulum), and an appropriately located stop codon (added in the antisense PCR primer). This gene, under the control of the HCMV major IE promoter, was subcloned into an Ad transfer vector similar to pΔE1sp1A *(25)*. The transfer vector supplies the expression cassette with flanking sequence homology from either side of the Ad E1 gene

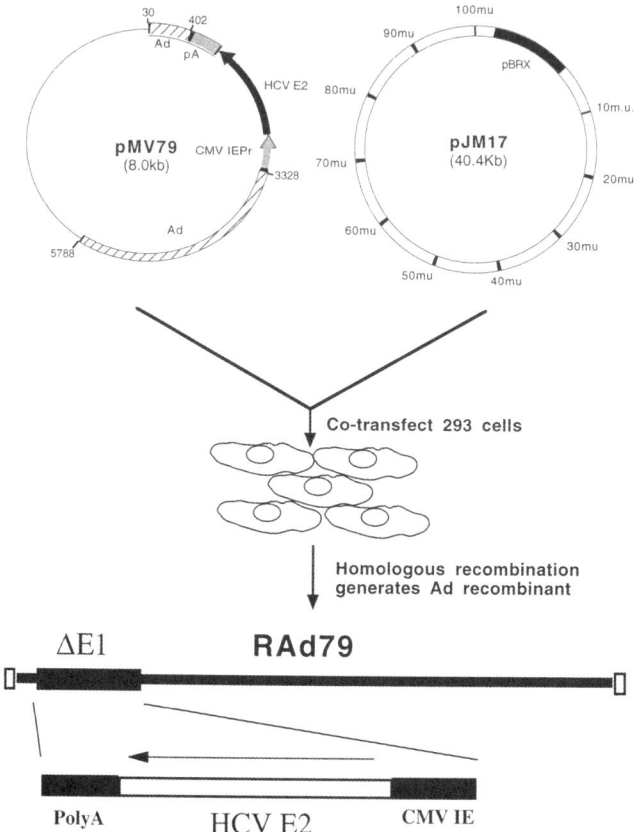

Fig. 2. Generation of an RDAd recombinant. In this example, HCV E2 sequences were amplified by PCR, with in-frame translational start and stop codons being added by incorporation into the PCR primers. The HCV E2 was cloned into the transfer vector under the control of the HCMV major IE promoter and with a downstream polyadenylation signal also derived from the HCMV major IE gene. The expression cassette was flanked with Ad sequences from upstream (30–402 bp) and downstream (3328–5788) of the E1 gene region. The plasmid pMV79 was cotransfected with pJM17 into 293 cells. pJM17 contains the entire Ad5 *dl*309 genome. Homologous recombination between the two plasmids generated an Ad recombinant in which the E1 gene region was replaced with the IEPr/E2 expression cassette to generate the recombinant virus RAd79.

region. The orientation of insertion into this vector will, in turn, control the orientation of insertion into the Ad genome. The orientation of the expression cassette in the E1 locus, however, does not significantly affect the level of expression.

3.2. Generation of Recombinant Virus

To generate a recombinant virus, the Ad transfer vector containing the expression cassette is cotransfected with pJM17 into 293 cells. Although pJM17 contains the complete Ad5 *dl*309 genome, the presence of additional prokaryotic vector sequences (pBRX inserted in E1) makes pJM17 DNA too large to package into Ad particles. Thus, transfection of pJM17 alone normally does not generate replicating virus. However, following homologous recombination, the E1 gene and prokaryotic sequences are replaced with the expression cassette, which reduces the overall size of the viral genome to one that can be efficiently packaged into the Ad particles (**Fig. 2**). A major feature of this system, designed by Graham and coworkers *(14,28)*, is that all the progeny of the transfection should theoretically contain the desired inserts; and this is normally the case in practice. Thus, although it is still necessary to confirm the identity of the recombinant, there is no need to screen for positive plaques (*see* **Note 5**).

1. 25-cm^2 tissue-culture flasks should be seeded with 293 cells the day before transfection (<40% confluency). Best transfection efficiencies are obtained when cells are evenly dispersed and virus plaques appear more rapidly in growing cells.
2. Ten micrograms of DNA (5 µg of transfer vector containing transgene + 5 µg pJM17) are dissolved in 210 µL of TEP buffer in a polypropylene Falcon tubes (12 × 75 mm).
3. Thirty microliters CaCl are added dropwise to DNA tube with vortexing. It aids transfection if vortexing is kept extremely vigorous.
4. DNA-CaCl$_2$ mixture is added dropwise to a second tube containing 240 µL of 2X HBS, again with vigorous vortexing.
5. The precipitate is allowed to form for 30 min.
6. Fresh media are added to the 293 cells in 25-cm^2 tissue-culture flasks. The transfection mixture is added directly the tissue-culture media on the 293 cells.
7. DNA is left on the cells for 16 h by which time a fine precipitate should be present on the cells when viewed using an inverted microscope. Cells are washed once with 5 mL PBS, once with 5 mL complete media, and then fresh media are added. The transfection process should not induce toxicity to the 293 cells.
8. Fresh media are added every 3 d or more frequently if necessary.
9. Plaques can be detected between 6 and 8 d and can be allowed to spread through the monolayer. Cultures should be retained and inspected for virus growth as long as the monolayer remains intact, since some recombinants can be slow-growing (*see* **Note 6**). All manipulations involving virus cultures are performed in an appropriate microbiological safety cabinet.
10. It is advisable to plaque-purify the recombinant (conventionally three times) to ensure that the virus stock is derived from a single entity.

3.3. Preparation of Virus Stock

By its nature, RDAd recombinants will not replicate in targets cells that do not contain a complementing E1 helper function. Because each target cell has to be infected with at least one virus particle to express the transgene, it is usually necessary to produce reasonably large stocks of virus.

Preparation of virus stocks requires the scale-up of 293 cells. Ad has no specific mechanism to lyse infected cells in vitro, and thus, the majority of virus remains cell-associated. Virus can be released by rupturing from cells by three rounds of freeze–thawing and then centrifugation of cell debris. However, we give details here of the method for generating a stock of virus partially purified by extraction with the fluorocarbon Arklone P. Where there is a need for highly purified virus, then stocks must be further purified by a CsCl gradient.

1. Routinely, 293 cells are grown up in 175-cm^2 flasks of 293 cells to 80% confluence. Two hundred ninety-three cells are difficult to grow on roller bottles, but can be grown on microcarriers and suspension cultures (less preferable) for extremely large-scale growth *(29)*. 293N3S cells have been adapted to grow in suspension *(30)*. Aspirate the media from the flasks and inoculate each with at a multiplicity of infection (MOI) of 0.1 or less in 25 mL of media or PBS. The inoculum is removed after 90 min, and fresh media added.
2. Media are replenished after 2 d and again whenever necessary. A clear cytopathic effect (CPE) will spread rapidly through the monolayer (*see* **Note 6**). Once 100% of the monolayer is exhibiting a gross CPE, cells will readily detach from the monolayer, and this can be assisted by tapping the flask gently. Infected cells are recovered by centrifugation at 500g for 5 min and the supernatant discarded. In case of leakage or tube failure, detachable centrifuge buckets with sealable caps should be used. Tubes should be removed from centrifuge buckets inside an appropriate microbiological safety cabinet. Discard the supernatant to approved disinfectant.
3. Cells can be stored at −70°C at this stage or resuspended in PBS at a concentration of 2×10^7 cells/mL. Add an equal volume of Arklone P to the cell suspensions, and mix vigorously. Centrifuge at 1000g for 5 min, and then remove the aqueous (top) phase. To maximize yields, the interface can be re-extracted with PBS. Virus can either be aliquoted immediately and used as a stock after titration, or further purified by CsCl gradient centrifugation before aliquoting into stocks (*see* **Notes 7** and **8**).

3.4. CsCl Purification of Virus

The virus stock prepared by Arklone P extraction is still relatively crude. Further purification from remaining cellular debris by centrifugation through cesium chloride gradient is required for many applications (*see* **Note 8**). Virus is extracted from the cells of at least 10×175 cm^2 flasks to ensure sufficient material to generate a visible band following centrifugation.

Adenovirus Recombinants

1. 1.6 mL of CsCl solution (1.45 g/mL) is first pipeted into 14 × 89 mm Ultra-Clear Beckman centrifuge tubes (cat. no. 344059) for an SW41 Ti rotor and then 3 mL of a less-dense CsCl solution (1.33 g/mL in 1 mM EDTA, 5 mM Tris-HCl, pH 7.8) and gently layered on top. The tube is then filled to 2.5 mm from the top with the aqueous phase of Arklone-P-extracted virus. Tubes are filled and loaded into an SW41 Ti rotor in a suitable microbiological safety cabinet.
2. Samples are centrifuged at 90,000g for 2 h at room temperature.
3. The virus appears an opalescent layer between the higher- and lower-density CsCl solutions. A second band higher up and resting on the top of the low-density CsCl solution is derived from cellular components. The virus is harvested in a suitable microbiological safety cabinet by puncturing the tube with a 19-gage needle and gently pulling the band into a 2-mL syringe.
4. The harvested virus is pooled together and diluted with equal volume of 10 mM Tris-HCl, pH 7.8.
5. The second round of centrifugation also uses the SW41 Ti Beckman rotor. Two milliliters of the high-density CsCl solution (1.45 g/L) are first pipeted into the 114 × 89 mm Ultra-Clear Beckman centrifuge tubes, and then 3 mL of the low-density CsCl solution (1.33 g/mL) are layered on top. Tubes are then filled to within 2.5 mm of the top with the diluted sample taken as the first CsCl gradient.
6. Samples are centrifuged for 16 h at 100,000g at room temperature. The virus again can be detected as an opalescent band at a density of 1.34–1.35 g/mL. The virus band is harvested puncturing the tube with a 19-gage needle and gently pulling the band into a 2 mL syringe.
7. The purified virus is then dialyzed against 1 mM MgCl$_2$, 135 mM NaCl, and 10 mM Tris, pH 7.8, containing 10% glycerol with two changes of buffer at 4 h periods.
8. Virus is aliquoted and stored at –70°C. Freeze–thawing of the Ad stock is to be avoided.

4. Notes
4.1. Plasmids

1. It is essential that plasmid DNA must be of good quality (pure) to provide efficient DNA transfection. Although DNA that has been twice purified by CsCl gradient centrifugation is recommended, good results have also been obtained using DNA purified in Qiagen affinity columns (Qiagen Inc., Chatsworth, MA).
2. The plasmids used in these experiments tend to be relatively large, e.g., pJM17 is 40.4 kb. The *E. coli* carrying this plasmid, not surprising, grows slowly and yields can be low. To compensate for this problem, we scale up the volume of bacterial cells used to make plasmid DNA from 200 mL to 2 L. pJM17 can also be unstable in *E. coli* presumably as a consequence of its large size, so the restriction endonuclease profile of pJM17 should be confirmed.
3. Maintain a glycerol stock of pJM17 in *E. coli* to avoid the need to retransform the plasmid. In our hands, pJM17 is stable in *E. coli* strain JM109.

4. Cloning into the transfer vector is relatively inefficient. The size of the vector (in excess of 6 kb) is larger than that of an average vector and is responsible for a poor transformation efficiency in *E. coli*.

4.2. Transfection

5. Efficient transfection is required to generate a recombinant virus and can be monitored by including an appropriate control in experiments. Transfection with the plasmid pFG140 alone should result in the efficient production of virus plaques, or alternatively, a plasmid encoding *LacZ* under the control of a constitutive promoter may be used to measure directly the number of transfected cells (following staining of transfected monolayers with X-gal). Surprisingly, up to 80% of 293 cells will express a transgene using the $CaPo_4$ transfection method describe. In our hands, when the transfection efficiency is below ~20%, it becomes difficult to generate Ad recombinants. Lipofection has been used successfully to generate Ad recombinants, but is not recommended.
6. Productive Ad infection characteristically causes a CPE in which cells round up to form "grape-like" clusters and detach from the monolayer. With practice, plaques are easily recognized and will rapidly increase in size to spread through the monolayer. To give time for plaques to develop, 293 cell monolayers have to be maintained for 1–3 wk. Two hundred ninety-three cells consequently overgrow, and routinely clumps of cells detach. The resultant "hole" in the monolayer can be mistaken for a plaque.

4.3. Virus Stocks

7. Virus can be titrated on 293 cells by using a standard plaque *(28,31)* or $TCID_{50}$ assays *(32)*. Although a standard virus quantification can be made on permissive cells, the ability of the virus to infect different cells varies enormously, being largely dependent on the level of surface expression of the Ad receptor *(19)* and the expression of integrins required for virus internalization *(33)*. Such barriers to infection can partially be overcome by using a higher MOI or the addition of agents that will promote virus uptake, such as 2 μM DEAE-dextran *(29)*. Once a virus stock has been generated, an aliquot should also be routinely tested on a cell line lacking an E1 helper function, such as HeLa cells, to test for the presence of any contaminating replication competent virus.
8. CsCl centrifugation-ultracentrifugation is a specialized technique using expensive equipment. To be used safely, ultracentifuges and ultracentrifuge rotors must be correctly handled and maintained. Individuals who are not experienced with the equipment must seek appropriate training before attempting to use the apparatus.
9. Additional point: A number of techniques have been developed to generate Ad recombinants. This chapter has highlighted the vector system supplied by Microbix, because it is both efficient and commercially available. We note that Quantum Biotechnologies Inc., 230 Bernard-Belleau, Suite 100, Laval, Quebec H74 4A9 (http://www.qbi.com/)also now market a human RDAd expression system.

Acknowledgments

The authors are grateful to F. L. Graham for his encouragement and invaluable advice, which enabled the Ad vector system in this laboratory. G. W. and C. R. received support from the Welsh Scheme for the Development of Health and Social Science.

References

1. Li, Q., Kay, M. A., Finegold, M., Stratford-Perricaudet, L. D., and Woo, S. L. C. (1993) Assessment of recombinant adenoviral vectors for hepatic gene therapy. *Hum. Gene Ther.* **4,** 403–409.
2. Smith, T. A. G., Mehaffey, M. G., Kayda, D. B., Saunders, J. M., Yei, S., Trapnell, B. C., et al. (1993) Adenovirus mediated expression of therapeutic plasma levels of human factor IX in mice. *Nature Genet.* **5,** 397–402.
3. Yang, Y., Ertl, H. C. J., and Wilson, J. M. (1994) MHC class I-restricted cytotoxic T lymphocytes to viral antigens destroy hepatocytes in mice infected with E1-deleted recombinant adenoviruses. *Immunity* **1,** 433–442.
4. Yang, Y. and Wilson, J. M. (1995) Clearance of adenovirus-infected hepatocytes by MHC class I-restricted CD4+ CTLs in vivo. *J. Immunol.* **155,** 2564–2570.
5. Kaneko, S., Hallenbeck, P., Kotani, T., Nakabayashi, H., McGarrity, G., Tamaoli, T., et al. (1995) Adenovirus-mediated gene therapy of hepatocellular carcinoma using cancer-specific gene expression. *Cancer Res.* **55,** 5283–5287.
6. Wilkinson, G. W. G. (1994) Gene therapy and viral vectors. *Rev. Med. Microbiol.* **5,** 97–106.
7. Makimura, M., Miyake, S., Akino, N., Takamori, K., Matsuura, Y., Miyamura, T., et al. (1996) Induction of antibodies against strucutral proteins of hepatitis C virus in mice using recombinant adenovirus. *Vaccine* **14,** 28–34.
8. BrunaRomero, O., Lasarte, J. J., Wilkinson, G., Grace, K., Clarke, B., Borras-Cuesta, F., et al. (1997) Induction of cytotoxic T-cell response against hepatitis C virus structural antigens using a defective recombinant adenovirus. *Hepatology* **25,** 470–477.
9. Lieber, A., He, C.-Y., Polyak, S. J., Gretch, D. R., Barr, D., and Kay, M. A. (1996) Elimination of hepatitis C virus RNA in infected human hepatocytes by adenovirus-mediated expression of ribozymes. *J. Virol.* **70,** 8782–8791.
10. Shenk, T. (1996) Adenoviridae: The viruses and their replication, in *Fields Virology* (Fields, B. N., Knipe, D. M., and Howley, P. M., eds.), Lippincott-Raven, Philadelphia, pp. 2111–2148.
11. Jacobs, S. C., Stephenson, J. R., and Wilkinson, G. W. G. (1992) High-level expression of the tick-borne encephalitis virus NS1 protein by using an adenovirus-based vector: protection elicited in a murine model. *J. Virol.* **66,** 2086–2095.
12. Wilkinson, G. W. G. and Akrigg, A. (1992) Constitutive and enhanced expression from the CMV major IE promoter in a defective adenovirus vector. *Nucleic Acids Res.* **20,** 2233–2239.

13. Fooks, A. R., Schadeck, E., Liebert, U. G., Dowsett, A. B., Rima, B. K., Steward, M., et al. (1995) High level expression of the measles nucleocapsid protein by using a replication-deficient adenovirus vector: induction of an MHC-1-restricted CTL response and protection in a murine model. *Virology* **210**, 456–465.
14. McGrory, W. J., Bautista, D. S., and Graham, F. L. (1988) A simple technique for the rescue of early region 1 mutants into infectios adenovirus type 5. *Virology* **163**, 614–617.
15. Yang, Y., Nunes, F. A., Berencsi, K., Gonczol, E., Engelhardt, J. F., and Wilson, J. M. (1994) Inactivation of E2a in recombinant adenovirus improves the prospect of gene therapy in cystic fibrosis. *Nature Genetics* **7**, 362–369.
16. Parks, R. J., Chen, L., Anton, M., Sanakr, U., Rudnichi, M. A., and Graham, F. L. (1996) A helper-dependent adenovirus vector system: removal of helper virus by Cre-mediated excision of viral packaging signal. *Proc. Natl. Acad. Sci. USA* **93**, 13,565–13,570.
17. Ruether, J. E., Maderious, A., Lavery, D., Logan, J. S. M. F., and Chen-Kiang, S. (1986) Cell-type-specific synthesis of murine immunoglobulin m RNA from an adenovirus vector. *Mol. Cell. Biol.* **6**, 123–133.
18. Krasnykh, V. N., Mikheeva, G. V., Douglas, J. T., and Curiel, D. T. (1996) Generation of recombinant adenovirus vectors with modified fibers for altering cell tropism. *J. Virol.* **70**, 6839–6846.
19. Wickham, T. J., Roelvink, P. W., Brough, D. E., and Kovesdi, I. (1996) Adenovirus targeted to heparin-containing receptors increase its gene delivery efficiency to multiple cell types. *Nature Biotechnol.* **14**, 1570–1573.
20. Davidson, D. and Hassell, J. A. (1987) Overproduction of polyomavirus middle t antigen in mammalian cells through use of an adenovirus vector. *J. Virol.* **61**, 1226–1239.
21. Quantin, B., Perricaudet, L. D., Tajbakhsh, S., and Mandel, J. L. (1991) Adenovirus as a vector in muscle cells. *Proc. Natl. Acad. Sci. USA* **89**, 2581–2584.
22. Chartier, C., Degryse, E., Gantzer, M., Dieterle, A., Pavirani, A., and Mehtali, M. (1996) Efficient generation of recombinant adenovirus by homologous recombination in *Eschericia coli*. *J. Virol.* **70**, 4805–4810.
23. Lochmuller, H., Jani, A., Huard, J., Prescott, S., Simoneau, M., Massie, B., et al. (1994) Emergence of early region 1-containing replication competent adenovirus in stocks of replication-defective adeovirus recombinants ($\Delta E1+\Delta E3$) during multiple passages in 293 cells. *Hum. Gene Ther.* **5**, 1485–1491.
24. Fallaux, F. J., Kranenburg, O., Cramer, S. J., Houweling, A., Van Ormondt, H., Hoeben, R. C., et al. (1996) Characterization of 911: a new helper cell line for the titration and propagation of early region 1-deleted adenovirus vectors. *Hum. Gene Ther.* **7**, 215–222.
25. Bett, A. J., Haddara, W., Prevac, L., and Graham, F. L. (1994) An efficient and flexible system for construction of adenovirus vectors with insertions or deletions in early regions 1 and 3. *Proc. Natl. Acad. USA* **91**, 8802–8806.
26. Bett, A. J., Krougliak, V., and Graham, F. L. (1995) DNA sequence of the deletion/insertion in early region 3 of Ad5 *dl*309. *Virus Res.* **39**, 75–82.

27. Graham, F. L., Smiley, J., Russell, W. C., and Nairn, R. (1977) Characteristics of a human cell line transformed by DNA from human adenovirus type 5. *J. Gen. Virol.* **36,** 59–72.
28. Graham, F. L. and Prevec, L., eds. (1991) Manipulation of adenovirus vectors, in *Methods in Molecular Biology, vol. 7: Gene Transfer and Expression Protocols* (Murray, E. J., ed.), Humana, Clifton, NJ, pp. 109–128.
29. Fooks, A. R., Warnes, A., Racher, A. J., Stephenson, A., Jr., Dowsett, A. B., and Wilkinson, G. W. G. (1995) Analysis of conditions required for scaled up production of replication-deficient adenovirus recombinants, in *Proceeding of 13th ESACT Meeting* (Spier, R. E., Griffiths, J. B., and Berthold, W., eds.), Butterworth-Heinemann Ltd., pp. 21–26.
30. Graham, F. L. (1987) Growth of 293 cells in suspension culture. *J. Gen. Virol.* **68,** 937–940.
31. Precious, B. A. R. W. C. (1985) Growth, purification and titration of adenoviruses, in *Virology: A Practical Approach* (Mahy, B. W. J., ed.), IRL, Oxford, pp. 193–205.
32. Lowenstein, P. R., Shering, A. F., Bain, D., Castro, M. G., and Wilkinson, G. W. G. (1996) How to examine the interactions between adenoviral gene transfer vectors and different identified target brain cell types in vitro, in *Gene Transfer into Neurones: Towards Gene Therapy of Neurological Disorders* (Lowenstein, P. R. and Enquist, L. W., eds.), Wiley, Chichester, UK, pp. 93–114.
33. Wickham, T. J., Mathias, P., Cheresh, D. A., and Nemerow, G. R. (1993) Integrins $\alpha v \beta 3$ and $\alpha v \beta 5$ promote adenovirus internalization but not virus attachment. *Cell* **73,** 309–319.

52

Generation of Recombinant Herpes Simplex Virus Amplicons

Zhi Hong and Ann D. Kwong

1. Introduction

The herpes simplex virus type 1 (HSV-1) amplicon has been developed as a novel eukaryotic expression vector, which contains an HSV-1 *ori* for DNA replication and a *pac* signal for cleaving/packaging genomes into viral capsids *(1–4)*. As shown in **Fig. 1**, amplicon vector can be amplified into head-to-tail concatemers and then packaged into defective HSV-1 viral particles up to one genome size (~150 kb) in the presence of HSV-1 helper viruses. The helper viruses provide all necessary proteins and enzymes for amplicon DNA replication/packaging and for the assembly of defective amplicon viruses *(1)*. One of the applications of this defective amplicon virus system is to transfer efficiently high copy numbers of foreign genes into a broad range of mammalian cells for high-level expression and gene therapy *(4,5)*. We have utilized the amplicon system to produce high levels of HCV NS3/4A complexes in mammalian cells *(6)*. Our results have demonstrated that the amplicon system provides a potential to study the expression of HCV proteins in a broadspectrum of mammalian cell lines, especially in those of human hepatocyte origin that may be biologically more relevant to HCV infection. In this chapter, methods for using the amplicon expression system will be described in three subsections:

1. Generation of high-titer defective HSV-1 amplicon virus stocks.
2. Determination of the titers of amplicon viruses.
3. Expression of HCV NS3/4A complexes using the defective amplicon viruses.

It is not our intent to review the biology of the amplicon system as well as its development from naturally occurring defective viruses, which have been discussed in recent reviews *(4,7–9)*. We assume that the genes of interest have

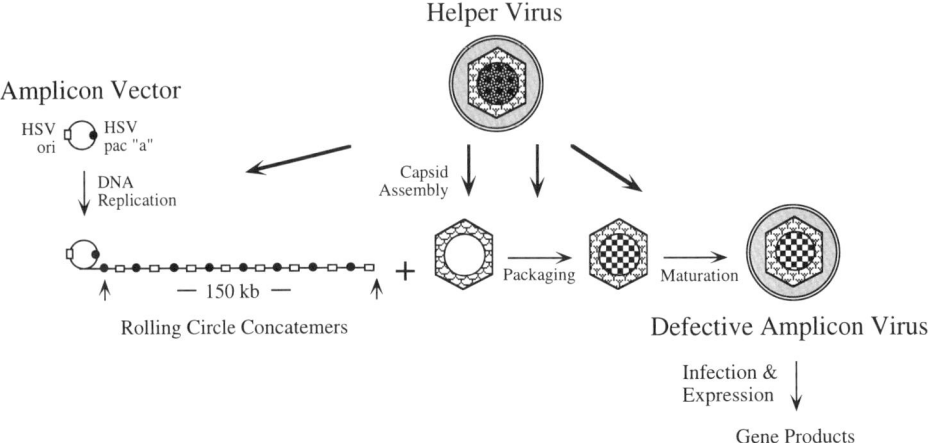

Fig. 1. Illustration of HSV-1 amplicon expression system.

been cloned into the amplicon vector for expression driven by appropriate promoters. We are not going to describe protocols for basic molecular biology and virology techniques involved in this system, such as cloning, virus plaque assays, and gel electrophoresis. We also assume that proper aseptic techniques will be rigorously enforced in order to avoid accidental contamination of cell cultures. All of the cell-culture experiments must be carried out in certified biohazard hoods under sterile conditions. Our protocols will focus on the generation of the defective amplicon viruses, titration of the amplicon stocks, and expression in mammalian cells using the amplicon viruses.

2. Materials
2.1. Reagents

The following media, buffers, cells, and virus should be ordered or prepared before working with the HSV-1 amplicon system:

1. DME: Dulbecco's Modified Eagle's Medium (JRH BioSciences).
2. EMEM: Minimum Essential Medium with Earle's balanced salts (JRH BioSciences).
3. M199: Medium 199 (199/EBSS) (JRH BioSciences).
4. FBS: Fetal bovine serum (BioWhittaker).
5. HEPES: 1 M solution (JRH BioSciences).
6. L-Gln: 200 mM L-glutamine solution in saline (JRH BioSciences).
7. Pen–Strep: Penicillin–streptomycin solution containing 10,000 U/mL penicillin G sodium and 10,000 µg/mL Streptomycin sulfate in 0.85% saline (Gibco-BRL).
8. MEM amino Acids: 100X solution in saline (JRH BioSciences).

9. MEM vitamins: 100X solution in saline (JRH BioSciences).
10. NaHCO$_3$: 7.5% solution (JRH BioSciences).
11. Versene: 1X solution in saline containing 53 mM EDTA (0.2 g/L) (Gibco-BRL).
12. DPBS: Dulbecco's phosphate-buffered saline without calcium and magnesium (JRH BioSciences).
13. PCIA: Phenol:chloroform:isoamyl alcohol (25:24:1, v/v) (Gibco-BRL).
14. RSC: Rabbit skin cells were obtained from Bernard Roizman, University of Chicago. RSC are maintained in DME + 10% FBS (*see* **Note 1**).
15. HEp-2: Human epidermoid 2 cells were also from Bernard Roizman, University of Chicago. HEp-2 cells are maintained in EMEM + 10% FBS.
16. Vero: African Green Monkey kidney cells were obtained from the American Type Culture Collection (CCL 81). Vero cells are maintained in M199 + 5% FBS.
17. Helper virus: The HSV-1 helper virus *tsk* is a temperature-sensitive ICP4 mutant obtained from H. S. Marsden at the MRC Virology Unit, Institute of Virology, Glasgow, UK. However, any self-replicating HSV-1 virus can be used as a helper virus (*see* **Note 2**).

2.2. Reagents for Generation of High-Titer Defective Amplicon Virus Stocks

2.2.1. Media

1. DME + 2% FBS: Supplement 1 L of DME with 20 mL of FBS, 10 mL of 1 M HEPES, 10 mL of Pen–Strep, and 20 mL L-Gln.
2. DME + 6% FBS: Same as above, except for adding 60 mL of FBS.
3. DME + 10% FBS: Same as above, except for adding 100 mL of FBS.
4. EMEM + 10% FBS: Supplement 1 L of EMEM with 100 mL of FBS, 10 mL of 1 M HEPES, 10 mL of Pen–Strep, and 20 mL L-Gln.
5. M199 + 1% IFBS: To 1 L of JRH M199 complete medium, add 10 mL Pen–Strep, 20 mL 0.2 M L-Gln, 10 mL 1 M HEPES and 10 mL inactivated FBS (IFBS, inactivated by incubating at 56°C for 1 h).
6. M199 + 5% FBS: Same as above except for adding 50 mL FBS (5%).

2.2.2. Buffers and Solutions

1. HeBS: 21 mM HEPES, pH 7.05, 0.7 mM Na$_2$HPO$_4$, 5 mM KCl, 137 mM NaCl and 5.6 mM glucose.
2. 2.0 M CaCl$_2$.

2.3. Reagents for Titration of the Defective Amplicon Virus Stocks

2.3.1. Media

1. MEM-PO$_4$: To make 1 L of MEM-PO$_4$ medium, first dissolve 0.1 g CaCl$_2$, 0.2 g KCl, 3.2 g NaCl, 0.096 g MgSO$_4$.7H$_2$O, 2.25 g D-glucose and 1.5 mL 0.5% phenol red (Gibco-BRL) in 900 mL of Milli-Q water. Supplement the solution with 10 mL Pen–Strep, 5 mL 0.2 M L-gln, 15 mL 7.5% NaHCO$_3$, 5 mL 100X MEM

amino acids, 5 mL 100X MEM vitamins, 8.5 mL 1 M HEPES, and 10 mL IFBS (1%). Adjust the pH to 6.8, bring the volume to 1 L with Milli-Q water, and sterilize the solution using a 0.2 μm filter (Nalgene Filterware).
2. DME + 10% FBS: To 1 L of DME medium, add 10 mL Pen–Strep, 20 mL 0.2 M L-Gln, 10 mL 1 M HEPES, pH 7.3 and 100 mL FBS (10%).
3. M199 + 1% IFBS: To 1 L of M199, add 10 mL Pen–Strep, 20 mL 0.2 M L-Gln, 10 mL 1 M HEPES, pH 7.3 and 10 mL IFBS (1%).
4. ^{32}P labeling medium: Add ^{32}P-orthophosphate (Amersham, cat. no. PBS13, 10 mCi/mL) to MEM-PO$_4$ medium to a final concentration of 50 μCi/mL.

2.3.2. Buffers and Solutions

1. Lysis buffer-SDS: 10 mM Tris-HCl, pH 8.0, 10 mM EDTA, and 100 mM NaCl.
2. DNA lysis solution: 25 mL lysis buffer-SDS, 0.2 mL 20% SDS and 2.5 mg proteinase K (Boehringer Mannheim). The lysis solution should be made fresh.
3. DPBS: Dulbecco's phosphate-buffered saline without calcium and magnesium (JRH BioSciences).
4. TE buffer: 10 mM Tris-HCl, pH 7.5, and 1 mM EDTA.

2.4. Reagents for Expression in Mammalian Cells Using the Amplicon Viruses

2.4.1. Media

1. DME-Met: Dissolve 10 g Dulbecco's Modified Eagle medium powder (1 package, Gibco-BRL formula #78-5382) in 800 mL milli-Q H$_2$O. Add 10 mL Pen–Strep, 20 mL 0.2 M L-Gln, 10 mL 7.5% NaHCO$_3$, 10 mL 1 M HEPES, and 10 mL IFBS (1%). Bring the final volume to 1 L and filter the medium using a 0.2-μm filter (Nalgene Filterware).
2. DME + 10% FBS: Same as described in **Subheading 2.1**.
3. M199 + 1% IFBS: Same as described in **Subheading 2.1**.
4. M199 + 5% FBS: Same as described in **Subheading 2.1**.
5. ^{35}S labeling medium: DME-Met medium supplemented with 1% of M199 + 1% IFBS medium and 50 μCi/mL ^{35}S-Met (Amersham, cat. no. SJ 1515, 15 mCi/mL).

2.4.2. Buffers and Solutions

1. Protein lysis buffer: 25 mM HEPES, pH 7.3, 25 mM NaCl, 1 mM EDTA, 2 mM DTT, 1% Nonidet P-40, 300 nM antipain, 200 nM leupeptin, and 10% glycerol.

3. Methods

3.1. Generation of High-Titer Defective Amplicon Virus Stocks

3.1.1. Transfection of Rabbit Skin Cells (RSC) with the Amplicon DNA

1. Seed RSC in DME + 10% FBS in a T-25 flask (FALCON tissue-culture flask, 25 cm^2 with canted neck) and use at about 90% confluency (check the cells under a light microscope).

HSV Amplicons

2. Check HeBS before adding the plasmid DNA by gently mixing 30 μL of 2 M $CaCl_2$ with 0.5 mL of HeBS. A light milky white color should form.
3. For each transfection in the T-25 flask, 10 μg of amplicon DNA (pF'$_1$CMV vector or pF'$_1$CMV-HCV-NS3/4A) were gently mixed with 0.5 mL of HeBS in a 15-mL conical tube.
4. Add 30 μL of 2 M $CaCl_2$ to each tube, and mix gently. A milky white color should form at room temperature after about 12 min.
5. Meanwhile, remove the medium, and wash the RSC monolayer twice with 4 mL of warm Versene solution (~37°C) and then twice with 4 mL of warm HeBS. Be sure to remove all of the residual HeBS after the second wash.
6. Add the HeBS/$CaCl_2$/DNA precipitate mixtures gently to the RSC monolayer and incubate the T-25 dish at room temperature or 37°C on a rocker platform for 30 min (*see* **Notes 4** and **5**).
7. Overlay the cells with 4 mL of DME + 2% FBS gently. Place the dish in a 37°C incubator (5% CO_2) for 4 h.
8. Remove the medium, and wash the cell monolayer three times with 4 mL of warm DME + 6% FBS. Incubate the cells in 4 mL of DME + 6% FBS overnight at 37°C.

3.1.2. Superinfection of Transfected RSC with the Helper Virus tsk

1. On the morning after transfection, remove the medium from the transfected cell culture completely.
2. Infect the cells with helper viruses (*tsk*) at an MOI of 0.1 in 1 mL of M199 + 1% IFBS. Rock the cells at room temperature on a rocker platform for 2 h.
3. Remove the viral inoculum, and wash with 4 mL of M199 + 1% IFBS. Overlay with 4 mL of M199 + 1% IFBS and incubate the cells at 33°C for 2–3 d.
4. Check cells for CPE after 2–3 d and freeze the cell culture at –70°C when it is fully infected. It usually takes about 3 d for the cells to be fully infected.

3.1.3. Amplification of the Amplicon Virus Stock Through Serial Passages

1. Seed HEp-2 cells in EMEM + 10% FBS in a T-75 flask (FALCON tissue-culture flask, 75-cm^2 with canted neck), and use at about 90% confluency (*see* **Note 6**).
2. Freeze and thaw the transfected/infected RSC culture three to four times to lyse the cells, and release the viruses. The viral stock at this step contains both helper *tsk* virus and the defective amplicon virus, and is designated as P_0 (passage # 0) stock.
3. Take 3 mL of the P_0 stock (from a total volume of 4 mL), and infect the HEp-2 cells in the T-75 flask at room temperature for 2 h. This is a 1:4 dilution which means that the lysate from one infected RSC cell is used to infect four uninfected HEp-2 cells in the next passage.
4. Remove the inoculum and rinse the HEp-2 monolayer twice with warm M199 + 1% IFBS.
5. Add 12 mL of fresh M199 + 1% IFBS to the infected HEp-2 cells, and incubate the cells at 33°C for 3–4 d. Check the cells for CPE to see if they are fully infected. If so, freeze the cell culture at –70°C.

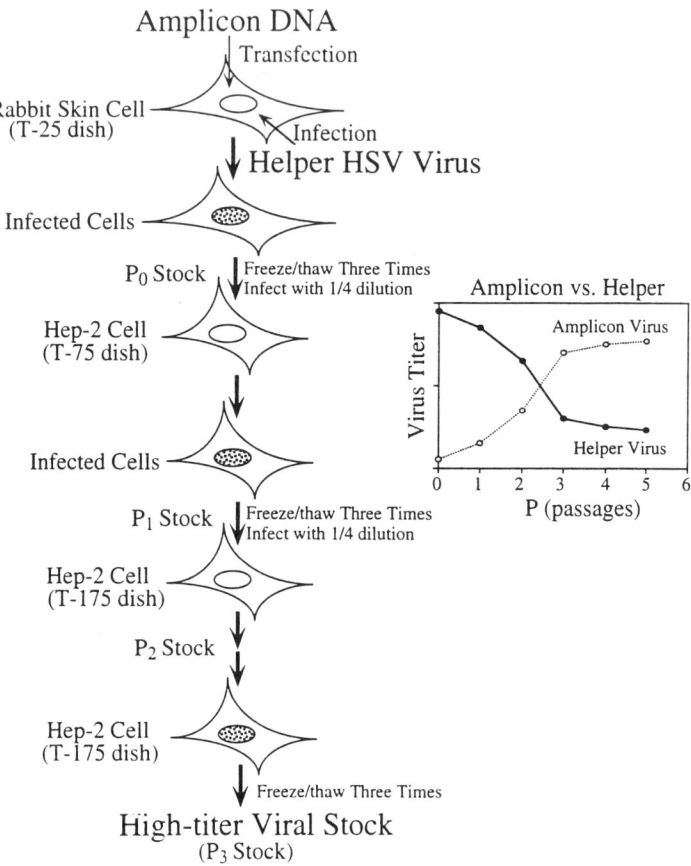

Fig. 2. Flowchart for generation of high-titer HSV-1 amplicon stocks. Infected cells are indicated by solid dots in the nuclei of the cells. The inserted graph simply depicts the trend of amplifying the amplicon viruses in the presence of decreasing amount of helper viruses.

6. Repeat the infection from **steps 1–5** using infected cell lysates, and amplify the amplicon viral stock by at least three serial passages as shown in **Fig. 2**. Freeze the final infected cell cultures (P_3 stock) at $-70°C$.

3.2. Determination of the Defective Amplicon Virus Titer

The defective amplicon viruses cannot replicate by themselves in the cells and will not form plaques on the cell monolayer. Thus, they are not quantifiable using a common plaque assay. To determine the titer of a defective amplicon virus stock, both amplicon DNA and helper virus DNA are labeled by ^{32}P-orthophosphate, and the relative amounts of amplicon DNA and helper virus DNA are measured. The amplicon titer can thus be estimated by first determining the ratio of amplicon DNA vs the helper virus DNA and then comparing to the helper virus titer. The following formula can be used to calculate the amplicon titers:

$$T_a = \frac{C_a/N}{C_h} \times T_h \qquad (1)$$

T_a and T_h represent the titers of the amplicon virus and the helper virus, respectively, while C_a and C_h represent the radioactivity (cpm) of an amplicon DNA fragment and a helper virus DNA fragment respectively (**Subheading 3.2., step 14**). N is the number of head-to-tail tandem repeats of the amplicon DNA in one HSV-1 genome unit (~150 kb) packaged in one virus capsid. For example, if the size of the amplicon DNA is 10 kb, there should be about 15 tandem repeats ($N = 15$) in each amplicon virus particle.

1. Determine the titer of the helper virus *tsk* in the amplicon stock after the final passage at 33°C using common plaque assays as described elsewhere *(10,11)*.
2. Seed Vero cells in M199 + 5% FBS in a T-25 dish and incubate the cells at 37°C (5% CO_2). The cells are ready for infection at about 90–95% confluency.
3. Infect cells with 1 mL of the amplicon viral stock in M199 + 1% IFBS and place the dish on a rocker platform at room temperature for 2 h.
4. Aspirate off the inoculum, and rinse the monolayer twice with 4 mL of MEM-PO_4. Incubate the cell cultures at 33°C in 4 mL MEM-PO_4 for an additional 2 h to deplete cellular phosphates
5. Remove the MEM-PO_4 and add 2 mL of ^{32}P labeling medium (containing ^{32}P-orthophosphate at 50 µCi/mL). Incubate the cells at 33°C for 18–24 h after infection until the cells are rounded owing to CPE, yet not detached from the plate.
6. Remove the ^{32}P labeling medium and gently rinse the cell monolayer twice with 4 mL of ice-cold DPBS.
7. Add 1 mL of the DNA lysis solution to each dish. Incubate the dish overnight at 37°C.
8. Transfer the cell lysate to a FALCON 15-mL conical tube. Add 6 vol of PCIA (phenol/chloroform/isoamyl alcohol), and mix by inverting the tubes five times.
9. Transfer the upper aqueous phase to a new 15-mL tube and add 5 vol of isopropanol. Gently mix by inverting the tube, and observe the formation of cotton-like DNA precipitates.
10. Spool out the DNA precipitate with a glass rod, and air-dry the DNA after removing excessive liquid with Kim Wipes (*see* **Note 7**). Do not dry the DNA too long, or it will be hard to dissolve in solution.
11. Dissolve DNA in 300 µL of TE buffer in a FALCON 6-mL tube by swirling the glass rod until the DNA precipitate goes into solution. Tap the tube to dissolve the DNA. You may need to incubate the tube at 50°C for 1 h to dissolve the DNA completely.
12. Take a 5-µL aliquot of the DNA solution, and set up a restriction enzyme digestion in 50 µL reaction volume using 20 U of *Hin*dIII.

13. Separate the digested DNA fragments on a 0.8% agarose gel, and dry the gel on a gel drier. Analyze the autoradiograph of the gel on an X-ray film.
14. Locate one amplicon fragment that is similar in size to another DNA fragment from the helper virus DNA. Quantify the amounts of both fragments by using an autoradiographic imager or by simply excising both bands and determining the radioactivity using a scintillation counter (*see* **Note 8**).
15. Determine the ratio of the amplicon DNA vs helper virus DNA and calculate the amplicon virus titer using the formula described above (*see* **Note 9**).

3.3. Expression of HCV NS3/4A in Mammalian Cells Using the Amplicon Viruses

1. Seed Vero cells in M199 + 5% FBS in a six-well dish (FALCON six-well tissue-culture dish), and incubate the cell culture at 37°C (5% CO_2) in M199 + 5% FBS. The cells are ready for infection at 90–95% confluency.
2. Remove the medium, and rinse the monolayer twice with 2 mL of M199 + 1% IFBS.
3. Infect cells with the amplicon viruses at an *MOI* of 1–3 in 0.5 mL M199 + 1% IFBS. Place the dish on a rocker platform at room temperature for 2 h.
4. Remove the inoculum, rinse the monolayer twice with 1 mL of M199 + 1% IFBS, and incubate the cells in 1 mL of M199 + 1% IFBS at 33°C.
5. At 6 h postinfection, remove the medium, and gently rinse the monolayer three times with 2 mL of DME-Met. Overlay the monolayer with 1 mL of ^{35}S-labeling medium (containing ^{35}S-Met at 50 µCi/mL) and incubate the cell culture at 33°C or 37°C for 1–2 d.
6. Aspirate off the ^{35}S-labeling medium, and rinse the cell monolayer three times with 2 mL of cold DPBS.
7. Add 0.5 mL cold protein lysis buffer to each well. Freeze and thaw three times to lyse the cells.
8. Transfer the cell lysate to an Eppendorf tube, and spin down nuclei and cellular debris at 10,000 rpm for 2 min. Transfer the supernatant to a new Eppendorf tube, and take a 10-µL aliquot of each lysate to count the radioactivity (~10^5–10^6 cpm). Store the sample at –80°C immediately.
9. Take an aliquot (~10 µL) of the supernatant, and analyze the protein on a 10–20% SDS-PAGE gradient gel by autoradiography as shown in **Fig. 3**.

4. Notes

1. The choice of cell lines is completely empirical based on the titers of the final amplicon stocks and the ratio of amplicon virus vs helper virus. Although RSC is a better cell line for efficient transfection and quicker superinfection to generate the initial amplicon viruses, HEp-2 cells are a better choice for amplification of the amplicon viruses. If HEp-2 cells are not available, Vero cells can be substituted for the amplification of amplicon virus stock.
2. The choice of helper viruses is critical in the expression level of a foreign gene. It has been demonstrated that a mutation in the virion host shutoff (vhs) function of the helper virus increases the expression level of a foreign gene *(3)*, suggesting

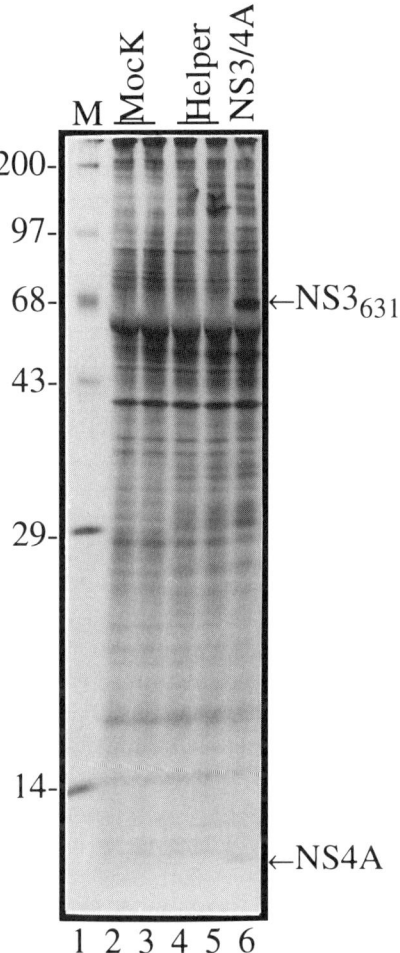

Fig. 3. Expression of HCV-NS3/4A in mammalian cells (Vero). ^{35}S-Met-labeled cell lysates were analyzed on a 10–20% SDS-PAGE gel, and the autoradiograph is shown here. Lane 1, mol wt markers; lanes 2 and 3, cell lysates from a mock infection; lanes 4 and 5, cells infected with helper viruses and amplicon viruses containing the amplicon vector pF'1CMV, which serve as a helper virus control; lane 6, cells infected with amplicon viruses containing pF'1CMV-HCV-NS3/4A in the presence of mutant tsk helper viruses.

that the wild-type vhs function decreases the expression levels by promoting the degradation of both host and viral mRNAs. Another viral factor that may affect the amplicon expression level is the function of ICP27, which inhibits normal host mRNA splicing activities *(12)*. A mutant virus without ICP27 may be a good choice as a helper virus. The mutant virus *tsk* described in this chapter has a temperature-sensitive mutation in ICP4, which is a major regulatory protein that controls the gene expression of HSV-1. When expressed at a nonpermissive temperature (37–39°C), *tsk* helper virus should have reduced interference with the host expression machinery and increase the expression level of HCV NS3/4A. It is very likely that a mutant virus with mutated vhs, ICP4, and ICP27 functions is the best choice as the helper virus. In addition, a helper-free amplicon system was recently developed for expression and gene therapy, which will greatly reduce the cytotoxicity of the amplicon system when used to infect mammalian cells *(13)*.

3. The size limitation of the amplicon DNA is a function of the packaging capacity of HSV-1 *(2)*. Since the genome size of HSV-1 is about 153 kb, the size of amplicon multiplied by the number of tandem repeats in one viral particle should be close to 153 kb. For example, if the amplicon plasmid is about 15 kb in size, 10 tandem repeats of the amplicon will be 150 kb, which is very close to the genome size and can thus be packaged efficiently. However, if the size of amplicon is 20 kb in size, eight tandem repeats are about 160 kb, which is too large to be packaged; although seven repeats are about 140 kb, which is too small to be packaged. Theoretically, amplicons of 30 or 50 kb can be packaged efficiently. However, such large amplicon plasmids will be difficult to be propagated in bacterial cells.

4. The pH of HeBS is very critical for optimal transfection of the amplicon DNA into mammalian cells. It has to be 7.05 exactly. This can be easily tested by mixing 30 µL 2.0 M $CaCl_2$ with 0.5 mL HeBS and observing the formation of a light milky white color after about 12 min at room temperature. It is easier to observe the fine precipitate in a clear glass tube. The pH has to be readjusted slightly around 7.05 if no precipitate or large heavy white flaky precipitate is formed.

5. The choice of transfection method is flexible. We have traditionally used the calcium phosphate method. However, other methods, such as DEAE-dextran transfection with or without glycerol shock, liposome-mediated transfection, and electroporation, also work with superinfection of helper viruses.

6. Cell-culture contamination can be a major problem when working with the amplicon system owing to extensive transfer of cell cultures during serial passages. It is a good practice to set aside an aliquot (1/4–1/2) of the infected cell culture at each passage. In case of an accidental contamination later on, you can always go back to an earlier uncontaminated passage without starting from the beginning.

7. The glass rod can be easily made to spool out the ^{32}P-labeled viral and amplicon DNA. To do that, the tip of a 9-in. Pasteur capillary pipet is flamed, so that the small opening is sealed and a small round tip is formed. The DNA precipitate will be spooled around and stay on the tip. Sometimes, it is hard to see the precipitate on the tip. It can simply be checked by pointing the tip of the pipet at a Geiger counter, which can also be used to check if the DNA on the tip is dissolved in TE buffer.

8. To compare accurately the relative amounts of amplicon DNA vs helper virus DNA, two DNA bands representing each DNA should be located. The helper virus DNA band can be easily identified by comparing to DNA from a helper virus only control. The sizes of both bands should be close so that a direct comparison can be made.
9. Alternative methods can be used to determine the amplicon virus titers. Reporter genes, such as *LacZ*, can be cloned into the amplicon DNA. Thus, the amplicon titers can be determined by histochemical staining for the expression of the *LacZ* gene product, β-galactosidase *(5,14)*. The black plaque ELISA can also be used to determine the amplicon virus titer *(11)* if an antibody is available for the gene product produced by the amplicon system. The cells infected with the amplicon viruses will be stained black and the titer can thus be determined.

References

1. Spaete, R. R. and Frenkel, N. (1982) The herpes simplex virus amplicon: a new eucaryotic defective-virus cloning-amplifying vector. *Cell* **30,** 295–304.
2. Kwong, A. D. and Frenkel, N. (1984) Herpes simplex virus amplicon: effect of size on replication of constructed defective genomes containing eucaryotic DNA sequences. *J. Virol.* **51,** 595–603.
3. Kwong, A. D. and Frenkel, N. (1985) The herpes simplex virus amplicon IV. Efficient expression of chimeric chicken ovalbumin gene amplified within defective virus genomes. *Virology* **142,** 421–425.
4. Kwong, A. D. and Frenkel, N. (1995) Biology of herpes simplex virus (HSV) defective viruses and development of the amplicon system in *Viral Vectors* (Kaplitt, M. G. and Loewy, A. D., eds.), Academic, New York, pp. 25–42.
5. Kaplitt, M. G., Kwong, A. D., Kleopoulos, S. P., Mobbs, C. V., Rabkin, S. D., and Pfaff, D. W. (1994) Preproenkephalin promoter yields region-specific and long-term expression in adult brain after direct *in vivo* gene transfer via a defective herpes simplex viral vector. *Proc. Natl. Acad. Sci. USA* **91,** 8979–8983.
6. Hong, Z., Ferrari, E., Wright-Minogue, J., Chase, R., Risano, C., Seelig, G., et al. (1996) Enzymatic characterization of hepatitis C virus NS3/4A complexes expressed in mammalian cells using the herpes simplex virus amplicon system. *J. Virol.* **70,** 4261–4268.
7. Frenkel, N., Singer, O., and Kwong, A. D. (1994) Minireview: the Herpes Simplex virus amplicon-A versatile defective virus vector. *Gene Ther.* **Feb. Suppl.,** S40–S46.
8. Geller, A. I. (1993) Herpesviruses: expression of genes in postmitotic brain cells. *Curr. Opinion Genet. Dev.* **3,** 81–85.
9. Kennedy, P. G. E. and Steiner, I. (1993) The use of herpes simplex virus vectors for gene therapy in neurological disease. *Q. J. Med.* **86,** 697–702.
10. Burleson, F. G., Chambers, T. M., and Wiedbrauk, D. L. (1992) *Virology: A Laboratory Manual*. Academic, San Diego.
11. Killington, R. A. and Powell, K. L. (1985) Growth, assay and purification of herpesviruses, in *Virology: A Practical Approach* (Mahy, B. M. J., ed.), IRL, Oxford, pp. 207–236.

12. Hardy, W. R. and Sandri-Goldin, R. M. (1994) Herpes simplex virus inhibits host cell splicing, and regulatory protein ICP27 is required for this effect. *J. Virol.* **68**, 7790–7799.
13. Fraefel, C., Song, S., Lim, F., Lang, P., Yu, L., Wang, Y., et al. (1996) Helper virus-free transfer of herpes simplex virus type 1 plasmid vectors into neural cells. *J. Virol.* **70**, 7190–7197.
14. Kaplitt, M. G., Pfaus, J. G., Kleopoulos, S. P., Mobbs, C. V., Rabkin, S. D., and Pfaff, D. W. (1991) Expression of a functional foreign gene in adult mammalian brain following in vivo transfer via a herpes simplex virus type 1 defective viral vector. *Mol. Cell. Neurosci.* **2**, 320–330.

53

Construction of Recombinant Sindbis-Based Expression Vectors for the Study of HCV Genes and Their Products

Brett D. Lindenbach, Ilya Frolov, and Charles M. Rice

1. Introduction

There are currently no methods for propogating hepatitis C virus (HCV) in culture useful for the analysis of viral proteins. Therefore, we have utilized Sindbis virus-based vectors to express and study HCV genes and their products.

Sindbis virus is the prototype Alphavirus, a genus of over 20 positive-sense ssRNA viruses *(1)*. The 11.7 kb genome is capped at the 5'-end and polyadenylated at the 3'-end. The 5' two-thirds of the genome are translated as a large polyprotein. which is processed into the nonstructural proteins essential for viral RNA replication (**Fig. 1**). Replication occurs in the cytoplasm of infected cells and proceeds through a (–) strand intermediate. The remaining one-third of the genome is transcribed from (–) strand RNA as a subgenomic RNA encoding the virion structural proteins.

The ability to recover viruses from transcribed genome-length RNA *(2)* has greatly facilitated the exploration of Sindbis molecular genetics. In turn, understanding of Sindbis molecular biology has led to the development of very useful tools for the expression of heterologous genes *(3–5)*. We have employed several strategies utilizing Sindbis vectors to drive expression of foreign genes. However, this protocol will focus on the widely useful and available SINrep5 system *(4)*. For a recent review of similar methods and variations, *see* **ref. 5**. The basis of the SINrep5 vector is a cloned cDNA of the Sindbis genome, which can be (run-off) transcribed in vitro using SP6 RNA polymerase to generate infectious RNA (**Fig. 2**). Immediately downstream of the subgenomic promoter, we have replaced the Sindbis structural genes with a selection of cloning sites for inserting foreign genes of interest. On transfection into a host

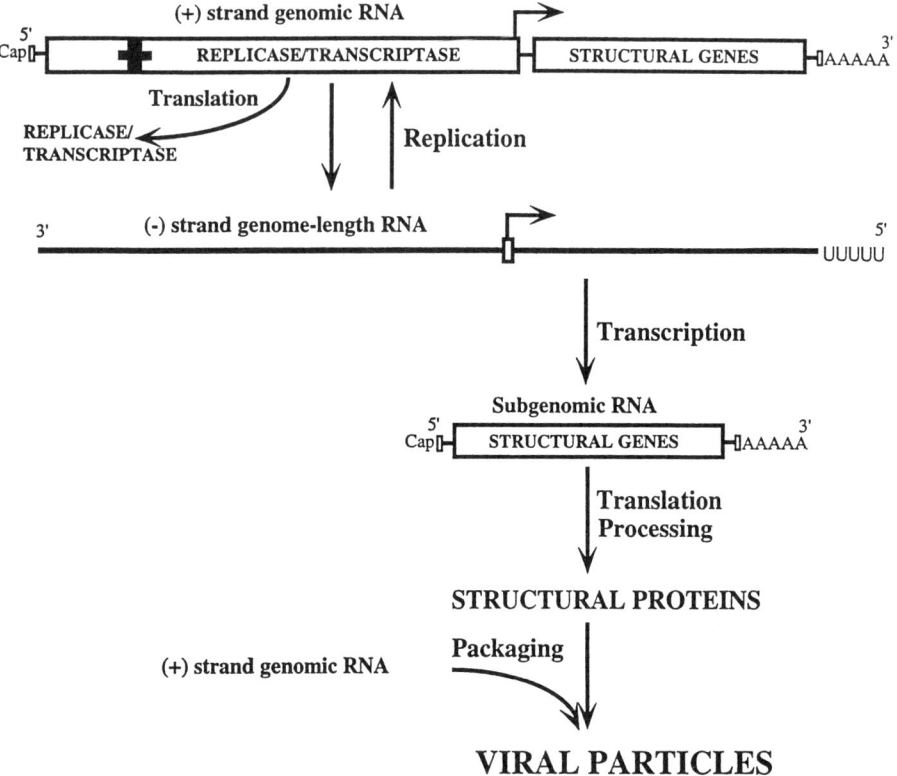

Fig. 1. Sindbis virus replication strategy. The 5' two-thirds of genomic ([+]strand) RNA is translated into components of the viral replication and transcription machinery. Genomic RNA is replicated via a (−) strand intermediate. This intermediate also serves as template for transcription of the subgenomic RNA, which encodes the viral structural genes.

cell, these self-replicating RNAs (replicons) are propagated to high levels and drive transcription of the foreign gene. Owing to the accumulation of the subgenomic RNA, as well as viral sabotage of the host translation machinery, large amounts of the foreign protein are synthesized.

The SINrep system was rendered more versatile through the development of packaging systems *(4)* to derive high-titer stocks of packaged replicons. This allows for the study of gene expression in poorly transfected cell types and greatly improves the yield of protein for analysis from a given amount of SP6 transcript. Essentially, the packaging system we use here involves cotransfection of the vector with a defective helper RNA (DH-BB[5'SIN]) that encodes the Sindbis structural proteins and is amplified by the Sindbis

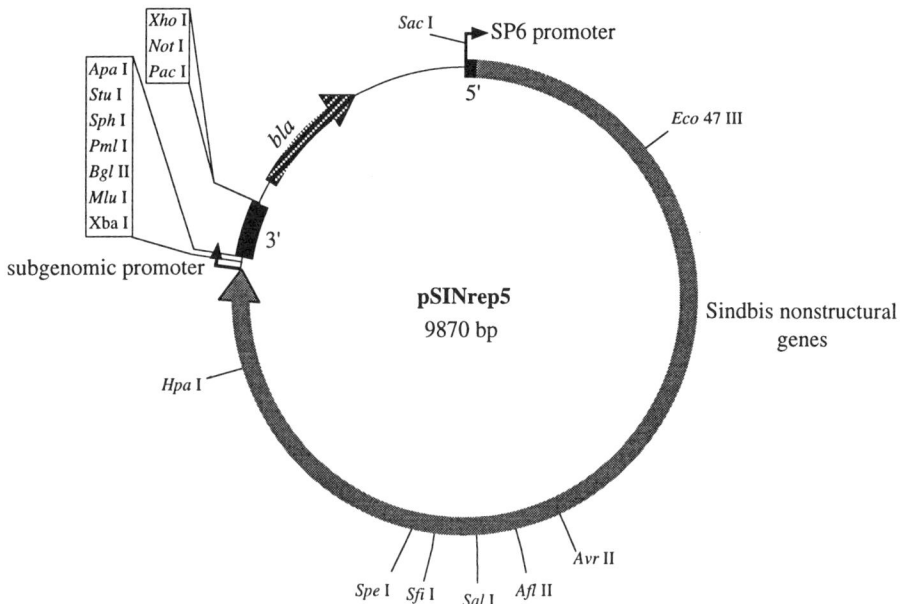

Fig. 2. Map of the SINrep5 vector. Shown are the SP6 promoter for in vitro transcription, nonstructural proteins, the Sindbis subgenomic promoter, multicloning sites (*Xba*I–*Apa*I), and sites for run off transcription (*Pac*I–*Xho*I).

replicase (**Fig. 3**). Although this RNA supplies virion components *in trans*, it is itself packaged much less efficiently than replicon RNA, and produces virion stocks that can infect cell populations, but are unable to spread. Once packaged replicons are obtained, typical expression studies commence with infection of a suitable cell type.

The advantages of the SINrep5 system for the study of HCV genes include:

1. Tractable methods for manipulating the SINrep genome to derive recombinant replicons.
2. The ease of rescuing packaged replicon stocks. It is quite feasible to go from pSINrep5 DNA to packaged stocks in 2 d.
3. High-titer, packaged replicons allow for many experiments to be performed from a minimum of setup. Titers usually exceed 10^7 infectious U/mL.
4. Very high levels of gene expression allow for many experiments from a small amount of cells and virus stock.
5. Cytoplasmic expression. Since it is believed that HCV, like other *Flaviviridae*, are replicated in the cytoplasm, potential processing of "cryptic" splice-donor and splice-acceptor sites within HCV genes is circumvented.

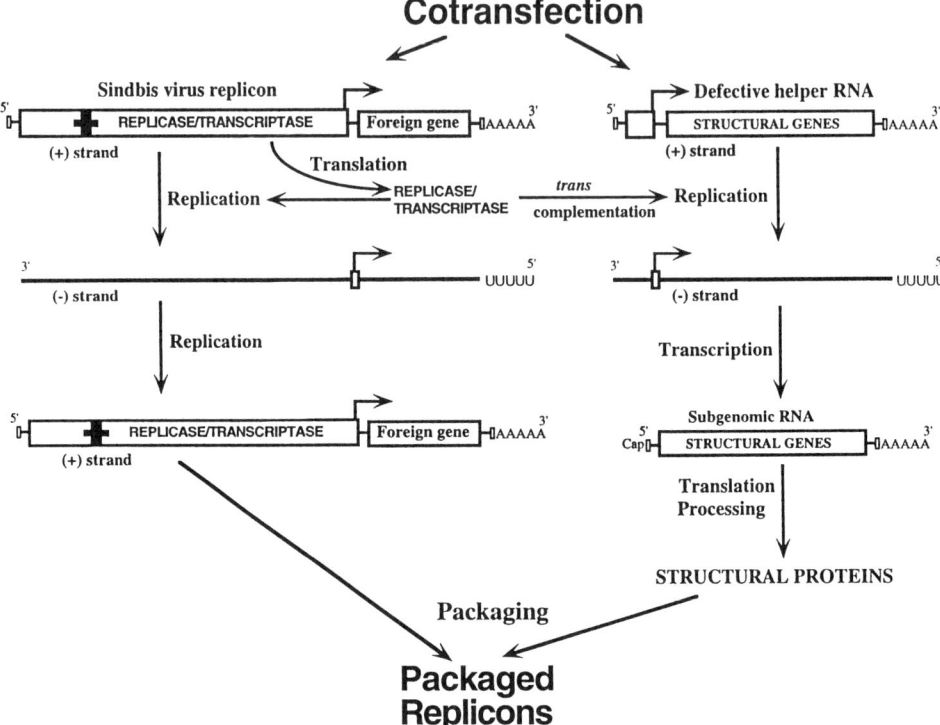

Fig. 3. Replicon packaging strategy. Transfection of replicon with helper RNAs leads to replication of both and selective packaging of replicon RNAs containing a packaging signal (+).

6. The ability to infect a variety of animal cell types of mammalian (including human), avian, and arthropod origin.

Careful application of the Sindbis expression system requires attention to the limitations of this system. These include:

1. Limited insert size. Although we have been able to express inserts of up to 6 kb, the entire HCV genome is too large for the Sindbis replication and/or packaging system. Therefore, we have focused on expressing several overlapping regions of the HCV genome.
2. Replicon stability. RNA viruses, including Sindbis-based replicons, are subject to great genetic plasticity. It is therefore somewhat common for recombination events to occur between replicon and helper RNA, generating full-length Sindbis viruses. However, these events rarely interfere with the analysis of foreign gene expression under controlled conditions.
3. Cytopathic effect. SINrep replication decimates infected cells typically within 24 h. Thus, expression studies must be planned appropriately.

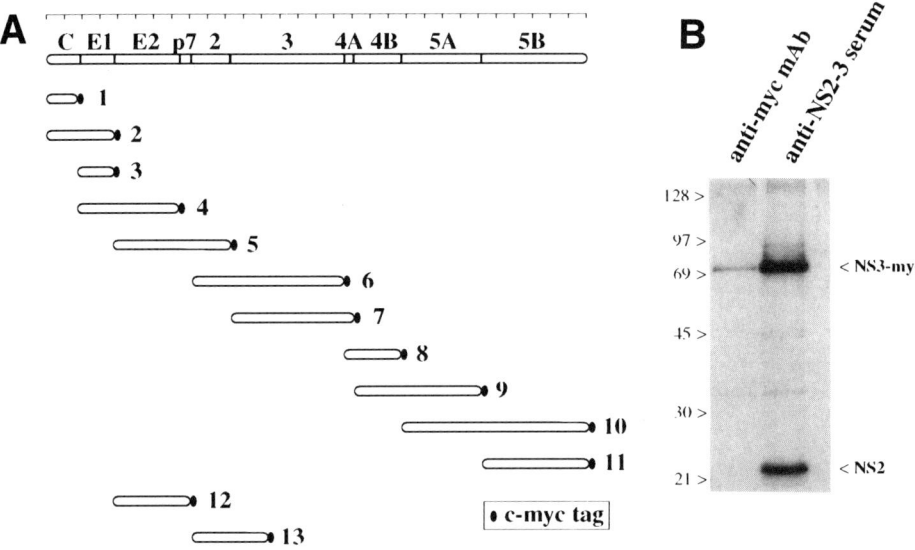

Fig. 4. Expression of HCV gene products using SINrep5. **(A)** Design of overlapping HCV cassettes inserted in SINrep5. Specific genomic regions are identified in **Table 1**. HCV genes were amplified by PCR and subcloned into a modified SINrep vector, fused to a c-*myc* tag. Tick marks represent 100 nt. **(B)** Example of expression using packaged SINrep5/HCV785-1657-*myc* (insert #6). BHK-21 cells were infected at MOI of 10, labeled with ^{35}S-Met, and lysed. Viral proteins were immunoprecipitated with an anti-*myc* MAb or rabbit anti-NS2/3 serum. Numbers refer to location of standards (in kDa).

4. Choice of permissive host cells. Although SINrep vectors can be used in primary fibroblasts and fibroblast lines, macrophage, and hepatocyte lines, as well as neural cell types, we have thus far been unable to infect efficiently human lymphocytic cell lines for studies on antigen processing and presentation.

SINrep/HCV replicons proved to be useful in defining a novel processing event in the C-terminus of the E2 glycoprotein to generate a small (approx 7 kDa) protein, p7 *(6)*. Since this polypeptide is rather hydrophobic and probably poorly immunogenic, examination of p7 was facilitated by the addition of an epitope tag (c-*myc*) at the predicted C-terminus of the expressed protein. Similarly, SINrep/HCVreplicons aided in the characterization of HCV-E1/E2 heterodimers and their intracellular localization *(7)*.

We have also derived a comprehensive bank of SINrep/HCV derivatives containing an overlapping set of inserts derived from cloned cDNA of the HCV-H strain (**Fig. 4** and **Table 1**). These were generated by PCR amplification and cloning into SINrep5. To aid in verifying proper gene expression and

Table 1
Details of HCV Regions Cloned into SINrep5[a]

Construction	HCV aa	Genomic region
1	1–176	Truncated capsid
2	1–379	Capsid, truncated E1
3	171–379	E1-signal peptide, truncated E1
4	171–723	E1-signal peptide, E1, truncated E2
5	370–1026	E2-signal peptide, E2, p7, NS2
6	785–1657	NS2-signal peptide, NS2, NS3
7	1027–1710	NS3, NS4A
8	1658–1971	NS4A, NS4B
9	1712–2419	NS4B, NS5A
10	1973–3011	NS5A, NS5B
11	370–802	E2-signal peptide, E2, truncated p7
12	785–1207	NS2 signal peptide, NS2, NS3 protease domain

[a]Amino acids are numbered corresponding to the HCV-H strain.

analysis of proteins for which we had no antibodies, this cloning was designed to generate HCV gene products fused to a c-*myc* epitope tag at their C-terminus.

The following protocol will be divided into:

1. Construction of recombinant vectors and generation of replicon RNA.
2. Rescue of packaged replicons.
3. Expression of HCV proteins using SINrep vectors.

2. Materials

2.1. Construction of Recombinant Vectors and Generation of Replicon RNA

1. HCV cDNA. These may be derived from previously cloned cDNAs or generated via RT-PCR of viral RNA.
2. Vector system DNAs, pSINrep5 and pDH-BB(5'SIN).
3. SP6 transcription components:
   a. RNase-free water.
   b. 5X transcription buffer: 200 mM Tris-HCl (pH 7.9), 30 mM MgCl$_2$, 10 mM spermidine-[HCl]$_3$.
   c. NTP mixture: 4 mM of each: UTP, ATP, CTP, GTP (Pharmacia).
   d. 10 mM CAP (^{m7}G[5']ppp[5']G) analog (New England Biolabs).
   e. 400 mM DTT.
   f. RNasin (40 U/µL, Promega).
   g. SP6 RNA Polymerase (50 U/µL, Epicentre Technologies).

h. [5,6-^{3}H]-UTP, 1.0 mCi/mL, 35–50 Ci/mmol (DuPont NEN).
i. (Optional) RNase-free DNase RQ1 (Promega).

2.2. Rescue of Packaged Replicons

1. BHK-21 cells (*see* **Subheading 4.**).
2. Complete BHK medium: α-MEM with glutamine (Gibco-BRL), 10% fetal calf serum, (optional) vitamins, (optional) 100 U/mL penicillin, and streptomycin.
3. Electroporator (Gene-Pulser, Bio-Rad; or similar) and 2 mm gap cuvettes.
4. RNase-free phosphate-buffered saline (PBS): 8 mM Na$_2$HPO$_4$, 3 mM KH$_2$PO$_4$, 147 mM NaCl, 5.4 mM KCl.
5. 2X MEM: sterile-filtered in 500 mL: 1 package (for 1 L) of powdered MEM (Gibco-BRL), 2.2 g NaHCO$_3$, 1 mM HEPES, pH 7.6, 4% fetal calf serum.
6. 1.5% (w/v) agarose in H$_2$O (Sea-Kem, FMC), autoclaved.
7. 5% (v/v) Formaldehyde.
8. 1% (w/v) Crystal violet in 20% ethanol.

2.3. Expression of HCV Genes

1. BHK-21 (or other cell type suitable for expression).
2. Metabolic label, such as Expre^{35}S^{35}S Protein Label Mix (DuPont, NEN).
3. Appropriately deficient media (Gibco-BRL).
4. Equipment and solutions for protein analysis, such as SDS-PAGE.

3. Methods

3.1. Construction of Recombinant Vectors and Generation of Replicon RNA

1. HCV genes are inserted into pSINrep5. Various strategies for generating these constructions may be employed, but we find it most straightfoward to amplify the region of interest using appropriately designed primers for directional cloning. For instance, we utilized a 5' (coding) primer that included a nontemplated *Xba*I site and an ATG codon for initiation and a 3' (noncoding) primer that included a *Mlu*I site for in-frame fusion to the epitope tag (other investigators may want to include a stop codon in this primer).
2. Helper and pSINrep/HCV derivatives are prepared in sufficient quantity and quality by alkaline lysis and CsCl banding *(8)*. Yields are generally high (0.2–0.5 mg/200 mL culture).
3. Five to ten micrograms of plasmid DNAs are linearized with an appropriate restriction enzyme. pDH-BB(5'SIN) is conveniently linearized with *Xho*I or *Eco*RI. *Xho*I, *Not*I, and *Pac*I sites are available at the 3'-end of the replicon genome. However, the choice of enzyme should consider the sequence of the insert. Our HCV-H cDNA clone contains a single *Not*I and 3 *Xho*I sites, so these are not used for constructs containing these inserts. *Pac*I may also be used although we find this enzyme to cleave poorly occasionally. It is important to digest the plasmids completely, so we generally overdigest 20-fold.

4. Following digestion, reactions are phenol-extracted, ethanol-precipitated, and resuspended to 0.2 µg/mL in RNase-free H_2O.
5. Assemble in vitro transcription reactions at room temperature:
    4 µL 5X SP6 buffer.
    1.2 µL 10 mM CAP analog.
    5 µL NTP mix (4 mM each).
    0.5 µL 400 mM DTT.
    0.5 µL ^{3}H-UTP (0.5 µCi).
    H_2O to 19.2 µL.
    0.4 µL RNasin (16 U).
    0.4 µL SP6 RNA Polymerase (20 U).
    0.2–1µg linearized DNA (add last).
    Incubate 60 min at 37 or 41°C.
6. Analyze yield of RNAs. Remove three aliquots of 0.5 µL: load one on a standard 0.8% agarose/TAE gel with loading buffer containing 0.01% DEPC, and spot the others on DE-81 papers to measure tritium incorporation. This is accomplished by washing one DE-81 paper 5X (5 min each) in 0.5 M Na_2HPO_4, once in H_2O, once in ethanol, and air-drying. The % incorporation is calculated as the ratio: $cpm_{washed}/cpm_{unwashed}$. Since the reaction started with 4 mM total nucleotide, the concentration of transcribed RNA is 1.2 × % incorporation (in µg/µL). On staining with ethidium bromide, the RNA should appear as an intense, sharp band of greater mobility than template DNA. Smearing below the RNA is indicative of RNase degradation, and reaction conditions should be corrected. Typical yields are 20–25 µg of RNA from 20-µL reactions. Store RNAs in 5 µg aliquots at –70°C.
7. (Optional; *see* **Note 1**) DNA templates may be digested by adding 0.4 µL of RNase-free RQ1 DNase to the reactions and incubating for an additional 10 min at 37°C. RNAs are then phenol-extracted, ethanol-precipitated, resuspended at 1 µg/µL, and aliquoted as above.

3.2. Rescue of Packaged Replicons

1. Grow BHK-21 cells in complete BHK medium (*see* **Note 2**). For efficient electroporation, they must be maintained subconfluent. You will need 1 × 10^7 cells/sample, which is the approximate yield of one 150 mm tissue-culture dish at 80% confluency (*see* **Note 3**).
2. Mix (on ice) 2.5 µg of SINrep RNA with 2.5 µg of helper RNA in a 1.6 mL sterile, RNase-free Eppendorf tube.
3. Aspirate medium, wash cells with PBS, and trypsinize (2 mL/150 mm) for 5 min at 37°C.
4. Resuspend in 8 mL complete medium and transfer to a 50 mL Falcon tube.
5. Centrifuge cells for 3 min at 1000g, aspirate supernatant, and resuspend in 10 mL ice-cold RNase-free PBS. Keep on ice.
6. Remove a small aliquot of cells and determine yield with a hemocytometer.
7. Wash cells again (repeat **step 5**).
8. Centrifuge cells again, and resuspend cells to 2.0 × 10^7/mL in RNase-free PBS.

9. Mix 0.5 mL of the cell suspension with the RNA, and transfer to a 2-mm gap electroporation cuvet. It is best to perform this step quickly, yet thoroughly. Three passes through a pipet tip should suffice.
10. Immediately pulse cells twice with 1.5 kV, 25 µF, infinite resistance.
11. Rest cells for 10 min at 25°C.
12. Transfer cells to a 100-mm tissue-culture dish containing 10 mL complete medium, and incubate at 37°C/5%CO_2 for 24–36 h. At this point, the cells should exhibit cytopathic effect: cells bodies will be rounded with spindly processes, ultimately losing adherence. It may be useful to compare transfectants to cells electroporated without RNA.
13. Collect supernatant, and clarify by 5000g for 10 min. Aliquot virus in 0.5-mL portions, and store at –70°C.
14. Determine the titer of packaged replicons. One useful way to estimate this is to determine the dilution (1:10, 1:40, 1:160, 1:640, 1:2560) required to destroy a monolayer of 5×10^5 cells. Because low-level packaging of helper RNA or generation of recombinant virus will lead to spread, a semisolid overlay is used. This is conveniently performed by infecting cells (with 0.2 mL PBS/2% FCS inoculae) in a six-well culture dish by occasional rocking for 1 h at 37°C. Pre-equilibrate 2X MEM and boiled 1.5% agarose to 43°C. Combine these 1:1 and replace inoculum with 2 mL/well. Allow to solidify (10 min at room temperature), and incubate at 37°C/5% CO_2 for 16–18 h. Examine cells and estimate the percentage of dead cells in each well. If desired, fix cells for 10 min in 5% formaldehye, remove overlays with a quick flick of a spatula, stain for 30 min with 1% crystal violet in 20% ethanol, and wash with water. The titer of recombinants in the stock are revealed as plaque-forming units, and should be >10^4-fold lower than the titer of infectious U/mL (*see* **Notes 4** and **5**).

3.3. Expression of HCV Gene Products

1. Seed the appropriate number of cells for the experiment. For most work 5×10^5 BHK-21 cells on a 35-mm dish is sufficient.
2. Infect cells with virus at a multiplicity of around three to five infectious U/cell in a volume of 0.2 mL/dish by rocking occasionally for 1 h. Replace medium and incubate at 37°C/5% CO_2.
3. At 8–12 h postinfection, wash cells with PBS, and label using 25 µCi/mL ^{35}S-Met/Cys or other label, in appropriately deficient medium, for 1 h.
4. Lyse cells in SDS-PAGE sample buffer, boil for 5 min, and analyze by SDS-PAGE.
5. If a specific antiserum is available, cell lysates may be used for immunoprecipitation and/or Western blotting.
6. Since SINrep directs the downregulation of host transcription and translation, the only proteins that will be labeled are those translated from SINrep messages. Expect to see a large quantity of the labeled HCV gene product over a small background of Sindbis nonstructural proteins. Packaged stocks containing large amounts of packaged helper RNA or recombinant viruses may also show a background of Sindbis structural proteins, particularly the capsid, which migrates at 34 kDa.

4. Notes

1. We do not find it necessary to remove the template DNA by DNase digestion.
2. We have been successful in packaging replicons in BHK-21 cells obtained from the ATCC. Some subcultures of this line, derived by laboratory passage, demonstrate increased growth rates and improved recovery from electroporation. It is therefore advisable to test a given BHK line for its transfectability.
3. Other methods of RNA transfection may used, including DEAE-dextran or cationic liposomes (Lipofectin, Gibco-BRL). Optimize transfection conditions with a helper-free SINrep5/LacZ or SINrep5/GFP replicon. We have also used the BTX Square-Porator system to electroporate BHK-21 cells using 5 pulses at 860 V of 99-µ length.
4. Other packaging systems are available that significantly reduce the occurence of recombination events between replicon and helper *(5)*.
5. Immunoflorescence is another useful method of titering SINrep stocks, although this requires specific antisera to Sindbis or the expressed gene product.

References

1. Strauss, J. H. and Strauss, E. G. (1994) The alphaviruses: gene expression, replication, evolution. *Microbiol. Rev.* **58**, 491–562.
2. Rice, C. M., Levis, R., Strauss, J. H., and Huang, H. V. (1987) Production of infectious RNA transcripts from Sindbis virus cDNA clones: Mapping of lethal mutations, rescue of a temperature-sensitive marker, and *in vitro* mutagenesis to generate defined mutants. *J. Virol.* **61**, 3809–3819.
3. Xiong, C., Levis, R., Shen, P., Schlesinger, S., Rice, C., and Huang, H. V. (1989) Sindbis virus: an efficient, broad host range vector for gene expression in animal cells. *Science* **243**, 1188–1191.
4. Bredenbeek, P. J., Frolov, I., Rice, C. M., and Schlesinger, S. (1993) Sindbis virus expression vectors: Packaging of RNA replicons by using defective helper RNAs. *J. Virol.* **67**, 6439–6446.
5. Frolov, I., Hoffman, T. A., Prágai, B. M., Dryga, S. A., Huang, H. V., Schlesinger, S., et al. (1996) Alphavirus-based expression systems: strategies and applications. *Proc. Natl. Acad. Sci. USA* **93**, 11,371–11,377.
6. Lin, C., Lindenbach, B. D., Prágai, B. M., McCourt, D. W., and Rice, C. M. (1994) Processing of the hepatitis C virus E2-NS2 region: identification of p7 and two distinct E2-specific products with different C termini. *J. Virol.* **68**, 5063–5073.
7. Dubuisson, J., Hsu, H. H., Cheung, R. C., Greenberg, H. B., Russell, D. G., and Rice, C. M. (1994) Formation and intracellular localization of hepatitis C virus envelope glycoprotein complexes expressed by recombinant vaccinia and Sindbis viruses. *J. Virol.* **68**, 6147–6160.
8. Sambrook, J., Fritsch, E., and Maniatis, T. (1989) *Molecular Cloning: A Laboratory Manual.* Cold Spring Harbor Laboratory, Cold Spring Harbor, NY.

X

IN VIVO MODELS

54

The Chimpanzee Model

Contributions and Considerations

Elizabeth Muchmore

1. Introduction

Chimpanzees *(Pan troglodytes)* became established as invaluable models for the study of human viral hepatitis after it was discovered, in 1967, that the chronic hepatitis B antigen carrier state existed in a naturally infected member of this species *(1–3)*. They were instrumental in the development of hepatitis B serologic marker assays and vaccines, and in safety testing human blood products for inactivation of this virus. In 1974, after hepatitis B-positive donor blood was no longer used, it was suggested that there were one or more unknown viral agents causing posttransfusion hepatitis *(4,5)* and chimpanzees were the most likely candidates for testing this hypothesis. By 1978 there were already three published reports that chimpanzees gave conclusive evidence of disease transmission after inoculation with putatively infectious materials from human patients with the newly named non-A, non-B hepatitis (NANBH) *(6–8)*.

Public sentiment against using animals in research is strong, especially for chimpanzees, so attempts were made to infect other primate and nonprimate species with human hepatitis viruses. Other animals proved to be suitable models for studying hepatitis A, D, E, and G, but chimpanzees are the only available animal models that can be reliably infected with hepatitis B and C *(9–11)*.

Infection studies, which are essential for obtaining information about previously unknown etiologic agents, cannot be done in human subjects, so many chimpanzees were infected to provide materials for isolation, identification, and characterization of the agent(s) of NANBH, to answer basic questions about transmission, epidemiology, pathology, and immunology of hepatitis C virus (HCV) infection, and to establish the chimpanzee infectious dose (CID_{50})

of inocula for use as standardized challenge material *(12)*. They were also employed for safety testing therapeutic human blood products for removal of NANBH infectivity *(13–16)*. All of these studies provided important information about the natural history of HCV infection and confirmed the potential of this model for simulating human conditions.

In 1989 it was reported that materials from chimpanzees had made possible the isolation of clones and development of serologic assays for detection of what is now known as HCV *(17,18)*. This opened the door for definitive new studies, vaccine development efforts, and retrospective analysis of stored samples from previous studies.

2. Attributes of the Animal Model

Chimpanzees infected with hepatitis viruses A–E are comparable to human patients, with two important differences. They experience such mild, anicteric, asymptomatic infection that the occurrence of illness in a chimpanzee following inoculation with hepatitis B virus *(19)* and a cluster of severe anemia cases in juvenile chimpanzees chronically infected with NANBH *(20)* were reportable. This fortunate coincidence makes possible the performance of frequent technical procedures, including plasmapheresis and liver biopsy, even during the acute phase of disease, without harm. It is advantageous that NANBH infection produces characteristic intracellular ultrastructural changes in chimpanzee hepatocytes *(21–24)*. This discovery made possible detection of infection before serologic assays were developed, even if enzyme elevation was insignificant and histopathology was equivocal.

The size of chimpanzees may be a disadvantage with respect to housing and handling, but it is an asset for obtaining biological materials. Even 2-yr-old chimpanzees are large ($\approx$10 kg) in comparison to most other laboratory animals, so it is possible to obtain relatively large quantities of whole blood (up to 10 mL/kg/mo) without harm and to harvest plasma by plasmapheresis at crucial times during the course of disease. Plasmapheresis by continuous flow centrifugation can be performed on animals weighing $\geq$35 kg, and adult chimpanzees (50–90 kg) can provide up to 1500 mL of plasma/week for several months without deleterious effect *(25)*.

Percutaneous punch liver biopsies can be performed up to twice/wk without causing significant elevation of liver enzymes. Six healthy animals that were biopsied on Mondays and Thursdays for 8 mo had slightly higher, but statistically insignificant, enzyme levels on Thursdays than on Mondays, and the Monday levels remained essentially constant *(26)*. When biopsy tissue is inadequate, liver wedges can be obtained via laparotomy. Liver wedges were often obtained preinoculation and during both acute and convalescent phases during early studies to provide material for absorption. Intestinal adhesions were the most deleterious effect noted. Current federal regulations permit only one "recovery" surgery/animal, unless a protocol requesting multiple operations is approved by the Institutional Animal Care and Use Committee (IACUC) before the study begins.

Serum levels of liver enzymes rise and fall after HCV challenge in chimpanzees, but the peaks are lower than those usually seen in human patients *(6,27)*, so empirical cutoff levels of significance for each individual are calculated from baseline mean levels. There is considerable normal variation in alanine aminotransferse (ALT) activity in chimpanzees, 60% of which has been explained by detection of a major gene by complex segregation analysis. Genetic analysis of change in ALT activity in HCV-infected chimpanzees indicated that 30% of the variation in response may also be attributable to genetic factors *(28)*. Aspartate aminotransferase (AST) levels are subject to wide fluctuations, unrelated to hepatitis *(29)*, so γ-glutamyl transpeptidase (GGT) is frequently monitored in conjunction with ALT to provide an additional indicator. Levels of GGT may rise before the ALT and persist after ALT returns to normal. Persistent GGT elevation is often the only biochemical indicator of long-term chronic infection *(30)*.

Unlike hepatitis B, which has been found in chimpanzees with no possible laboratory exposure *(31)*, hepatitis C has been found only in chimpanzees at facilities where HCV research was being conducted, and the incidence in animals without intentional exposure is negligible *(32,33)*. Vertical transmission of HCV in chimpanzees has not been reported, but the case of a female that was challenged with HCV during the second trimester of pregnancy and delivered a negative infant was described. The mother, who became a chronic carrier, showed electronmicroscopic liver changes indicative of infection 1 wk after challenge, but had no enzyme elevation until after birth of the infant *(34)*. This apparent suppression of liver damage during gestation is consistent with the immunosuppression of pregnancy seen in women *(35)*, which may be responsible for the low incidence of vertical transmission, and supports the concept that liver damage in hepatitis C infection is related to immune response *(36)*.

3. Research

Early infection studies showed that the iv route was as efficient in producing infection as the intrahepatic route, and that serum or plasma was as infectious as homogenized liver tissue *(8)*. It is reported that the HCV genome was not found in human body fluids, other than serum, by polymerase chain reaction (PCR) *(37)*, but NANBH was transmitted to a chimpanzee by iv inoculation of saliva from an NANBH-infected chimpanzee *(38)*. Chimpanzees given fecal material from a chimpanzee in the acute phase of NANBH, by the oral or iv route, did not become infected *(39)*. These early studies established the viral nature of the agent, because many of the challenge inocula had been passed through bacteria-retaining filters *(40)*.

Naive animals simultaneously exposed to hepatitis B and NANBH showed early evidence of NANBH infection and delayed serologic evidence of hepatitis B infection *(41)*.

Reinfection studies suggested that there were at least two NANBH agents, because chimpanzees that had apparently recovered from infection with one isolate could be reinfected with another, and repeatedly develop biochemical and histologic signs of hepatitis *(42,43)*. These findings were compatible with the observation of human patients with multiple attacks of viral hepatitis *(44)*. However, chimpanzees rechallenged with the same inoculum also developed apparent reinfection, and continuing surveillance of NANBH-infected animals showed recrudescence of disease in some that had apparently recovered and had not been rechallenged *(45)*. These studies supported the concept of chronic infection with reactivation of acute disease, and passage studies confirmed the presence of persistent viremia *(46)*. Later, PCR and anti-HCV analyses showed that the weak immunity after HCV infection enables reinfection of HCV carriers and recovered chimpanzees with identical virus *(47)*, and that some animals with high levels of antibody also have high titers of circulating virus *(48)*.

Sequential superinfection of HCV carrier chimpanzees with HCV of different genotypes showed that the newly introduced HCV replaces or expels the predecessor, and that each rechallenge resulted in reappearance of viremia and an episode of liver injury *(49,50)*.

Long term surveillance of chimpanzees chronically infected with HCV has shown that they develop hepatocellular carcinoma, without cirrhosis or elevated serum α-fetoprotein levels *(51–53)*. Genetic drift was documented in chimpanzees followed for years *(54)*. The GOR autoepitope, which appears to have an immunopathogenic role in hepatitis C infection *(36)*, was originally isolated from a chimpanzee infected with HCV *(55)*, but others have reported no reactivity to GOR in chimpanzees *(56)*.

The efficacy of postexposure prophylaxis for prevention of HCV infection was tested in two chimpanzees: one given anti-HCV-negative iv immune globulin (IVIG) and the other given HCV immune globulin (HCIG) 2 h after challenge. Both test animals and a positive control became infected, but the postexposure HCIG treatment markedly prolonged the incubation period of acute hepatitis C *(57)*.

In vitro neutralization of hepatitis C acute-phase human plasma, previously titered for chimpanzee infectivity, was attempted with plasma obtained 2 yr and 13 yr postacute phase from the same chronically infected patient. Evaluation of residual infectivity in chimpanzees showed that the 2-yr plasma neutralized infectivity, but the 13-yr plasma did not. Genetic mapping showed significant divergence in the patient, even at two years, and one chimpanzee infected with acute-phase plasma showed the same pattern. These data show that HCV infection elicits neutralizing antibody response in humans, suggest that the antibodies are isolate-specific, and confirm that HCV is present in vivo as a quasispecies *(58)*.

In spite of the weak humoral immune response seen in experimentally infected chimpanzees, seven animals vaccinated with both E1 and E2 envelope glycoproteins of HCV developed a strong humoral immune response. The five highest responders showed complete protection against iv challenge with homologous virus (HCV-1, genotype 1a) *(59)*.

Cellular immunity studies have shown that HCV establishes a persistent infection in humans and chimpanzees despite the presence of virus-specific, class I major histocompatibility complex-restricted $CD8^+$ cytotoxic T-lymphocytes (CTLs) in the liver. CTLs directed against a conserved epitope in the HCV nonstructural 3 protein persisted in the liver of a chronically infected chimpanzee for at least 2 yr after infection. However, these CTLs did not recognize the HCV quasispecies present in the plasma of this animal at wk 16 postinfection or at later time-points. Escape was facilitated by a mutation. These results strongly support the concept that CTL responses can select for variant viruses with an enhanced ability to persist in a host, and have important implications for vaccine design *(60)*. The fact that orthologous chimpanzee and human MHC class I loci are so alike that the differences are similar to those between HLA class I antigen presentation in different human populations or individual, contributes to the value of chimpanzees for studying HCV infection and development of vaccines for diverse human populations *(61)*.

A highly strand specific method of reverse transcriptase-polymerase chain reaction (RT-PCR) that will detect both positive and negative strands of HCV detected no negative-strand HCV RNA, which is indicative of replication, in HCV-infected human or chimpanzee peripheral blood mononuclear cells (PBMC). The ability to evaluate human necropsy tissues is limited by the impact of handling and storage conditions necessary for detection of HCV-RNA *(62)*.

Euthanasia of a chimpanzee because of kidney failure, which may have been owing to his long-term HCV carrier state, provided the opportunity to preserve the cellular RNA by snap-freezing tissues in liquid nitrogen at the time of death. Positive-strand HCV RNA was detected in serum and all tissues examined (spleen, muscle, lymph node, pancreas, kidney, bone marrow), but negative-strand HCV RNA was found only in the liver *(63)*.

Cultivation of HCV in primary chimpanzee hepatocytes now provides an in vitro test system that can be used to evaluate the effects of antiviral compounds and vaccine candidates *(64)*. Although chimpanzees are needed to provide cells for primary cultures, this minimizes the numbers of animals that will be needed for definitive in vivo studies.

4. Supply

The demand for chimpanzees to study hepatitis B prompted the National Institutes of Health National Heart Lung and Blood Institute (NHLBI) to fund a program for the importation and breeding of chimpanzees in 1974. The US signed the Convention on International Trade in Endangered Species (CITES) in 1973, and the US Fish and Wildlife Service designated wild chimpanzees as endangered and those in captivity as threatened in 1977, so no chimpanzees were legally imported after 1976. Breeding became the only source of naive animals, and adequate numbers for judicious use were provided through the efforts of independent and government-supported breeding programs.

In January 1995, the International Species Inventory System (ISIS) database listed 2572 chimpanzees in captivity worldwide, two-thirds of which were housed in US biomedical research laboratories *(65)*. The chimpanzees now available for biomedical research in the US are maintained by six institutions: Yerkes Regional Primate Research Center of Emory University in Atlanta, GA; University of Southwestern Louisiana New Iberia Research Center in New Iberia, LA; Southwest Foundation for Biomedical Research (SFBR) in San Antonio, TX; University of Texas M. D. Anderson Science Park in Bastrop, TX; Primate Foundation of Arizona in Tempe, AZ; and the Coulston Foundation, with facilities in Alamogordo, NM.

5. Cost

Maintenance and monitoring of chimpanzees in a research setting have always been expensive, because they are large, late-maturing, long-lived, behaviorally complex animals, whose husbandry and caging are costly. Pressure from animal rights groups has resulted in US Department of Agriculture (USDA) regulations that enlarged spatial requirements, increased the difficulty of handling the animals for technical procedures, and added man hours for psychological enrichment.

The responsibilities of owning endangered/threatened species make it unreasonable for them to change hands for short-term research, so facilities retain ownership of chimpanzees and charge assignment or leasing fees for their use. In 1990, at a nongovernment facility, it cost approx $50,000 for one chimpanzee on a 1-yr hepatitis study protocol. This included usage fee and maintenance per diem plus weekly technical procedures for blood drawing, percutaneous liver biopsy, plasmapheresis, and liver enzyme determinations.

The financial problem is compounded by the fact that the killing of chimpanzees is not condoned unless it is in the true sense of euthanasia to relieve suffering. The life-span of chimpanzees in captivity is considered to be 55 yr for males and 60 yr for females *(65)*. There are now hundreds of chimpanzees, chronically infected with hepatitis viruses and/or the human immunodeficiency virus (HIV), that must be held under conditions dictated by the USDA in a humane manner that will not pose a hazard to handlers. Since there is little research employment for such animals, the option of retirement facility development is under consideration in many sectors. However, under existing conditions, their maintenance costs must be borne by the working animals in each colony, by retirement endowment fees charged to investigators, or federal funding.

Future costs of maintaining just the chimpanzees that were in US research institutions at the beginning of 1995, assuming no new births, was calculated on the basis of $25/d in 1995 dollars with 4% inflation and using detailed long-term actuarial projections and mortality statistics. This study estimates an annual expenditure of $13–15 million/yr for 20 yr before dropping toward the $30,000 estimated for the 60th yr *(65)*.

6. Summary

There is reluctance to use chimpanzees as experimental animals, in spite of their demonstrated value, and the reasons are twofold: public sentiment and cost. This is unfortunate because the chimpanzee is an excellent model for studies of human hepatitis A–E. Although chimpanzees do not typically exhibit clinical illness, these animals do develop definitive evidence of the viral infection: elevated serum liver enzyme levels, light and electron microscopic histopathology found in acute and chronic disease, and development of specific antiviral antibodies.

The chimpanzee has been essential to isolation and characterization of the hepatitis viruses. These animals provide high-quality resource reagents (antigens, antibodies, viruses), and make possible studies of virus–host interactions during the course of acute and chronic infections *(66–68)*. They provide a model for development of vaccines and effective antiviral therapeutic agents, as well as for safety testing vaccines, prophylactic immunoglobulins, plasma-derived coagulation products, and disinfectant and sterilization reagents and methods. With careful and judicious use, the chimpanzee will continue to provide support for studies of human infectious diseases.

References

1. Prince, A. M. (1968) An antigen detected in the blood during the incubation period of serum hepatitis. *Proc. Natl. Acad. Sci. USA* **60,** 814–821.
2. Hirschman, R. J., Shulman, N. R., Barker, L. F., and Smith, K. O. (1969) Virus-like particles in sera of patients with infectious and serum hepatitis. *JAMA* **208,** 1667–1670.
3. Lichter, E. A. (1969) Isoprecipitins to macroglobulins in chimpanzees. *Ann. NY Acad. Sci.* **162,** 202–204.

4. Prince, A. M., Brotman, B., Grady, G. F., Kuhns, W. J., Hazzi, C., Levine, R. W., et al. (1974) Long incubation post-transfusion hepatitis without serological evidence of exposure to hepatitis B virus. *Lancet* **2**, 241–246.
5. Feinstone, S. M., Kapikian, A. Z., Purcell, R. H., Alter, H. J., and Holland, P. V. (1975) Transfusion associated hepatitis not due to viral hepatitis type A or B. *N. Engl. J. Med.* **292**, 767–770.
6. Alter, H. J., Purcell, R. H., Holland, P. V., and Popper, H. (1978) Transmissible agents in non-A, non-B hepatitis. *Lancet* **1**, 459–463.
7. Tabor, E., Gerety, R. J., Drucker, J. A., Seef, L. B., Hoofnagle, J. H., Jackson, D. R., et al. (1978) Transmission of non-A, non-B hepatitis from man to chimpanzee. *Lancet* **1**, 463–465.
8. Hollinger, F. B., Gitnick, G. L., Aach, R. D., Szmuness, W., Mosley, J. W., Stevens, C. E., et al. (1978) Non-A, non-B hepatitis transmission in chimpanzees: A project of the Transfusion-Transmitted Viruses Group. *Intervirology* **10**, 60–68.
9. Tabor, E., Seef, L. B., and Gerety, R. J. (1979) Lack of susceptibility of marmosets to human non-A, non-B hepatitis. *J. Infect. Dis.* **140**, 794–797.
10. Feinstone, S. M., Alter, H. J., Dienes, H. P., Shimizu, Y., Popper, H., Blackmore, D., et al. (1981) Non-A, non-B hepatitis in chimpanzees and marmosets. *J. Infect. Dis.* **144**, 588–598.
11. Abe, K., Kurata, T., Teramoto, Y., Shiga, J., and Shikata, T. (1993) Lack of susceptibility of various primates and woodchucks to hepatitis C virus. *J. Med. Primatol.* **22**, 433,434.
12. Tabor, E., Purcell, R. H., and Gerety, R. J. (1983) Primate animal models and titered inocula for the study of human hepatitis A, hepatitis B, and non-A, non-B hepatitis. *J. Med. Primatol.* **12**, 305–318.
13. Hollinger, F. B., Dolana, G., Thomas, W., and Gyorkey, F. (1984) Reduction in risk of hepatitis transmission by heat treatment of a human factor VIII concentrate. *J. Infect. Dis.* **150**, 250–262.
14. Heldebrant, C. M., Gomperts, E. D., Kasper, J. S., McDougal, J. S., Friedman, A. E., Hwang, D. S., et al. (1985) Evaluation of two viral inactivation methods for the preparation of a safer factor VIII and Factor IX concentrates. *Transfusion* **25**, 510–515.
15. Louie, R. E., Galloway, C. J., Duman M. L., Wong, M. F., and Mitra, G. (1994) Inactivation of hepatitis C virus in low pH intravenous immunoglobulin. *Biologicals* **22**, 13–19.
16. Biswas, R. M., Nedjar, S., Wilson, L. T., Mitchell, F. D., Snoy, P. J., Finlayson, J. S., et al. (1994) The effect on the safety of intravenous immunoglobulin of testing plasma for antibody to hepatitis C. *Transfusion* **34**, 100–104.
17. Choo, Q.-L., Kuo, G., Weiner, A. J., Overby, L. R., Bradley, D. W., and Houghton, M. (1989) Isolation of a cDNA clone derived from a blood-borne non-A, non-B viral hepatitis genome. *Science* **244**, 359–362.
18. Kuo, D., Choo, Q.-L., Alter, H. J., Gitnick, G. L., Redeker, A. G., Purcell, R. H., et al. (1989) An assay for circulating antibodies to a major etiologic virus of human non-A, non-B hepatitis. *Science* **244**, 362–364.

19. Sly, D. L., London, W. T., and Purcell, R. H. (1979) Illness in a chimpanzee inoculated with hepatitis B virus. *J. Am. Vet. Med. Assoc.* **75,** 987,988.
20. Muchmore, E. (1983) Anemia in chimpanzees on hepatitis studies, in *Viral and Immunological Diseases in Nonhuman Primates* (Kalter, S. S., ed.), Liss, New York, pp. 225–229.
21. Shimizu, Y. K., Feinstone, S. M., and Purcell, R. H. (1979) Ultrastructural evidence for two agents in experimentally infected chimpanzees. *Science* **205,** 197–200.
22. Jackson, D., Tabor, E., and Gerety, R. J. (1979) Acute non-a, non-B hepatitis, Specific ultrastructural alterations in endoplasmic reticulum of infected hepatocytes. *Lancet* **1,** 1249,1250.
23. Pfeifer, U., Thomssen, R., Legler, K., Böttcher, U., Gerlich, W., Weinmann, E., et al. (1980) Experimental non-A, non-B hepatitis, Four types of cytoplasmic alteration in hepatocytes of infected chimpanzees. *Virchows Arch. B (Cell Pathol.)* **33,** 233–243.
24. Schaff, Z., Tabor, E., Jackson, D. R., and Gerety, R. J. (1984) Ultrastructural alterations in serial liver biopsy specimens from chimpanzees experimentally infected with a human non-A, non-B hepatitis agent. *Virchows Arch. B (Cell Pathol.)* **45,** 301–312.
25. Muchmore, E. and Valenza, F. (1983) Plasmapheresis of chimpanzees on hepatitis studies by continuous flow centrifugation. Read at 34th Annual Session of the American Association for Laboratory Animal Science, San Antonio, TX, Nov. 7–11.
26. Muchmore, E. and Shapiro, M. (1981) Effect of liver biopsies on chimpanzee serum aspartate and alanine aminotransferases (AST, ALT). Read at 32nd Annual Session of the American Association for Laboratory Animal Science, Salt Lake City, UT, Sept. 20 25.
27. Valenza, F. P. and Muchmore, E. (1982) The clinical chemistry of chimpanzees, I. Determination of aminotransferase baseline values for hepatitis studies. *J. Med. Primatol.* **11,** 342–351.
28. Williams-Blangero, S., Blangero, J., Murthy, K. K., and Lanford, R. E. (1996) Genetic analysis of serum alanine transaminase activity in normal and hepatitis C virus-infected chimpanzees, An application of research-oriented genetic management. *Lab. Anim. Sci.* **46,** 26–30.
29. Muchmore, E. and Valenza, F. P. (1984) Serum enzyme elevation in chimpanzees caused by stress and factors other than viral hepatitis. Read at 35th Annual Session of the American Association for Laboratory Animal Science, Cincinnati, OH, Oct. 28–Nov. 2.
30. Valenza, F. P. and Muchmore, E. (1985) The clinical chemistry of chimpanzees, II. Gamma glutamyl transferase levels in hepatitis studies. *J. Med. Primatol.* **14,** 305–315.
31. Zuckerman, A. J., Thornton, A., Howard, C. R., Tsiquaye, K. N., Jones, D. M., and Brambell, M. R. (1978) Hepatitis B outbreak among chimpanzees at the London Zoo. *Lancet* **2,** 652–654.
32. Lanford, R. E., Notvall, L., Barbosa, L. H., and Eichberg, J. W. (1991) Evaluation of a chimpanzee colony for antibodies to hepatitis C virus. *J. Med Virol.* **34,** 148–153.

33. Suzuki, E., Kaneko, D., Udono, T., Tanoue, T., Hayashi, Y., Yoshihara, N., et al. (1993) Absence of nonpercutaneous transmission of hepatitis C virus in a colony of chimpanzees. *J. Med. Virol.* **39,** 286–291.
34. Muchmore, E. and Peterson, D. A. (1987) NANB hepatitis in pregnant chimpanzee and offspring, A case report, in *Viral Hepatitis and AIDS, Proceedings of the International Symposium on Viral Hepatitis and AIDS* (Villarejos, V. M., ed.), Trejos Hnos. San José, Costa Rica, pp. 401–403.
35. Siiteri, P. K. and Stites, D. P. (1982) Immunologic and endocrine interrelationships in pregnancy. *Biol. Reprod.* **26,** 1–14.
36. Quiroga, J. A., Pardo, M., Navas, S., Martin, J., and Carreno, V. (1996) Patterns of immune response to the host-encoded GOR and hepatitis C virus core-derived epitopes with relation to hepatitis C viremia, genotypes and liver disease severity. *J. Infect. Dis.* **173,** 300–305.
37. Hsu, H. H., Wright, T. L., Luba, D., Martin, M., Feinstone, S. M., Garcia, G., et al. (1991) Failure to detect hepatitis C virus genome in human secretions with the polymerase chain reaction. *Hepatology* **14,** 763–767.
38. Abe, K., Kurata, T., Shikata, T., Sugitani, M., and Oda, T. (1987) Experimental transmission of non-A, non-B hepatitis by saliva. *J. Infect. Dis.* **153,** 1078,1079.
39. Brotman, B., Prince, A. M., Huima, T., Richardson, L., and van den Ende, M. C. (1983) Blood-borne non-A, non-B hepatitis: Lack of infectivity of feces from chimpanzees infected with a strain producing cytoplasmic tubular alterations. *J. Infect. Dis.* **147,** 535–539.
40. Prince, A. M. and Brotman, B. (1994) The biology of hepatitis C virus infection, Lessons learned from chimpanzees, in *Hepatitis C Virus. Current Studies in Hematology and Blood Transfusion* (Reesink, H. D., ed.), Karger, Basel, Switzerland, pp. 195–207.
41. Mimms, L. T., Mosely, J. W., Hollinger, F. B., Aach, R. D., Stevens, C. D., Cunningham, M., et al. (1993) Effect of concurrent acute infection with hepatitis C virus on acute hepatitis B virus infection. *Br. Med. J.* **307,** 1095–1097.
42. Bradley, D. W., Maynard, J. E., Cook, E. H., Ebert, J. W., Gravelle C. R., Tsiquaye, K. N., et al. (1980) Non-A, non-B hepatitis in experimentally infected chimpanzees, Cross-challenge and electron microscopic studies. *J. Med. Virol.* **6,** 185–201.
43. Yoshizawa, H., Itoh, Y., Iwakziri, S., Kitajima, D., and Tanaka, A. (1981) Demonstration of two different types of non-A, non-B hepatitis by reinjection and cross-challenge studies in chimpanzees. *Gastroenterology* **81,** 107–113.
44. Mosley, J. W., Redeker, A. G., Feinstone, S. M., and Purcell, R. H. (1977) Multiple hepatitis viruses in multiple attacks of acute viral hepatitis. *N. Engl. J. Med.* **296,** 75–78.
45. Bradley, D. W., Krawczynski, K., Cook, E. H., Gravelle, C. R., Ebert, J. W., and Maynard, J. E. (1983) Recrudescense of non-A, non-B hepatitis in persistently infected chimpanzees, in *Viral Hepatitis-Proceedings of Second International Hepatitis Workshop, Edinburgh, Scotland,* Nuclear Enterpises, pp. 43–48.

46. Bradley, D. W., Maynard, J. E., Popper, H., Ebert, J. W., Cook, E. H., Fields, H. A., et al. (1981) Persistent non-A, non-B hepatitis in experimentally infected chimpanzees. *J. Infect. Dis.* **143,** 210–218.
47. Prince, A. M. (1994) Immunity in hepatitis C virus infection [review]. *Vox Sang.* **67 Suppl. 3,** 227–228.
48. Bradley, D. W., Krawczynski, K., Ebert, J. W., McCaustland, K. A., Choo, Q.-.L., Houghton, M., et al. (1990) Parenterally transmitted non-A, non-B hepatitis, virus-specific antibody response patterns in hepatitis C virus-infected chimpanzees. *Gastroenterology* **99,** 1054–1060.
49. Okamoto, H., Mishiro, S., Tokita, H., Tsuda, F., Miyakawa, Y., and Mayumi, M. (1994) Superinfection of chimpanzees carrying hepatitis C virus of genotype II/1b with that of genotype III/2a or I/1a. *Hepatology* **20,** 1131–1136.
50. Farci, P., Alter, H. J., Govindarajan, S., Wong, D. C., Engle, R., Lesniewski, R. R., et al. (1992) Lack of protective immunity against reinfection with hepatitis C virus. *Science* **258,** 135–140.
51. Muchmore, E., Popper, H., Peterson, D. A., Miller, M. F., and Lieberman, H. M. (1988) Non-A, non-B hepatitis-related hepatocellular carcinoma in a chimpanzee. *J. Med. Primatol.* **17,** 235–246.
52. Muchmore, E., Socha, W. W., and Krawczynski, K. (1990) HCC in chimpanzees, in *Viral Hepatitis and Hepatocellular Carcinoma,* (Sung, J.-L. and Chen, D.-S., eds.), Excerpta Medica Asia, Hong Kong, pp. 698–702.
53. Tabor E., Hsia, C. C., and Muchmore, E. (1994) Histochemical and immunohistochemical similarities between hepatic tumors in two chimpanzees and man. *J. Med. Primatol.* **23,** 271–279.
54. Okamoto, H., Kojima, M., Okada, S., Yoshizawa, H., Iizuka, H., Tanka, T., et al. (1992) Genetic drift of hepatitis C virus during an 8.2 year infection in a chimpanzee, variability and stability. *Virology* **190,** 894–899.
55. Mishiro, S., Hoshi, Y., Takeda, K., Yoshikawa, A., Gotanda, T., Takahashi, K., et al. (1990) Non-A, non-B hepatitis specific antibodies directed at host derived epitope, implication for an autoimmune process. *Lancet* **2,** 1400–1403.
56. Wang, Y. F., Brotman, B., Andrus, L., and Prince, A. M. (1996) Immune response to epitopes of hepatitis C virus (HCV) structural proteins in HCV-infected humans and chimpanzees. *J. Infect. Dis.* **173,** 808–821.
57. Krawczynski, K., Alter, H. J., Tankersley, D. L., Beach, M., Robertson, B. H., Lambert, S., et al. (1996) Effect of immune globulin on the prevention of experimental hepatitis C virus infection. *J. Infect. Dis.* **173,** 822–828.
58. Farci, P., Alter, H. J., Wong, D. C., Miller, R. H., Govindarajan, S., Engle, R., et al. (1994) Prevention of hepatitis C virus infection in chimpanzees after antibody-mediated in vitro neutralization. *Proc. Natl. Acad. Sci. USA* **91,** 7792–7796.
59. Choo Q.-L., Kuo, G., Ralston, R., Weiner, A., Chien, D., VanNest, G., et al. (1994) Vaccination of chimpanzees against infection by the hepatitis C virus. *Proc. Natl. Acad. Sci. USA* **91,** 1294–1298.
60. Weiner, A., Erickson, A. L., Kansopon, J., Crawford, K., Muchmore, E., Hughes, A. L., et al. (1995) Persistent hepatitis C virus infection in a chimpanzee is associ-

ated with emergence of a cytotoxic T lymphocyte escape variant. *Proc. Natl. Acad. Sci. USA* **92,** 2755–2759.
61. Kowalski, H., Erickson, A. L., Cooper, S., Domena, J. D., Parham, P., and Walker, C. M. (1996) Patr-A and B, the orthologues of HLA-A and B, present hepatitis C virus epitopes to CD8+ cytotoxic T cells from two chronically infected chimpanzees. *J. Exp. Med.* **183,** 1761–1775.
62. Lanford, R. E., Chavez, D., Chisari, F. V., and Sureau, C. (1995) Lack of detection of negative-strand hepatitis C virus RNA in peripheral blood mononuclear cells and other extrahepatic tissues by the highly strand-specific rTth reverse transcriptase PCR. *J. Virol.* **69,** 8079–8083.
63. Halfon, P., Khiri, H., Gerolami, V., Bourliere, M., Feryn, J. M., Reynier, P., et al. (1996) Impact of various handling and storage conditions on quantitative detection of hepatitis C virus RNA. *J. Hepatol.* **25,** 307–311.
64. Lanford, R. E., Sureau, C., Jacob, J. R., White, R., and Fuerst, T. R. (1994) Demonstration of in vitro infection of chimpanzee hepatocytes with hepatitis C virus using strand-specific RT/PCR. *Virology* **202,** 608–614.
65. Dyke, B., Williams-Blangero, S., Mamelka, P. M., and Goodwin, W. J. (1995) Future costs of chimpanzees in U. S. Research Institutions. *Ilar J.* **37,** 193–198.
66. Abe, K., Inchauspe, G., Shikata, T., and Prince, A. M. (1992) Three different patterns of hepatitis c virus infection in chimpanzees. *Hepatology* **15,** 690–695.
67. Beach, M. J., Meeks, E. L., Mimms, L. T., Vallari, D., DuCharme, L., Spelbring, J., et al. (1992) Temporal relationships of hepatitis C virus RNA and antibody responses following experimental infection of chimpanzees. *J. Med. Virol.* **36,** 226–237.
68. Shindo, M., DiBisceglie, A. M., Biswas, R., Mihalik, K., and Feinstone, S. M. (1992) Hepatitis C virus replication during acute infection in the chimpanzee. *J. Infect. Dis.* **166,** 424–427.

55

Liver Transplantation as a Model to Study Hepatitis C Virus Infection

Howayda M. Hassoba and Teresa L. Wright

1. Introduction

Hepatitis C virus-associated end-stage liver disease is a leading diagnosis in patients undergoing liver transplantation, accounting for approx 25% of patients transplanted at major medical centers in the United States, and for 5–15% of those transplanted worldwide *(1)*. Although HCV infection in the early posttransplantation period usually results in indolent disease, the full clinical consequences may not be seen for five or more years after transplantation, when progressive liver failure and even hepatocellular carcinoma can develop. Orthotopic liver transplantation (OLT) provides a unique opportunity to study HCV infection for the following reasons:

1. The exact timing of infection is known (shortly after liver transplantation).
2. Possible source(s) of infection can be identified (pretransplantation infection and/or infection from the organ donor or from blood products transfused in the perioperative period).
3. Serial serum samples are often available, since these patients are typically followed in a single center.
4. Multiple liver biopsies are typically performed, which facilitates study of the histological evolution of HCV-associated liver disease.

These four points contrast to the study of HCV in non-transplant patients in whom:

1. The timing of initial infection is often difficult to determine accurately, since acute infection is typically subclinical.
2. The source of infection is frequently unknown with 40% of patients with HCV infection giving no clear risk factor for infection.

3. The duration of followup is typically short, and longitudinal serum sampling is infrequent.
4. Histological evaluation is often available at only one or two time-points, which limits the ability to study histological evolution of disease.

In this chapter, we will review the literature of HCV infection in patients undergoing liver transplantation, and attempt to demonstrate how the liver transplant model has enhanced our understanding of the natural history and pathogenesis of HCV-related liver disease.

1.1. Structure of the HCV Genome

A detailed description of the HCV genome is beyond the scope of this chapter and is described elsewhere in this book. However, a brief description is necessary to understand the role of this virus in patients undergoing liver transplantation. HCV is the prototype of a third genus of the flaviviridae family, with the other two genera being pestiviruses and flaviviruses. The HCV genome is a positive-polarity, single-stranded RNA viruses of approx 9400 nucleotides with 5'- and 3'-noncoding (NC) regions *(2)*. After translation, the polyprotein is cleaved into three structural proteins at the amino-terminal end and six nonstructural (NS) proteins at the carboxyl-terminal end *(3)*. The complete function of these non-structural proteins is still unclear, but certain functions have been identified: the amino-terminus region of the NS3 protein is a viral serine protease necessary for posttranslational cleavage of the long viral polyprotein; the activity of this protease is enhanced by a viral cofactor, NS4a. The carboxyl-end of NS3 functions as a helicase, necessary for unwinding of viral RNA during replication. The NS5b protein is a virallyencoded RNA polymerase essential for synthesis of the new viral genome. The function of the NS5a protein is unknown, but recent observations have linked mutations in this region to both sensitivity to interferon therapy and low levels of virus, observations that suggest that the protein plays a role in the regulation of replication *(4)*.

The 5'NC region and the core region are the most conserved parts of the HCV genome (5). The sequences encoding the two envelope proteins (E1 and E2) are very heterogeneous among different HCV isolates, whereas the nonstructural proteins demonstrate differing degrees of heterogeneity *(6)*. These viral sequences and the proteins they encode have the following relevance to patients undergoing liver transplantation: the hypervariable region of E2 was sequenced in one of the first descriptions of HCV recurrence after liver transplantation, in which the specific sequence was used to "track" HCV in the peritransplantation period, and prove that the virus responsible for pretransplantation infection was identical to that responsible for posttransplantation infection *(7)*. The hypervariable region of E2 has been used more recently to determine whether certain viral species dominate prior to transplantation and whether these species, if propagated after transplantation, are associated with severe liver disease *(8)*. Other viral proteins may have indirect effects on patients undergoing liver transplantation. For example, HCV RNA levels reliably increase under posttransplantation immuno-suppression *(9)*, owing either to increased viral polymerase activity under immuno-suppression and/or impaired immune function, which enhances viral replication directly. Inhibitors of the NS3 protein (viral protease) are being sought intensively as potential drugs for the treatment of this disease, and if developed, will likely be important for treatment of HCV infection prior to and/or following liver transplantation. Inhibitors of the viral polymerase (NS5b) are also being sought as potential therapies against HCV.

1.2. Heterogeneous Nature of HCV

The HCV genome exhibits significant genetic heterogeneity as a result of mutations that occur during viral replication. The RNA-dependent RNA polymerase, which is a viral enzyme pivotal to replication, is prone to error and lacks either proofreading ability or an effective RNA repair mechanism *(10)*. The genetic heterogeneity of HCV can be addressed under two headings: quasispecies and genotypes. Both genotypes responsible for infection and the diverse nature of HCV may be relevant to the patient undergoing liver transplantation for HCV (*see* **Subheadings 3.2.3.** and **3.3.1.**) *(8,11,12)*.

2. Background and Natural History

An estimated 3.6 million people in the United States are infected with HCV. Annually, 8000–10,000 infected patients die of liver-related complications and approx 1000 undergo transplantation. HCV is currently a major cause of end-stage liver disease in patients requiring liver transplantation in North America and in Europe, where the majority of liver transplants take place *(13)*. Between 1987 and 1994, the United Network for Organ Sharing (UNOS) estimated that 19,947 liver transplants were performed in 17,475 recipients at 108 medical center in the US. The remaining 2472 transplants represent cases of retransplantation for second, third, fourth, and fifth grafts. According to UNOS data, the number of centers performing liver transplantation increased by 74% between 1988 and 1994, and the number of surgical procedures had doubled in the same period. Since 1993, one-quarter of all patients undergoing liver transplantation have HCV infection (either alone or in combination with hepatitis B infection [HBV] or alcoholic liver disease [ALD]).

When the patient is infected at the time of transplantation, persistent HCV infection following transplantation is the rule *(14)*. However, at least with medium-term follow-up, not all infections result in serious disease *(15)*. The source of persistent virus after transplantation includes circulating virions present in the patient's blood at the time of transplantation, which presumably derive from the recipient's liver and/or virus from other extrahepatic sites. The virus may be acquired in those without evidence of viral infection prior to transplantation from infected organ donors, blood and/or blood products, and by nosocomial acquisition of virus during the transplant hospitalization. The risk of acquiring HCV infection in the peritransplantation period depends not only on the prevalence of HCV in the blood and in organ donors, but also, on the efficacy of current screening tests to detect HCV in these sources *(7,16)*. Transmission of HCV by organ donors is discussed in detail elsewhere *(17)*. Whether the presence of HCV in the recipient is protective against further infection with HCV from blood or organ donors remains to be determined, but animal studies would suggest that prior infection does not necessarily protect against subsequent infection with either heterologous or even homologous strains of HCV *(18)*.

In patients undergoing liver transplantation for HCV, histological hepatitis is present in the majority of patients with recurrent HCV infection, even in those with prolonged periods of normal ALT. The degree of hepatic inflammation tended to be greater in those with than in those without elevated ALT, but the degree of hepatic fibrosis was comparable in the two groups. A minority of patients (16%) have normal transaminases and little hepatic inflammation *(19)*.

Two patterns of HCV infection post-transplantation have been identified: (1) recurrent HCV infection in the allograft by endogenous virus present prior to transplantation *(14,20)*, and (2) primary HCV infection which may be acquired from different sources in the peritransplantation period *(7,16,17)*.

2.1. Recurrence of HCV Infection

2.1.1. Sources of the Virus

Removal of native liver at the time of transplantation does not lead to eradication of infection, since the virus persists in the blood and can subsequently infect the new liver *(21)*. Feray et al. using nucleotide sequencing of the hypervariable domain coding for the putative envelope protein of HCV (E2/NS1 region) demonstrated that reinfection of the graft by the pretransplant strain can occur *(7)*. Extrahepatic sites may act as a reservoir of replicating viruses leading to infection of the new liver, although there are more than enough virions circulating in blood at the time of transplantation, to account for reinfection in most instances *(22)*. Moreover, a recent study showed that when the liver is removed after transplantation, HCV RNA levels decline rapidly, beginning during the anhepatic phase of transplantation. The fall was so precipitous

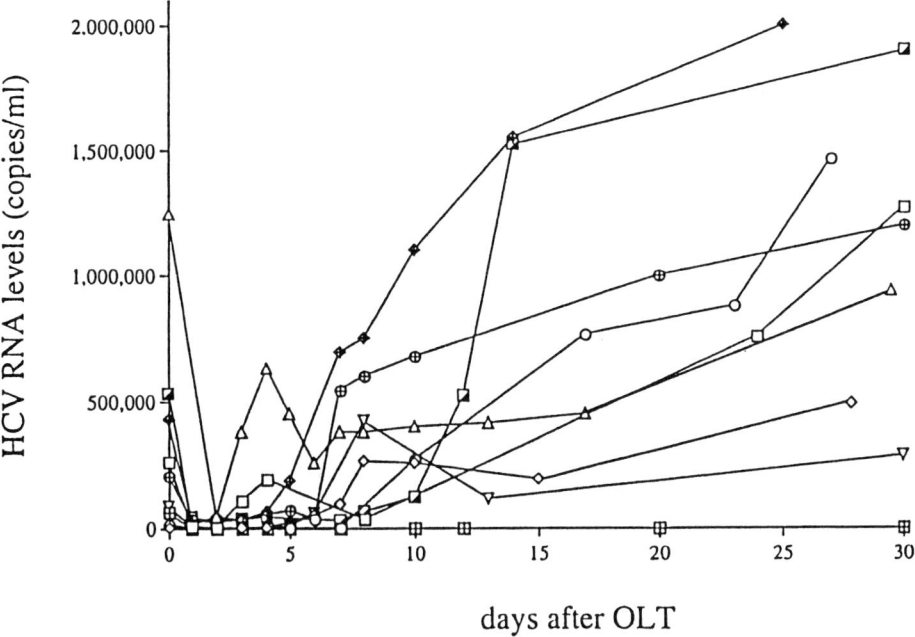

Fig. 1. Serum HCV-RNA levels in nine patients 1 d before OLT (d 0) and at various time points for up to 30 d after OLT (data from **ref.** *23*).

that the authors concluded that there is little contribution from extrahepatic sources to the circulating viral pool in plasma (**Fig. 1** *[23]*).

2.1.2. HCV RNA Levels and Course

Although hyperimmunoglobulin and antiviral therapy have reduced and delayed the recurrence of HBV significantly, no such strategies are available for the prevention of HCV. Recurrence of HCV viremia following liver transplantation for HCV cirrhosis is almost universal with virus detectable in virtually all patients within a few weeks of transplantation *(7,14)*. In a recent study, significant viral replication was observed as early as the third postoperative day, exceeding pretransplantation levels by the eighth postoperative day *(23)*. Several studies have demonstrated that HCV RNA levels rise following transplantation *(9,24)*. In one study, posttransplantation HCV RNA levels were 16-fold higher than pretransplantation levels, and posttransplantation levels tended to be higher in patients with high pretransplantation levels. No significant differences in HCV RNA levels have been observed in patients with recurrent and acquired HCV infection *(9)*. In a prospective study HCV RNA levels were measured serially 1 d prior to transplantation and daily for 30 d after transplantation *(23)*. A marked decline in the HCV RNA levels was observed (from $3.1 \pm 1.3 \times 10^5$ copies/mL preoperatively to $0.15 \pm 0.6 \times 10^5$ copies/mL and $0.16 \pm 0.6 \times 10^5$ copies/mL at 1 and 2 d posttransplantation, respectively), before levels rose to values higher than those observed prior to transplantation. From the changes of HCV RNA, these authors concluded that the mean half-life of a hepatitis C virion in plasma is 4 h *(23)*.

The relationship between the level of virus in serum and the degree of liver injury is controversial. An initial crosssectional study was unable to show a correlation between level of viremia and histological evidence of hepatitis, and indeed in some patients, very high levels of virus have been observed in the absence of liver injury *(9)*. However, other studies have shown that severe liver injury tends to be associated with higher levels of virus than mild liver injury. Higher levels of virus at 1 and 2 wk posttransplantation have been observed in those patients who subsequently developed active hepatitis at 1 yr posttransplantation than in those without subsequent liver injury *(24)*. A second prospective study demonstrated increased levels of virus in association with a peak of serum alanine aminotransferase level at 3 mo posttransplantation *(15)*. In this later study, the relation between serum aminotransferase levels and histologic evidence of liver injury was not investigated, so that the pathogenetic importance of these findings is questionable. To summarize, HCV RNAs levels clearly rise under immunosuppression, and high levels are associated with severe liver injury, but not all patients with high levels have clinically significant liver disease.

2.1.3. Recurrent Infection vs Recurrent Disease

Recurrent "infection" is defined as persistence of virus detected by molecular techniques, such as polymerase chain reaction (PCR) whereas, recurrent "disease" is defined as evidence of end-organ damage (histological evidence of hepatitis). Recurrent disease occurs in the majority (up to 70%) of transplant recipients by 1 yr after transplantation, although a subset remain viremic without biochemical or histological evidence of liver injury *(9,14,20)*.

2.1.4. Short- and Long-Term Outcome

Despite the discrepancies in the reported incidence of post-transplantation HCV hepatitis, short term survival rates (for the first 2–4 yr after transplantation) are comparable to those without infection, and the natural history is similar to the early benign course seen in immunocompetent patients with posttransfusion hepatitis *(20,25)*. Of the 50–70% of transplant recipients who have histological liver injury, the majority have mild hepatitis, with <10% having significant fibrosis or cirrhosis at 1 yr *(14,26,27)*. Demonstration of cirrhosis and even graft failure developing within 1 yr of infection of the new liver does suggests however that the natural history of infection in immunosuppressed patients may be "truncated" *(28)*, since progression to cirrhosis is rarely observed in immunocompetent patients infected with HCV.

The long-term outcome of recurrent HCV infection is less clear. Certainly, with extended follow-up, progressive liver injury has been observed *(15,29)*. In one series, HCV-related disease was responsible for 26% of all hospital readmissions in liver transplant recipients during the first postoperative year *(19)*. The extent of the influence of HCV infection itself on patient and graft survival is difficult to ascertain, since many pre- and posttransplantation factors may alter the outcome (i.e., age of the patient, severity of initial liver disease, type and amount of post-transplant immunosuppression, and so on), and few investigators have included these variables in the analysis. In a study that evaluated posttransplantation survival at 1, 2, and 3 yr, rates were similar in patients with HCV infection (94, 89, and 87%, respectively) to rates in patients with cryptogenic cirrhosis (84, 84, and 73%, respectively) *(20)*. However, the numbers of patients included in this study was insufficient to detect minor differences in outcome (differences in survival of 10% or less), so that the negative findings of this study do not necessarily prove the absence of difference in survival between the two groups. A larger study from the University of Pittsburgh found that the survival of 157 HCV-infected patients was significantly worse than that of 644 nonviral control patients ($p = 0.0002$ at 3 yr). Graft survival at 3 yr was also worse in HCV-infected recipients than in the controls ($p = 0.00001$) *(30)*. Moreover, the rate of retransplantation was higher in the HCV-infected group than in the control group ($p = 0.01$) *(30)*.

A study of the long-term survival of 61 patients with post-transplantation HCV infection showed that cumulative survival at 2, 5, and 10 yr was the same as in 474 patients without HCV (**Fig. 2** *[19]*). Unfortunately, this study is difficult to interpret, because patients with hepatitis B infection were included in the control group (which could potentially adversely bias survival of the controls), and patients with hepatocellular carcinoma were included in HCV group, but not in the control group. The authors concluded that the natural history of HCV infection is comparable to that of other patient groups, but that within the HCV study group, the presence of pretransplantation hepatocellular carcinoma is the single most important predictor of a poor outcome (**Fig. 3** *[19]*).

2.2. Acquired HCV Infection *(De Novo Infection)*

Acquired HCV infection after liver transplantation is presumably transmitted by an infected organ and/or blood or blood products *(21,31,32)*. The early reports about the incidence of *de novo* HCV infection were conflicting as a result of the different sensitivities of the methods used to diagnose HCV infection. The incidence of 35% from our group was an overestimate resulting

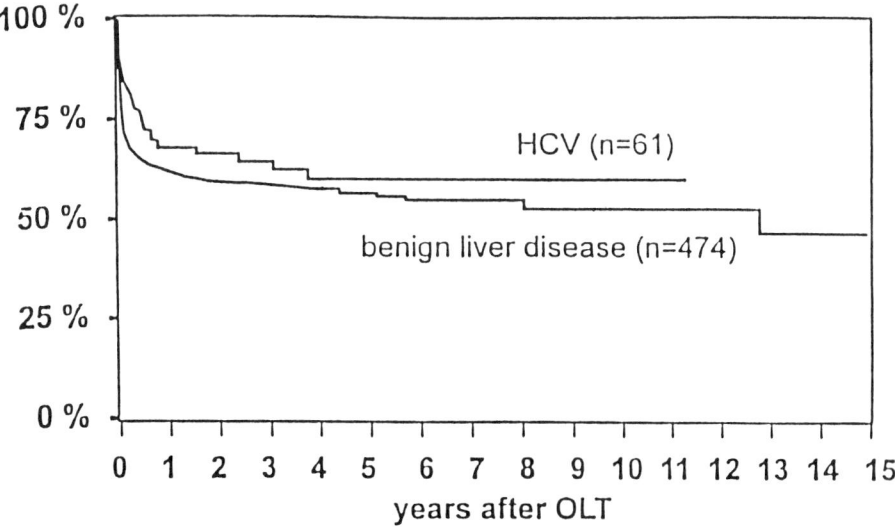

Fig. 2. Cumulative survival of patients transplanted for hepatitis C-related disease vs patients transplanted for other nonmalignant indications. Patients with hepatitis B-related disease are included in the nonmalignant indication group and survival was the same as in the control group; $p = 0.25$ (log rank test) (data from **ref. 19**).

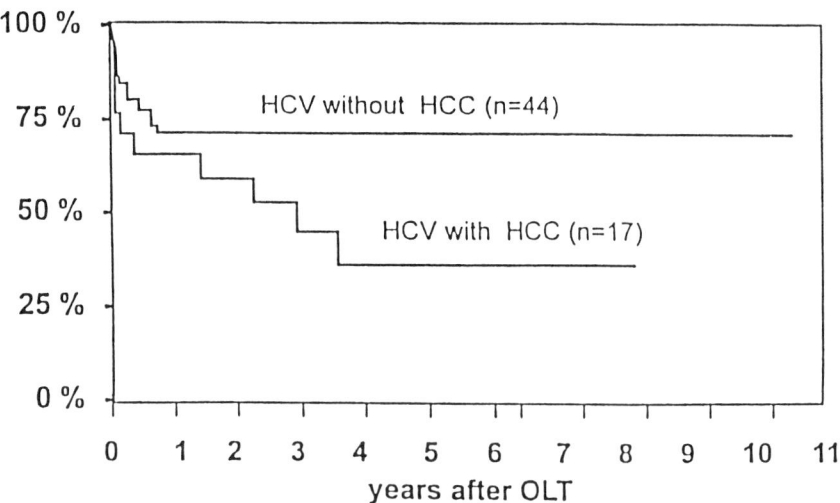

Fig. 3. Cumulative survival of HCV-infected patients with and without HCC at transplantation. Survival was adversely effected by the presence of HCC ($p = 0.049$ by log rank test) (data from **ref. 19**).

from the relative insensitivity of EIA1 in excluding pretransplantation HCV infection *(14)*. Using virological techniques to detect HCV RNA and EIA2, a second study reported the incidence of acquired HCV to be 2.5% *(33)*. This second study, but not the first, was conducted after the introduction of screening of blood products for HCV infection, screening which would be predicted to reduce the acquisition of HCV *(16)*. The natural history of acquired HCV has been investigated. Renal transplant recipients of HCV-infected donors have a 4.4-fold higher risk of posttransplantation HCV-related liver disease than recipients of anti-HCV-negative donors *(17)*. Although HCV-RNA can be documented in 100% of recipients of such organs, clinical hepatitis and posttransplantation liver disease occurs in only 45 and 48%, respectively *(31,32)*. The policy regarding use of seropositive organs in situations of need (such as an HCV-infected patient with end-stage liver disease) is discussed elsewhere.

In conclusion, whether HCV infection is recurrent or acquired, short-term survival in those with posttransplantation infection is not different from those with other causes of end-stage liver disease. Nevertheless, infection has clearly been linked to cirrhosis and early allograft failure, but fortunately this is rare. Because evidence of allograft damage may be delayed, the true effect of HCV on the graft will only be apparent after long term followup *(15)*.

3. Diagnosis of HCV Infection After Liver Transplantation

3.1. Serological Diagnosis

Molecular characterization and cloning of HCV has led to the development of serological and virological diagnostic assays. The first-generation enzyme-linked immunoassay (EIA) incorporated c100-3 polypeptide from the NS4 region of the genome, but it lacked sensitivity and specificity, both of which have been improved in subsequent assays. The use of viral proteins that are well conserved between different HCV strains, such as core protein (C), NS3, and NS4, has ensured a broadly reactive and sensitive diagnostic assay.

In the immunocompetent patient, the presence of antibody usually, but not always signifies ongoing infection. Depending on the population under study, seropositivity may also indicate resolved HCV infection, passive antibody transfer, or false reactivity *(34)*. Serologic evidence of HCV infection can be demonstrated in 33% of patients undergoing liver transplantation. Anti-HCV develops in a subset of recipients who were seronegative prior to transplantation, with a seroconversion rate of 10–15% after a mean follow-up period of 18 mo *(27)*. In liver transplant recipients, immunosuppressive therapy delays or suppresses antibody response to infection so that serologic tests underestimate the presence of infection *(35)*. For example, the sensitivity of second-generation recombinant immunoblot assay (RIBA-2) drops following liver transplantation from 81 to 64% in patients with documented viremia *(28)*.

In evaluating serologic vs virologic methods for detection of HCV in the transplant setting, Gretch et al. compared first- and second-generation anti-HCV assays with reverse transcripterase polymerase chain reaction (RT-PCR). HCV-RNA was found in 30% of their patients at the time of transplantation, and all of them were seroreactive by second-generation assays, whereas, only 82% were seropositive by first-generation assays *(33)*. However, second-generation assays are limited in their ability to identify HCV infection after organ transplantation, since immunosuppression inhibits antibody formation *(31)* In conclusion, current serologic assays underestimate the presence of both recurrent and acquired HCV infection after liver transplantation. Accurate diagnosis of infection requires use of virological methods.

3.2. Virological Diagnosis

3.2.1. HCV RNA Detection

Recent developments in nucleic acid detection techniques (e.g., the PCR Chiron Corp. [Emeryville, CA] and branched-chain DNA [bDNA] assay) have enabled us to identify HCV infection in patients undergoing liver transplantation with a high degree of accuracy *(14)*. PCR in the transplant setting can be useful for:

1. Documentation of the presence of the virus early prior to the development of detectable antibodies.
2. Diagnosis of infection in patients with hepatitis who are seronegative.
3. Stimation of the true incidence of de novo HCV infection post-transplant.

3.2.2. HCV RNA Quantitation

Commercially available methods of HCV RNA quantitation include signal amplification (Quantiplex bDNA by Chiron Corporation) and target amplification (Roche Monitor). Independent laboratories have developed quantitative RNA assays that have been validated against commercial assays *(36)*. Quantitative tests of HCV-RNA have been used to assess the relationship between level of virus and degree of liver injury (*see* **Subheading 2.1.2.**). In the posttransplant setting, commercially available RNA assays (such as bDNA) may also be used for diagnosis. The limitation in sensitivity of bDNA is less critical in liver transplant patients in whom levels of virus are higher than those in immunocompetent patients *(9)*. To determine the best method for HCV detection in liver transplant recipients, four diagnostic assays were compared in 101 liver transplant recipients. HCV RNA was detected by PCR and DNA signal amplification, and HCV antibody was tested by second-generation EIA and recombinant immunoblot assay. "True" positives were defined as the detection of HCV infection by two independent assays. Of the true positives, 98% were positive by PCR, 88% by bDNA, 88% by EIA, and 63% by RIBA. Nine percent of serologically negative recipients had virus detected by both methods. Sixty-nine percent of patients negative by RIBA showed detectable levels of HCV RNA, perhaps owing to the limited sensitivity of RIBA for diagnosis. In conclusion, measurement of HCV RNA is the best way to diagnose HCV viral infection in liver transplant recipients *(37)*.

3.2.3. Tracking of HCV Quasispecies

The role of HCV quasispecies in pathogenesis of liver disease is uncertain, although viral diversity may explain viral persistence after acute infection, through mechanisms of antibody escape. There are conflicting results of studies that have related the degree of viral diversity to the severity of liver disease *(38)*. In immunocompetent patients with HCV, transplantation of uninfected liver allograft provides the opportunity to study the quasispecies in a new host. There is little information regarding the relationship of HCV diversity and disease in patients following OLT. The pattern of HCV quasispecies before and after liver transplantation has been investigated in five patients who were transplanted for HCV-related disease. Three had severe recurrent liver disease, whereas the other two had asymptomatic high-titer viremia. In those with recurrent disease, the pretransplant quasispecies major variants were efficiently propagated immediately after liver transplantation, whereas, for the asymptomatic patients, consensus sequences of the pretransplant major variants were not detectable at any time after transplantation. Instead, there was a dramatic reduction in HCV viremia during the first week after surgery, followed by the emergence of a new quasispecies major variant 1 mo after liver transplantation. This new viral species was likely derived from a minor variant present prior to transplantation. These emergent quasispecies, despite their high rate of replication, were unable to induce hepatitis. Possible explanations for this include attenuation of these variants as a result of mutation and reduction in hepatotropism of these quasispecies *(8)*. These preliminary findings are intriguing, but conclusive results of the relationship between HCV quasispecies and disease will require further investigation.

3.2.4. Detection of HCV Antigens in Liver Tissue

Immunocompetent patients with severe hepatitis have increased detection of HCV antigens in liver tissue compared to those with mild hepatitis *(39)*. Results for three liver transplant recipients suggest this is also true in the setting of immunosuppression *(24)*.

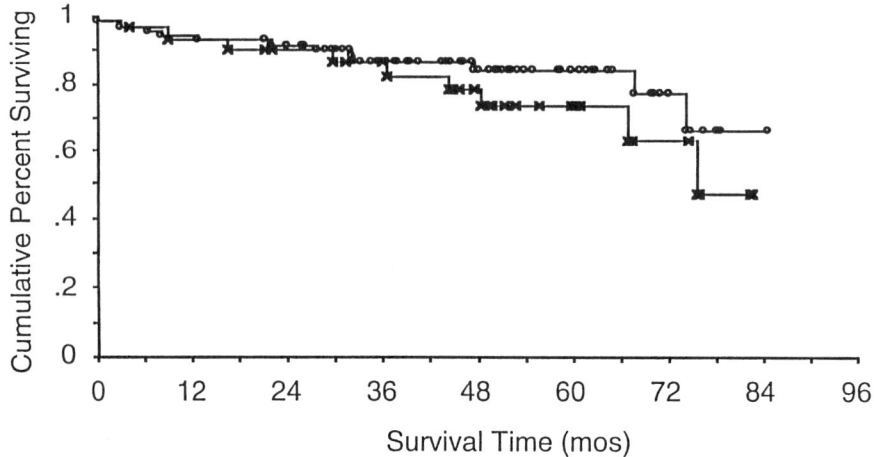

Fig. 4. Actuarial graft survival by genotype (type 1 vs non-1 type). The actuarial survival following transplantation (in months) was compared between patients infected with HCV types 1a and 1b (—x—) ($n = 72$) and with those infected with non-1 genotypes (- - - x - - -) ($n = 40$). There was no significant difference in survival ($p = 0.48$, Gehan's Wilcoxon test) (data from **ref. 12**). Survival was independent of the infection genotype.

3.3. Pathogenesis of Posttransplantation Liver Disease

3.3.1. Role of HCV Genotype

In the immunocompetent patient, the relationship between genotype responsible for infection and severity of disease associated with infection is controversial *(40)*. This is also true for patients undergoing liver transplantation. Some studies have shown that infection with genotype 1b is associated with rapidly progressive liver disease *(11,15)*. Possible explanations for this association are as follows: (a) high levels of HCV viremia in type 1b infection, which lead to early recurrence and, hence, severe liver disease, and (b) enhanced cytopathic effect of genotype 1b on liver cells. Other studies have been unable to demonstrate an association between disease severity and genotype 1b *(12,19)* (**Fig. 4** *[12]*). There are several explanations for these discrepant results:

1. The difference in methods used for genotyping in the different studies.
2. The definition and methods of assessing disease severity.
3. The confounding effect of the different lengths of histological follow-up.
4. The presence of other unmeasured factors that may contribute to disease severity (i.e., amount of immunosuppression).
5. The difference in geographical distribution of HCV genotypes.

3.3.2. Role of Donor–Recipient HLA Match/Mismatch

In contrast to kidney and heart, liver transplantation does not seem to benefit from HLA matching in most patients. Furthermore, lower graft survival rates have been reported in association with HLA compatibility between donor and recipient *(41)*. A dualistic role of HLA in liver transplantation has been proposed: HLA-matching reduces the risk of acute cellular rejection. However, HLA-matching augments other mechanisms of allograft injury mediated by major histocompatibility complex-restricted lymphocytes, mechanisms that are pertinent to the patient with viral infection *(42)*.

The role of HLA matching/mismatching in the recurrence of HCV hepatitis has been studied. The incidence of recurrence has been reported to be significantly higher for HLA-B-compatible liver transplant recipients than for those without an HLA-B antigen match ($p < 0.05$) after a follow up period of 18–24 mo. One or two HLA-B antigen matches between donor and recipient increases the relative risk of recurrent hepatitis 2.8 times. HLA-B sharing between donor and recipient may promote liver injury associated with HCV infection by facilitating recognition of viral peptides presented by class I antigens to $CD8^+$ cells *(43)*.

3.3.3. Immune Response

In contrast to the blunted immune response to HCV, after liver transplantation, humoral immunity to other common pathogens, such as CMV, EBV, and HIV, appears to be intact. Antibodies to the core peptide of HCV appear to be reduced specifically with immunosuppression, whereas antibody response to other viral peptides remains intact *(27,44)*.

3.4. Complications of Posttransplantation HCV Disease

3.4.1. Risk for Other Infection

Recurrence of HCV infection has been associated with an increased risk of fungal, but not bacterial infections compared to noninfected controls *(45)*. Increased risk of infection appears to be greater after 6 mo posttransplantation than in the early posttransplantation period. Increased risk of serious infections in OLT recipients with recurrent HCV is suggestive of an HCV-induced suppression of cell-mediated immunity *(45)*.

3.4.2. Risk of Rejection

Acute rejection episodes occur in up to 60% of liver transplant recipients, usually within the first few weeks after transplantation *(46)*. Since histological features of rejection and HCV recurrence overlap, and HCV recurrence may also occur in the early posttransplantation period, distinguishing between these two entities may be difficult for both the clinician and the pathologist. The risk of allograft rejection has been reported to be higher in patients undergoing liver transplantation for HCV than for HBV infection or ALD *(47)*. Multiple episodes of rejection have been associated with a high incidence and early presentation of recurrent hepatitis C *(48)*.

3.4.3. Risk of Graft Loss

The spectrum of allograft injury related to HCV recurrence ranges from no evidence of biochemical or histological injury to graft failure requiring retransplantation *(26,28)*. Some studies had suggested that graft survival in patients retransplanted for severe HCV in the primary graft may be poorer than those retransplanted for other causes *(49)*. However, a recent study denoted that despite the high frequency of recurrent histologic evidence of HCV, graft failure attributable solely to HCV is an infrequent finding (<3%) *(50)*. It is probable that multiple mechanisms are implicated in determining the severity of allograft injury, pointing to the importance of long-term follow-up to determine the ultimate rate of graft loss owing to HCV recurrence.

3.5. Liver Transplantation in Children

Little is known about the risks and clinical presentation of hepatitis C in children undergoing liver transplantation. HCV is much a less common indication for liver transplantation in this population than in adults, and thus, posttransplantation HCV is less of a problem for children *(51)*. Moreover, since the volume of blood product exposure is lower in children than in adults, one would predict that acquired HCV would also be less common in the former than in the latter group *(51)*. Very few studies have looked at liver transplantation for HCV related disease in the pediatric population. In one study of 149 children who underwent liver transplantation, six (4%) were positive for HCV markers (anti-HCV and/or HCV RNA) before and after liver transplantation, whereas eight (5.4%) acquired HCV in the peritransplant period. Of the six children with pretransplantation infection, only two had histological recurrence of disease, whereas two other patients had recurrent viremia, without biochemical evidence of liver injury. The remaining two patients lost virus by PCR technique despite immunosuppression. In those children who acquired HCV, exposure to blood and blood products was the same as those who did not acquire infection. Liver biopsies are performed much less commonly in children than in adults after liver transplantation, so that there is little information on the histological progression of HCV in children. However, biochemical abnormalities with HCV infection are highly variable, ranging from normal ALT or permanent increases in ALT to marked fluctuation in ALT *(52)*. As in adults, knowledge of the impact of HCV infection in children will require evaluation of large numbers of patients followed for a prolonged duration.

3.6. Treatment

So far, limited success has been achieved in preventing HCV infection or in reducing severity of recurrent disease after transplantation. In most studies, presence of virus alone is considered insufficient reason to initiate therapy. There are four possible approaches to the management of HCV infection in liver transplant recipients:

1. Treatment with effective antivirals prior to transplantation in an attemp to prevent further decompensation and/or to eradicate virus, which may in turn prevent reinfection.
2. Prophylactic therapy to all patients who are viremic at the time of transplantation in an effort to prevent reinfection of the new allograft. This approach has been successfully used with HBsAg-positive patients undergoing liver transplantation *(53)*.
3. Early treatment of patients in the post-transplantation period when they are viremic but before the development of histological recurrence.
4. Treatment of the patients only when they develop recurrent histological disease.

In patients with HBV infection undergoing liver transplantation, prophylactic therapy has been successful owing to effective neutralization of HBV by hepatitis B immunoglobulin. Unfortunately, the neutralizing humoral immune response to HCV infection is weak, and effective therapeutic neutralizing antibodies are unavailable. Treatment options for HCV infection are very limited. Interferon is the only approved drug for this disease. Two agents, interferon-α and ribavirin have been studied in several small case series after transplantation.

1. Interferon-α: Preliminary studies showed a transient biochemical response rate of 12–28% of liver transplant recipients treated with interferon, which is lower than that typically observed in immunocompetent patients *(54)*. HCV RNA levels also decrease significantly on treatment even in those with persistently abnormal liver function *(54)*. However, sustained clearance of virus is rare, and serum ALT and HCV RNA levels tend to return to pretreatment levels when interferon is stopped. No significant change in histology with treatment was observed.
2. Ribavirin: In a pilot study of ribavirin monotherapy in nine liver transplant recipients with persistently elevated liver enzymes, complete normalization of liver enzymes was observed transiently in four patients. However, there was no significant reduction in viral RNA. Biochemical relapse was observed in all patients with an initial response, and histological improvement was not demonstrated (**Fig. 5** *[55]*). Though data are limited, ribavirin monotherapy does not appear to be beneficial in the treatment of posttransplantation hepatitis.
3. Combination therapy: In the immunocompetent patient with HCV infection, combination therapy with interferon and ribavirin appears to be promising *(56)*. Controlled trials of combination therapy in liver transplant recipients are awaited.

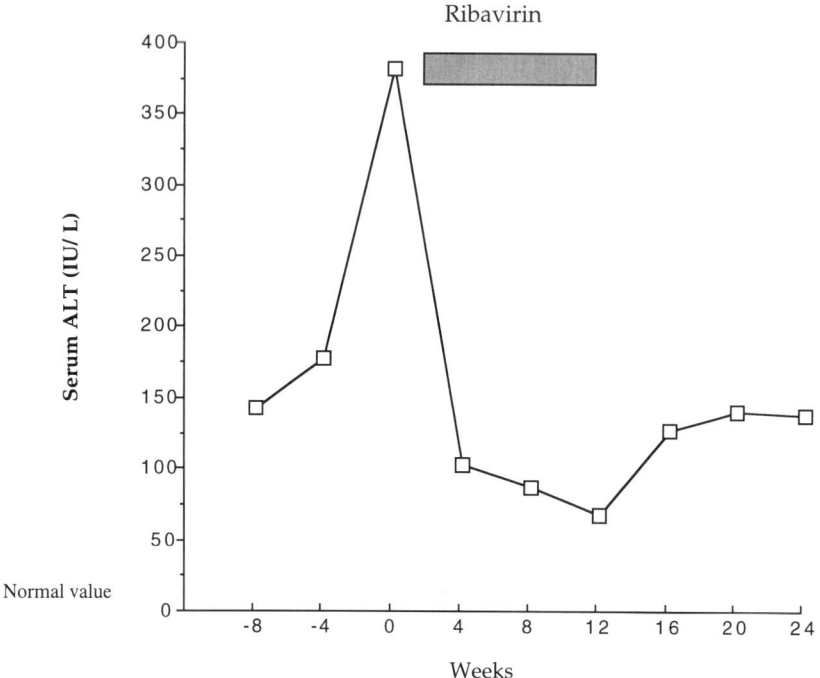

Fig. 5. Serum alanine aminotransferase activities in 9 liver transplant recipients treated with ribavirin (mean + standard deviation) (data from **ref. 55**).

4. Summary

Liver transplantation provides a unique model to study HCV infection in a new host. The intensive study of HCV infection in the transplant setting has increased our understanding of the natural history of disease and the mechanisms by which HCV causes liver injury. Recurrence of HCV is the rule following liver transplantation in those with HCV infection before transplantation. HCV RNA levels increase as early as the first week after transplantation. Levels of virus appear to be related to the degree of histologic liver damage, with severe liver injury observed in some, but not all patients with high levels of virus in serum. Viral factors (pretransplant level of viremia, size of the inoculum, HCV genotype, and quasispecies) may influence the progression of liver disease in the new liver, but these results are preliminary. Moreover, the role of host factors (age of the patient at time of transplantation, gender, possible risk factor[s] for acquiring the original disease, duration of illness, clinical course of the disease prior to liver transplantation, and the type and amount of posttransplant immunosuppression) on the severity of liver injury is unknown. Effective prevention and treatment of posttransplantation HCV disease is needed.

References

1. Fishman, J. A., Rubin, R. H., Koziel, M. J., and Periera, B. J. (1996) Hepatitis C virus and organ transplantation. *Transplantation* **62,** 147–154.
2. Choo, Q., Kuo, G., Weiner, A., Overby, L., Bradley, D., and Houghton, M. (1989) Isolation of a cDNA derived from a blood-borne non-A, non-B viral hepatitis genome. *Science* **244,** 359–362.
3. Hijikata, M., Kato, N., Ootsuyama, Y., Nakagawa, M., and Shimotohno, K. (1991) Gene mapping of the putative structural region of the hepatitis C virus genome by in vitro processing analysis. *Proc. Natl. Acad. Sci. USA* **88,** 5547–5551.
4. Enomoto, N., Sakuma, I., Asahina, Y., Kurosaki, M., Murakami, T., Yamamoto, C., et al. (1996) Mutations in the nonstructural protein 5A gene and response to interferon in patients with chronic hepatitis C virus 1b infection. *N. Eng. J. Med.* **334,** 77–81.
5. Okamoto, H., Okada, S., Sugiyama, Y., Yotsumoto, S., Tanaka, T., Yoshizawa, H., et al. (1990) The 5'-terminal sequence of the hepatitis C virus genome. *Jpn. J. Exper. Med.* **60,** 167–177.
6. Okamoto, H., Kurai, K., Okada, S., Yamamoto, K., Lizuka, H., Tanaka,T., et al. (1992) Full length sequence of a hepatitis C virus genome having poor homology to reported isolates: a comparative study of four distinct genotypes. *Virology* **188,** 331–341.
7. Feray, C., Samuel, D., Thiers, V., Gigou, M., Pichon, F., Bismuth, A., et al. (1992) Reinfection of liver graft by hepatitis C virus after liver transplantation. *J. Clin. Invest.* **89,** 1361–1365.
8. Gretch, D. R., Polyak, S. J., Wilson, J. J., Carithers, R. L., Jr., Perkins, J. D., and Corey, L. (1996) Tracking hepatitis C virus quasispecies major and minor variants in symptomatic and asymptomatic liver transplant recipients. *J. Virol.* **70,** 7622–7631.
9. Chazouilleres, O., Kim, M., Combs, C., Ferrell, L., Bacchetti, P., Roberts, J., et al. (1994) Quantitation of hepatitis C virus RNA in liver transplant recipients. *Gastroenterology* **106,** 994–999.
10. Bukh, J., Miller, R., and Purcell, R. (1995) Genetic heterogeneity of hepatitis C virus: quasispecies and genotypes. *Semin. Liver Dis.* **15,** 41–63.
11. Feray, C., Gigou, M., Samuel, D., Paradis, V., Mishiro, S., Maertens, G., et al. (1995) Influence of the genotypes of hepatitis C virus on the severity of recurrent liver disease after liver transplantation. *Gastroenterology* **108,** 1088–1096.
12. Zhou, S., Terrault, N. A., Ferrell, L., Hahn, J. A., Lau, J. Y., Simmonds, P., et al. (1996) Severity of liver disease in liver transplantation recipients with hepatitis C virus infection: relationship to genotype and level of viremia. *Hepatology* **24,** 1041–1046.
13. Gretch, D., Corey, L., Wilson, J., Dela Rosa, C., Wilson, R., Carithers, R., et al. (1994) Assessment of hepatitis C virus RNA levels by quantitative competitive RNA polymerase chain reaction: high-titer viremia correlates with advanced stage of disease. *J. Infect. Dis.* **169,** 1219–1225.

14. Wright, T., Donegan, E., Hsu, H., Ferrell, L., Lake, J., Kim, M., et al. (1992) Recurrent and acquired hepatitis C viral infection in liver transplant recipients. *Gastroenterology* **103,** 317–322.
15. Gane, E., Naoumov, N., Qian, K., Mondelli, M., Maertens, G., Portmann, B., et al. (1996) A longitudinal analysis of hepatitis C virus replication following liver transplantation. *Gastroenterology* **110,** 167–177.
16. Donahue, J., Munoz, A., Ness, P., Brown, D., Yawn, D., McAllister, H., et al. (1992) The declining risk of post-transfusion hepatitis C virus infection. *N. Engl. J. Med.* **327,** 369–373.
17. Pereira, B., Wright, T., and Schmid, C. (1995) A controlled study of hepatitis C transmission by organ transplantation. The New England Organ Bank Hepatitis C Study Group. *Lancet* **345,** 484–487.
18. Farci, P., Alter, H. J., Govindarajan, S., Wong, D. C., Engle, R., Lesniewski, R. R., et al. (1992) Lack of protective immunity against reinfection with hepatitis C virus. *Science* **258,** 135–140.
19. Boker, K., Dalley, G., Bahr, M., Maschek, H., Tillmann, H., Trautwein, C., et al. (1997) Long-term outcome of hepatitis C virus infection after liver transplantation. *Hepatology* **25,** 203–210.
20. Ascher, N., Lake, J., Edmond, J., and Roberts, J. (1994) Liver transplantation for hepatitis C virus-related cirrhosis. *Hepatology* **20,** 24S–27S.
21. Randhawa, P. S. and Demetris, A. J. (1995) Hepatitis C virus infection in liver allografts. *Pathol. Ann.* **30 pt. 2,** 203–226.
22. Bouffard, P., Hayashi, P. H., Acevedo, R., Levy, N., and Zeldis, J. B. (1992) Hepatitis C virus is detected in a monocyte/macrophage subpopulation of peripheral blood mononuclear cells of infected patients. *J. Infect. Dis.* **166,** 1276–1280.
23. Fukumoto, T., Berg, T., Ku, Y., Bechstein, W. O., Knoop, M., Lemmens, H. P., et al. (1996) Viral dynamics of hepatitis C early after orthotopic liver transplantation: evidence for rapid turnover of serum virions. *Hepatology* **24,** 1351–1354.
24. Gretch, D. R., Bacchi, C. E., Corey, L., dela Rosa, C., Lesniewski, R. R., Kowdley, K., et al. (1995) Persistent hepatitis C virus infection after liver transplantation: clinical and virological features. *Hepatology* **22,** 1–9.
25. Seeff, L., Buskell-Bales, Z., Wright, E., Durako, S., Alter, H., Iber, F., et al. (1992) Long-term mortality after transfusion-associated non-A, non-B hepatitis. *N. Engl. J. Med.* **327,** 1906–1911.
26. Ferrell, L., Wright, T., Roberts, J., Ascher, N., and Lake, J. (1992) Hepatitis C viral infection in liver transplant recipients. *Hepatology* **16,** 865–876.
27. Hsu, H., Wright, T., Tsao, S., Combs, C., Donets, M., Feinstone, S., et al. (1994) Antibody response to hepatitis C virus infection after liver transplantation. *Am. J. Gastroenterol.* **89,** 1169–1174.
28. Martin, P., Munoz, S., Di Bisceglie, A., Rubin, R., Waggoner, J., Armenti, V., et al. (1991) Recurrence of hepatitis C virus infection following orthotopic liver transplantation. *Hepatology* **13,** 719–721.
29. Feray, C., Gigou, M., Samuel, D., Paradis, V., Wilber, J., David, M. F., et al. (1994) The course of hepatitis C virus infection after liver transplantation. *Hepatology* **20,** 1137–1143.

30. Casavilla, A., Mateo, R., Rakela, J., Irish, W., Starzl, T., and Fung, J. (1995) Impact of hepatitis C viral infection on survival following primary transplantation under FK506. AASLD Single Topic Symposium, Reston, VA.
31. Pereira, B., Milford, E., Kirkman, R., Quan, S., Sayre, K., Johnson, P., et al. (1992) Prevalence of hepatitis C virus RNA in organ donors positive for hepatitis C antibody and in the recipients of their organs. *N. Engl. J. Med.* **327**, 910–915.
32. Pereira, B., Milford, E., Kirkman, R., and Levey, A. (1991) Transmission of hepatitis C virus by organ transplantation. *N. Engl. J. Med.* **325**, 454–460.
33. Gretch, D., dela Rosa, C., Perkins, J., Corey, L., and Carithers, R. (1992) HCV infection in liver transplant recipients: Chronic reinfection is universal, de novo acquisition rare. [Abstract] *Hepatology* **16**, 45A.
34. McFarlane, I. G., Smith, H. M., Johnson, P. J., Bray, G. P., Vergani, D., and Williams, R. (1990) Hepatitis C virus antibodies in chronic active hepatitis: pathogenetic factor or false-positive result? *Lancet* **335**, 754–757.
35. Alter, H. J. (1992) New kit on the block: evaluation of second-generation assays for detection of antibody to the hepatitis C virus [Editorial; Comment]. *Hepatology* **15**, 350–353.
36. Gretch, D. R., dela Rosa, C., Carithers, R. L., Jr., Willson, R. A., Williams, B., and Corey, L. (1995) Assessment of hepatitis C viremia using molecular amplification technologies: correlations and clinical implications. *Ann. Intern. Med.* **123**, 321–329.
37. Donegan, E., Wright, T. L., Roberts, J., Ascher, N. L., Lake, J. R., Neuwald, P., et al. (1995) Detection of hepatitis C after liver transplantation. Four serologic tests compared. *Am. J. Clin. Pathol.* **104**, 673–679.
38. Honda, M., Kaneko, S., Sakai, A., Unoura, M., Murakami, S., and Kobayashi, K. (1994) Degree of diversity of hepatitis C virus quasispecies and progression of liver disease. *Hepatology* **20**, 1144–1151.
39. Hiramatsu, N., Hayashi, N., Haruna, Y., Kasahara, A., Fusamoto, H., Mori, C., et al. (1992) Immunohistochemical detection of hepatitis C virus-infected hepatocytes in chronic liver disease with monoclonal antibodies to core, envelope, and NS3 regions of the hepatitis C virus genome. *Hepatology* **16**, 306–311.
40. Benvegnu, L., Pontisso, P., Cavalletto, D., Noventa, F., Chemello, L., and Alberti, A. (1996) Lack of correlation between hepatitis C virus genotypes and clinical course of hepatitis C virus-related cirrhosis. *Hepatology* **25**, 211–215.
41. Yagihashi, A., Kobayashi, M., Noguchi, K., Konno, A., Yoshida, Y., Terasawa, K., et al. (1992) HLA matching effect in liver transplantation. *Transplant. Proc.* **24**, 2432–2433.
42. Markus, B. H., Duquesnoy, R. J., Gordon, R. D., Fung, J. J., Vanek, M., Klintmalm, G., et al. (1988) Histocompatibility and liver transplant outcome. Does HLA exert a dualistic effect? *Transplantation* **46**, 372–377.
43. Manez, R., Mateo, R., Tabasco, J., Kusne, S., Starzl, T. E., and Duquesnoy, R. J. (1995) The influence of HLA donor-recipient compatibility on the recurrence of HBV and HCV hepatitis after liver transplantation. *Transplantation* **59**, 640–642.

44. Lok, A., Chien, D., Choo, Q., Chan, T., Chiu, E., Cheng, I., et al. (1993) Antibody response to core, envelope and nonstructural hepatitis C virus antigens: Comparison of immunocompetent and immunosuppressed patients. *Hepatology* **18**, 497–502.
45. Singh, N., Gayowski, T., Wagener, M. M., and Marino, I. R. (1996) Increased infections in liver transplant recipients with recurrent hepatitis C virus hepatitis. *Transplantation* **61**, 402–406.
46. Lautenschlager, I., Nashan, B., Schlitt, H. J., Hoshino, K., Ringe, B., Tillmann, H. L., et al. (1994) Different cellular patterns associated with hepatitis C virus reactivation, cytomegalovirus infection, and acute rejection in liver transplant patients monitored with transplant aspiration cytology. *Transplantation* **58**, 1339–1345.
47. Farges, O., Saliba, F., Farhamant, H., Samuel, D., Bismuth, A., Reynes, M., et al. (1996) Incidence of rejection and infection after liver transplantation as a function of the primary disease: possible influence of alcohol and polyclonal immunoglobulins. *Hepatology* **23**, 240–248.
48. Sheiner, P., Schwartez, M., Mor, E., Schluger, L., Theise, N., Kolesnikov, V., et al. (1995) Severe or multiple rejection episodes are associated with early recurrence of hepatitis C after orthotopic liver transplantation. *Hepatology* **21**, 30–34.
49. Feray, C., Habsanne, A., Samuel, D., Farges, O., Reynes, M., and Bismuth, H. (1995) Poor prognosis of patients retransplanted for recurrent liver disease due to hepatitis C virus. *Hepatology* **22**, 135A.
50. Rosen, H., O'Reilly, P., Shackleton, C., McDiarmid, S., Holt, C., Busuttil, R., et al. (1996) Graft loss following liver transplantation in patients with chronic hepatitis C. *Transplantation* **62**, 1773–1776.
51. Nowicki, M. J., Ahmad, N., Heubi, J. E., Kuramoto, I. K., Baroudy, B. M., and Balistreri, W. F. (1994) The prevalence of hepatitis C virus (HCV) in infants and children after liver transplantation. *Dig. Dis. Sci.* **39**, 2250–2254.
52. Dussaix, E., de Paillette, L., Laurent-Puig, P., Martres, P., Lykavieris, P., Bernard, O., et al. (1993) Hepatitis C virus infection in pediatric liver transplantation. *Transplantation* **55**, 795–798.
53. Terrault, N., Zhou, S., Combs, C., Hahn, J., Lake, J., Roberts, J., et al. (1996) Prophylaxis in liver transplant recipients using a fixed dosing schedule of hepatitis B immunoglobulin. *Hepatology* **24**, 1327–1333.
54. Wright, T., Combs, C., Kim, M., Ferrell, L., Bacchetti, P., Ascher, N., et al. (1994) Interferon-alpha therapy for hepatitis C virus infection after liver transplantation. *Hepatology* **20**, 773–779.
55. Cattral, M. S., Krajden, M., Wanless, I. R., Rezig, M., Cameron, R., Greig, P. D., et al. (1996) A pilot study of ribavirin therapy for recurrent hepatitis C virus infection after liver transplantation. *Transplantation* **61**, 1483–1488.
56. Lai, M. Y., Kao, J. H., Yang, P. M., Wang, J. T., Chen, P. J., Chan, K. W., et al. (1996) Long-term efficacy of ribavirin plus interferon alfa in the treatment of chronic hepatitis C. *Gastroenterology* **111**, 1307–1312.

Index

A

AAV, 533
AAV particle quantification
  PCR assay
    rAAV construction, 537
Adeno-associated virus, 533
Ad recombinants, 539–548
  transcriptional mapping, 540f
Agarose gel control
  HCV genotyping, 194
Agarose gel electrophoresis
  HCV NS5B, 367–369
  PCR product analysis, 297
Aluminum boat method, 272, 273
AmpErase
  HCV RNA detection, 59
Amplicon expression system
  HCV-1, 554 560
AMPLICOR HCV tests
  HCV RNA detection, 55–68
    laboratory safety, 66–68
    performance characteristics, 65, 66
    processes, 58, 59
Amplified PCR product visualization
  RFLP, 178
Animal model
  attributes, 578, 579
Anti-body-mediated supershift analysis
  HCV-specific RNA binding proteins, 398, 399
Anti-GOR antibody detection
  HCV infection, 3–8
Anti-HCAg
  HCV antigens *in situ* detection, 253

Assay controls
  PCR laboratory, 85, 86
Assay performance validation
  PCR laboratory, 93–95
ATPase assay
  HCV NS3 helicase domain, 356, 359, 361, 362
Auto-LIA system
  HCV antibody confirmation, 19
Auto-LiPA system
  HCV genotyping, 190
Autologous target cell preparation
  $CD8^+$ cytotoxic T-cells, 433, 434
Autoradiography
  discistronic vector
    HCV IRES quantitation, 322
  HCV NS5B, 369, 370

B

B-cell cloning procedure
  HCV-positive patients, flowchart, 454f
B-cell immune response
  HCV infection, 411
bDNA assay
  HCV RNA quantification, advantages, 121, 122
  liver tissue
    HCV RNA quantification, 119–128
bDNA technology
  HCV RNA quantification, 71–77
  laboratory safety, 76
  schematic representation, 72f
Binding site titration
  HCV NS3 helicase domain, 356, 359, 360, 362

Branched DNA technology
  HCV RNA quantification, 71–77
Branched peptides
  serotyping assay, 200
Bulk-expanded CTL assay
  $CD8^+$ cytotoxic T-cells, 433, 435

C

$CD8^+$ cytotoxic T-cells
  HCV determination in liver, 431–437
  HCV measurement
    europium release assay, 423–428
    peptide stimulation, 425t
  preparation, 432–434
$CD4^+$ T-cells
  activity determination, 413, 414
  HCV determination, 414–418
    PBMC, 413–421
    phenotypic characterization, 418
$CD4^+$ T-cells response
  T-helper cell, 410
Cell culture systems
  HCV infection detection, 483–487
Cell extracts of liver biopsy specimens, 75
Cell-free translation
  HCV NS2 protease, 337, 339
Cell harvesting
  HCV replication, 491, 492
Cell lysis
  HCV proteins
    Vaccinia virus/T7 expression system, 308, 311
Cellular immune response
  HCV infection, 410
Chemical RNA modification
  negative strand RNA
    HCV, 465–470
Chimpanzee hepatocytes
  cultivation method
    HCV replication, 501–513
Chimpanzee model, 577–583
  attributes, 578, 579
  cost, 582, 583
  research, 579–581
  supply, 582
Chomczynski's solution
  HCV RNA detection, 48
Chromium release assay
  $CD8^+$ cytotoxic T-cells, 433
Cloning
  $CD4^+$ T-cells, 416–418
  genotype-specific HCV RNA
    transcript preparation, 102, 104, 105
Cloning procedure
  B-cell
    HCV-positive patients, 454f
Cloning transgene
  RDAd recombinants generation, 543, 544
Column-purified RNA
  genotype-specific HCV RNA
    transcript preparation, 110
Contamination control
  PCR laboratory, 83–85
Cryopreservation
  hepatocyte
    primary human hepatocytes
      culture, 497, 498
CsCl purification
  RDAd recombinants generation, 546, 547
CTL assay
  $CD8^+$ cytotoxic T-cells, 433, 435
Cultivation method
  chimpanzee hepatocytes, 504–510
Cytopathic
  HCV infection, 411
Cytotoxicity assay
  HCV $CD8^+$ cytotoxic T-cells, 428
  HCV CTL characterization, 444
Cytotoxic T-cells
  viremia, 409
Cytotoxic T-lymphocytes, 423
  HCV characterization
    liver, 439–448

Index

D

DE81 analysis
  genotype-specific HCV RNA
    transcript preparation, 107
DE81 chromatography
  genotype-specific HCV RNA
    transcript preparation, 106–108
Defective amplicon virus stock, high-titer
  HCV-1 amplicon expression system, 555–558
Defective amplicon virus stock titration
  HCV-1 amplicon expression system, 556, 558–560
Detection reaction
  HCV RNA detection, 64
Discistronic vector
  HCV IRES quantitation, 315–324
DNA amplification
  strand-specific RT-PCR
    chemical RNA modification, 468, 469
DNA purification and digestion
  genotype-specific HCV RNA
    transcript preparation, 103
DNA stock preparation
  Vaccinia virus/T7 expression system, 306–309
DNA synthesis
  RT in situ PCR
    hepatitis C, 263, 264
DNA template linearization
  HCV NS2 protease, 336, 338
DNA transcription
  genotype-specific HCV RNA
    transcript preparation, 105
DNA transfection and RDAd recombinant generation, 547, 548

E

EIA procedure
  anti-GOR antibody detection, 6
Electrophoresis
  HCV RNA detection, 49, 51
  HCV typing protocol, 160f
  SSCP and HCV quasispecies
    heterogeneity detection, 217
Electrophoretic mobility shift assay
  HCV-specific RNA-binding proteins, 392–394
ELISA techniques
  HCV antibody confirmation, 12
  NS4 protein, 201–203
EMSA
  HCV-specific RNA-binding proteins, 392–394
  vs UV-crosslinking, 398
Epitope cluster
  HCV antibody confirmation, 17
Epitope mapping
  HCV CTL characterization, 441, 444–446, 448
  NS4 protein, 200
Epstein-Barr virus transformation
  HCV CTL characterization, 441, 443, 447
Escherichia coli
  HCV antibody confirmation, 14
Europium release assay
  HCV $CD8^+$ cytotoxic T-cells
    measurement, 424–428
  HCV measurement
    $CD8^+$ cytotoxic T-cells, 423–428

F

Fermentation and the HCV NS3
  helicase domain, 355–358, 361
Flaviviridae, 11, 294, 303, 407
Fluorography solutions
  discistronic vector
    HCV IRES quantitation, 319, 321

G

Gel electrophoresis
  genotyping systems
    HCV determination, 161
Gel reagents
  rTth RT-PCR, 474

Genotype identification
  RFLP, 179
Genotype-specific HCV RNA transcript preparation
  HCV detection and quantification, 99–110
Genotyping systems
  HCV determination, 160, 161
  HCV types 1–6, 159
GOR, 3
GOR peptide
  immunoassays, 3, 4

H

HBV
  hepatocyte entry modes, 502, 503
HCV
  history, 134, 135
  immune response, 407–411
  immunoelectron microscopic characterization, 279–284
  molecular phylogenetic trees, 154–157
  primary human hepatocytes culture, 495–500
  in situ detection, 237–244
  in situ hybridization, 238–241
  types and subtypes, 11, 133–140
HCV, 3'-end detection and cloning, 373–380
  characteristics, 373
HCV antibody confirmation, 14–20
  line immunoassay INNO-LIA HCV Ab III, 11–23
HCV antibody screening, 11, 12
HCV antigen detection
  virological diagnosis
    liver transplantation, 599
HCV antigens
  in situ detection, 249–256
    flow diagram, 253f
HCV $CD8^+$ cytotoxic T-cells
  generation, 426, 427

HCV cDNA clone libraries, 289–300
HCV characterization
  cytotoxic T-lymphocytes
    liver, 439–448
  hMAb production, 451–459
HCV core protein
  dimerization and expression
    Escherichia coli, 325–330
  HCV antibody confirmation, 14
HCV core protein crosslinking
  Escherichia coli, 327, 328
HCV core protein expression
  Escherichia coli, 326–328
HCV CTL characterization, 441–446
HCV detection
  hepatocytes and RT-PCR, 498, 499
HCV detection and quantification
  genotype-specific HCV RNA transcript preparation, 99–110
HCV determination
  $CD8^+$ cytotoxic T-cells
    liver, 431–437
  $CD4^+$ T-cells, 420
    phenotypic characterization, 418
  specific $CD4^+$ T-cells
    PBMC, 413–421
HCV epitopes
  HCV antibody confirmation, 17
HCV expression
  HCV-1 amplicon expression system, 556, 560
HCV gene expression, 571–573
  recombinant vaccinia virus construction, 519–531
HCV genome
  genetic heterogeneity, 591
  structure, 590, 591
HCV genotype determination
  RFLP, 175–181
HCV genotype role
  liver transplantation, 600
HCV genotypes, 133–231
  characteristics, 135–137

Index 613

serological differences, 137
typing assays, 137, 138
variations, 138, 139
HCV genotyping
  line probe assay, 183–191
  RFLP, 178, 179
  type-specific primers
    NS5 region PCR based, 165–171
HCV HTA, 220–231
HCV infection
  B-cell immune response, 411
  cellular immune response, 410
  cytopathic, 411
  host-cell response, 408t
  nonspecific immune response, 408, 409
  orthotopic liver transplantation, 589
  specific immune response, 409
  T-cells' response, 410
HCV infection detection
  cell culture systems, 483–487
HCV infection diagnosis
  liver transplantation, 597–604
HCV IRES quantitation
  discistronic vector, 315–324
HCV isolates
  genotyping, 185, 186
HCV isolates analysis, 184, 185
HCV measurement
  $CD8^+$ cytotoxic T-cells
    europium release assay, 423–428
HCV NS5B, 370
  polymerase, 365–370
HCV NS3 helicase domain
  biochemical domains, 353
  expression and characterization, 353–363
HCV NS2 protease expression and characterization, 331–341
HCV NS3 protease
  expression and characterization, 343–350
HCV peptide-sensitized target cells preparation, 427

HCV protein analysis
  Vaccinia virus/T7 expression system, 308, 311
HCV protein expression
  Vaccinia virus/T7 expression system, 307, 310
HCV quasispecies determination, 209
  cloning and sequencing, 207–210
HCV quasispecies heterogeneity detection
  singlestrand conformational polymorphism, 213–219
HCV quasispecies tracking
  virological diagnosis
    liver transplantation, 599
HCV replication
  applications, 490t
  liver-derived cell lines, 489–493
HCV RNA
  positive-strand
    analysis, 479f
    rTth RT-PCR, 480f
HCV RNA-dependent RNA polymerase, 365–370
HCV RNA detection, 30–41, 52
  AMPLICOR HCV tests, 55–68
  HCV replication, 492
  liver tissue
    RT-PCR, 115–119
  (RT)-PCR, 29–43
  RT-PCR, 47–52, 115, 116
    laboratory safety, 116
  virological diagnosis
    liver transplantation, 598
HCV RNA genotype-specific transcript preparation
  HCV detection and quantification, 99–110
HCV RNA *in situ* hybridization, 257–261
HCV RNA isolation, 290
HCV RNA levels
  liver transplantation, 593, 594

HCV RNA quantification
  bDNA assay, 123–128
  bDNA technology, 71–77
  liver tissue
    bDNA assay, 119–128
HCV RNA quantitation
  bDNA technology, 76
  virological diagnosis
    liver transplantation, 598, 599
HCV RNA stability, 381–383
HCV sequences, 159
HCV-specific RNA binding proteins, 385–401
  electrophoretic mobility shift assay, 392–394
  mechanisms, 386
  protein preparations, 391, 392
  RNA UV-crosslinking, 395–397
  schematic model, 387f
HCV types 1–6
  type-specific primer genotyping, 159–163
HCV typing protocol, flow chart, 160f
HDV
  hepatocytes
    entry modes, 502, 503
HeLa cells
  Xenopus oocytes, 381
Helicase assay
  HCV NS3 helicase domain, 356, 357, 360, 362, 363
Hepatitis C
  in situ PCR, 263–277
Hepatitis-specific primers, 273t
Hepatocyte
  HCV detection
    RT-PCR, 498, 499
  primary human hepatocytes culture
    cryopreservation, 497, 498
    isolation, 496, 497
    plating and monitoring, 497
Hepatocyte cultivation
  chimpanzee, 505, 506

Hepatocyte isolation
  chimpanzee, 504, 505, 507–510
Hepatocytes
  entry modes
    HBV and HDV, 502, 503
Herpes simplex virus amplicons
  generation, 553–563
Heteroduplex tracking assay
  HCV, 220–231
High-titer defective amplicon virus stock
  HCV-1 amplicon expression system, 555–558
hMAb production
  HCV characterization, 451–459
Host-cell response
  HCV infection, 408t
HPV 16-specific sequence, 273t
HSV-1 amplicon expression system, 554–560
HSV-1 amplicon generation, 553–563
HTA
  applications, 221, 222
  HCV, 220–231
  RT-PCR primers, 222t
Human monoclonal antibody production
  HCV characterization, 451–459
Hybridization
  HCV HTA, 229
  rTth RT-PCR, 474, 477
Hybridization, *in situ*
  HCV protein detection, 238–241
Hybridization reaction
  HCV RNA detection, 63, 64
Hyperchromicity
  genotype-specific HCV RNA transcript preparation, 108–110
  analysis, 104

I

Immune response
  B-cells and HCV infection, 411
  cellular HCV infection, 410

HCV, 407–411
HCV infection
  nonspecific, 408, 409
  specific, 409
liver transplantation, 601
Immunoelectron microscopic characterization
  HCV, 279–284
Immunohistochemistry
  HCV protein detection, 241–243
Immunoprecipitation
  HCV proteins
    Vaccinia virus/T7 expression system, 308, 311
    RNA protein crosslinked, 397, 398
Incubations
  HCV NS5B, 368
INNO-LIA HCV Ab III
  HCV antibody confirmation, 12, 13
  schematic representation, 14f
INNO-LiPA HCV II
  HCV genotyping, 183–191
  test principle, 186–188
Inocula
  HCV infection detection, 485t
Internal ribosomal entry site
  function, 315
Intrahepatic T-lymphocyte isolation
  HCV CTL characterization, 441, 442, 446, 447
Isoelectrofocusing
  HCV hMAb, 457f
Isotopic tracer analysis
  genotype-specific HCV RNA transcript preparation, 103, 104

K

Kuppfer cells, 274, 277

L

LIA
  HCV antibody confirmation, 12
LIA III strip interpretation
  HCV antibody confirmation, 19

LIA-Scan system
  HCV antibody confirmation, 21f
Linear epitope
  HCV hMAb, 458f
Line immunoassay INNO-LIA HCV Ab III
  HCV antibody confirmation, 11–23
Line probe assay
  HCV genotyping, 183–191
LiPA
  HCV genotyping, 186
LiPA II strip interpretation
  HCV genotyping, 190, 191
Liver biopsy specimens
  cell extracts, 75
Liver tissue
  HCV RNA detection
    RT-PCR, 115–119
  HCV RNA quantification
    bDNA assay, 119–128
Liver tissue homogenization
  HCV RNA quantification, 126, 127
Liver transplantation
acquired HCV infection, 595–597
  background and history, 591, 592
  children, 602
  HCV infection, 589–604
  HCV infection diagnosis, 597–604
  HCV infection recurrence, 592–595
  outcomes, 594, 595
  posttransplantation liver disease, 600, 601
    complications, 601, 602
    pathogenesis, 600, 601
  recurrent infection vs recurrent disease, 594
  treatment, 603

M

Major histocompatability complex
  class II antigens, 413
Maximum likelihood method
  phylogenetic tree construction, 153, 154

Mispriming
  in situ PCR
    hepatitis C, 266
ML method
  phylogenetic tree construction, 153, 154
Molecular evolutionary analysis
  HCV, 147–157
Molecular phylogenetic trees
  HCV, 154–157
Monoclonal antibodies
  HCV antigens *in situ* detection, 254
Mutant RNAs
  use and preparation
    HCV-specific RNA binding proteins, 399–402

N

NAP-25 chromatography
  genotype-specific HCV RNA transcript preparation, 103, 107
Negative strand HCV RNA
  detection, 492
Negative strand RNA
  HCV
    chemical RNA modification, 465–470
Neighbor joining method
  phylogenetic tree construction, 153, 154
Nested PCR
  HCV HTA, 227, 228
NJ method
  phylogenetic tree construction, 153, 154
Nonspecific immune response
  HCV infection, 408, 409
NS4A region
  HCV antibody confirmation, 16, 17
NS5A region
  HCV antibody confirmation, 17
NS4B region
  HCV antibody confirmation, 16, 17

NS3 helicase region
  HCV antibody confirmation, 15, 16
NS4 protein
  epitope mapping, 200
NS5 region PCR based
  type-specific primers
    HCV genotyping, 165–171
Nucleotides
  types, 147
Nucleotide substitution estimation
  methods
    phylogenetic tree construction, 153, 154
    rational, 153
Nucleotide substitutions
  estimation, 147, 148

O

Oligonucleotides
  amplification
    HCV cDNA clone libraries, 292t
One-parameter method
  anti-GOR antibody detection, 7
  nucleotide substitution estimation, 148–150
Orthotopic liver transplantation
  HCV infection, 589

P

PBMC
  $CD4^+$ T-cells
    HCV determination, 413–421
PCR
  genotyping systems
    HCV determination, 161
  HCV cDNA clone libraries, 291–293, 296, 297
  HCV typing protocol, 160f
  laboratory
    amplification and detection controls, 88
    amplification conditions, 91
    assay controls, 85, 86
    assay performance validation, 93–95

Index

equipment, 80
equipment calibration and
   maintenance, 95
internal control, 86, 87
operation, 80–83
polymerases, 89–91
primers, 88, 89
quality control, 83–85
reaction mixture composition, 92
specimen processing controls, 87
techniques and practices, 81, 82
thermal cycling parameters, 92
work area design, 80–83
primers
   sequencing and genotyping, 162t
quality control, 79–96
PCR, *in situ*
hepatitis C, 263–277
PCR amplification
HCV RNA detection, 31, 32, 61–63
RFLP, 178
PCR assembling
HCV cDNA clone libraries, 293, 294
PCR fragments
assembling, 298
cDNA cloning, 294
cloning, 298, 299
PCR primers and HCV quasispecies
   heterogeneity detection, 217t
PCR product analysis
agarose gel-electrophoresis, 297
purification, 297, 298
PCR reagents
rTth RT-PCR, 474
PCR technique, *in situ*
HCV protein detection, 243, 244
PEPSCSAN analysis
HCV hMAb, 458f
Peptide stimulation
$CD8^+$ cytotoxic T-cells, 425t
Peptide handling
anti-GOR antibody detection, 7
Pestiviruses, 11

Phenol extraction
genotype-specific HCV RNA
   transcript preparation, 108
Phosphate analysis
genotype-specific HCV RNA
   transcript preparation, 108, 109
Phosphate determination
genotype-specific HCV RNA
   transcript preparation, 104, 109
Phylogenetic tree construction
nucleotide substitution estimation
   methods, 153, 154
Phylogenetic trees, 147
^{32}P-labeled HCV RNA probes
generating method
   HCV-specific RNA-binding
   proteins, 390, 391
Plasmid construction
VV/HCV recombinant generation,
   524–527
Plasmids
rAAV construction, 534
RDAd recombinants generation, 547,
   548
Polymerase assay
HCV NS5B, 366, 368
Positive-strand HCV RNA
analysis, 479f
Primary human hepatocytes culture
HCV, 495–500
Primer-dependent DNA synthesis and
   in situ PCR hepatitis C, 266–271
Primer dimerization and *in situ* PCR
   hepatitis C, 266–268
Primer extension experiment
HCV, 3'-end detection and cloning,
   374, 377
Primer-independent DNA synthesis
in situ PCR
   hepatitis C, 264–266
Primers
PCR sequencing and genotyping, 162t
PCR laboratory, 88, 89

Probe labeling
  HCV RNA detection, 30, 31
Probe preparation
  HCV RNA detection, 36
Proliferation assays and HCV determination of CD4+ T-cells, 416
Protease digestion time
  optimal, 270
  RT *in situ* PCR, 269–271
  suboptimal, 270
Proteinase K digestion, 290
Protein complexes
  RNA UV-crosslinking, 394, 395
Protein preparation methods
  RNA-binding studies
    HCV-specific RNA-binding proteins, 392
Protein preparations of HCV-specific RNA-binding proteins, 391, 392
Protein purification
  HCV NS3 protease, 345, 346
Proteins translated immunoprecipitation
  HCV NS2 protease, 337, 339, 340
Proteolytic cleavage assay
  HCV NS3 protease, 345, 347

Q

Quantiplex
  HCV RNA quantification, 76, 77

R

Radiolabeled liquid hybridization
  HCV RNA detection, 29–43
Radiolabeled RNA probes
  HCV-specific RNA-binding proteins
  use and preparation, 389, 390
Recombinant adeno-associated virus construction, 533–538
Recombinant herpes simplex virus amplicons
  generation, 553–563
Recombinant sindbis-based expression vector and construction of HCV genes, 565–574

Recombinant vaccinia virus construction
  HCV gene expression, 519–531
Recombinant vector construction
  HCV genes, 571, 572
Recombinant virus generation
  RDAd recombinants generation, 545, 548
  VV/HCV recombinant generation, 524, 525, 527, 528
Recombinant virus selection
  VV/HCV recombinant generation, 525, 526, 528, 529
Recombinant virus transfection
  VV/HCV recombinant generation, 525, 527, 528
Refolding
  HCV NS3 protease, 345, 346
Replication-deficient adenovirus recombinant production, 539–548
Restriction fragment length polymorphism
  genotyping systems, 159
Reverse transcriptase-PCR
  HCV RNA detection, 29–43
Reverse transcriptase reaction
  RFLP, 179
RFLP
  genotyping systems, 159
  HCV genotype determination, 175–181
  advantages, 175
  HCV genotyping, 192
RNA digestion
  genotype-specific HCV RNA transcript preparation, 104, 108, 109
RNA extraction
  genotyping systems
    HCV determination, 161
  HCV genotyping
    type-specific primers, 167, 170
  HCV HTA, 226
  HCV RNA detection, 31, 37, 47, 48, 50, 60, 61

HCV RNA quantification, 74–75
RFLP, 179
SSCP
   HCV quasispecies heterogeneity
      detection, 215, 216
   strand-specific RT-PCR
      chemical RNA modification, 468
RNA isolation
   HCV RNA quantification, 126, 127
RNA ligation experiment
   HCV, 3'-end detection and cloning,
      375, 377–380
RNA purification
   HCV cDNA clone libraries, 290,
      295, 296
   rTth RT-PCR, 475, 476
RNA quantitation
   HCV RNA detection, 65
RNA synthesis and rTth RT-PCR, 474
RNA transcription
   genotype-specific HCV RNA
      transcript preparation, 103
   HCV NS2 protease, 336, 338, 339
RNA UV crosslinking
   HCV-specific RNA-binding proteins,
      395–397
   protein complexes, 394, 395
RT
   avian myeloblastosis virus, 290, 291
   genotyping systems
      HCV determination, 161
   HCV quasispecies determination
      cloning and sequencing methods, 208
   HCV typing protocol, 160f
   RT-nested PCR and 3'-end detection
      and cloning of, 375–377
   HCV RNA detection, 48, 49
   RT PCR and *in situ* PCR of hepatitis C,
      272, 273
   RT-PCR and genotype-specific HCV
      RNA transcript preparation, 102,
      104, 105
   HCV, 3'-end detection and cloning, 374

   HCV RNA detection, 38, 39, 47–52,
      61
   liver tissue, 115–119
hepatocyte
   HCV detection, 498, 499
RT-PCR assay
   SSCP
      HCV quasispecies heterogeneity
         detection, 216, 217
RT RNA
   HCV genotyping
      type-specific primers, 167
rTth RT-PCR
   HCV replication analysis, 471–481
   protocol, 476, 477

S

SDS-PAGE
   discistronic vector
      HCV IRES quantitation, 318–321
SDS solubilization, 290
Self-seal method, 272, 273
Sephadex G-25
   HCV RNA detection, 30
Serological diagnosis
   liver transplantation, 597, 598
Serological genotyping
   NS4 protein, 201–204
      advantages, 200, 201
   synthetic peptides
      NS4 derivation, 199–204
Serotyping assay
   branched peptides, 200
Serum-free medium
   chimpanzee hepatocyte, 505–507
   supplements, 507t
Sindbis virus replication strategy, 566f
Single-strand conformational
   polymorphism
   HCV quasispecies heterogeneity
      detection, 213–219
Single-stranded probes
   HCV HTA, 228, 229

SINrep5 system and HCV genes, 570–573
  advantages, 567, 568
  limitations, 568, 569
Six-parameter method
  nucleotide substitution estimation, 152
Solid phase peptide coating
  anti-GOR antibody detection, 5, 6
Solution hybridization
  HCV RNA detection, 33, 39
Specific cytotoxicity, 436
Specific immune response
  HCV infection, 409
Specimen collection
  HCV RNA detection, 35, 36
Specimen handling
  HCV RNA detection, 35, 36
SSCP
  experimental approach, 214f
  HCV quasispecies heterogeneity detection, 213–219
  optimization conditions, 214t
  requirements, 213
ssDNA
  HCV HTA, 228, 229
    production protocol, 231
    radiolabeling, 229
Strand-specific RT-PCR
  chemical RNA modification, 468, 469
  flowchart, 467f
Strand-specific rTth RT-PCR
  HCV replication analysis, 471–481
  advantages, 473
  schematic diagram, 472f
Synthetic peptides, NS4 derivation and serological genotyping of, 199–204

T

Tail-PCR/rTth assay
  negative strand HCV RNA, 492
    experimental outline, 490f
Target-specific amplification
  primer-dependent DNA synthesis
    hepatitis C *in situ* PCR, 268, 269

T-cells
  categories, 413
T-cells' response
  HCV infection, 410
T-helper cell
  $CD4^+$ T-cells responses, 410
Thermal cycling parameters
  PCR laboratory, 92
Thymine, 147
T4 Kinase
  HCV RNA detection, 30
TLC analysis
  genotype-specific HCV RNA transcript preparation, 109
TNT T7-coupled reactions
  discistronic vector
    HCV IRES quantitation, 319
Transcription reactions
  genotype-specific HCV RNA transcript preparation, 106, 107
Transfection
  RDAd recombinants generation, 548
Transfer vector
  RDAd recombinants generation, 543, 544
Two-parameter method
  nucleotide substitution estimation, 151, 152
Type-specific primer genotyping
  HCV types 1–6, 159–163
Type-specific primers
  HCV genotyping, 165–170
    NS5 region PCR based, 165–171

U

Unweighted pair grouping method with arithmetic mean
  phylogenetic tree construction, 153, 154
UPGMA method
  phylogenetic tree construction, 153, 154

UV-crosslinking
vs EMSA, 398

V

Vaccinia virus, 519
Vaccinia virus/T7 expression system
HCV protein processing, 303–312
Viral clearance, 411
Viral pathogenesis
stages, 407, 408
Viremia
cytotoxic T-cells, 409
Visualization
HCV RNA detection, 39–41

VTF7-3 stock preparation
Vaccinia virus/T7 expression
system, 307, 309, 310
VV/HCV recombinant generation, 524–529

W

Western blotting
HCV hMAb, 456, 459
HCV NS3 helicase domain, 356, 358, 361

X

Xenopus oocytes
HeLa cells, 381